COGNITIVE ELECTROPHYSIOLOGY
OF ATTENTION

COGNITIVE ELECTROPHYSIOLOGY OF ATTENTION

Signals of the Mind

GEORGE R. MANGUN

AMSTERDAM • BOSTON • HEIDELBERG • LONDON
NEW YORK • OXFORD • PARIS • SAN DIEGO
SAN FRANCISCO • SINGAPORE • SYDNEY • TOKYO
Academic Press is an Imprint of Elsevier

Academic Press is an imprint of Elsevier
525 B Street, Suite 1800, San Diego, CA 92101-4495, USA
32 Jamestown Road, London NW1 7BY, UK
225 Wyman Street, Waltham, MA 02451, USA

Notice
No responsibility is assumed by the publisher for any injury and/or damage to persons, or property as a matter of products liability, negligence or otherwise, or from any use or, operation of any methods, products, instructions or ideas contained in the material herein. Because of rapid advances in the medical sciences, in particular, independent verification of diagnoses and drug dosages should be made.

British Library Cataloguing-in-Publication Data
A catalogue record for this book is available from the British Library

Library of Congress Cataloging-in-Publication Data
A catalog record for this book is available from the Library of Congress

ISBN: 978-0-12-398451-7

For information on all Academic Press publications
visit our website at elsevierdirect.com

Typeset by TNQ Books and Journals Pvt Ltd
www.tnq.co.in

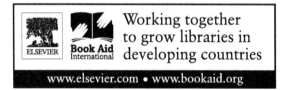

Working together
to grow libraries in
developing countries

www.elsevier.com • www.bookaid.org

Dedication

This book is dedicated to Tamara, Alex, and Nick, as well as to all the loved ones of the authors. It is written in honor of Steven A. Hillyard, scientist, scholar, teacher, and friend, as well as loving husband, father and grandfather.

Contents

Preface

The *Cognitive Electrophysiology of Attention: Signals of the Mind* was a labor of love, for all of the contributors. First, all are passionate about their work and wanted to provide concise reviews and cutting edge data and models. Second, however, and more importantly, the book is a tribute to the life, work and accomplishments of Professor Steven A. Hillyard, one of the founding fathers of cognitive neuroscience, who helped lead the charge to study human higher mental function using physiological methods. In his case, this largely means the methods of cognitive electrophysiology, which are recordings of the electroencephalogram (EEG) and event-related potentials (ERPs), but has also included studies in patients with focal brain damage and remarkable medical cases such as split-brain patients, as well as the futuristic (to us from the last generation) neuroimaging methods like functional magnetic resonance imaging (fMRI).

The book follows, but is not wholly derivative of the 2011 conference in Professor Hillyard's honor, which was held in San Francisco, California in April, 2011, as a satellite symposium of the Cognitive Neuroscience Society annual meeting. There, many of the authors of this volume presented their latest work to honor the mentor, colleague, and friend who taught them how to turn their curiosity into science. The conference gave life to this volume, but the current authors include several of Professor Hillyard's students, trainees, and colleagues who were unable to attend the conference, providing a current view of the cognitive neuroscience of attention and related higher mental functions.

The book includes much of the most current electrophysiology, but also includes studies using fMRI and other modern methods. The quality of the papers presented not only attests to the scientific impact that Professor Hillyard has had through his training and mentoring of generations of scholars, but also to the love they have for him personally, and the respect they have for his immense intellectual contributions to cognitive neuroscience.

George R. Mangun
Davis, California, USA
2013

Foreword

The history of cognitive neuroscience is replete with examples of scientific insights that led to paradigm-shifting new knowledge and the birth of new models and theories. One such story is the struggle to understand how attention influences our perceptions of the world, and hence, shapes our experience. It was indeed a struggle, because two strongly and dogmatically opposed theoretical positions were vigorously advocated by teams of scholars lining up to defend their faith, with data and experiment, of course. What was the nature of this battle for understanding? In its simplest form it was the question of whether or not focused selective attention could alter early sensory processes. Although we all now know the answer, for decades this question was hotly contested. Some argued that it was inopportune for the nervous system to alter sensory inputs until those inputs were fully analyzed, whereupon attentional processes could begin to filter the relevant from the irrelevant. Others took the position that simple sensory cues could be used to bias the processing of incoming information in favor of relevant information, thereby preventing information overload, and possibly analytic failures at higher decision stages. Straightforward question, complicated answer.

This so-called "early versus late selection debate" was foreshadowed in the thinking and writing of late 19th century scholars. William James, the great American psychologist and philosopher, extensively wrote about attention in his seminal *Principles of Psychology* (1890). James believed that attention was multifaceted, and that top-down effects of attention could be directed to different types of information, including sensory information and information stored in memory. For James, attention was a high-level mental operation. His contemporary, Hermann Von Helmholtz, the inspirational physicist and a forefather of psychophysics, speculated that attention might involve interactions with sensory processes (Von Helmholtz, 1909–1911). Neither James nor Von Helmholtz could really test different models of the attention mechanisms: that was to come later with refinements in psychophysics, experimental psychology, and physiology.

In the 1950s, physiologists like Raul Hernández-Peón, the Mexican physiologist, and his colleagues hypothesized that attention might influence early sensory processing (Hernández-Peón et al., *Science*, 1956). Working at UCLA, they recorded from subcortical auditory

relays while a cat was quietly resting or being attracted by mice in a jar. They reported that the auditory responses to clicks were larger in amplitude in the cat's cochlear nucleus when the animal was passively listening than when distracted to pay attention to the mice. Hernández-Peón and colleagues suggested that this was evidence that attention could affect early subcortical sensory processing via inhibition of unattended signals.

At about the same time, Robert Galambos, David Hubel, and their colleagues working at the Walter Reed Army Institute for Research in Washington D.C., were also interested in the effects of attention, but this time on cortical activity. They recorded from auditory cortex neurons in a cat that was awake. They found that neurons that could not be reliably driven to respond by clicks, tones, or speaker noise would respond when the stimuli were more interesting, such as a human voice, a tap on the table, and so on. They concluded that these neurons were putative 'attention' neurons, in that they only responded when the sounds were relevant to the animals. In summing up, they also made the observation that: *"Unfortunately, attention is an elusive variable that no one has yet been able to quantify"* (Hubel et al., *Science*, 1959).

This type of evidence seemed at the time to very clearly indicate that attention affected sensory processing. But a theoretical problem was soon recognized, which led to the appreciation of some important experimental concerns with these early studies. It was understood that the study of attention was confounded with general behavioral arousal. That is, a cat presented with mice is in a different aroused state than one resting quietly. Although it is interesting to understand how arousal might affect neural processing, it is subtly but importantly different from understanding the nature of selective attention: attending to one source of inputs while simultaneously ignoring other distracting ones. This theoretical distinction was made clear in influential writings by Risto Näätänen, the distinguished Finnish psychologist and psychophysiologist (e.g., Näätänen, 1975). Näätänen clearly articulated the distinction between arousal and selective attention and argued for key experimental controls that would be necessary to demonstrate selective attention while controlling nonspecific behavioral arousal.

These arguments were not lost on his colleagues, and in 1973, Steven A. Hillyard (a former student of Robert Galambos) and his coworkers at UC San Diego performed a seminal study that warmed the hearts of not only Finns, but all researchers interested in attention. Recording from electrodes on the scalp of healthy humans, they both controlled for nonspecific arousal and sensory signal intensity, in a study of auditory selective attention (Hillyard et al., *Science*, 1973). The finding was that a cortical-evoked response, gleaned from the ongoing EEG by signal averaging methods, was larger in amplitude for attended than ignored stimuli, convincingly demonstrating for the first time that selective attention modulated sensory processing. This volume, edited by George R. Mangun (one of Hillyard's many students and colleagues), now carries us into the present with a series of chapters presenting detailed information about what has happened in studies of human attention in the ensuing 40 years.

The book is organized into three sections that cover topics in spatial attention, feature and object attention, and higher-order aspects of attention. The authors are the students and colleagues of Hillyard, as well as their students and trainees. One of the first things to appreciate is the tremendous impact of Hillyard's contributions as reflected in the who's who of authors. From his lab, a spectacular array of leading scholars has continuously emerged, and they provide concise and cutting edge information about the state of studies of attention and cognition. It is beyond the scope of the foreword to give an exhaustive summary of the works contained herein, but I would point to some highlights.

In the first section, the chapter by Risa Sawaki and Steven J. Luck presents a model for how the brain prevents orienting to irrelevant events. They describe an event-related potential (ERP) that they have shown to be part of an active suppression mechanism. The idea is that preventing unwanted shifts of attention involves, in part, inhibiting information from salient events at irrelevant spatial locations. This is a critical elaboration on attention models because rather than focusing on the differential facilitation versus inhibition for relevant and irrelevant events, respectively, the model includes a separate mechanism to avert unwanted shifts of attention.

In the second section on feature and object attention, the chapter by Ariel Schoenfeld and Christian Stoppel is a scholarly and comprehensive review of the neural mechanisms of feature attention. They incorporate work in animals and humans to lay out a view of how attention to stimulus features is managed in the human brain.

The authors draw on work from single neuron recording, ERPs, and functional imaging to tell the tale, reviewing some of their own elegant work.

Finally, in the third section, Robert Knight and his colleagues, Boaz Sadeh and Sara Szczepanski, take us on a tour of some new work in the basic neurophysiology of cognition. Their chapter describes cross-frequency coupling of neuronal oscillations, an area of heightened interest in recent years. They recount the evidence from multiple sources, including their fascinating work in human intracranial recordings, where Knight's team recently discovered high-frequency signals that provide a new view of neural function.

The foregoing are merely a taste of some of the many interesting chapters in this book, including some by Hillyard and his colleagues, which I chose not to mention in order to highlight the work of his former students and colleagues, but are nonetheless impressive contributions and worth the read.

In closing, let me place this history and current book in its place in the science of the mind. Over the past 50 years, we have seen the growth of a new field known as cognitive neuroscience. The work of Steven A. Hillyard and his many students and colleagues have played a major role in the development of the field, and studies of attention are among the clearest examples of how neuroscience and psychology have come together to solve basic questions about how the brain gives rise to the mind.

Michael S. Gazzaniga
Santa Barbara
2013

References

Von Helmholtz, H. (1909–1911). *Handbuch der Physiologischen Optik [Treatise on Physiological Optics]*. Leipzig, Germany: L. Vos. (Translated in Warren R. M. & Warren R. P., Helmholtz on Perception: Its Physiology and Development. New York: Wiley, 1968.).

Hernández-Peón, R., Scherrer, H., & Jouvet, M. (1956). Modification of electrical activity in cochlear nucleus during attention in unanesthetized cats. *Science, 123*, 331–2.

Hillyard, S. A., Hink, R. F., Schwent, V. L., & Picton, T. W. (1973). Electrical signs of selective attention in the human brain. *Science, 182*, 177–80.

Hubel, D. H., Henson, C. O., Rupert, A., & Galambos, R. (1959). Attention units in the auditory cortex. *Science, 129*, 1279–80.

James, W. (1890). *Principles of Psychology*. New York: Holt.

Näätänen, R. (1975). Selective attention and evoked potentials in humans: a critical review. *Biological Psychology, 2*, 237–307.

Contributors

David E. Anderson   Department of Psychology, University of Oregon, Eugene, OR, USA

Antonio Arjona   Human Psychobiology Lab, Experimental Psychology Department, University of Seville, Seville, Spain

Edward Awh   Department of Psychology, University of Oregon, Eugene, OR, USA

David L. Barack   Center for Cognitive Neuroscience, Duke University, Durham, NC, USA; Department of Psychology & Neuroscience, Duke University, Durham, NC, USA; Department of Philosophy, Duke University, Durham, NC, USA

Carsten N. Boehler   Department of Experimental Psychology, Ghent University, Ghent, Belgium

Vincent P. Clark   Department of Psychology, University of New Mexico, Albuquerque, NM, USA; Psychology Clinical Neuroscience Center, University of New Mexico, Albuquerque, NM, USA; Mind Research Network and LBERI, Albuquerque, NM, USA

Brian A. Coffman   Department of Psychology, University of New Mexico, Albuquerque, NM, USA; Psychology Clinical Neuroscience Center, University of New Mexico, Albuquerque, NM, USA; Mind Research Network and LBERI, Albuquerque, NM, USA

Tanya J. D'Avanzo   Department of Psychology, Rehabilitation Hospital of the Pacific, Honolulu, HI, USA

Francesco Di Russo   Department of Human Movement, Social and Health Sciences, University of Rome "Foro Italico", Rome, Italy; Neuropsychological Unit, Santa Lucia Foundation IRCCS, Rome, Italy

Sean P. Fannon   Department of Psychology, Folsom Lake College, Folsom, CA, USA

Adam Gazzaley   Department of Neurology, Physiology and Psychiatry, Sandler Neurosciences Center, University of California, San Francisco, San Francisco, CA, USA

Carlos M. Gómez   Human Psychobiology Lab, Experimental Psychology Department, University of Seville, Seville, Spain

Marcia Grabowecky   Department of Psychology and Interdepartmental Neuroscience Program, Northwestern University, Evanston, IL, USA

Steven A. Hackley   University of Missouri, Columbia, MO, USA

Joseph A. Harris   Center for Cognitive Neuroscience, Duke University, Durham, NC, USA; Department of Psychology & Neuroscience, Duke University, Durham, NC, USA

Karen Hebert   University of Missouri, Columbia, MO, USA

Hans-Jochen Heinze   Leibniz Institute for Neurobiology, Magdeburg, Germany; Department of Neurology, Otto-von-Guericke University, Magdeburg, Germany

Steven A. Hillyard   Department of Neurosciences, University of California, San Diego, La Jolla, CA, USA

Jens-Max Hopf   Leibniz Institute for Neurobiology, Magdeburg, Germany; Department of Neurology, Otto-von-Guericke University, Magdeburg, Germany

Jorge Iglesias   Cuban Center for Neuroscience, Havana, Cuba

Vicente J. Iragui   Department of Neurosciences, University of California, San Diego, La Jolla, CA, USA

Robert T. Knight   Helen Wills Neuroscience Institute, University of California, Berkeley, Berkeley, CA, USA; Department of Psychology, University of California, Berkeley, Berkeley, CA, USA

Marta Kutas   Department of Neurosciences, University of California, San Diego, La Jolla, CA, USA; Department of Cognitive Science, University of California, San Diego, La Jolla, CA, USA

Steven J. Luck   Department of Psychology and Center for Mind and Brain, University of California, Davis, Davis, CA, USA

George R. Mangun   Departments of Psychology and Neurology and Center for Mind and Brain, University of California, Davis, Davis, CA, USA

Antígona Martínez   Department of Neurosciences, School of Medicine, University of California, San Diego, La Jolla, CA, USA; Nathan Kline Institute for Psychiatric Research, Orangeburg, NY, USA

Hiroaki Masaki   Waseda University, Tokyo, Japan

John J. McDonald   Department of Psychology, Simon Fraser University, Burnaby, BC, Canada

Alex R. McMahon   Center for Cognitive Neuroscience, Duke University, Durham, NC, USA

Katsumi Minakata   North Dakota State University, Fargo, ND, USA

Jyoti Mishra   Department of Neurology, Physiology and Psychiatry, Sandler Neurosciences Center, University of California, San Francisco, San Francisco, CA, USA

Stephen R. Mitroff   Center for Cognitive Neuroscience, Duke University, Durham, NC, USA; Department of Psychology & Neuroscience, Duke University, Durham, NC, USA

Matthias M. Müller   Department of Psychology, University of Leipzig, Germany

Yu-Qiong Niu   Department of Neurology, University of California, Davis, Sacramento, CA, USA; Center for Mind and Brain, University of California, Davis, Davis, CA, USA

John M. Olichney   Department of Neurology, University of California, Davis, Sacramento, CA, USA; Center for Mind and Brain, University of California, Davis, Davis, CA, USA

Ken A. Paller Department of Psychology and Interdepartmental Neuroscience Program, Northwestern University, Evanston, IL, USA

Michael A. Pitts Department of Psychology, Reed College, Portland, OR, USA

Sabrina Pitzalis Department of Human Movement, Social and Health Sciences, University of Rome "Foro Italico", Rome, Italy; Neuropsychological Unit, Santa Lucia Foundation IRCCS, Rome, Italy

Boaz Sadeh Helen Wills Neuroscience Institute, University of California, Berkeley, Berkeley, CA, USA; Department of Psychology, University of California, Berkeley, CA, USA

David P. Salmon Department of Neurosciences, University of California, San Diego, La Jolla, CA, USA

Risa Sawaki Department of Psychology and Center for Mind and Brain, University of California, Davis, Davis, CA, USA

Mircea Ariel Schoenfeld Department of Neurology, Otto-von-Guericke-University, Magdeburg, Germany; Leibniz-Institute for Neurobiology, Magdeburg, Germany; Kliniken Schmieder, Allensbach, Germany

Christian Michael Stoppel Department of Neurology, Otto-von-Guericke-University, Magdeburg, Germany

Viola S. Störmer Harvard University, Vision Sciences Laboratory, Cambridge, MA, USA

Satoru Suzuki Department of Psychology and Interdepartmental Neuroscience Program, Northwestern University, Evanston, IL, USA

Sara M. Szczepanski Helen Wills Neuroscience Institute, University of California, Berkeley, Berkeley, CA, USA; Department of Psychology, University of California, Berkeley, Berkeley, CA, USA

Wolfgang A. Teder 41114th street south, Moorhead, MN, USA

Rosario Torres Neurodevelopment Department, Cuban Center for Neuroscience, Havana, Cuba

Nelson Trujillo-Barreto Neuroinformatics Department, Cuban Center for Neuroscience, Havana, Cuba

Michael C.S. Trumbo Department of Psychology, University of New Mexico, Albuquerque, NM, USA; Psychology Clinical Neuroscience Center, University of New Mexico, Albuquerque, NM, USA

Mitchell Valdes-Sosa Cuban Center for Neuroscience, Havana, Cuba

Fernando Valle-Inclán University of La Coruña, La Coruña, Spain

Cyma Van Petten Department of Psychology, Binghamton University, State University of New York, Binghamton, NY, USA

Edward K. Vogel Department of Psychology, University of Oregon, Eugene, OR, USA

Ashley R. Wegele Department of Psychology, University of New Mexico, Albuquerque, NM, USA; Ronald E. McNair Post-Baccalaureate Achievement & Research Opportunity Program, University of New Mexico, Albuquerque, NM, USA

Jennifer C. Whitman Department of Psychology, Simon Fraser University, Burnaby, BC, Canada

Marty G. Woldorff Center for Cognitive Neuroscience, Duke University, Durham, NC, USA; Department of Psychology & Neuroscience, Duke University, Durham, NC, USA; Department of Psychiatry, Duke University, Durham, NC, USA; Department of Neurobiology, Duke University, Durham, NC, USA

Jin-Chen Yang Department of Neurology, University of California, Davis, Sacramento, CA, USA; Center for Mind and Brain, University of California, Davis, Davis, CA, USA

Lin Zhang Department of Neurology, University of California Davis, Sacramento, CA, USA

Marla Zinni Department of Neurosciences, University of California, San Diego, La Jolla, CA, USA

Acknowledgments

My love and thanks to my wife Tamara Swaab and our boys Alexander and Nicholas for their support and encouragement of this volume. My editorial assistant, Molly Allison-Baker, was invaluable in completing this project in a timely fashion. One could not ask for a better colleague. The contributors to this volume also deserve my thanks for working on a tight timeline and meeting all the deadlines to produce such a lovely set of chapters to honor Steven A. Hillyard. Deep gratitude also goes to my students and scientific colleagues who have contributed directly and indirectly to the research presented in this book. I would like to acknowledge the National Institute of Mental Health, National Science Foundation, and the University of California, Davis, for their support. Mica Haley, my publisher at Elsevier, has been a great source of encouragement and advice, and I truly enjoyed working with her on this project. I would also like to acknowledge her staff, especially April Graham. They were just fantastic, and I cannot thank them enough. Lastly, I want to express my deep, sincere, and heartfelt thanks to Steven A. Hillyard, who has been my teacher, mentor, and friend.

SPATIAL ATTENTION

Quick over here.
Don't turn your head, don't look.
Just look with your mind's eye or ear
get ready to see or hear or feel, more -
sensitivity galore.
Just focus that attentional spotlight
brightly in your head and use it instead
of any observable movement of the behavioral kind.
Trust your mind – don't peek.
Seek to fixate from behind that pate from within.
Use those various and sundry
distributed frontal and parietal nooks
and you'll be able to know
everybody's biz like they were open books
that you need not confess that you actually ever read.

By Marta Kutas

Profiling the Spatial Focus of Visual Attention

Jens-Max Hopf[1,2], *Hans-Jochen Heinze*[1,2], *Carsten N. Boehler*[3]

[1]Leibniz Institute for Neurobiology, Magdeburg, Germany, [2]Department of Neurology, Otto-von-Guericke University, Magdeburg, Germany, [3]Department of Experimental Psychology, Ghent University, Ghent, Belgium

INTRODUCTION

The observation that attention can be covertly focused in space dates back to seminal self-experiments by Helmholtz (Helmholtz, 1896) who reported "that one is able to focus attention onto the sensation of a selected part of our peripheral nervous system by means of a form volitional intention, without eye movements, without changing accommodation […]" ("*dass man durch eine willkuerliche Art von Intention, auch ohne Augenbewegungen, ohne Änderung der Accomodation die Aufmerksamkeit auf die Empfindungen eines bestimmten Theils unseres peripherischen Nervensystems concentrieren, […] kann.*" p. 601). The following century of psychological research into the phenomenon of covert attentional focusing was essentially guided by thinking in metaphors like a search- or spotlight, or a zoom-lens, which can be used to scrutinize parts of a visual scene without moving the eyes (the "spotlight has a rich metaphoric reach"; LaBerge, Carlson, Williams, & Bunney, 1997). The implicit understanding of these metaphors was, in fact, very "analog" (Yantis, 1988). That is, the spatial focus of attention was envisioned to correspond to a unitary, spatially circumscribed enhancement of sensory processing, with spatial shifts of this focus between locations involving analog movements across the visual field (Posner, 1980; Shulman, Remington, & McLean, 1979; Tsal, 1983).

In contrast to this view, however, a large body of experimental evidence has mounted indicating that a simple direct mapping of those analog conceptualizations of the focus of attention is unlikely to be entirely correct. For example, the notion of a simple enhancement of neural processing corresponding with the attended region appears to be too simple under many conditions. It has been demonstrated that the spatial activity profile of the attended region in space may display a Mexican-hat profile, that is, a center-surround organization, where the activity enhancements at the region of relevant input is surrounded by a spatial zone of neural attenuation (Boehler, Tsotsos, Schoenfeld, Heinze, & Hopf, 2009; Hopf, Boehler, et al., 2006; Hopf, Boehler, Schoenfeld, Heinze, & Tsotsos, 2010; Muller & Kleinschmidt, 2004). Furthermore, there is data suggesting that analog movements of attention (moving-spotlight metaphor) may be an inappropriate notion, as the time lag of selecting subsequent locations was not found to scale with distance between locations (LaBerge et al., 1997; Remington & Pierce, 1984; Yantis, 1988). Finally, there is evidence that the concept of a unitary focus may not always be the appropriate conceptualization of attentional focusing in space (Drew, McCollough, Horowitz, & Vogel, 2009; Driver & Baylis, 1989; McMains & Somers, 2004; Morawetz, Holz, Baudewig, Treue, & Dechent, 2007; Niebergall, Khayat, Treue, & Martinez-Trujillo, 2011).

In view of the immense body and complexity of observations, it has been suggested that one should go beyond mere analogies and focus on more specific issues (Cave & Bichot, 1999). In addition, we think the experimental data discussed below suggests that for integrating the complex set of observations it may be helpful to change the perspective of construing spatial focusing. Traditional thinking about the mechanisms underlying spatial focusing of attention followed the implicit propensity to take analogies in a veridical sense and to expect them to be directly implemented in neural processing. However, as Yantis (1988) puts it: "we must keep in mind that the idea of a spotlight of attention is not a theory, but a heuristic metaphor." As we aim at emphasizing here, a potentially more revealing approach would be to understand the operation of spatial attention from the inner constraints of its implementation in neural processing (Tsotsos, 2011). Central to this approach is taking the hierarchical constraints on top-down directed selection in the visual cortex as the starting point—something that has been previously proposed (Ahissar & Hochstein, 2004; Hochstein & Ahissar, 2002) and which was explicitly implemented in computational models of visual attention (Tsotsos, 1990, 2005, 2011). As we lay out below, this approach may allow us to integrate seemingly independent or even conflicting observations and ideas. In particular, we will see that taking guidance by architecture-bound constraints will provide a useful framework for explaining conflicting observations regarding the spatial distribution of attention. While this approach has generally proved to be successful in accommodating a wide range of phenomena and mechanisms underlying attentional selection (Tsotsos, 2011; Tsotsos, Rodriguez-Sanchez, Rothenstein, & Simine, 2008), the following will focus on the spatial distribution of visual attention as a prime example. We will show that this perspective has, in fact, the potential to redefine the exploratory power of the spatial profile as a diagnostic of the inner workings of neural processing underlying attentional selection in the visual cortical processing hierarchy.

THE SPATIAL PROFILE OF VISUAL ATTENTION—CONFLICTING OBSERVATIONS

Behavioral and Neurophysiological Evidence Suggesting a Simple Gradient

A considerable body of data from different methodologies suggests that the spatial profile of visual attention shows a simple profile with enhanced sensory processing at the attended location gradually falling off with increasing distance. Behavioral evidence for such a simple gradient profile was provided by demonstrating with cued-orienting that the speed or accuracy of stimulus detection continuously drops with distance from the center of attention (Castiello & Umilta, 1990; Downing & Pinker, 1985; Henderson & Macquistan, 1993; LaBerge et al., 1997; Shulman, Wilson, & Sheehy, 1985). Other approaches documented such a gradient profile by showing that the interference effect of response-incompatible distractors on discrimination performance steadily falls off with distance from the target (Eriksen & James, 1986). Furthermore, spatial cuing effects on temporal-order judgments, the line motion illusion (Hikosaka, Miyauchi, & Shimojo, 1993a, 1993b), or on perceptual latency priming (Scharlau, 2004) were found to continuously decrease with distance from the focus of attention in line with a simple gradient model.

Also consistent with this notion were observations based on event-related potential (ERP)-recordings (Mangun & Hillyard, 1987, 1988). Mangun and Hillyard (1988) recorded ERPs while subjects focused their attention on one of three permanent placeholder-boxes at midline or 5.3° in the left or right visual field (VF) in order to detect occasional targets at this location. The attention-related amplitude enhancement of early sensory components (P135, N190) showed a graded decrease with increasing distance to the focus of attention. Likewise, Eimer (Eimer, 1997) reported that sensory ERP components (N1, Nd1, Nd2) elicited by items presented at unexpected locations were gradually attenuated with distance to the expected target location.

Behavioral Data Suggesting a Center-Surround Profile

In contrast to the above observations, many experimental reports suggest a more complex profile or topology of the distribution of spatial attention (Egly & Homa, 1984; Eimer, 2000; Muller & Hubner, 2002). Behavioral indices of attentional benefits were sometimes found to show a performance decrement in the immediate surround of the attentional focus even falling below performance measures at locations farther away from the focus (Bahcall & Kowler, 1999; Caputo & Guerra, 1998; Carr & Dagenbach, 1990; Cave & Zimmerman, 1997; Cutzu & Tsotsos, 2003; Fecteau & Enns, 2005; Krose & Julesz, 1989; McCarley & Mounts, 2007; Mihalas, Dong, von der Heydt, & Niebur, 2011; Mounts, 2000a, 2000b; Muller, Mollenhauer, Rosler, & Kleinschmidt, 2005; Steinman, Steinman, & Lehmkuhle, 1995). This was taken to suggest that the spatial profile of the focus of attention shows a more complex profile than a simple gradient, where a center enhancement is surrounded by a zone of relative attenuation. For example, Steinman and colleagues (Steinman et al., 1995) investigated effects of cued orienting on the line motion illusion (Hikosaka et al., 1993a) by varying the cue-to-line distance in a systematic way. They observed the previously described effect of attention producing the illusion of a line moving away from the attended location, but they also found an inversion of the direction of the illusion in the immediate surround of the cued location (illusory motion toward the attended location), suggesting that temporal priority perception is impeded in a zone immediately surrounding the cued location. (It should be noted that there is some evidence challenging the notion that the illusory line motion effect reflects a consequence of spatial attention (Downing & Treisman, 1997).)

The most comprehensive evidence for a center-surround profile was provided in visual search experiments. Cave and Zimmerman (1997) combined a letter-search task (circular search arrays) with a subsequent spatial probe-detection task at prior target or distractor locations. As expected, probe detection at the location of the target turned out to be faster than at distractor locations. However, probe-detection at distractor locations near to the target was slower than at distractor locations far from the target—an observation taken to index flanking inhibition of distractors close to the target. Similarly, Mounts (2000b) had subjects discriminate a feature-singleton in an array of shape-8 elements. A shape-probe was then unmasked by removing selected lines of one shape-8 element at varying distances from the feature-singleton (67 ms after array onset). Discrimination performance of the shape-probe turned out to be lower in the vicinity of the feature singleton as compared to item location farther away. Another approach for estimating the precise shape of the attentional focus is to assess target discrimination performance as a function of the spatial distance to interfering distractors. Caputo and Guerra (1998), for example, observed that distractor interference was strongest in the vicinity of the target. A related way to assess the spatial profile of visual attention is to analyze item-matching performance as a function of item-distance, which reveals that farther away items are better matched than items close to each other (Bahcall & Kowler, 1999; Cutzu & Tsotsos, 2003; Fecteau & Enns, 2005). Thus, taken together, there has been some behavioral support that the focus of attention has the form of a Mexican-hat profile, with evidence coming from a diverse set of experimental approaches.

Neurophysiological Data Suggesting a Center-Surround Profile

Schall et al. (Schall & Hanes, 1993; Schall, Hanes, Thompson, & King, 1995; Schall, Sato, Thompson, Vaughn, & Juan, 2004) recorded from frontal eye field (FEF) neurons while monkeys performed saccades to a search target among distractors. They observed that presaccadic firing (100 ms prior to saccade execution) to a distractor falling in the cell's response field was suppressed when the search target was near to the response field relative to when the target was farther away. This surround suppression in FEF was hypothesized to reduce the probability of saccades to irrelevant distractor locations that could be confused with the target's location. Sundberg, Mitchell, and Reynolds (2009) had monkeys perform a multiple-object-tracking (four objects) task while recording from V4 neurons. The firing response was compared for situations in which the tracked target appeared inside, outside but close, or away from the neuron's receptive fields (RF). They reported that stimulus configurations with an object simultaneously placed inside and near outside, the response was suppressed in comparison to a single object presented inside the RF (surround suppression effect). Importantly, this effect depended on the position of the focus of attention

relative to the RF, that is, surround suppression was substantially larger for attending an object close to the RF than attending the object inside the RF or the object distant from the RF. Along similar lines, using double-label deoxyglucose technique to visualize attention-related metabolic activity changes in macaque striate cortex, Vanduffel, Tootell and Orban (2000) documented a suppression of metabolic activity in a circumscribed region retinotopically corresponding with the surround of the attended stimulus.

Some neuroimaging evidence for a center-surround profile of the attentional focus has also been reported for humans (Boehler et al., 2009; Boehler, Tsotsos, Schoenfeld, Heinze, & Hopf, 2011; Heinemann, Kleinschmidt, & Muller, 2009; Hopf et al., 2010; Hopf et al., 2006; Muller & Kleinschmidt, 2004; Schwartz et al., 2005; Slotnick, Hopfinger, Klein, & Sutter, 2002). In one such study, functional magnetic resonance imaging (fMRI) in humans revealed evidence for neural suppression in regions of the striate visual cortex that are retinotopically consistent with the surround of attended locations (Muller & Kleinschmidt, 2004). Muller and Kleinschmidt used symbolic cuing to direct attention to one of four isoeccentric location-placeholder boxes in the upper visual field. Following the cue, four items were flashed into the placeholders and subjects had to discriminate the item in the attended box. This stimulation protocol was combined with retinotopic mapping to attain a specific analysis of the attention-related BOLD response as a function of distance (at, near, and far) from the cued location in retinotopic areas V1–V4. In areas V2–V4, a simple activation gradient falling off with distance was observed. V1, in contrast, showed a significant reduction of signal change in the location near as compared to far from the target, suggesting that in the primary visual cortex the activity modulation underlying spatial attention shows a center-surround profile.

Systematic evidence for such center-surround profile was recently provided in a series of visual search experiments using magnetoencephalographic (MEG) recordings in human observers (Boehler et al., 2009; Boehler et al., 2011; Hopf et al., 2006; Hopf et al., 2010). The general experimental approach in these studies was to combine a visual search task with a subsequent presentation of a task-irrelevant probe, with the probe serving to assess the passive responsiveness of the visual cortex as a function of its distance to the search target, i.e., the spatial focus of attention. Figure 1.1 shows the general stimulus setup (Hopf et al., 2006). To avoid stimulation confounds resulting from changing positions of the probe, the probe always appeared at a constant location in the right lower VF, while the search target varied its position and distance relative to the probe from trial to trial within the same visual quadrant (using only a single quadrant also avoided potential confounds between

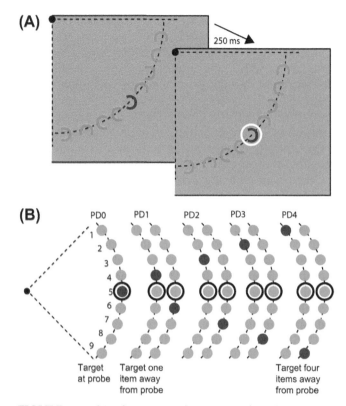

FIGURE 1.1 Stimulus setup and experimental conditions of the visual search experiment 1 reported in Hopf et al. (2006). Panel (A): Search frames always contained nine items (Cs with random gap-orientation) arrayed at an isoeccentric distance to fixation (black dot) in the right lower visual quadrant. The search target was a red C among eight blue distractor Cs, which randomly appeared at any of the nine item positions. On 50% of the trials, a small white ring (the probe) was flashed for 50 ms around the middle item position 250 ms after search frame onset. If presented, the probe always appeared at this middle position and was task irrelevant. This yielded five probe-to-target distance conditions (PD0 through PD4), permitting us to assess the size of the brain response to the probe as a function of its distance to the search target, i.e., to the focus of attention. *Source: Adapted from Hopf et al. (2006).* Panel (B) illustrates all possible probe-to-target distance conditions. Note the dashed lines in panel (A) are shown for illustration purposes and were not visible during the experiment.

spatial distance and stimulated hemisphere). Figure 1.1(B) illustrates all possible probe-target distance conditions. Note that corresponding probe-distance (PD) conditions toward the vertical and horizontal meridian (shown as pairs in Figure 1.1(B)) were collapsed for data analysis. The primary goal of the experimental setup was to assess and quantify the passive brain response to the probe proper, rather than measuring the attention-related modulation of the brain response to the target. To this end, a probe followed a search frame (**frame-probe (FP-) trials**) on only 50% of the trials; on the other trials the search frame appeared without a subsequent probe (**frame-only (FO-) trials**). The passive cortical response to the probe could then be isolated by subtracting the response to FO-trials from that of FP-trials (**FP-minus-FO-difference**). Importantly,

this subtraction was separately done for each target location, which (additivity assumed) should not only eliminate the response to the search frame (including the effect of attending the target), but also cancel the potentially confounding effect of the target changing its position relative to the probe. It is important to avoid such stimulus-location confounds, because the sensory MEG response varies with spatial position, which would contaminate the amplitude variation reflecting the spatial profile of attention in an unpredictable way. In fact, a number of previous studies have afforded such confounds which rendered their conclusions somewhat vague.

As shown in Figure 1.1(A), search frames were composed of nine items (letter C) presented at an isoeccentric distance in the right lower visual quadrant. The gap of the items randomly varied along the horizontal (left, right) and vertical (up, down) directions. The subjects' task was to report the gap-orientation of the color singleton (the red C among eight blue Cs), which randomly appeared at one of nine fixed item positions. The probe (a small white ring), if presented, was always flashed (50 ms stimulus duration) around the C at the center position. During most of the experiments reviewed below, the probe was presented with an SOA of 250 ms after search frame onset. Both, the location of the target singleton, and whether a probe was presented or not, was unpredictable. As sketched in Figure 1.1(B), from the nine item positions, the following five probe-to-target distances (in short: **PD**) were defined: the target appeared at the probe position (**PD0**), the target appeared at the positions one item away next to the probe (**PD1**), the target appeared two (**PD2**), three (**PD3**), or four item positions away from the probe (**PD4**).

Figure 1.2(A) shows the size of the probe-response (FP-minus-FO-difference) at the different PDs toward the vertical and horizontal meridian of experiment 1 reported in Hopf et al. (2006). The probe-response was found to be largest at the focus of attention (PD0), but it showed a substantial attenuation at PD1 not only relative to PD0, but also relative to the amplitudes elicited by probes with larger distances to the target (PD2–PD4). Hence, the passive responsivity of the cortex at the spatial focus of attention does not show a simple monotonic gradient that gradually falls off with distance from the center. Instead, the activity profile shows a small center enhancement with an annulus of reduced responsivity surrounding the attended item resembling a Mexican-hat profile.

Although this experimental setup controls for many potential confounds through its use of a constant probe position and the FP-minus-FO subtraction, it does not fully rule out a potential issue, which is illustrated in Figure 1.3. The experimental design entails that on FP-trials the probe is flashed around a blue item on 8/9 cases

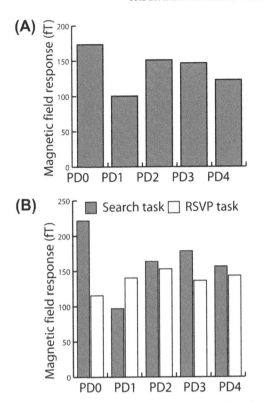

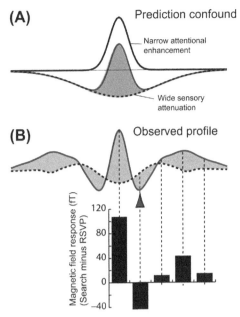

FIGURE 1.2 Panel (A): Results of experiment 1 and experiment 2 (B) in Hopf et al. (2006) demonstrating the center-surround profile of the focus of attention in visual search. The barplots show the size of the probe-related, event-related magnetic field (ERMF) response (FP-minus-FO-trials) for the different PD conditions. Surround attenuation is visible as significant reduction of the ERMF response to the target position next to the probe (PD1, gray bars) relative to PD0 and farther away positions. Panel (B): Results of experiment 2 in Hopf et al. (2006). The gray bars show the size of the probe-response as a function of PD when subjects attended to the search target (search task), the white bars show the size of the probe-response when subjects attended away from the search items and performed the rapid serial visual presentation task (RSVP task) at fixation. *Source: Adapted from Hopf et al. (2006).*

FIGURE 1.3 Panel (A): Illustration of a possible confound producing a center-surround profile caused by sensory interactions due to a frequency-imbalance of the target and the distractor color at and close to the probe location. Assuming this imbalance gives rise to a wide Gaussian-like attenuation (dashed black bar) and focal attention elicits a narrower positive enhancement (solid black bar), a combination of both would appear as a center-surround profile (red bar). Panel (B) sketches the results of experiment 2 in Hopf et al. (2006), which addressed this confound by comparing the profile during visual search with an attend-away condition where subject performed a demanding RSVP task at fixation while ignoring the search items. As visible, the attenuation at PD1 is much stronger in the visual search task than in the RSVP task (red arrowhead), which rules out the confound illustrated in panel (A).

while it appears around a red item in 1/9 cases. Furthermore, in 2/9 cases the probe is flanked by a red item, while on the majority of trials the probe is flanked by a blue item. This frequency imbalance of color-contrast may violate the assumption that the search frame and the probe do not interact in a spatially-specific manner (which is a prerequisite for a successful subtraction) by causing some low-level sensory modulation of the cortical responsiveness, resulting in an attenuated response to the probe. If we assume as illustrated in Figure 1.3(A) (prediction confound) that this sensory attenuation has a wider spatial extent (black dashed negative Gaussian) than the enhancement peak due to attention (black positive Gaussian), both effects could combine to a center-surround profile (red trace) that does not reflect the operation of focal attention. One way to address this issue is to assess whether such color-frequency related

low-level sensory attenuation effect actually arises in the experimental setup used here, and if yes, whether the size and extension of the attenuation would explain the observed profile. This was done by extending the experimental setup shown in Figure 1.1 by adding a rapid serial visual presentation (RSVP) task at fixation to effectively draw attention away from the peripheral search items. Subjects performed this RSVP task on half of the trial blocks. The search items and the probe were still presented as before, but subjects had to ignore the peripheral items. On the other half of the trial blocks, subjects performed the search task as before but ignored the RSVP stream at fixation. The data of the RSVP-blocks were analyzed analogous to the data of the visual search blocks, which should reveal the profile of cortical responsiveness arising from imbalances of sensory stimulation, in particular of the color-contrast between the color singleton and the probe. The observations are shown in Figure 1.2(B). The profile of the RSVP-blocks indeed shows a slight dip of responsiveness at PD0 and PD1, which, however, cannot account for the attenuation at PD1 seen when attention is focused onto the search target. If the center-surround profile arises from a confound as sketched in Figure 1.3(A), we would predict that for any PD the attenuation seen in the visual search task would never fall below the attenuation seen in the RSVP task. However, as illustrated in Figure 1.3(B), the attenuation at PD1 is substantially stronger when subjects performed the visual search task than the RSVP task (red arrowhead). Hence, surround attenuation shown in Figure 1.2 is a true effect of focusing attention onto the target during visual search.

THE SPATIAL PROFILE OF VISUAL ATTENTION VARIES WITH DEMANDS ON FEEDFORWARD AND FEEDBACK PROCESSING IN VISUAL CORTEX

As outlined above, despite the large set of data on spatial attention amounted by different methodological approaches, a clear characterization of the spatial profile of attention remains controversial. Many observations suggest spatial attention to show a simple gradient profile while others clearly demonstrate the presence of a more complex center-surround profile. Notably, past research has mainly focused on demonstrating one or the other profile with little emphasis on answering the more fundamental question of what may be the basis for a specific profile to appear. The issue seems to defy easy clarification from available experimental evidence as experimental designs and stimulus materials are very heterogeneous. Nonetheless, a few studies addressed the issue more explicitly and converged on a possible solution. As we will see, the solution lends itself to an explanation in terms of constraints on and the direction of selection in the visual cortical hierarchy, a notion explicitly proposed by computational models of attention (Tsotsos, 1990, 2005, 2011; Tsotsos et al., 1995).

For example, McCarley and Mounts (2007) investigated the influence of the type of input discrimination on surround attenuation (in their terminology the amount of *localized attentional interference* (**LAI**)). Subjects were either asked to respond to the mere presence of a certain color in the display no matter whether one or two items were drawn in the target color (feature-detection task) or to respond when two items but not one item appeared with the target color (item-individuation task). The display could contain one or two items drawn in the target color. The separation between the targets on two-item trials was varied to quantify the effect of LAI. LAI was observed for the item-individuation task but not for the feature-detection task, suggesting that surround attenuation arises when individual item properties need to be resolved, but not during the mere detection of a feature which does not require scrutiny to individuate the target. Hence, it appears

that surround attenuation arises when the selection of item specific information requires increased spatial resolution.

Boehler et al. (2009) (experiment 2 in Boehler et al., 2009) explicitly addressed this possibility with MEG recordings. The experimental setup was analogous to the one in Hopf et al. (2006) illustrated in Figure 1.1 except that only PDs PD0 through PD2 were used. The experiment again combined a visual search for a color-popout target (a red or green C among blue distractor Cs) with the subsequent presentation of a task-irrelevant probe 250 ms after search frame onset on 50% of the trials. On half of the trial-blocks, subjects were instructed to report the gap-orientation of the target as in Hopf et al. (2006)—a task that requires spatial resolution to discriminate the position of the gap. On the other half of trial-blocks, subjects were required to just report the color of the color-popout target—a task that can be solved without spatial resolution (Evans & Treisman, 2005; Tsotsos et al., 2008). Figure 1.4(A) and (B) shows the size of the probe-response (FP-minus-FO difference) as a function of probe-to-target distance for (A) the color and (B) the orientation task. Confirming our prediction, surround attenuation appeared for the orientation task, that is, when spatial scrutiny is critical for solving the task, whereas a simple gradient appeared for the color task where spatial scrutiny is not required. One may object that the color task was easier to perform than the orientation task, which may be an uncontrolled source of influence potentially relevant for whether surround attenuation arises or not. This is unlikely in view of some other experimental observations (Hopf et al., 2010). Specifically, we observed that increasing the difficulty of discrimination while keeping the spatial scale of discrimination constant did not influence the size of surround attenuation in an experimental setup analogous to the one shown in Figure 1.1.

A further notable observation in Boehler et al. (2009) was made when comparing the color and the orientation task with respect to the current source activity underlying target selection in visual cortex. Figure 1.4(C) shows the distribution of current source density estimates during four subsequent time-periods after search frame onset (FO-trials only) for the color task (upper row) and the orientation task (lower row). Apparently, the initial source activity in early striate (a) and extrastriate cortex (b) up to ~100 ms is comparable between the two experimental tasks. In contrast, later recurrent (presumably feedback) activity occurring between 200 and 300 ms in early visual cortex (c, the exact time-range is indicated by the red horizontal bar) is much stronger in the orientation than in the color task, suggesting that the center-surround profile is indeed associated with increased recurrent processing in visual

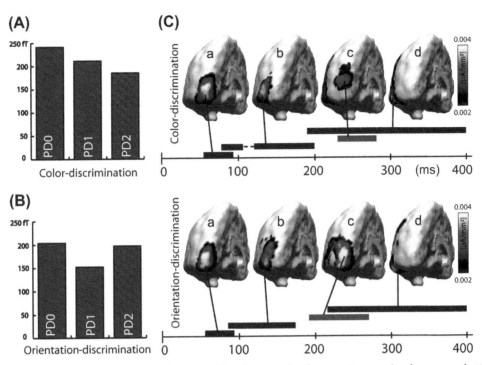

FIGURE 1.4   Results of experiment 2 in Boehler et al. (2009) addressing the role of recurrent processing for surround attenuation to appear. Panels (A) and (B) show the size of the probe-related event-related magnetic field response (FP-minus-FO-trials) as a function of PD (PD0 through PD2) for the color- and orientation-discrimination task, respectively. Note, in this experiment only PDs PD0 through PD2 were used, which is sufficient to characterize surround suppression. Panel (C) shows the current source density distribution underlying the magnetic field response elicited by frame-only (FO-) trials of the color- (upper row) and orientation task (lower row) during four subsequent time ranges after search frame onset (a–d). The red bar highlights the time-range of recurrent activity in early visual cortex areas. *Source: Adapted from Boehler et al. (2009).*

cortex. Notably, for the orientation task, the enhancement of recurrent source activity in early visual cortex appeared between 190 and 270 ms after search frame onset, that is shortly before and around the onset of the probe at 250 ms. Given that the cortical response to the probe takes roughly another 50 ms to reach the primary visual cortex (Foxe & Simpson, 2002), this top-down modulation will clearly appear prior to the probe-elicited feedforward in early visual cortex.

A further observation suggesting that surround attenuation arises from recurrent processing in visual cortex was provided by another experiment in which the FP SOA was varied in order to obtain a more detailed analysis of the time course of the surround attenuation effect (experiment 1 in Boehler et al., 2009). The experimental setup was again analogous to the one in Hopf et al. (2006) except that on FP-trials the probe randomly followed the search frame at one of five different SOAs (100, 175, 250, 325, and 400 ms). It was observed that surround attenuation was not present until 175 ms. At 250 ms surround attenuation was clearly the prominent feature of the probe-response, while at 325 ms the effect already tapered off and was not significant anymore. Hence, surround attenuation is a delayed and transient effect that takes more than 175 ms to build up in the type of search experiments we

used here. Importantly, such delay is consistent with the typical delay of attention-driven recurrent processing in visual cortex in response to an onset stimulation (Di Russo, Martinez, & Hillyard, 2003; Hopf, Heinze, Schoenfeld, & Hillyard, 2009; Martinez et al., 2001; Noesselt et al., 2002). Taken together, the delayed onset of surround attenuation (beyond 175 ms), the fact that it appeared for a discrimination task requiring recurrent processing but not for a task that does not depend on recurrent processing, strongly suggests that surround attenuation arises as a consequence of recurrent processing in visual cortex.

Such a direct link between recurrent processing in visual cortex and the occurrence of surround attenuation represents a key notion of the selective tuning model (STM) of visual attention (Tsotsos, 1990, 2011; Tsotsos et al., 1995). In the STM, it is proposed that surround attenuation arises as a consequence of iterative level-by-level selection of target information in reverse direction through the visual cortical hierarchy. The recurrent selection process starts at the highest level of representation from the unit corresponding to the winner of the competition for item salience during the initial feedforward sweep of processing through the visual hierarchy. As the spatial resolution of selectivity at a given hierarchical level corresponds with the size of the RFs at this level, it is coarsest at the highest level. Figure 1.5 illustrates this for a simplified three-layer hierarchy where the highest level is represented by level (n) and

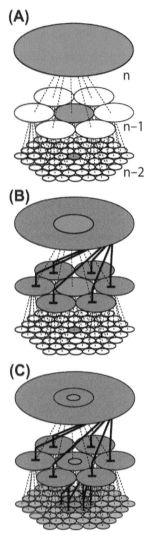

FIGURE 1.5 Illustration of how recurrent top-down processing increases the spatial resolution of discrimination in a simple three-layer model of the visual cortical processing hierarchy. Hierarchical levels are indexed by n with layer n−2 representing the lowest level. The ellipses denote processing units at each level, the size of the ellipses refers to the size of RFs. Note, the illustration provides only a simplified version of hierarchical selection in visual cortex as suggested by the selective tuning model (STM) of visual attention (Tsotsos, 2011). Only forward-converging projections (dashed lines) are considered. Blue indicates an activated unit best corresponding with the input (winner). Gray highlights units whose projections are attenuated. Panel (A) shows the state of activation in the hierarchy after the initial feed-forward sweep of processing reached the highest level of representation where RF size is large and the resolution of discrimination low. Panel (B) shows an intermediate state where the resolution of discrimination is increased to match the RF size at layer n−1, brought about by top-down pruning (solid black lines) forward connections from nonwinning units at layer (n−1) to the winner at (n). Panel (C) shows the final state where selection has propagated a further level down in the hierarchy and reached the input layer n−2. At this state of top-down selection the spatial scale of discrimination is adjusted to the highest resolution of the input-level.

the subsequent lower levels represented by n−1 and n−2. The ellipses illustrate the size of RFs at a given hierarchical level. Panel (A) shows the situation after the feedforward sweep of processing has just reached the top level (n). At this moment, the resolution of discrimination in the processing hierarchy is very low as it corresponds with the size of the RFs at level (n). To increase the resolution of selection, STM proposes a winner-take-all (WTA) process iteratively propagating to lower levels in the hierarchy where RF size becomes progressively smaller and better suited for the discrimination of small-scale item properties. The downward selection from level-to-level is suggested to operate by identifying a winning unit at the next lower level that is inside the forward projection zone of RFs to the winner at the next level. The lower-level winner (the blue unit at level n−1 in (A)) is then selected by pruning away connections inside the projection zone not projecting from the lower-level winner as illustrated in panel (B). This WTA propagates downward in the hierarchy until the input layer is reached as shown in panel (C) (see Tsotsos (2011) for details of implementation).

A consequence of the downward propagating WTA and pruning process is that the spatial resolution of discrimination progressively increases with each level downward in the hierarchy, such that the effective RF size and location at the top level is shrunk to the size and location of the lowest-level units representing the visual input (situation in panel (C)). Another inherent consequence of pruning projections from nontarget units inside the projection zones is that cortical excitability is attenuated in a circumscribed zone of retinotopic cortex that corresponds to the immediate surround of the target location. Hence, in STM surround attenuation is an inherent consequence of recurrent processing that serves to increase the spatial resolution of discrimination. The observations in Boehler et al. (2009) provide direct support for this notion by showing that the center-surround profile appeared for the gap-orientation task but not the color task. The former required that spatial resolution increases to enable the gap discrimination. The color discrimination task instead does not require spatial resolution as the task can be performed without precise localization of the target. Here, STM predicts that discrimination can be performed by relying on the initial feedforward pass of information through the hierarchy—an operation referred to as forward-binding in STM (Tsotsos et al., 2008). In fact, in the framework of the feature integration theory and related accounts (Evans & Treisman, 2005; Treisman & Gelade, 1980; Treisman & Gormican, 1988; Wolfe & Cave, 1999), the color task would be assumed to not require exact spatial binding of the target color and could be solved already with the feedforward sweep of processing. Finally, surround attenuation in early visual cortex areas turns out to arise with a delay relative to the initial feedforward response in visual cortex consistent with the additional time necessary for top-down modulations from higher-level visual areas to modify (tune) neural processing in progressively lower-level areas.

SURROUND ATTENUATION AND THE ROLE OF DISTRACTORS IN VISUAL SEARCH

The experimental evidence discussed so far suggests that surround attenuation arises as a consequence of recurrent processing in visual cortex, which serves to increase the spatial resolution of discrimination. A formal implementation is provided by the STM of visual attention, in which the increase in resolution is brought about by a top-down pruning process that eliminates forward projections from units representing the distractors in the immediate surround of the target. An obvious interpretation would be that surround attenuation serves to eliminate the input noise that is spatially most interfering with the target information. Hence, spatial resolution may be a welcome consequence of recurrent processing but not its driving force. Instead, the need to individuate the target by eliminating the interference from surrounding distractors may be the primary cause. In principle, target individuation by distractor elimination and increasing the resolution of discrimination could be equivalent operations, but it could also be that the latter is independent and not bound to the elimination of distractors. The issue was recently addressed with MEG recordings in human observers (Boehler et al., 2011). Specifically, it was asked whether surround attenuation would also appear when the target is not surrounded by distractors (experiment 2 in Boehler et al., 2011). The experimental setup was analogous to the one in Hopf et al. (2006). Visual search for a color-popout was combined with the presentation of a task-irrelevant probe 250 ms after search frame onset. The probe appeared on 50% of the trials at a constant location at the center position of the search array. Subjects had to report the gap-orientation of the target-popout. In contrast to Hopf et al. (2006), during one type of trial-blocks the target was randomly presented at the different item positions in complete isolation without distractors. During other trial-blocks, the target appeared together with distractors as in Hopf et al. (2006). As visible in Figure 1.6 surround attenuation was observed no matter whether the target was surrounded by distractors or not, indicating that distractor elimination per se may not be its primary cause. Instead, the observations in Boehler et al. (2011) support the notion that surround attenuation arises as a consequence of the need to increase the spatial resolution of discrimination.

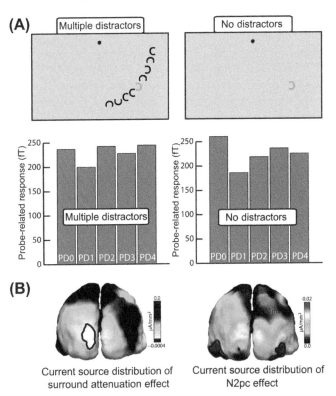

FIGURE 1.6 Example search arrays and results of experiment 2 (A) in Boehler et al. (2011) addressing the influence of distractors on surround attenuation. The barplots show the size of the probe-related event-related magnetic field response (FP-minus-FO-trials) as a function of probe-to-target distance (PD0 through PD4) for the multiple (left) and the no distractor condition (right). Panel (B, left) shows the distribution of attenuated source activity derived by estimating the PD1-minus-PD2 ERMF difference of the multiple distractor condition in Boehler et al. (2011) (experiment 1). The maps show grand average source density estimates (over subjects) computed with, and rendered onto, the 3D-surface of the MNI-brain (Montreal Neurological Institute, average 152 T1-weighted stereotaxic volumes of the ICBM project, ICBM152). The right map shows the corresponding current source distribution of brain activity underlying the N2pc response (collapsed over multiple and the single distractor conditions). The black bars outline cortical regions with maximum source activity. *Source: Adapted from Boehler et al. (2011).*

This observation seems to be relevant for discussing earlier behavioral findings (McCarley & Mounts, 2007). As reviewed above, McCarley and Mounts (2007) observed behavioral effects of surround attenuation LAI when subjects were required to individuate items drawn in the target color but not when they had to report the mere presence of a target color. Their observations were taken to indicate that LAI is a consequence of the demand to "resolve properties of individual stimuli"—a notion in line with the results in Boehler et al. (2009, 2011). However, the experiments using LAI as an index of surround attenuation cannot be specific as to whether surround attenuation relates to resolving the competition between items that are close to each other, or to the requirement to increase the spatial resolution of discrimination to detect a separation between the items. McCarley and Mounts (2007) seem to prefer the former interpretation and emphasize that their data lines up with the biased competition account of visual attention (Desimone & Duncan, 1995). In view of Boehler et al. (2011), however, it seems that the mere requirement to attain high spatial resolution for stimulus discrimination, independent of whether the discrimination competes with distractors, is the actual cause of surround attenuation to arise.

Note, item competition per se has been shown to be reflected by the amplitude of the N2pc—an ERP/ERMF component known to index attentional focusing onto the target item in visual search in humans (Eimer, 1996; Hopf, Boehler, Schoenfeld, & Heinze, 2011; Hopf, Boelmans, Schoenfeld, Heinze, & Luck, 2002; Hopf et al., 2000; Luck & Hillyard, 1994a, 1994b; Woodman & Luck, 1999; Woodman & Luck, 2003) and monkeys (Cohen, Heitz, Schall, & Woodman, 2009; Cohen, Heitz, Woodman, & Schall, 2009; Heitz, Cohen, Woodman, & Schall, 2010; Woodman, Kang, Rossi, & Schall, 2007). An increase of competition between target and distractor items in visual search was found to be associated with an increase of the N2pc amplitude, suggesting that the N2pc reflects distractor attenuation in visual search (Boehler et al., 2011; Hopf et al., 2002; Luck, Girelli, McDermott, & Ford, 1997; see also Hickey, Di Lollo, & McDonald, 2009). In Boehler et al. (2011) (experiment 1), we used a modified version of the task with bilateral search arrays in order to be able to assess the N2pc response. The latter is derived by subtracting the brain response to trials with the target in one visual hemifield from trials with the target appearing in the opposite hemifield. Notably, the amplitude of the N2pc, but not surround attenuation, was influenced by the number of distractors in the search array. Source localization analyses revealed that current source activity underlying the N2pc arises from higher and midlevel cortical areas of the ventral visual cortex. When the target was flanked by distractors in its immediate surround, additional source activity was found in hierarchically lower-level extrastriate cortex as compared to when only one distant distractor was presented in the opposite visual field. Notably, source activity at the lower hierarchical level appeared with a delay (~20 ms) relative to the initial N2pc current source in higher-level ventral extrastriate cortex. Lower-level visual areas are progressively better suited to resolve the competition between closely spaced items because of smaller RF size. The observation was therefore taken to suggest that the current origin of the N2pc reflects the spatial scale of item competition (RF size) in visual cortex (see Hopf et al., 2006 for analogous observations). In contrast, localization analyses of the surround attenuation effect invariably revealed a maximum of attenuation in early visual cortex, presumably in the primary visual cortex (V1) (Boehler et al., 2011; Hopf

et al., 2006). Typical localization results are illustrated in Figure 1.6(B). The distribution of attenuated source activity underlying the surround attenuation effect (source density estimates of the PD1-minus-PD2 event-related magnetic field (ERMF) difference) is shown together with the distribution of source activity underlying N2pc of the multiple distractor condition of experiment 1 reported in (Boehler et al., 2011). Such maximal surround attenuation in early visual cortex is a direct prediction of STM in which the number of attenuated units shows a progressive increase toward lower hierarchical levels. For neural population measures, like magneto- and electroencephalography, this means that correlates of surround attenuation become more and more apparent the lower the hierarchical level of cortical representation is. On the contrary, as detailed in Boehler et al. (2011) in the framework of the STM, the N2pc is suggested to reflect a top-down biasing operation at the hierarchical level where competition between units arises due to large RFs typically covering target and distractor input. As RF size and competition increase with hierarchy, the N2pc as a population measure of biasing competition (Luck et al., 1997) will become most prominent at corresponding levels of representation. Importantly, the amount of modulation needed to bias competition in favor of the unit representing the target at a given hierarchical level may differ and therefore be mirrored by changes of the N2pc amplitude. Once competition is resolved and a winning unit is identified, the spatial extent and number of units being subsequently pruned by the downward propagating WTA process (units that give rise to surround attenuation, see Figure 1.5) will be independent of the amount of prior biasing involved to resolve competition in favor of that winner. Hence, surround attenuation and the N2pc index functionally independent operations during top-down attentional selection.

To conclude, surround attenuation turns out to not reflect the resolution of competition between items. Instead, it rather reflects the requirement to increase spatial resolution for precise item localization or discrimination. As detailed above, increasing the spatial resolution of discrimination is suggested to involve top-down directed, coarse-to-fine processing in the visual cortical hierarchy—an integral notion of influential theories of attentional selection in visual cortex (Deco & Schurmann, 2000; Deco & Zihl, 2001; Hochstein & Ahissar, 2002; Tsotsos, 1990, 2011; Tsotsos et al., 1995; Tsotsos et al., 2008). According to STM, this top-down process operates by attenuating forward projections not contributing to the representation of the target input. The attenuation of cortical excitability in the target's surround is not an explicit goal of selection but comes as an inherent byproduct of tuning top-down selection for higher spatial resolution of discrimination.

SUMMARY

The reviewed experimental data clearly indicate that the spatial focus of attention does not have a fixed uniform distributional profile. The profile turns out to qualitatively change in response to different requirements on target discrimination, and it rapidly varies during the process of stimulus selection on the order of a few tens of milliseconds after stimulation onset. In this chapter, we characterize one critical distinction of task requirements that we and others found to determine whether the spatial focus takes a simple monotonic gradient or a more complex center-surround profile. Specifically, we show that the center-surround profile arises when target discrimination requires spatial resolution and/or precise item localization. In contrast, when the selection of task-relevant information is largely independent of the spatial resolution of discrimination, e.g. when feature information can be discriminated without precise item localization, the focus of attention displays a simple gradient profile.

Importantly, this distinction in terms of requirements on the spatial resolution of discrimination maps onto the fundamental distinction between feedforward and feedback processing in the visual cortical processing hierarchy as suggested by computational accounts like the STM of visual attention (Tsotsos et al., 2008). According to STM, the complex center-surround profile arises as a consequence of recurrent top-down selection after the initial feedforward sweep of processing passed upward the visual processing hierarchy and reached the highest levels of representation. At the latter, the spatial resolution of discrimination is very coarse due to the on average large size of RFs. An important function of the subsequent top-down directed selection is to adjust the low spatial resolution of discrimination at higher levels in the processing hierarchy (large RF size) to the higher resolution of lower levels with smaller RFs. This is the case if the resolution of the initial feedforward sweep of processing is too coarse to permit a discrimination of task-relevant information. If coarse resolution is sufficient, discrimination can be performed without recurrent selection. The spatial distribution of attention will accordingly reflect the forward spread of activation in the processing cascade, which would resemble a simple gradient. The important point is that this account, in terms of hierarchical constraints on feedforward and feedback cortical selection, not only accommodates the observation of a varying profile, but also explains why surround attenuation takes additional time beyond the typical time-range of the initial feedforward sweep of processing in order to appear. Moreover, it explains why surround attenuation is independent of the presence of distractors in the target's surround. For spatial selection, the essential goal of recurrent top-down processing is to increase the resolution of the visual hierarchy, that is, to "shrink" the effective size of RF at hierarchically higher levels to the size of lower levels where RF size matches the spatial scale of discrimination. This is accomplished by eliminating the forward-projection of units toward the higher-level units, something that is involved independent of whether the target is surrounded by distractors or not. In sum, an explanation that starts from the cortical architecture and its hierarchical constraints on forward and recurrent processing (as e.g., STM) appears to be powerful in explaining many of the spatio-temporal characteristics of attentional selection in space, and links outwardly controversial observations.

This brings us back to our initial remarks. Research into the distribution of spatial attention was guided by thinking in analogies and metaphors for more than a century now. As outlined above, while considerable experimental data was gathered, the issue of the spatial profile remained controversial. The evidence from electromagnetic recordings reviewed above may be taken to highlight the fact that for future research it may be valuable to built predictions based on the inner architectural constraints of cortical selection rather than following the intuitive appeal of metaphoric analogies (Yantis, 1988). For example, the architecture of selection as suggested by STM would predict that movements of the focus of attention are not analogue as often conceptualized (Posner, 1980; Shulman et al., 1979; Tsal, 1983), but that they reflect the cycle-time of the recurrent top-down selection, resulting in a quantized stepping rather than a smooth movement across the visual field. In fact, there is some evidence suggesting that attention operates on a "periodic regime" (VanRullen, Carlson, & Cavanagh, 2007). Furthermore, it may turn out that conflicting evidence against or in favor of the ability to split the spatial focus of attention may be accounted for by differing notions of the focus of attention in terms of feedforward vs feedback defined distributions.

To conclude, we believe that understanding visual attentional from the perspective of architecture-bound cortical selection as outlined above proves to be a successful and promising approach. It has the potential to accommodate a heterogeneous body of experimental observations, which defies clarification in terms of mere metaphorical notions and analogies. Of course, much experimental work is left to be done in order to evaluate its full explanatory reach.

References

Ahissar, M., & Hochstein, S. (2004). The reverse hierarchy theory of visual perceptual learning. *Trends in Cognitive Sciences*, 8(10), 457–464.

Bahcall, D. O., & Kowler, E. (1999). Attentional interference at small spatial separations. *Vision Research*, 39(1), 71–86.

Boehler, C. N., Tsotsos, J. K., Schoenfeld, A., Heinze, H. -J., & Hopf, J. M. (2009). The center-surround profile of the focus of attention arises from recurrent processing in visual cortex. *Cerebral Cortex*, *19*(4), 982–991.

Boehler, C. N., Tsotsos, J. K., Schoenfeld, M. A., Heinze, H. J., & Hopf, J. M. (2011). Neural mechanisms of surround attenuation and distractor competition in visual search. *Journal of Neuroscience*, *31*(14), 5213–5224.

Caputo, G., & Guerra, S. (1998). Attentional selection by distractor suppression. *Vision Research*, *38*(5), 669–689.

Carr, T. H., & Dagenbach, D. (1990). Semantic priming and repetition priming from masked words: evidence for a center-surround attentional mechanism in perceptual recognition. *Journal of Experimental Psychology: Learning, Memory, and Cognition*, *16*(2), 341–350.

Castiello, U., & Umilta, C. (1990). Size of the attentional focus and efficiency of processing, [Research Support, Non-U.S. Gov't]. *Acta Psychologica*, *73*(3), 195–209.

Cave, K. R., & Bichot, N. P. (1999). Visuo-spatial attention: beyond a spotlight model. *Psychonomic Bulletin and Review*, *6*, 204–223.

Cave, K. R., & Zimmerman, J. M. (1997). Flexibility in spatial attention before and after practice. *Psychological Science*, *8*(5), 399–403.

Cohen, J. Y., Heitz, R. P., Schall, J. D., & Woodman, G. F. (2009). On the origin of event-related potentials indexing covert attentional selection during visual search. *Journal of Neurophysiology*, *102*(4), 2375–2386.

Cohen, J. Y., Heitz, R. P., Woodman, G. F., & Schall, J. D. (2009). Neural basis of the set-size effect in frontal eye field: timing of attention during visual search. *Journal of Neurophysiology*, *101*(4), 1699–1704.

Cutzu, F., & Tsotsos, J. K. (2003). The selective tuning model of attention: psychophysical evidence for a suppressive annulus around an attended item. *Vision Research*, *43*(2), 205–219.

Deco, G., & Schurmann, B. (2000). A hierarchical neural system with attentional top-down enhancement of the spatial resolution for object recognition. *Vision Research*, *40*(20), 2845–2859.

Deco, G., & Zihl, J. (2001). A neurodynamical model of visual attention: feedback enhancement of spatial resolution in a hierarchical system. *Journal of Computational Neuroscience*, *10*(3), 231–253.

Desimone, R., & Duncan, J. (1995). Neural mechanisms of selective visual attention. *Annual Review of Neurosciences*, *18*, 193–222.

Di Russo, F., Martinez, A., & Hillyard, S. A. (2003). Source analysis of event-related cortical activity during visuo-spatial attention. *Cerebral Cortex*, *13*(5), 486–499.

Downing, P. E., & Pinker, S. (1985). The spatial structure of visual attention. In M. I. Posner & O. S. Marin (Eds.), *Attention and performance XI* (pp. 171–188). Hillsdale, NJ: Erlbaum.

Downing, P. E., & Treisman, A. M. (1997). The line-motion illusion: attention or impletion? *Journal of Experimental Psychology: Human Perception and Performance*, *23*(3), 768–779.

Drew, T., McCollough, A. W., Horowitz, T. S., & Vogel, E. K. (2009). Attentional enhancement during multiple-object tracking. *Psychonomic Bulletin and Review*, *16*(2), 411–417.

Driver, J., & Baylis, G. C. (1989). Movement and visual attention: the spotlight metaphor breaks down. *Journal of Experimental Psychology: Human Perception and Performance*, *15*(3), 448–456.

Egly, R., & Homa, D. (1984). Sensitization of the visual field. *Journal of Experimental Psychology: Human Perception and Performance*, *10*(6), 778–793.

Eimer, M. (1996). The N2pc component as an indicator of attentional selectivity. *Electroencephalography and Clinical Neurophysiology*, *99*(3), 225–234.

Eimer, M. (1997). Attentional selection and attentional gradients: an alternative method for studying transient visual-spatial attention. *Psychophysiology*, *34*, 365–376.

Eimer, M. (2000). An ERP study of sustained spatial attention to stimulus eccentricity. *Biological Psychology*, *52*(3), 205–220.

Eriksen, C. W., & James, J. D. S. (1986). Visual attention within and around the field of focal attention: a zoom lens model. *Perception and Psychophysics*, *40*(4), 225–240.

Evans, K. K., & Treisman, A. (2005). Perception of objects in natural scenes: is it really attention free? *Journal of Experimental Psychology: Human Perception and Performance*, *31*(6), 1476–1492.

Fecteau, J. H., & Enns, J. T. (2005). Visual letter matching: hemispheric functioning or scanning biases? *Neuropsychologia*, *43*(10), 1412–1428.

Foxe, J. J., & Simpson, G. V. (2002). Flow of activation from V1 to frontal cortex in humans. A framework for defining "early" visual processing. *Experimental Brain Research*, *142*(1), 139–150.

Heinemann, L., Kleinschmidt, A., & Muller, N. G. (2009). Exploring BOLD changes during spatial attention in non-stimulated visual cortex. *PloS One*, *4*(5), e5560.

Heitz, R. P., Cohen, J. Y., Woodman, G. F., & Schall, J. D. (2010). Neural correlates of correct and errant attentional selection revealed through N2pc and frontal eye field activity. *Journal of Neurophysiology*, *104*(5), 2433–2441.

Helmholtz, H. v (1896). *Handbuch der physiologischen Optik*. Hamburg und Leipzig: Verlag von Leopold Voss.

Henderson, J. M., & Macquistan, A. D. (1993). The spatial distribution of attention following an exogenous cue. *Perception and Psychophysics*, *53*(2), 221–230.

Hickey, C., Di Lollo, V., & McDonald, J. J. (2009). Electrophysiological indices of target and distractor processing in visual search. *Journal of Cognitive Neuroscience*, *21*(4), 760–775.

Hikosaka, O., Miyauchi, S., & Shimojo, S. (1993a). Focal visual attention produces illusory temporal order and motion sensation. *Vision Research*, *33*(9), 1219–1240.

Hikosaka, O., Miyauchi, S., & Shimojo, S. (1993b). Voluntary and stimulus-induced attention detected as motion sensation. *Perception*, *22*(5), 517–526.

Hochstein, S., & Ahissar, M. (2002). View from the top: hierarchies and reverse hierarchies in the visual system. *Neuron*, *36*(5), 791–804.

Hopf, J. M., Boehler, C. N., Luck, S. J., Tsotsos, J. K., Heinze, H. -J., & Schoenfeld, M. A. (2006). Direct neurophysiological evidence for spatial suppression surrounding the focus of attention in vision. *Proceedings of the National Academy of Sciences of the United States of America*, *103*(4), 1053–1058.

Hopf, J. -M., Boehler, C. N., Schoenfeld, M. A., & Heinze, H. J. (2011). Attentional selection in vision: insights from electromagnetic brain activity. In G. R. Mangun (Ed.), *Neuroscience of attention* (pp. 3–29). Oxford University Press.

Hopf, J. -M., Boehler, C. N., Schoenfeld, M. A., Heinze, H. -J., & Tsotsos, J. K. (2010). The spatial profile of the focus of attention in visual search: insights from MEG recordings. *Vision Research*, *50*(14), 1312–1320.

Hopf, J. -M., Boelmans, K., Schoenfeld, A. M., Heinze, H. -J., & Luck, S. J. (2002). How does attention attenuate target-distractor interference in vision? Evidence from magnetoencephalographic recordings. *Cognitive Brain Research*, *15*(1), 17–29.

Hopf, J. -M., Heinze, H. J., Schoenfeld, M. A., & Hillyard, S. A. (2009). Spatio-temporal analysis of visual attention. In M. S. Gazzaniga (Ed.), *The cognitive neurosciences IV* (pp. 235–250). Cambridge, MA: MIT Press.

Hopf, J. -M., Luck, S. J., Boelmans, K., Schoenfeld, A., Boehler, N., Rieger, J. W., et al. (2006). The neural site of attention matches the spatial scale of perception. *Journal of Neuroscience*, *26*(13), 3532–3540.

Hopf, J. -M., Luck, S. J., Girelli, M., Hagner, T., Mangun, G. R., Scheich, H., et al. (2000). Neural sources of focused attention in visual search. *Cerebral Cortex*, *10*, 1233–1241.

Krose, B. J., & Julesz, B. (1989). The control and speed of shifts of attention. *Vision Research*, *29*(11), 1607–1619.

LaBerge, D., Carlson, R. L., Williams, J. K., & Bunney, B. G. (1997). Shifting attention in visual space: tests of moving-spotlight models versus an activity-distribution model. *Journal of Experimental Psychology: Human Perception and Performance*, *23*(5), 1380–1392.

Luck, S. J., Girelli, M., McDermott, M. T., & Ford, M. A. (1997). Bridging the gap between monkey neurophysiology and human perception: an ambiguity resolution theory of visual selective attention. *Cognitive Psychology, 33,* 64–87.

Luck, S. J., & Hillyard, S. A. (1994a). Electrophysiological correlates of feature analysis during visual search. *Psychophysiology, 31,* 291–308.

Luck, S. J., & Hillyard, S. A. (1994b). Spatial filtering during visual search: evidence from human electrophysiology. *Journal of Experimental Psychology: Human Perception and Performance, 20*(5), 1000–1014.

Mangun, G. R., & Hillyard, S. A. (1987). The spatial allocation of visual attention as indexed by event-related brain potentials. *Human Factors, 29,* 195–211.

Mangun, G. R., & Hillyard, S. A. (1988). Spatial gradients of visual attention: behavioral and electrophysiological evidence. *Electroencephalography and Clinical Neurophysiology, 70,* 417–428.

Martinez, A., DiRusso, F., Anllo-Vento, L., Sereno, M. I., Buxton, R. B., & Hillyard, S. A. (2001). Putting spatial attention on the map: timing and localization of stimulus selection processes in striate and extrastriate visual areas. *Vision Research, 41*(10–11), 1437–1457.

McCarley, J. S., & Mounts, J. R. (2007). Localized attentional interference affects object individuation, not feature detection. *Perception, 36*(1), 17–32.

McMains, S. A., & Somers, D. C. (2004). Multiple spotlights of attentional selection in human visual cortex. *Neuron, 42*(4), 677–686.

Mihalas, S., Dong, Y., von der Heydt, R., & Niebur, E. (2011). Mechanisms of perceptual organization provide auto-zoom and auto-localization for attention to objects. *Proceedings of the National Academy of Sciences of the United States of America, 108*(18), 7583–7588.

Morawetz, C., Holz, P., Baudewig, J., Treue, S., & Dechent, P. (2007). Split of attentional resources in human visual cortex, [Research Support, Non-U.S. Gov't]. *Visual Neuroscience, 24*(6), 817–826.

Mounts, J. R. (2000a). Attentional capture by abrupt onsets and feature singletons produces inhibitory surrounds. *Perception and Psychophysics, 62*(7), 1485–1493.

Mounts, J. R. (2000b). Evidence for suppressive mechanisms in attentional selection: feature singletons produce inhibitory surrounds. *Perception and Psychophysics, 62*(5), 969–983.

Muller, M. M., & Hubner, R. (2002). Can the spotlight of attention be shaped like a doughnut? Evidence from steady-state visual evoked potentials. *Psychological Science, 13*(2), 119–124.

Muller, N. G., & Kleinschmidt, A. (2004). The attentional 'spotlight's' penumbra: center-surround modulation in striate cortex. *Neuroreport, 15*(6), 977–980.

Muller, N. G., Mollenhauer, M., Rosler, A., & Kleinschmidt, A. (2005). The attentional field has a Mexican hat distribution. *Vision Research, 45*(9), 1129–1137.

Niebergall, R., Khayat, P. S., Treue, S., & Martinez-Trujillo, J. C. (2011). Multifocal attention filters targets from distracters within and beyond primate MT neurons' receptive field boundaries. *Neuron, 72*(6), 1067–1079.

Noesselt, T., Hillyard, S., Woldorff, M., Schoenfeld, A., Hagner, T., Jancke, L., et al. (2002). Delayed striate cortical activation during spatial attention. *Neuron, 35*(3), 575–587.

Posner, M. I. (1980). Orienting of attention. *Quarterly Journal of Experimental Psychology, 32,* 3–25.

Remington, R., & Pierce, L. (1984). Moving attention: evidence for time-invariant shifts of visual selective attention. *Perception and Psychophysics, 35*(4), 393–399.

Schall, J. D., & Hanes, D. P. (1993). Neural basis of saccade target selection in frontal eye field during visual search. *Nature, 366,* 467–469.

Schall, J. D., Hanes, D. P., Thompson, K. G., & King, D. J. (1995). Saccade target selection in frontal eye field of macaque. I. Visual and premovement activation. *Journal of Neuroscience, 15*(10), 6905–6918.

Schall, J. D., Sato, T. R., Thompson, K. G., Vaughn, A. A., & Juan, C. H. (2004). Effects of search efficiency on surround suppression during visual selection in frontal eye field. *Journal of Neurophysiology, 91*(6), 2765–2769.

Scharlau, I. (2004). The spatial distribution of attention in perceptual latency priming. *The Quarterly Journal of Experimental Psychology, 57*(8), 1411–1436.

Schwartz, S., Vuilleumier, P., Hutton, C., Maravita, A., Dolan, R. J., & Driver, J. (2005). Attentional load and sensory competition in human vision: modulation of fMRI responses by load at fixation during task-irrelevant stimulation in the peripheral visual field. *Cerebral Cortex, 15*(6), 770–786.

Shulman, G. L., Remington, R. W., & McLean, J. P. (1979). Moving attention through visual space. *Journal of Experimental Psychology: Human Perception and Performance, 5*(3), 522–526.

Shulman, G. L., Wilson, J., & Sheehy, J. B. (1985). Spatial determinants of the distribution of attention. *Perception and Psychophysics, 37*(1), 59–65.

Slotnick, S. D., Hopfinger, J. B., Klein, S. A., & Sutter, E. E. (2002). Darkness beyond the light: attentional inhibition surrounding the classic spotlight. *Neuroreport, 13*(6), 773–778.

Steinman, B. A., Steinman, S. B., & Lehmkuhle, S. (1995). Visual attention mechanisms show a center-surround organization. *Vision Research, 35*(13), 1859–1869.

Sundberg, K. A., Mitchell, J. F., & Reynolds, J. H. (2009). Spatial attention modulates center-surround interactions in macaque visual area v4. *Neuron, 61*(6), 952–963.

Treisman, A., & Gelade, G. (1980). A feature-integration theory of attention. *Cognitive Psychology, 12,* 97–136.

Treisman, A., & Gormican, S. (1988). Feature analysis in early vision: evidence from search asymmetries. *Psychological Review, 95*(1), 15–48.

Tsal, Y. (1983). Movements of attention across the visual field. *Journal of Experimental Psychology: Human Perception and Performance, 9*(4), 523–530.

Tsotsos, J. K. (1990). Analyzing vision at the complexity level. *Behavioral and Brain Sciences, 13,* 423–469.

Tsotsos, J. K. (2005). The selective tuning model for visual attention. In L. Itti, G. Rees & J. K. Tsotsos (Eds.), *Neurobiology of attention* (pp. 562–569). San Diego, CA: Elsevier.

Tsotsos, J. K. (2011). *A computational perspective on visual attention.* Cambridge, MA: The MIT Press.

Tsotsos, J. K., Culhane, S. M., Wai, W. Y. K., Lai, Y., Davis, N., & Nuflo, F. (1995). Modeling visual attention via selective tuning. *Artificial Intelligence, 78,* 507–545.

Tsotsos, J. K., Rodriguez-Sanchez, A. J., Rothenstein, A. L., & Simine, E. (2008). The different stages of visual recognition need different attentional binding strategies. *Brain Research, 1225,* 119–132.

Vanduffel, W., Tootell, R. B. H., & Orban, G. A. (2000). Attention-dependent suppression of metabolic activity in early stages of the macaque visual system. *Cerebral Cortex, 10,* 109–126.

VanRullen, R., Carlson, T., & Cavanagh, P. (2007). The blinking spotlight of attention. *Proceedings of the National Academy of Sciences of the United States of America, 104*(49), 19204–19209.

Wolfe, J. M., & Cave, K. R. (1999). The psychophysical evidence for a binding problem in human vision. *Neuron, 24,* 11–17.

Woodman, G. F., Kang, M. S., Rossi, A. F., & Schall, J. D. (2007). Nonhuman primate event-related potentials indexing covert shifts of attention. *Proceedings of the National Academy of Sciences of the United States of America, 104*(38), 15111–15116.

Woodman, G. F., & Luck, S. J. (1999). Electrophysiological measurement of rapid shifts of attention during visual search. *Nature, 400,* 867–869.

Woodman, G. F., & Luck, S. J. (2003). Serial deployment of attention during visual search. *Journal of Experimental Psychology: Human Perception and Performance, 29*(1), 121–138.

Yantis, S. (1988). On analog movements of visual attention. *Perception and Psychophysics, 43*(2), 203–206.

2

How the Brain Prevents and Terminates Shifts of Attention

Risa Sawaki, Steven J. Luck

Department of Psychology and Center for Mind and Brain, University of California, Davis, Davis, CA, USA

INTRODUCTION

Our environment is filled with a vast amount of information to be perceived, whereas our capacity to process this information is severely limited. Attentional control processes therefore play a fundamental role in cognition. For example, if you are trying to find a teaspoon in the scene shown in Figure 2.1, it is not sufficient to have a mechanism that simply enhances processing of visual inputs that have features in common with a teaspoon; it is also necessary to have a mechanism that can prevent attention from being directed to the highly salient but task-irrelevant objects, such as the tomato. Furthermore, it is important to have a mechanism that can terminate attention after it has been focused on an item that is similar to the target, but turns out not to be the target, such as a tablespoon when you are searching for a teaspoon. Moreover, once the teaspoon has been attended and then perceived, some mechanism must terminate this episode of attention so that the visual system can move on to other tasks.

Attention may shift from object to object 10 times per second (Woodman & Luck, 1999, 2003), and a salient distractor object can be suppressed within 150ms of stimulus onset (Sawaki & Luck, 2010). The event-related potential (ERP) technique is the only noninvasive neural method with the temporal resolution to track this fast time course. The N2-posterior-contralateral (N2pc) component has been used extensively over the past 20 years to understand the mechanisms by which attention is focused toward visual objects (see, e.g., Luck, 2012; Luck & Hillyard, 1994a, 1994b; also Eimer, 1996; Eimer & Kiss, 2008; Hickey, McDonald, & Theeuwes, 2006; Kiss, Jolicœur, Dell'acqua, & Eimer, 2008; Leblanc, Prime, & Jolicoeur, 2008; Lien, Ruthruff, Goodin, & Remington,

2008; Rodríguez Holguín, Doallo, Vizoso, & Cadaveira, 2009; Woodman & Luck, 1999, 2003). Almost two decades after the first observation of N2pc component (Luck & Hillyard, 1990), Hickey, Di Lollo, and McDonald (2009) described in detail the Pd (distractor positivity) component, which appears to reflect an attentional suppression process that is the mirror image of the attentional focusing mechanism reflected by N2pc. Since then, the Pd component has been used to investigate the active suppression process that is used to prevent and terminate attention (Sawaki & Luck, 2010, 2011, 2013; Sawaki, Geng, & Luck, 2012). The primary goal of this chapter is to review studies that explore this newly discovered attentional suppression mechanism.

BASICS OF N2pc AND Pd

The N2pc component is a sensitive index of the covert deployment of visual attention (Luck, 2012; Luck & Hillyard, 1994a, 1994b). This component is observed as a more negative voltage at contralateral scalp sites than at ipsilateral scalp sites relative to the position of an attended item in a visual search display (Figure 2.2 (A)-left). That is, the voltage over the right hemisphere is more negative for left visual field (LVF) targets than for right visual field (RVF) targets from approximately 175–300ms, and the voltage of the left hemisphere is more negative for RVF targets than for LVF targets during this period. Many studies demonstrate that the N2pc is associated with the focusing of attention onto an object (reviewed by Luck, 2012). The neural generators of the N2pc component have been identified using combined magnetoencephalogram (MEG) and electroencephalogram (EEG) recordings (e.g., Hopf, Boelmans,

Schoenfeld, Luck, & Heinze, 2004; Hopf et al., 2006; Hopf et al., 2000). In the study of Hopf et al. (2000), for example, participants searched for a specific color bar (red or green) among blue distractor bars, and they responded whether the target bar was vertical or horizontal. These MEG-EEG simultaneous recording studies demonstrated that the N2pc component has a magnetic analog and the N2pc component appears to be generated in intermediate and high levels of the ventral visual processing pathway, including area V4 and the lateral occipital complex

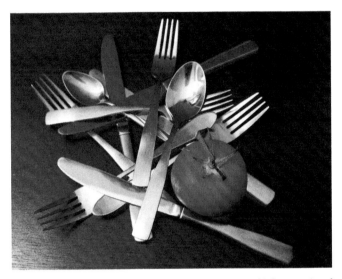

FIGURE 2.1 Example of a natural scene in which attentional enhancement and suppression are required to find a target (e.g., a teaspoon).

(see especially Hopf et al., 2006). This is quite close to the estimated location of the generator of the late portion of the visual P1 wave (Di Russo, Martinez, Sereno, Pitzalis, & Hillyard, 2002).

In contrast, the Pd component is an electrophysiological marker of attentional suppression (Hickey et al., 2009). This component is observed as a more positive voltage at contralateral scalp sites than at ipsilateral scalp sites relative to the position of a suppressed item. It begins approximately 150–250 ms after the onset of the stimulus presentation (Figure 2.2(A)-right). The N2pc and Pd components have similar topographies, with maximal voltage at lateral occipital-temporal electrode sites, and differ mainly in polarity (Figure 2.2(B)).

The Pd component was first isolated from the N2pc component by Hickey et al. (2009). In their study, participants viewed visual search arrays containing one green square or diamond that was brighter than the background and one short or long red line that was isoluminant with the background (Figure 2.3(A)). The square was target and the line was the distractor, or vice versa, depending on the task instruction. Individual stimuli could be presented at one of six locations (locations on the vertical meridian and locations at 60°, 120°, 240°, 300° off vertical). Critical trials were when the bright green square was presented on the vertical meridian and the isoluminant red line was presented on a lateralized location: any ERP activity corresponding to the vertical item was neither ipsilateral nor contralateral to a given electrode, and any lateralized ERP activity must reflect the processing of the

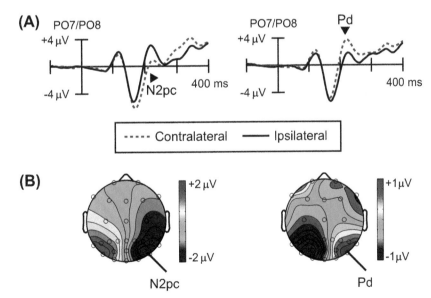

FIGURE 2.2 Example of N2pc and Pd waveforms (A) and topographic maps (B). Separate waveforms are shown for contralateral and ipsilateral sites, relative to the target (N2pc) and the distractor (Pd); the contralateral waveform for the target is the average of the left-hemisphere electrode when the target is in the right visual field, and the right-hemisphere electrode when the target is in the left visual field; the ipsilateral waveform for the target is the average of the left-hemisphere electrode when the target is in the left visual field, and the right-hemisphere electrode when the target is in the right visual field. The N2pc and the Pd are defined as the difference between these contralateral and ipsilateral waveforms.

lateral item. As shown in Figure 2.3(B), when the lateralized red line was the target and the midline green square was the distractor, a contralateral negativity (N2pc) was elicited by the red line. In contrast, when the lateralized red line was the distractor and the midline green square was the target, a contralateral positivity (Pd) was elicited by the red line.

The N2pc and Pd components make it possible to track attentional enhancement and suppression with millisecond-level temporal resolution. Note that, because these components have opposite polarities and similar scalp distributions, they will cancel each other if they are both equally strong at a given moment in time. The average ERP waveform therefore indicates the relative balance of enhancement and suppression at a given moment in time. However, given that attention operates mainly on the basis of competitive interactions, the balance of enhancement and suppression is often the key factor (Sawaki & Luck, 2011).

ACTIVE SUPPRESSION OF A SALIENT DISTRACTOR

A longstanding debate in the attention literature focuses on how top-down control mechanisms interact with bottom-up sensory factors to determine whether a salient nontarget stimulus will capture attention. The findings of previous studies have led to differing hypotheses about whether attentional capture by salient

distractors can be purely stimulus-driven (the *bottom-up saliency hypothesis*; e.g., Theeuwes, 1991; Theeuwes & Burger, 1998) or if it depends entirely on the *attentional set* that is induced by task demands (the *contingent involuntary orienting hypothesis*; e.g., Bacon & Egeth, 1994; Folk, Remington, & Johnston, 1992; Folk, Remington, & Wright, 1994). These alternative hypotheses have led to many interesting experiments, but 20 years of research has not led to a resolution of this controversy.

We have proposed an alternative hypothesis that attempts to resolve the controversy by blending elements of the bottom-up saliency hypothesis and the contingent involuntary orienting hypothesis and adding a third factor, attentional suppression (Sawaki & Luck, 2010). Like the bottom-up orienting hypothesis, we propose that salient singletons (i.e., stimuli that contain a unique feature value in an otherwise homogeneous scene) are always detected and generate a priority signal (an "attend-to-me" signal). In the absence of top-down control, this priority signal will cause a shift of attention to the salient object. However, like the contingent involuntary orienting hypothesis, we propose that top-down control plays an important role. Specifically, the priority signal can be suppressed (canceled) before attention is actually shifted. We call this the *signal suppression hypothesis* to indicate that the salient object generates a signal, but that this signal can be suppressed.

It may be difficult to obtain direct evidence of the suppression process with behavioral measures. That is, participants may fail to orient to a salient item because

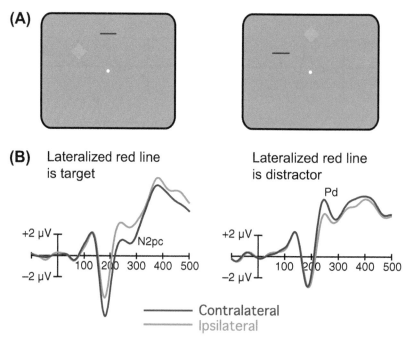

FIGURE 2.3   Example stimulus displays (A) and grand average ERPs (B) from the study of Hickey et al. (2009). Each array contained a bright green square or diamond along with a short or long red line that was isoluminant with the background. When the lateralized red line was the target, an N2pc was elicited by the red line. In contrast, when the lateralized red line was the distractor, a Pd was elicited by the red line.

the item never generated a priority signal, and this might lead to the same behavioral output that would result from a priority signal that is rapidly suppressed. However, the N2pc and Pd components provide a means of covertly monitoring attentional focusing and attentional suppression. We therefore used these components in a series of experiments to test the signal suppression hypothesis (Sawaki & Luck, 2010). In these experiments, participants searched for a specific letter (e.g., "A"; Figure 2.4(A)-left), which was sometimes accompanied by a salient distractor (a color singleton; e.g., "Y" in Figure 2.4(A)-right). It should be noted that the target was not a singleton along any dimension so that the participants had no motivation to use an attentional set that emphasizes singletons.

The bottom-up orienting hypothesis predicts that attention will be automatically deployed toward the salient singleton distractor, leading to an N2pc component (as has been found many times when color singletons were targets; see, e.g., Luck & Hillyard, 1994a, 1994b). In contrast, the contingent involuntary orienting hypothesis predicts that the salient singleton distractor will simply not generate any kind of attentional priority signal, leading to no significant lateralized ERP activity. The signal suppression hypothesis predicts yet a different pattern, in which the salient singleton distractor generates an attentional priority signals that is then suppressed to prevent actual attentional capture, producing a Pd component. The results confirmed the predictions of the signal suppression hypothesis. Whereas the targets elicited an N2pc component, that salient distractors did not elicit an N2pc, but instead elicited a Pd (Figure 2.4(B)). The Pd effect was small but very reliable (and it exceeded a *Hillivolt*, which is defined either as 0.1 μV or the thickness of the lines used to draw the waveforms).

These findings suggest that salient singletons automatically produce an attend-to-me signal, irrespective of top-down control settings, but this signal can be overridden by an active suppression mechanism to prevent the actual capture of attention. Similar findings have been observed by other researchers (e.g., Kiss, Grubert, Petersen, & Eimer, 2012). It should be noted that these studies have focused on salience that is determined by the interrelationships among the items in the scene (e.g., a letter of one color among letters of another color) rather than by the intrinsic properties of the individual items

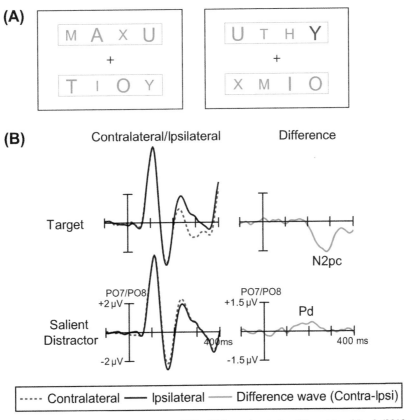

FIGURE 2.4 Example stimulus displays (A) and grand average ERPs (B) from the study of Sawaki and Luck (2010; Experiment 1). Each stimulus display consisted of eight letters. All letters were the same color (either green or red) except for the salient distractor (red if other letters were green or vice versa). ERPs for the target and the salient distractor are shown for contralateral and ipsilateral PO7/PO8 electrode sites, along with the difference between the contralateral and ipsilateral waveforms (which isolates the N2pc and Pd components). An N2pc component can be observed for the target. In contrast, a Pd component can be observed for the salient distractor.

(e.g., an onset). Further research is needed to determine whether the same mechanisms apply to other salient signals.

One might wonder whether it is possible to suppress a priority signal without first attending to it. However, it is not difficult to imagine a mechanism by which priority signals, arising from a given feature dimension, will trigger a suppression process. This would not require any of the perceptual selection or gain control mechanism that are ordinarily associated with attention. Of course, one could define the term *attention* broadly enough such that any controlled brain activity would fall within this definition, but such a broad definition of attention would not be very useful.

SENSORY CONFOUNDS AND THE HILLYARD PRINCIPLE

Sensory confounds can be a significant problem in ERP studies of attention. Over the years, Steve Hillyard and his colleagues have developed attention paradigms that eliminate the possibility of sensory confounds (e.g., Hillyard, Hink, Schwent, & Picton, 1973; Hillyard & Münte, 1984; Van Voorhis & Hillyard, 1977). In general, sensory confounds can be avoided by following the "Hillyard Principle", which states that "To avoid sensory confounds, you must compare ERPs elicited by exactly the same physical stimuli, varying only the psychological conditions" (Luck, 2005). However, this is not generally possible in ERP studies of bottom-up attentional control, because bottom-up salience by definition requires manipulations of the physical stimuli. For example, studies using peripheral cues face sensory confounds because the target on a valid trial is immediately preceded by a cue in the same location, whereas the target on an invalid trial is preceded by a cue in a different location. Short-term adaptation or refractory processes may lead to different sensory responses in these situations, irrespective of attention, and this must be taken into account when interpreting studies using peripheral cues (see, e.g., Handy, Jha, & Mangun, 1999; Hopfinger & Mangun, 1998).

There are two potential sensory confounds in the study shown in Figure 2.4. First, the salient distractor was the only item of its color in the display, and lateral inhibition between the other items could potentially lead to a smaller response from these items, and a relatively larger response from the singleton. Second, a given non singleton item was usually preceded by an item of the same color in the same location on the previous trial, whereas the color singleton was usually preceded by an item of a different color. This may have led to less adaptation for the singleton color, again leading to a larger sensory response for the singleton (Luck & Hillyard, 1994b).

If the priority signal produced by a color singleton is truly automatic, then it is impossible to eliminate this by means of a simple instructional manipulation. That is, there was no way to satisfy the Hillyard Principle in the study shown in Figure 2.4. As an alternative, we conducted control experiments that were designed to show that any sensory differences between the singleton and non singleton items were not sufficient to produce the observed ERP results. In one control experiment (Sawaki & Luck, 2010; Experiment 4), the differential adaptation confound was eliminated by randomly intermixing trials in which the singleton was red and the other items were green, and trials in which the singleton was green and the other items were red. Red and green were therefore equally adapted, and yet we still observed an N2pc for targets and a Pd for the salient singleton distractors. Thus, these effects were not a consequence of adaptation. To rule out the lateral inhibition confound, we conducted an additional control experiment in which the stimuli from the main task were combined with additional tiny stimuli near the fixation point (Sawaki & Luck, 2010; Experiment 3). Participants ignored the stimuli from the main task and instead performed a very demanding visual search task with the foveal stimuli. This eliminated the N2pc and Pd effects for the stimuli from the main task, showing that these effects are not caused by a pure sensory confound. That is, if spatial attention is sufficiently focused, the attend-to-me signal can be prevented. Previous research has shown that very demanding tasks of this nature can also eliminate attentional capture by sudden onsets (Yantis & Jonides, 1990), which is ordinarily strong.

ACTIVE SUPPRESSION OF A MEMORY-MATCHING DISTRACTOR

Several studies have proposed that items matching the contents of visual working memory automatically have an advantage in attentional priority (Desimone, 1998; Desimone & Duncan, 1995). However, there has been mixed evidence about whether memory-matching items inevitably capture attention (e.g., Carlisle & Woodman, 2011; Downing, 2000; Soto et al., 2005, 2008; Woodman & Luck, 2007), perhaps because the memory-driven attentional priority can be overcome by attentional suppression. We tested this hypothesis by asking whether a memory-matching item elicits an N2pc (indicating that it captured attention) or a Pd (indicating that it was actively suppressed; Sawaki & Luck, 2011).

The task was designed so that participants would store the color of a *sample* stimulus in working memory, and we would then assess the processing of a task-irrelevant *probe* stimulus that matched or mismatched the color in memory. The design was complicated, however, by the need to follow the Hillyard Principle. For example, any effect of the match between the color of the task-irrelevant probe and the color of the sample stimulus could reflect a sensory interaction rather than an interaction with memory. In addition, we wanted to eliminate the possibility that participants would have a strategic reason to attend to the color of the probe.

As shown in Figure 2.5(A), we addressed the sensory confound issue by using pairs of stimuli, only one of which was task relevant, and the relevant item was determined by the task instructions. Each trial sequence consisted of a cue stimulus, a sample array, a probe array, and a test array. The cue stimulus indicated that the participant should direct attention to either the upper or lower half of the display on that trial (indicated by dark gray side of the cue for half of the participants and by the light gray side for the other half). The sample array consisted of two rectangles, one above and one below the fixation point. One rectangle was red and the other was green, with the color at each location varied randomly across trials. To eliminate the strategic use of color in the

task, participants were instructed to remember the orientation of the rectangle in the cued region and to ignore the orientation of the rectangle in the uncued region. The color was task-irrelevant, but previous research has demonstrated that people will automatically encode all features of an object into working memory if instructed to remember only a single feature (Hollingworth & Luck, 2009; Hyun, Woodman, Vogel, Hollingworth, & Luck, 2009).

The probe array was presented during the retention interval of the memory task, and it consisted of two circles to the left and right of fixation. One circle was red and the other was green, and the color at each stimulus location varied randomly across trials. Therefore, one of the probe circles matched the color of the to-be-remembered rectangle for that trial (a *memory-matching probe*) and the other did not. Participants were explicitly instructed that the probe circles were not task relevant. The test array consisted of two rectangles, one above and one below fixation, and participants indicated which rectangle matched the orientation of the memory rectangle.

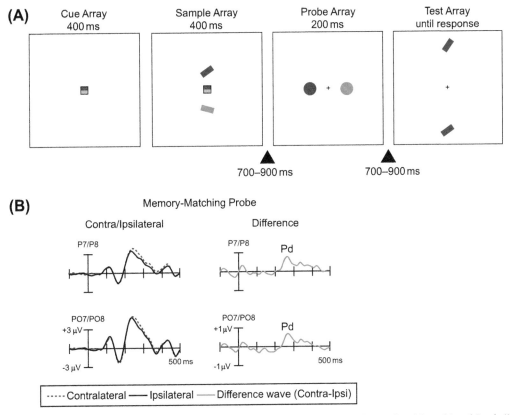

FIGURE 2.5 Example sequence of events in a trial (A) and grand average ERPs (B) from the study of Sawaki and Luck (2011). Half of the participants were instructed to attend to the region indicated by the dark half of the cue. In this example trial, these participants would store the upper rectangle in memory and compare it with the two rectangles shown in the test array, and the red circle would be the memory-matching probe item. For the other participants, who were instructed to attend to the region indicated by the light half of the cue, the lower rectangle would be stored in memory and the green circle would be the memory-matching probe item. ERPs are shown for memory-matching probe at contralateral vs. ipsilateral electrode sites, along with the difference between the contralateral and ipsilateral waveforms. The memory-matching probe on the probe array elicited a Pd component.

We found that task-irrelevant probes matching the contents of visual working memory elicited a Pd component rather than an N2pc component (Figure 2.5(B)). Thus, these results indicate that attention is not inevitably captured by an item that matches the contents of visual working memory. Instead, the finding of the Pd effect suggests that the memory-matching item was actively suppressed. This is the same pattern that we observed for task-irrelevant stimuli with high bottom-up salience (as described in the previous section).

Hollingworth, Matsukura, and Luck (2013) used a similar task with eye movement recordings and found that the eyes moved toward the memory-matching distractor on a significant proportion of trials (see especially Experiment 5). However, when a search target and a memory-matching distractor were simultaneously presented, the eyes moved to the target more often than to the memory-matching distractor. Together, the eye movement and ERP results suggest that a memory-matching distractor captures attention on a significant subset of trials, but it is actively suppressed on a majority of trials. For example, when top-down control is poor, subjects may fail to suppress the memory-matching item, leading to capture, but when top-down control is good, the memory-matching item is suppressed. If top-down control is good on a majority of trials, leading to suppression more often than capture, a Pd will be present in the average. Note that eye movements were not allowed in the ERP study, so a direct test of this explanation will require further experimentation.

A COMMON MECHANISM FOR PREVENTING AND TERMINATING ATTENTION

Active Suppression Follows Attentional Enhancement at a Target Location

Our visual environment is continuously changing, and attention systems operate to select different sources of information from moment to moment. After attention has facilitated perception at a location, does the focus of attention passively fade away? Or, is attention actively terminated after the completion of perception so that the brain can be prepared for upcoming information? We investigated this issue using a simple target detection task shown in Figure 2.6(A) (Sawaki et al., 2012). The target was a circle containing a particular color (e.g., red) at either of the lateral locations. Each lateral circle (red, blue, or green) had a notch on the top or the bottom, and the location of the notch on each lateral circle varied randomly across trials. Participants were instructed to respond when they detected a target circle, indicating the location of the notch on this circle.

We found that targets elicited an N2pc, followed by a Pd (Figure 2.6(B)). This general pattern can be seen in the waveforms in many previous studies that focused on the N2pc component (e.g., Brisson & Jolicœur, 2007; Carlisle & Woodman, 2011; Lien et al., 2008; Luck & Hillyard, 1994b), but the Pd was not formally analyzed in these studies. In the study shown in Figure 2.6(B), we developed a new analysis technique that was able to isolate the Pd from the N2pc by means of geometric area measures and permutation tests (see Sawaki et al., 2012 for details), demonstrating for the first time that the Pd following the N2pc was a statistically significant effect. This N2pc-Pd sequence indicates that attention was deployed toward the location of the target (N2pc) and then this episode of attention was actively terminated (Pd). This active termination process may enable people to efficiently prepare for upcoming information. Furthermore, these findings indicate that the same active suppression mechanism that is used to prevent the allocation of attention to salient and memory-matching distractors (Sawaki & Luck, 2010, 2011) is also used to terminate attention after it is no longer needed.

Linking Active Suppression with the Completion of Perception

Does the Pd reflect an active termination process, or is it a passive, automatic process that inevitably follows

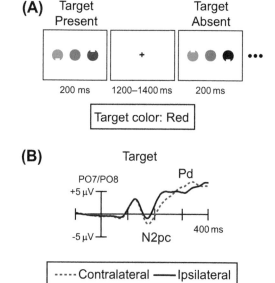

FIGURE 2.6 Example stimulus displays (A) and grand average ERPs (B) from the study of Sawaki et al. (2012, Experiment 1). The target was a circle of a specific color (red in this example) that could appear at either of the two lateral locations, and participants were asked to report whether the target had a notch on its top or bottom. ERPs for targets are shown at contralateral vs. ipsilateral electrode sites (averaged over PO7 and PO8). The target elicited an N2pc component, followed by a Pd component.

N2pc (e.g., some sort of ion equilibration processing)? To answer this question, we used a spatial cuing paradigm (Figure 2.7) in which attention was directed toward the cued location in advance of the onset of the discrimination array (as verified by an enhancement of the sensory response to the discrimination array at the cued location). In this experiment (Sawaki et al., 2012), a to-be-attended location (left or right) was precued on each trial by a pair of horizontal and vertical bars. To follow the Hillyard Principle, some participants were instructed to attend to the location indicated by the vertical bar in each pair, and others were instructed to attend to the location of the horizontal bar. After a delay, a *discrimination array* was presented that consisted of two colored circles. Participants were instructed to look for a specific color (e.g., red) at the cued location in this array. If this color appeared at the uncued location, it was to be treated as a nontarget; that is, the cue *defined* the target location rather than *predicting* the target location. There were three types of trials: target trials (target color present at the cued location and not at the uncued location); target color absent trials (target color absent from both locations); and target-color distractor trials (target color present at the uncued location but not at the cued location). We predicted that a target color presented at the cued location in the discrimination array would not elicit an N2pc, because attention was already focused on that location. Instead, we predicted that the target would elicit a Pd, reflecting the termination of attention after target detection processing was complete. In addition, we predicted that the Pd would be elicited even more rapidly when the target color was not present at the cued location, because perceptual processing would be completed even more rapidly on such trials. Note that, because the target location was precued with 100% validity in this experiment, it is extremely unlikely that a positivity contralateral to the target would be caused by an N2pc reflecting a shift of attention to the opposite location.

We found that the P1 elicited by the discrimination array was greater at contralateral sites than at ipsilateral sites relative to the cued location, equivalently for all three trial types (Figure 2.8(A)). This P1 effect demonstrates that attention had been shifted to the cued location prior to the onset of the discrimination array, and has been observed in several previous studies (Heinze, Luck, Mangun, & Hillyard, 1990; Luck, Heinze, Mangun, & Hillyard, 1990; Mangun, 1995; Mangun & Hillyard, 1988). Furthermore, when attention was already focused prior to the onset of the discrimination array, a Pd was triggered rapidly after the onset of this array (Figure 2.8(B)). This Pd began approximately 150 ms after the onset of the discrimination array when the target color was not present at the cued location, indicating that attention was rapidly terminated as soon as the visual system could determine that there was no need to maintain attention on the cued location. The Pd was delayed by approximately 60 ms when the target color was present at the cued location, presumably reflecting the continued processing of information at the cued location when the relevant color was perceived at this location (Figure 2.8(C)). These results demonstrate that the Pd is not an automatic and immediate consequence of a shift of attention, but instead reflect a controlled process that is triggered when attention is no longer needed.

Pd and N2pc Responses Correlate with Behavioral Performance

Although prior research has shown that Pd appears under conditions that would be expected to involve attentional suppression (Hickey et al., 2009; Sawaki & Luck, 2010, 2011), additional evidence is needed to demonstrate that Pd is related to behavioral measures of suppression. We therefore conducted an experiment to provide this link using the simple target detection task shown in Figure 2.9(A) (Sawaki et al., 2012). The target was a circle containing a particular color (e.g., red) at the central location, and a target-colored distractor was sometimes presented at a lateral location to attract attention (Figure 2.9(A)). Participants were instructed to respond on each trial to indicate whether the target was present or absent at the central location. Thus, a target absent response was required for trials where a lateral circle was the target color (i.e., target-color distractor).

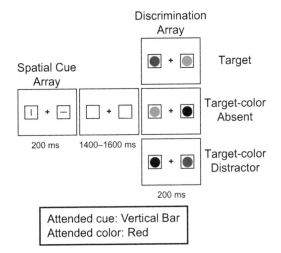

FIGURE 2.7 Example stimulus displays from the study of Sawaki et al. (2012; Experiment 2). Participants were asked to direct attention to the location indicated by the vertical (or horizontal) cue bar and make a button-press response to indicate whether the circle with the target color was present or absent at this location. In this example, the target color was red and the participant was instructed to attend to the location indicated by the vertical bar.

When the central target was absent, the degree of attentional capture by the lateralized target-color distractor should be reflected in the time it takes to make a "target absent" decision. That is, if attention is captured by a distractor on a given trial, the amount of time required to determine that the target is absent should be longer on that trial. Previous research demonstrates that attentional capture fluctuates from trial to trial (Geng & DiQuattro, 2010; Leber, 2010; Mazaheri, DiQuattro, Bengson, & Geng, 2011). Therefore, a robust N2pc should be observed for the target-color distractor on trials with relatively long reaction times (RTs). In contrast, if the participant is able to suppress attending to the target-color distractor on a given trial, the

amount of time required to determine that the target is absent should be decreased on that trial. Therefore, the target-color distractor should elicit a Pd on trials with relatively short RTs.

We found that when RT was short (meaning that capture was presumably avoided), the target-colored distractor elicited a large Pd (Figure 2.9(B)-left). In contrast, when RT was long (and attention was presumably captured), the target-colored distractor elicited a large N2pc (Figure 2.9(B)-right). This relationship between behavioral performance and ERP effects confirmed that the Pd component reflects a neural processing of attentional suppression, whereas the N2pc component reflects a neural processing of attentional deployment.

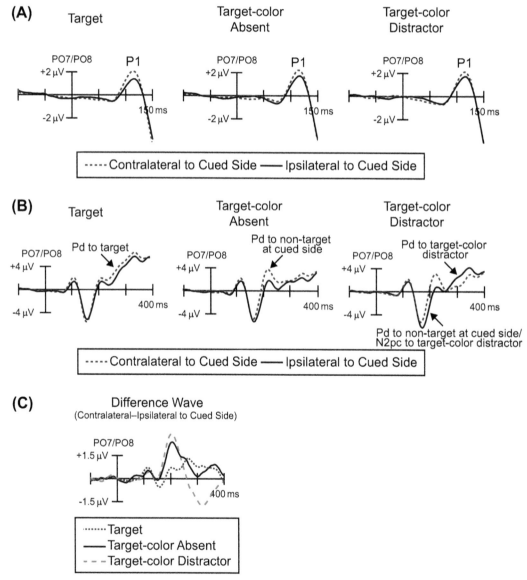

FIGURE 2.8   ERPs elicited by the discrimination array in Sawaki et al. (2012; Experiment 2). (A) Grand average waveforms at contralateral vs. ipsilateral electrode sites relative to the cued side (averaged over PO7 and PO8), shown with a short time scale to emphasize the early P1 component. (B) The same data as in (A), shown on a longer time scale to show the N2pc and Pd components. (C) Grand average difference waveforms obtained by subtracting the ipsilateral waveforms from the contralateral waveforms (average of PO7 and PO8).

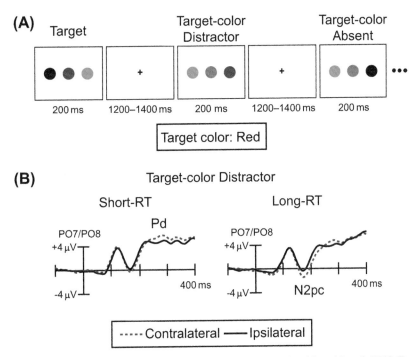

FIGURE 2.9 Example stimulus displays (A) and grand average ERPs (B) from the study of Sawaki et al. (2012; Experiment 3). The target was a central circle with the target color (red in this example). The target-color distractor was a circle that contained the target color but was presented at a lateral location. Participants were asked to report whether the central circle was the target color or not, ignoring the lateral circles. ERPs for the target-color distractor are shown at contralateral vs. ipsilateral electrode sites (averaged over PO7 and PO8). The ERPs were averaged separately for trials with fast RTs (presumably reflecting suppression of the salient distractor) and trials with slow RTs (presumably reflecting capture of attention by the salient distractor). A larger Pd can be observed for the target-color distractor in the short-RT trials. In contrast, a larger N2pc can be observed for the target-color distractor in the long-RT trials.

ACTIVE SUPPRESSION AFTER INVOLUNTARY CAPTURE OF ATTENTION

In some situations, attention is oriented toward an irrelevant item, and this shift of attention must presumably be canceled. Little is known about how the brain recovers from an involuntary shift of attention so that attention can be reoriented to a relevant item. One possibility is that an active suppression process is applied to terminate the shift of attention to the distractor, especially if attention is needed for a concurrent or upcoming target. We, therefore, conducted an additional experiment to assess the processes that occur during the transition from attentional capture by a distractor to attentional reorienting toward a target (Sawaki & Luck, 2013). We used a cuing capture paradigm in which a cue array was presented prior to a search array containing a target (Figure 2.10). The cue array consisted of four colored circles on 80% of trials and four gray circles on 20% of trials. Participants searched for an outlined square of a predefined target color (e.g., red) in the search array, and reported whether this object contained a top gap or a bottom gap. They were told to ignore the cue array. When the cue array contained four colors, one matched the color of the subsequent target, but the location of this target-color

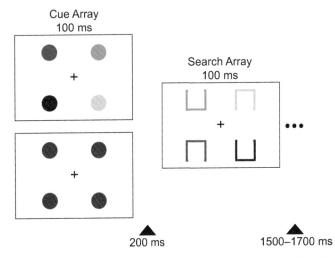

FIGURE 2.10 Example stimulus displays from the study of Sawaki and Luck (2013). The cue array consisted of four colored circles on 80% of trials and four gray circles on 20% of trials. Observers searched for an object of a predefined target color in the search array and reported whether this object contained a top gap or a bottom gap. They were told to ignore the cue array. When the cue array contained four colors, one matched the color of the subsequent target, but the location of this target-color cue was not predictive of the location of the target.

cue was not predictive of the location of the target. The combination of cues and targets led to five types of trials: same-quadrant trials (target-color cue and target in the same quadrant); vertical-quadrant trials (target-color cue and target directly across the horizontal meridian); horizontal-quadrant trials (target-color cue and target directly across the vertical meridian); diagonal-quadrant trials (target-color cue and target in diagonally opposed positions); and neutral trials (cue circles were gray).

In this paradigm, it is very difficult to avoid being captured by the target-color cue item, and many studies have found behavioral evidence of capture in this paradigm. We found the same pattern: the target in the search array was detected more rapidly when it was preceded by a target-color cue in the same quadrant (compared to the neutral trials), indicating that the cue captured attention. However, these behavioral results do not indicate the sequence of processes that happen between the capture of the attention by the cue and the response to the target. If attention passively fades after being captured by the target-color cue, followed by orienting of attention to the target, an N2pc component should be observed for the target-color cue, and then another N2pc component should be observed for the search target. If, however, an active suppression process is applied after attention is captured by the target-color cue, a Pd component should be observed after the N2pc to the target-color cue and before the N2pc to the search target.

Figure 2.11 shows the ERP waveforms from the same-quadrant, vertical-quadrant, and neutral trials. In both the same-quadrant and vertical-quadrant trials, the N2pc component was observed, beginning approximately 150 ms after the onset of cue array. This N2pc shows that attention was captured by the target-color cue. After the N2pc, a Pd component was also elicited, beginning approximately 400 ms after the onset of cue array. This result suggests that an active suppression process was applied to disengage attention from the distractor when attention was involuntary captured (note that, because the Pd effect began within 100 ms of search array onset, it is very unlikely that it could have been a response to the target within the search array). Consistent with this, no significant Pd was observed contralateral to the target when it was preceded by a neutral cue.

Following the Pd component, an N2pc component was observed contralateral to the search target, beginning approximately 480 ms from the onset of cue array (i.e., 180 ms from the onset of search array). Thus, attention was shifted back to the target location once the search display appeared. For the neutral trials, only the target-elicited N2pc component was observed, beginning at approximately 450 ms from the onset of cue array (i.e., 150 ms after the onset of search array), suggesting that attention was deployed toward the search target. Note that on horizontal-quadrant and diagonal-quadrant

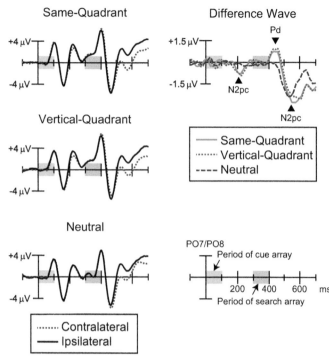

FIGURE 2.11 Grand average ERPs in the study of Sawaki and Luck (2013), time-locked to the onset of the cue array for same-quadrant trials, vertical-quadrant trials, and neutral trials, averaged over the PO7 and PO8 electrode sites. Separate waveforms are shown for contralateral vs ipsilateral electrode sites relative to the side of the target-color cue (which was also contralateral to the side of the target on these trials). Difference waveforms are also shown, obtained by subtracting the ipsilateral waveforms from the contralateral waveforms. The gray areas indicate the period of the cue array and the search array. For same-quadrant and vertical-quadrant trials, an N2pc component was elicited by the target-color cue in the cue array. This was followed by the Pd component, and this was then followed by the N2pc component to the target in the search array. In contrast, for neutral trials, only the target-elicited N2pc component was observed.

trials, the cue-elicited Pd and target-elicited N2pc were the same polarity, and therefore could not be isolated from each other. Consequently, these data were ambiguous and are not shown in Figure 2.11.

It should be noted that several studies have examined ERPs in similar contingent capture paradigms (Eimer & Kiss, 2008, 2010; Eimer, Kiss, Press, & Sauter, 2009; Leblanc et al., 2008; Lien et al., 2008), and some evidence of a Pd was observed in the post-cue portion of the waveforms in all of them. However, the Pd was not fully investigated in these studies because they were conducted before the Pd had been identified as a distinct ERP component and/or an active suppression process was not the main interest in these studies, and thus they did not use an optimal paradigm/analyses to test the Pd. Taken together, this pattern of results appears to be quite general, suggesting that the involuntary capture of attention is typically followed by an active suppression process.

THE SIGNAL SUPPRESSION HYPOTHESIS: COMPETITION BETWEEN THE ATTEND-TO-ME SIGNAL AND ACTIVE SUPPRESSION

On the basis of these findings, we propose that high-priority objects (i.e., perceptually salient objects or objects that partially match the attentional set) always generate an attend-to-me signal that is detected by brain. However, the actual deployment of attention is not always triggered because it can be overcome by an active suppression mechanism. This is the *signal suppression hypothesis* (Sawaki & Luck, 2010, 2011, 2013; Sawaki et al., 2012). In support of this hypothesis, we have demonstrated that the Pd component is observed for salient singleton distractors (Sawaki & Luck, 2010), distractors that match the current contents of working memory (Sawaki & Luck, 2010), and distractors that possess a target feature (Sawaki et al., 2012). Although these distractors are task-irrelevant items, they generate attend-to-me signals due to bottom-up and top-down bias signals, respectively. The Pd indicates that these attend-to-me signals were suppressed to prevent attentional deployment toward the distractors. In addition, the Pd component is observed following attentional deployment toward targets (Sawaki et al., 2012) and following involuntary capture by distractors (Sawaki & Luck, 2013). Therefore, the same suppression mechanism that is used to prevent the orienting of attention to distractors may also be used to terminate attention after it has been focused on an object.

Many models of attention propose that the brain maintains a priority map in which visual stimuli in the world are represented by activity that is proportional to their attentional priority, and attention is deployed toward the peak of the map (Bisley & Goldberg, 2003, 2010; Itti & Koch, 2000; Serences & Yantis, 2007; Treisman & Sato, 1990; Wolfe, 1994). The deployment of attention results in higher fidelity coding by sensory neurons that encode features of attended information (Kastner & Ungerleider, 2000; Luck, Chelazzi, Hillyard, & Desimone, 1997; Reynolds & Desimone, 2003; Serences & Yantis, 2006). It is possible that an attend-to-me signal is associated with a peak of the priority map in brain, and the active suppression mechanism indexed by Pd is used to minimize the priority of these items under some circumstances. The actual deployment of attention toward distractors can be avoided because the active suppression mechanism quashes the increased attentional priority at the location of the distractor. Furthermore, a voluntary shift of attention toward a target, and an involuntary capture by a distractor can be terminated by this same active suppression mechanism, resetting the attentional priority.

The neural source of the Pd component has not been identified, but several studies have shown that the N2pc component is generated mainly in area V4 and the lateral occipital complex (Hopf et al., 2000, 2004, 2006). It is possible that N2pc and Pd are associated with opposing attentional processes within the same neural source because their scalp distributions are similar (i.e., maximal voltage at lateral occipital-temporal electrode sites), their polarities are opposite (i.e., negative vs positive), and their roles in spatial attention are complementary (i.e., enhancement vs suppression). Additional research is needed to elucidate precise neural source of the Pd component and its relationship with the neural source of the N2pc component.

We assume that the actual deployment of attention is determined by competition between the attend-to-me signal (i.e., a peak of the priority map) and the active suppression mechanism. When a target is presented, it generates a strong attend-to-me signal, creating a very high peak in the priority map, and there is no interference from the active suppression mechanism until perception is completed. Therefore, attention is always deployed toward the target in the absence of strong competitors. In contrast, when a distractor is presented, its attend-to-me signal competes with active suppression control. Therefore, the actual deployment of attention is determined by the relative strengths of the attend-to-me signal and the active suppression mechanism. This hypothesis predicts that suppression will fail and capture will occur when the attend-to-me signal is stronger than the active suppression mechanism. Thus, the fact that distractors led to capture of attention in some previous studies but not in others may reflect differences across studies in the relative strengths of the attend-to-me signal and the active suppression mechanism. This fits with prior studies showing that attention capture is greater when top-down control mechanisms are impaired, whether by an interfering task or by individual differences in executive control abilities (Fukuda & Vogel, 2009, 2011; Lavie & De Fockert, 2005). Thus, the signal suppression hypothesis can potentially explain differences in attentional capture across studies and across individuals.

References

Bacon, W. F., & Egeth, H. E. (1994). Overriding stimulus-driven attentional capture. *Perception and Psychophysics, 55*, 485–496.

Bisley, J. W., & Goldberg, M. E. (2003). Neuronal activity in the lateral intraparietal area and spatial attention. *Science, 299*, 81–86.

Bisley, J. W., & Goldberg, M. E. (2010). Attention, intention, and priority in the parietal lobe. *Annual Review of Neuroscience, 33*, 1–21.

Brisson, B., & Jolicœur, P. (2007). Electrophysiological evidence of central interference in the control of visuospatial attention. *Psychonomic Bulletin and Review, 14*, 126–132.

Carlisle, N. B., & Woodman, G. F. (2011). When memory is not enough: electrophysiological evidence for goal-dependent use of working memory representations in guiding visual attention. *Journal of Cognitive Neuroscience, 23*, 2650–2664.

Desimone, R. (1998). Visual attention mediated by biased competition in extrastriate visual cortex. *Philosophical Transactions of the Royal Society of London. Series B, Biological Sciences*, 353, 1245–1255.

Desimone, R., & Duncan, J. (1995). Neural mechanisms of selective visual attention. *Annual Review of Neuroscience*, 18, 193–222.

Di Russo, F., Martinez, A., Sereno, M. I., Pitzalis, S., & Hillyard, S. A. (2002). Cortical sources of the early components of the visual evoked potential. *Human Brain Mapping*, 15, 95–111.

Downing, P. E. (2000). Interactions between visual working memory and selective attention. *Psychological Science*, 11, 467–473.

Eimer, M. (1996). The N2pc component as an indicator of attentional selectivity. *Electroencephalography and Clinical Neurophysiology*, 99, 225–234.

Eimer, M., & Kiss, M. (2008). Involuntary attentional capture is determined by task set: evidence from event-related brain potentials. *Journal of Cognitive Neuroscience*, 20, 1423–1433.

Eimer, M., & Kiss, M. (2010). Top-down search strategies determine attentional capture in visual search: behavioral and electrophysiological evidence. *Attention Perception and Psychophysics*, 72, 951–962.

Eimer, M., Kiss, M., Press, C., & Sauter, D. (2009). The roles of feature-specific task set and bottom-up salience in attentional capture: an ERP study. *Journal of Experimental Psychology: Human Perception and Performance*, 35, 1316–1328.

Folk, C. L., Remington, R. W., & Johnston, J. C. (1992). Involuntary covert orienting is contingent on attentional control settings. *Journal of Experimental Psychology: Human Perception and Performance*, 18, 1030–1044.

Folk, C. L., Remington, R. W., & Wright, J. H. (1994). The structure of attentional control: contingent attentional capture by apparent motion, abrupt onset, and color. *Journal of Experimental Psychology: Human Perception and Performance*, 20, 317–329.

Fukuda, K., & Vogel, E. K. (2009). Human variation in overriding attentional capture. *Journal of Neuroscience*, 29, 8726–8733.

Fukuda, K., & Vogel, E. K. (2011). Individual differences in recovery time from attentional capture. *Psychological Science*, 22, 361–368.

Geng, J. J., & Diquattro, N. E. (2010). Attentional capture by a perceptually salient non-target facilitates target processing through inhibition and rapid rejection. *Journal of Vision*, 10, 5.

Handy, T. C., Jha, A. P., & Mangun, G. R. (1999). Promoting novelty in vision: Inhibition of return modulates perceptual-level processing. *Psychological Science*, 10, 157–161.

Heinze, H. J., Luck, S. J., Mangun, G. R., & Hillyard, S. A. (1990). Visual event-related potentials index focused attention within bilateral stimulus arrays. I. Evidence for early selection. *Electroencephalography and Clinical Neurophysiology*, 75, 511–527.

Hickey, C., Di Lollo, V., & McDonald, J. J. (2009). Electrophysiological indices of target and distractor processing in visual search. *Journal of Cognitive Neuroscience*, 21, 760–775.

Hickey, C., McDonald, J. J., & Theeuwes, J. (2006). Electrophysiological evidence of the capture of visual attention. *Journal of Cognitive Neuroscience*, 18, 604–613.

Hillyard, S. A., Hink, R. F., Schwent, V. L., & Picton, T. W. (1973). Electrical signs of selective attention in the human brain. *Science*, 182, 177–179.

Hillyard, S. A., & Münte, T. F. (1984). Selective attention to color and location: an analysis with event-related brain potentials. *Perception and Psychophysics*, 36, 185–198.

Hollingworth, A., & Luck, S. J. (2009). The role of visual working memory (VWM) in the control of gaze during visual search. *Attention, Perception and Psychophysics*, 71, 936–949.

Hollingworth, A., Matsukura, M., & Luck, S. J. (2013). Visual working memory modulates rapid eye movements to simple onset targets. *Psychological Science*.

Hopf, J. M., Boelmans, K., Schoenfeld, M. A., Luck, S. J., & Heinze, H. J. (2004). Attention to features precedes attention to locations in visual search: evidence from electromagnetic brain responses in humans. *Journal of Neuroscience*, 23, 1822–1832.

Hopf, J. -M., Luck, S. J., Boelmans, K., Schoenfeld, M. A., Boehler, N., Rieger, J., et al. (2006). The neural site of attention matches the spatial scale of perception. *Journal of Neuroscience*, 26, 3532–3540.

Hopf, J. M., Luck, S. J., Girelli, M., Hagner, T., Mangun, G. R., Scheich, H., et al. (2000). Neural sources of focused attention in visual search. *Cerebral Cortex*, 10, 1233–1241.

Hopfinger, J. B., & Mangun, G. R. (1998). Reflective attention modulates processing of visual stimuli in human extrastriate cortex. *Psychological Science*, 9, 441–447.

Hyun, J. S., Woodman, G. F., Vogel, E. K., Hollingworth, A., & Luck, S. J. (2009). The comparison of visual working memory representations with perceptual inputs. *Journal of Experimental Psychology: Human Perception and Performance*, 35, 1140–1160.

Itti, L., & Koch, C. (2000). A saliency-based search mechanism for overt and covert shifts of visual attention. *Vision Research*, 40, 1489–1506.

Kastner, S., & Ungerleider, L. G. (2000). Mechanisms of visual attention in the human cortex. *Annual Review of Neuroscience*, 23, 315–341.

Kiss, M., Grubert, A., Petersen, A., & Eimer, M. (2012). Attentional capture by salient distractors during visual search is determined by temporal task demands. *Journal of Cognitive Neuroscience*, 24, 749–759.

Kiss, M., Jolicœur, P., Dell'acqua, R., & Eimer, M. (2008). Attentional capture by visual singletons is mediated by top-down task set: new evidence from the N2pc component. *Psychophysiology*, 45, 1013–1024.

Lavie, N., & De Fockert, J. (2005). The role of working memory in attentional capture. *Psychonomic Bulletin and Review*, 12, 669–674.

Leber, A. B. (2010). Neural predictors of within-subject fluctuations in attentional control. *Journal of Neuroscience*, 30, 11458–11465.

Leblanc, E., Prime, D. J., & Jolicoeur, P. (2008). Tracking the location of visuospatial attention in a contingent capture paradigm. *Journal of Cognitive Neuroscience*, 20, 657–671.

Lien, M., Ruthruff, E., Goodin, Z., & Remington, R. W. (2008). Contingent attentional capture by top-down control settings: Converging evidence from event-related potentials. *Journal of Experimental Psychology. Human Perception and Performance*, 34, 509–530.

Luck, S. J. (2005). *An Introduction to the Event-Related Potential Technique*. Cambridge: MIT Press.

Luck, S. J. (2012). Electrophysiological correlates of the focusing of attention within complex visual scenes: N2pc and related ERP components. In S. J. Luck & E. S. Kappenman (Eds.), *Oxford handbook of ERP components*. New York: Oxford University Press.

Luck, S. J., Chelazzi, L., Hillyard, S. A., & Desimone, R. (1997). Neural mechanisms of spatial selective attention in areas V1, V2, and V4 of macaque visual cortex. *Journal of Neurophysiology*, 77, 24–42.

Luck, S. J., Heinze, H. J., Mangun, G. R., & Hillyard, S. A. (1990). Visual event-related potentials index focused attention within bilateral stimulus arrays. II. Functional dissociation of P1 and N1 components. *Electroencephalography and Clinical Neurophysiology*, 75, 528–542.

Luck, S. J., & Hillyard, S. A. (1990). Electrophysiological evidence for parallel and serial processing during visual search. *Perception and Psychophysics*, 48, 603–617.

Luck, S. J., & Hillyard, S. A. (1994a). Electrophysiological correlates of feature analysis during visual search. *Psychophysiology*, 31, 291–308.

Luck, S. J., & Hillyard, S. A. (1994b). Spatial filtering during visual search: evidence from human electrophysiology. *Journal of Experimental Psychology. Human Perception and Performance*, 20, 1000–1014.

Mangun, G. R. (1995). Neural mechanisms of visual selective attention. *Psychophysiology*, 32, 4–18.

Mangun, G. R., & Hillyard, S. A. (1988). Spatial gradients of visual attention: behavioral and electrophysiological evidence. *Electroencephalography and Clinical Neurophysiology, 70,* 417–428.

Mazaheri, A., DiQuattro, N. E., Bengson, J., & Geng, J. J. (2011). Pre-stimulus activity predicts the winner of top-down vs. bottom-up attentional selection. *PLoS One, 6,* e16243.

Reynolds, J. H., & Desimone, R. (2003). Interacting roles of attention and visual salience in V4. *Neuron, 37,* 853–863.

Rodríguez Holguín, S., Doallo, S., Vizoso, C., & Cadaveira, F. (2009). N2pc and attentional capture by colour and orientation-singletons in pure and mixed visual search tasks. *International Journal of Psychophysiology, 73,* 279–286.

Sawaki, R., Geng, J. J., & Luck, S. J. (2012). A common neural mechanism for preventing and terminating the allocation of attention. *Journal of Neuroscience, 32,* 10725–10736.

Sawaki, R., & Luck, S. J. (2010). Capture versus suppression of attention by salient singletons: electrophysiological evidence for an automatic attend-to-me signal. *Attention Perception and Psychophysics, 72,* 1455–1470.

Sawaki, R., & Luck, S. J. (2011). Active suppression of distractors that match the contents of visual working memory. *Visual Cognition, 19,* 956–972.

Sawaki, R., & Luck, S. J. (2013). Active suppression after involuntary capture of attention. *Psychonomic Bulletin and Review, 20,* 296–301.

Serences, J. T., & Yantis, S. (2006). Selective visual attention and perceptual coherence. *Trends in Cognitive Sciences, 10,* 38–45.

Serences, J. T., & Yantis, S. (2007). Spatially selective representations of voluntary and stimulus-driven attentional priority in human occipital, parietal, and frontal cortex. *Cerebral Cortex, 17,* 284–293.

Soto, D., Heinke, D., Humphreys, G. W., & Blanco, M. J. (2005). Early, involuntary top-down guidance of attention from working memory. *Journal of Experimental Psychology: Human Perception and Performance, 31,* 248–261.

Soto, D., Hodsoll, J., Rotshtein, P., & Humphreys, G. W. (2008). Automatic guidance of attention from working memory. *Trends in Cognitive Sciences, 12,* 342–348.

Theeuwes, J. (1991). Exogenous and endogenous control of attention: the effect of visual onsets and offsets. *Perception and Psychophysics, 49,* 83–90.

Theeuwes, J., & Burger, R. (1998). Attentional control during visual search: the effect of irrelevant singletons. *Journal of Experimental Psychology: Human Perception and Performance, 24,* 1342–1353.

Treisman, A., & Sato, S. (1990). Conjunction search revisited. *Journal of Experimental Psychology: Human Perception and Performance, 16,* 459–478.

Van Voorhis, S. T., & Hillyard, S. A. (1977). Visual evoked potentials and selective attention to points in space. *Perception and Psychophysics, 22,* 54–62.

Wolfe, J. M. (1994). Guided search 2.0: a revised model of visual search. *Psychonomic Bulletin and Review, 1,* 202–238.

Woodman, G. F., & Luck, S. J. (1999). Electrophysiological measurement of rapid shifts of attention during visual search. *Nature, 400,* 867–869.

Woodman, G. F., & Luck, S. J. (2003). Serial deployment of attention during visual search. *Journal of Experimental Psychology: Human Perception and Performance, 29,* 121–138.

Woodman, G. F., & Luck, S. J. (2007). Do the contents of visual working memory automatically influence attentional selection during visual search? *Journal of Experimental Psychology: Human Perception and Performance, 33,* 363–377.

Yantis, S., & Jonides, J. (1990). Abrupt visual onsets and selective attention: voluntary versus automatic allocation. *Journal of Experimental Psychology: Human Perception and Performance, 16,* 121–134.

Neuronal and Neural-Population Mechanisms of Voluntary Visual-Spatial Attention

Satoru Suzuki, Marcia Grabowecky, Ken A. Paller

Department of Psychology and Interdepartmental Neuroscience Program, Northwestern University, Evanston, IL, USA

We have the ability to intentionally direct the mind's eye to a location in space in a covert way—without moving the eyes to foveate that location. This ability is useful, for instance, when we wish to surreptitiously monitor a person of interest without risking eye contact at a social gathering. Such use of voluntary visual-spatial attention was described at the turn of the nineteenth century by Jane Austin in her novel, *Pride and Prejudice* (Austin, 1813): "though he was not always looking at her mother, she was convinced that his attention was invariably fixed by her." When we voluntarily direct our visual-spatial attention to a specific location, we believe that we can detect, identify, and scrutinize things at that location with greater sensitivity, acuity, and speed. Many behavioral experiments have confirmed this intuition (e.g., Carrasco, 2011; Cheal & Lyon, 1991; Downing & Pinker, 1985; Ling & Carrasco, 2006; Posner, 1980; Posner & Cohen, 1984; Posner, Snyder, & Davidson, 1980; Sperling & Melchner, 1978).

The neural mechanisms of voluntary visual-spatial attention are the focus of this chapter. Before we begin our discussion of this one type of attention, we briefly discuss how it relates to other ways in which we can deploy visual attention. In particular, we can attend to a specific feature such as color (e.g., attending to red items while ignoring intermixed yellow items), motion (e.g., attending to leftward-moving dots while ignoring intermixed rightward-moving dots), shape (e.g., attending to a concave shape while ignoring a superimposed convex shape), or object (e.g., attending to a cat image while ignoring a superimposed guitar image) (e.g., Blaser, Sperling, & Lu, 1999; Carrasco, 2011; Cave & Bishot, 1999; Pastukhov, Fischer, & Braun, 2009; Suzuki, 2001, 2003). Whereas our discussion of neural mechanisms of voluntary visual-spatial attention focuses on visual neurons with receptive fields inside versus outside the attended region of space, analogous mechanisms may apply to feature-based attention. That is, feature-based attention may involve modulating activity of visual neurons preferentially tuned to the attended (e.g., vertical orientation) vs. ignored (e.g., other orientations) feature values.

Attention can also be captured, irrespective of our intention, by a salient or behaviorally relevant stimulus. We need not be aware of this attentional capture and we might even be intent on avoiding it. This phenomenon is typically referred to as stimulus-driven (or bottom-up) attention, and is often juxtaposed to voluntary (or top-down) attention (e.g., Carrasco, 2011; Cheal & Lyon, 1991; Eriksen & Collins, 1969; Hawkins et al., 1990; Hickey, McDonald, & Theeuwes, 2006; Hikosaka, Miyauch, & Shimojo, 1993; Jiang, Costello, Fang, Huang, & He, 2006; Nakayama & Mackeben, 1989; Pestilli & Carrasco, 2005; Posner, 1980; Posner & Cohen, 1984; Yantis, 1996; Yantis & Johnson, 1990; Yeshurun & Carrasco, 1998). The literature suggests that visual improvements at the attended location are qualitatively similar whether attention is intentionally allocated or captured by a salient stimulus (see Carrasco, 2011; Funes, Lupianez, & Milliken, 2005; Guzman-Martinez, Grabowecky, Palafox, & Suzuki, 2011, for reviews). On the one hand, stimulus-driven visual-spatial attention typically produces stronger, faster, and a greater variety of beneficial effects than does voluntary visual-spatial attention. On the other hand, the latter may play unique roles in improving texture segmentation at central locations (e.g., Yeshurun & Carrasco, 1998; Yeshurun, Montagna, & Carrasco, 2008) and in utilizing redundant information from multiple stimuli (e.g., Guzman-Martinez et al., 2011). It appears that the stimulus-driven and voluntary modes of visual-spatial attention are mediated by a combination of overlapping and distinct neural mechanisms (see Carrasco, 2011; Guzman-Martinez et al., 2011, for reviews).

The goal of this chapter is to provide an integrative perspective on the effects of voluntarily attending to a specific location in space. Relevant results concern a variety of mechanisms, both at the neuronal and neural-population levels, which we describe in early and later sections of the chapter, respectively. Accordingly, we present a view of attention wherein these mechanisms collectively support our ability to voluntarily enhance visual processing at a specific location under a variety of conditions.

EFFECTS OF VOLUNTARY VISUAL-SPATIAL ATTENTION ON NEURONAL SPIKE RATES

Roughly speaking, voluntarily attending to a specific location increases both spontaneous spike rates (in the absence of stimuli) and stimulus-evoked responses of visual neurons that have receptive fields for the attended region. These neuronal spike-rate enhancements occur in visual areas in both the ventral and dorsal pathways (e.g., Bushnell, Goldberg, & Robinson, 1981; Colby, Duhamel, & Goldberg, 1996; Luck, Chelazzi, Hillyard, & Desimone, 1997; Mountcastle, Motter, Steinmentz, & Setokas, 1987; Reynolds, Chelazzi, & Desimone, 1999; Spitzer & Richmond, 1991). Because quickly and accurately identifying a potentially important stimulus is the primary goal of attending, many studies have examined the effects of voluntary visual-spatial attention on neuronal responses in the ventral visual pathway thought to mediate pattern identification and categorization (e.g., Fang & He, 2005; Goodale & Westwood, 2004; Mishkin, Ungerleider, & Macko, 1983).

A general principle is that voluntary visual-spatial attention more strongly modulates neuronal spike rates in higher-level visual areas than in lower-level visual areas. Although attention modulates spike rates in primary visual cortex (V1), the modulation increases in V2 and V4, and the modulation can be nearly complete (a neuron responding only when its preferred stimulus is selectively attended) in inferotemporal cortex (IT), the highest-level ventral visual area where neurons respond to faces and familiar objects (e.g., Chelazzi, Duncan, Miller, & Desimone, 1998; Luck et al., 1997; McAdams & Maunsell, 1999a; Reynolds et al., 1999). Preferential amplification of the neuronal effect of voluntary visual-spatial attention in higher-level visual areas may be partly due to accumulation of attentional modulation in downstream visual areas through feedforward connections, and/or stronger feedback connections from frontal and parietal areas thought to mediate voluntary attention (e.g., Corbetta & Shulman, 2002; Desimone &

Duncan, 1995; Gregoriou, Gotts, Zhou, & Desimone, 2009; Kastner & Ungerleider, 2001; Moore & Armstrong, 2003; Moore & Fallah, 2004). However, a major contributing factor appears to be within-receptive-field input competition.

WHEN MULTIPLE STIMULI ARE PRESENTED WITHIN A NEURON'S RECEPTIVE FIELD

Because the spatial extent of neuronal receptive fields progressively increases along the cortical visual processing stream (e.g., see Suzuki, 2005, for a review of the animal literature, and Kastner & Ungerleider, 2001, for a review of human functional magnetic resonance imaging (fMRI) data), higher-level visual neurons are more likely to have competing stimuli falling within their receptive fields. When multiple stimuli fall within a visual neuron's receptive field, stimulus selection is critical. Without stimulus selection, the neuron is unlikely to respond strongly. Specifically, unless a particular stimulus is selected by attention, the neuron's spike rate to the combination of stimuli is approximately the average of the spike rates to the individual stimuli presented one at a time, thus lessening the impact of a preferred stimulus (e.g., Miller, Gochin, & Gross, 1993; Rolls & Tovee, 1995; Sato, 1989; Zoccolan, Cox, & DiCarlo, 2005). Consistent with this necessity for within-receptive-field stimulus selection, attentional modulation of neuronal spike rates is especially strong throughout the ventral visual pathway when multiple stimuli are presented within a neuron's receptive field (e.g., Chelazzi et al., 1998; Luck et al., 1997; Reynolds et al., 1999). In contrast, when one stimulus is within a neuron's receptive field and a competing stimulus outside the receptive field, attentional modulation of neuronal spike rates can be weak or unreliable (e.g., Moran & Desimone, 1985; Spitzer, Desimone, & Moran, 1988; Williford & Maunsell, 2006) even in higher-level visual areas such as IT (e.g., Chelazzi et al., 1998). For a subset of neurons, however, attentional modulation of responses to a single stimulus can be as large as a doubling of spike rates (McAdams & Maunsell, 1999a), if the stimulus is large relative to the receptive field and the scope of attention (see below).

How does attention strongly influence neuronal spike rates when multiple stimuli are simultaneously presented within a neuron's receptive field? The neurophysiological literature suggests that the strong attentional modulation arises from an engagement of input competition. Suppose a preferred stimulus is presented within a neuron's receptive field and a nonpreferred stimulus is presented outside it. When the preferred stimulus within the receptive field is attended, the spike-rate response would increase. When the nonpreferred stimulus outside of the receptive field is attended, the neuron would still respond well to the preferred stimulus presented within its receptive field except that the response would no longer be increased by attention. Thus, the attention effect (the difference between these two conditions) would be relatively modest. Now, suppose that a preferred stimulus and a nonpreferred stimulus are both presented within the neuron's receptive field. In this case, the inputs from the two stimuli, processed separately by lower-level visual neurons with smaller receptive fields, would compete to activate this downstream target neuron. When neither stimulus is attended (i.e., another stimulus outside the receptive field is attended), the neuron would respond at a spike rate that is approximately the average of its responses to the individual stimuli presented separately; that is, the preferred and nonpreferred inputs would equally contribute to the neuron's response in the absence of selective attention.[1] When the preferred stimulus is attended, the weight of the preferred input is increased while the weight of the nonpreferred input is reduced, so that the neuron would respond strongly almost as if the preferred stimulus were presented alone. When the nonpreferred stimulus is attended, the weight of the nonpreferred input is increased while the weight of the preferred input is reduced, so that the neuron would respond poorly almost as if the nonpreferred stimulus were presented alone. Thus, when multiple stimuli are presented within a neuron's receptive field, an attention effect can be as large as the effect of presenting a preferred vs nonpreferred stimulus.

ATTENTIONAL CONTRAST-GAIN AND THE BIASED-COMPETITION MODEL

How does attention modulate the weights of competing inputs? A variety of computational models have been proposed, but they all share the idea that visual neurons tuned to different locations (and/or different features) engage in dynamic competition for influence on downstream neurons, and that a relatively small top-down attentional signal can substantially bias the outcome of the competition in favor of the attended input (see Deco & Thiele, 2009, for a review). In an influential model in the domain of voluntary visual-spatial attention—the biased-competition model—it was postulated that attention increases the weight of the input from the attended

stimulus by increasing its effective luminance contrast—the attentional contrast-gain hypothesis (e.g., Desimone & Duncan, 1995; Reynolds & Chelazzi, 2004; Reynolds, Pasternak, & Desimone, 2000).

The attentional contrast-gain hypothesis was motivated by the fact that relative stimulus contrast influences within-receptive-field stimulus competition. Consider the case of simultaneously presenting a preferred stimulus and a nonpreferred stimulus within a neuron's receptive field, when both stimuli are of an intermediate visual contrast. If the preferred stimulus was of relatively greater contrast, then the neuron would respond strongly, as it is primarily driven by input from the preferred stimulus. If, alternatively, the nonpreferred stimulus was of relatively greater contrast, then the neuron would respond weakly, as it is primarily driven by the input from the nonpreferred stimulus. The attentional contrast-gain hypothesis postulates that visual-spatial attention mechanisms have exploited this tendency of a visual neuron to preferentially respond to the highest-contrast stimulus within its receptive field (Reynolds & Desimone, 2003). By increasing the effective contrast of the selected stimulus relative to ignored stimuli within the receptive field, attention can ensure that a visual neuron responds primarily to the attended stimulus.

Attentional weighting of within-receptive-field stimulus competition is indispensable for identifying features and objects. The relevant higher-level visual neurons encode increasingly complex features, such as contour curvatures, spatial relations of curved contours, shapes, objects, faces, and so on (see Orban, 2008; Suzuki, 2005, for reviews). These neurons have large receptive fields, and most importantly, they do not respond well to their preferred stimuli if other nonpreferred stimuli are also present within their receptive fields. For example, a face-tuned neuron would not strongly respond to a face if it were next to a soda can. However, the face-tuned neuron would strongly respond if the face were selectively attended. In other words, face recognition could not take place in a cluttered environment without attentional weighting of within-receptive-field stimulus competition. In this sense, selective attention is necessary for object recognition in general, because of the greater spatial integration (larger receptive fields) required for encoding complex visual patterns in higher-level visual processing, irrespective of any potential limitation of neural resources.

THE NORMALIZATION MODEL OF ATTENTION

The basic idea that visual-spatial attention enhances the effective contrast of the attended stimulus, however, required a few modifications. The attentional

---

[1]For neurons in middle temporal area (MT), however, preferred inputs are typically weighted higher than nonpreferred inputs, and the strength of attentional modulation is inversely related to this asymmetry. That is, attentional modulation is stronger for MT neurons for which the default weighting of their preferred inputs is lower (Ni, Ray, & Maunsell, 2012).

contrast-gain model makes a specific prediction about the effect of attention on neuronal spike rates as a function of stimulus contrast when only one stimulus is presented within a neuron's receptive field (i.e., when the within-receptive-field stimulus competition mechanisms are not engaged). Visual neurons have a finite dynamic range, so that their spike rates follow a sigmoidal shape as a function of stimulus contrast, saturating at high contrast; that is, if the stimulus contrast is sufficiently high, further increase in contrast does not increase the neuron's spike rate. Thus, if the effect of visual-spatial attention on neuronal spike rates is equivalent to increasing the input contrast, attention should be effective for low- to medium-contrast stimuli, but ineffective for high-contrast stimuli. This prediction was supported by some studies (e.g., Reynolds, Pasternak, & Desimone, 2000; Treue, 2004), but others showed that attention effects on neuronal spike rates were relatively independent of stimulus contrast or even stronger for higher-contrast stimuli (e.g., Thiele, Pooresmaeili, Delicato, Herrero, & Roelfsema, 2009; Williford & Maunsell, 2006).

A recent modification of the attentional contrast-gain model, the normalization model of attention (Reynolds & Heeger, 2009), resolves this seeming discrepancy by incorporating divisive normalization. Roughly, the model postulates that a visual neuron's spike rates follow a sigmoidal function of the contrast signal from the stimulus within its receptive field, with the contrast signal multiplied by attention and divided by a normalization factor proportional to the sum of responses from all neurons that respond to the stimulus. This type of normalization is consistent with the fact that a visual neuron typically responds strongly to a small high-contrast stimulus presented at the center of its receptive field (e.g., Cavanagh, Bair, & Movshon, 2002; Kapadia, Westheimer, & Gilbert, 1999; Sceniak, Ringach, Hawken, & Shapley, 1999); a small stimulus would activate fewer neighboring neurons, thereby incurring relatively weak divisive normalization.

The normalization model of attention predicts that whether attention is effective for low- to medium-contrast stimuli, high-contrast stimuli, or both, depends on stimulus size (relative to the receptive field) and the size of the spatial focus of attention. Here, we qualitatively illustrate the predictions of the normalization model in two distinct cases (see Reynolds & Heeger, 2009, for quantitative predictions). Suppose a small stimulus (small relative to the receptive field) is presented at the center of the receptive field of a visual neuron, and the focus of attention is large. The model then predicts that the neuron would receive the full signal from the stimulus (because of the large focus of attention) while the divisive normalization would be minimal because the small stimulus would minimally activate other neurons with their receptive-field centers elsewhere. When

the divisive normalization is minimal as in this case, attention would increase neuronal spike rates for low- to medium-contrast stimuli, but not for high-contrast stimuli due to response saturation. In contrast, suppose a large stimulus (large relative to the receptive field) is presented at the center of the receptive field of a visual neuron, and attention is narrowly focused within the stimulus. Then, the divisive normalization would be strong because the large stimulus would activate many neurons with neighboring receptive fields. Importantly, the strong divisive normalization would keep the neuron's response well below saturation even when the stimulus is high in contrast. At the same time, the small focus of attention would enhance the stimulus signal primarily for the target neuron (without also enhancing normalization), allowing attention to multiplicatively increase the neuron's response. Thus, the attention effect would be especially strong for high-contrast stimuli.

In this way, the normalization model of attention predicts strong attention effects for low- to medium-contrast stimuli when the stimulus is small and the focus of attention is large (relative to the receptive field), whereas it predicts strong attention effects for high-contrast stimuli when the stimulus is large and the focus of attention is narrow. The model predicts intermediate dependencies of attention effects on stimulus contrast, including equivalent attention effects for a broad range of stimulus contrast for intermediate combinations of stimulus size and the scope of attention. Reynolds and Heeger's (2009) review of the literature shows that these predictions reconcile previously discrepant results regarding how neuronal effects of attention depend on stimulus contrast.

We note in passing that the normalization model of attention also accounts for multiplicative enhancing of feature-tuning curves (e.g., McAdams & Maunsell, 1999a; Motter, 1993), making feature-tuning curves steeper. A steeper tuning curve at the focus of attention improves a neuron's ability to discriminate different values of a feature (e.g., different orientations) because attention increases stimulus-evoked neural responses more than it does response variability (McAdams & Maunsell, 1999b), and also because attention reduces locally correlated intrinsic noise (Mitchell, Sundberg, & Reynolds, 2009). The normalization model also accounts for the effects of feature-based attention (e.g., attending to a specific orientation) by incorporating neural tuning and attentional focus in a feature dimension as well as in space.

So far we have discussed how voluntary visual-spatial attention increases the effective contrast of a stimulus presented at an attended location, with the magnitude of the attentional enhancement of neuronal spike rates modulated by response saturation and divisive normalization. Attention effects are especially strong when multiple stimuli compete within a neuron's receptive field because attending to one stimulus strongly inhibits inputs from ignored stimuli. The biased-competition model (with its attentional contrast-gain hypothesis) postulates that this inhibition arises from attentional enhancement of the effective contrast of the attended stimulus because a visual neuron tends to preferentially respond to the highest-contrast stimulus within its receptive field. Recent neurophysiological results, however, have elucidated additional mechanisms by which attention may strongly inhibit inputs from ignored stimuli in the context of within-receptive-field stimulus competition.

RESOLVING WITHIN-RECEPTIVE-FIELD STIMULUS COMPETITION: ATTENTIONAL MODULATION OF FAST-SPIKING INHIBITORY INTERNEURONS AND FACILITATION OF GAMMA-BAND OSCILLATIONS OF NEURAL EXCITABILITY

In most studies investigating attention effects on neuronal spike rates, attention effects were not separately analyzed for different classes of neurons. Moreover, because attention is considered to be a gating mechanism, it is typically assumed that attention would primarily influence the responses of pyramidal neurons that transmit signals from one cortical area to another. Mitchell, Sundberg, & Reynolds (2007) discovered that the responses of both broad-spiking neurons, likely pyramidal neurons, and narrow-spiking neurons, likely inhibitory interneurons, in V4, were equivalently enhanced by attention in terms of the proportion of increase in their spike rates. Interestingly, attention more strongly increased raw spike rates for the inhibitory interneurons because they generated faster spikes than did the pyramidal neurons. Attention also increased the reliability of neuronal responses more strongly for the inhibitory interneurons than for the pyramidal neurons. These results suggest that strongly attention-dependent responses of fast-spiking inhibitory interneurons mediate the strong suppression of input from ignored stimuli during within-receptive-field stimulus competition.

Attentional modulation of fast-spiking inhibitory interneurons may additionally influence stimulus competition by modulating neural synchronization. Computational modeling has shown that top-down enhancement of a subset of fast-spiking inhibitory interneurons can make them synchronously oscillate in gamma-band frequencies (see Tiesinga, Fellous, & Sejnowski, 2008, for a review). Synchronously oscillating interneurons can generate an inhibitory rhythm so that the excitability of the pyramidal neurons in the vicinity (connected to the inhibitory interneurons) oscillates with the rhythm. This mechanism allows attention to establish a preferred communication channel for input selection.

If two groups of neurons are subjected to an inhibitory rhythm in the same frequency band, appropriately phase-shifted to compensate for the conduction delay between them (about 1–3 ms within a cortical area and about 5 ms across cortical areas; Fries, 2005; Womelsdorf et al., 2007), signal transmission between the two neuron groups should be facilitated because when one group transmits the signal in its low-inhibition phase, the other group receives the signal also in its low-inhibition phase, making it likely for the receiving group to respond to the signal. Suppose two stimuli, A and B, activate separate groups of V4 neurons with smaller receptive fields, but they both activate the same group of IT neurons with larger receptive fields. Attending to A would generate coherent inhibitory rhythms between the V4 neurons responding to A and the IT neurons, so that the IT neurons would respond well to signals from A, arriving at the low-inhibition phases of the IT neurons, but would respond less well to signals from B, that arrive randomly at low- and high-inhibition phases of the IT neurons. Similarly, attending to B would generate coherent inhibitory rhythms between the V4 neurons responding to B and the IT neurons, so that the IT neurons would optimally respond to signals from B but suboptimally to signals from A.

Such gamma-band synchronization-based facilitation of neural communication is hypothetical. Nevertheless, it has been shown that, in V4, attending to a stimulus increases gamma-band oscillations in local field potentials (LFPs) for neurons with their receptive fields covering the attended location—indicative of the inhibitory rhythm—and their spike trains in response to the attended stimulus are correlated with this LFP rhythm—indicative of modulation of neuronal excitability by the inhibitory rhythm (Fries, Reynolds, Rorie, & Desimone, 2001). There is also evidence suggesting that transient correlations between spike trains within cat area 17, within monkey areas V1 and V4, and across cat areas 17 and 21a—indicative of signal transmissions within and across cortical areas—tend to occur when gamma-band LFPs are appropriately aligned in phase among the interacting neural populations (Womelsdorf et al., 2007). It is therefore possible that one way in which voluntary visual-spatial attention resolves a within-receptive-field stimulus competition might be to generate a gamma-band-synchronized communication channel between the receiving downstream neurons and the afferent neurons whose receptive fields coincide with the focus of attention (via enhancing responses of a subset of fast-spiking inhibitory interneurons). In support of this possibility, a recent study (Bosman et al., 2012) has shown that attention selectively increases gamma-band synchronization between V4 neurons and the afferent V1 neurons that have receptive fields in the focus of attention. Furthermore, electroencephalography (EEG) studies with human observers have shown that attending to a stimulus increases long-range EEG phase synchronization in gamma-band (and alpha-band) frequencies in the contralateral scalp regions (e.g., Doesburg, Green, McDonald, & Ward, 2009; Doesburg, Roggeveen, Kitajo, & Ward, 2008).

ATTENTIONAL REDUCTION OF LATERAL INTERFERENCE IN LOW-LEVEL VISUAL AREAS

Using small static bars as stimuli, Chalk et al. (2010) have shown that attention reduces the power of gamma-band oscillation in V1 (cf. Bosman et al., 2012, found little effect of attention on V1 gamma-band oscillations for small drifting gratings). Why would attention reduce rather than increase gamma-band oscillations in V1 for small static stimuli? Because neuronal receptive fields are small in V1, it is rarely the case that two distinct objects fall within a V1 neuron's receptive field. Thus, stimulus competition in V1 may primarily involve interactions among neurons with neighboring receptive fields rather than within-receptive-field stimulus competition. Because reduced gamma-band oscillation suggests reduced activity of inhibitory interneurons, an attention effect on V1 neurons might be to reduce suppressive influences from the neighboring neurons to the neurons responding to the attended stimulus (Chalk et al., 2010).

Another mechanism by which attention reduces interference from neighboring distractors in V1 may be via top-down modulation of the cholinergic system (e.g., from the prefrontal cortex). Acetylcholine (ACh) suppresses the efficacy of intracortical synapses while it simultaneously increases the efficacy of feedforward thalamocortical input to V1. ACh could thus increase the effect of a stimulus within the classical receptive field while it simultaneously reduces the effect of distractor stimuli outside of the classical receptive field. Indeed, it has been shown that an application of ACh reduces spatial integration in V1 neurons (see Deco & Thiele, 2009, for a review of these effects of ACh). Thus, voluntary visual-spatial attention may increase spatial resolution by reducing spatial integration in V1 neurons via top-down release of ACh. Attentional reduction of lateral interference has also been found in V4 (Sundberg, Mitchell, & Reynolds, 2009).

While attention may generally reduce lateral interference in V1, it may facilitate specific lateral interactions that are behaviorally relevant. For example, when a vertical bar is presented in a V1 neuron's receptive field and a collinear vertical bar is presented adjacent to it, attending to the vertical bar within the receptive field increases the facilitative effect from the neighboring collinear bar (Ito & Gilbert, 1999). Attention may promote detection of contours by increasing the efficacy of collinearity-based grouping (see Field & Hayes, 2004; Hess, Hayes, & Field, 2003, for reviews).

INTERIM SUMMARY

Our review so far suggests that voluntary visual-spatial attention modulates neuronal spike rates in multiple ways (see Figure 3.1 for an illustration). When a visual scene is sparse and visual neurons in most visual areas process information from only a single object at a time, attention multiplicatively increases the effective contrast signal with divisive normalization (Figure 3.1(B)). When a visual scene is cluttered with many objects so that multiple objects fall within the receptive fields of mid- to high-level visual neurons that have relatively large receptive fields, attention suppresses input from ignored stimuli by increasing the activity of fast-spiking inhibitory interneurons (Figure 3.1(D)), which may directly inhibit inputs from ignored stimuli (Figure 3.1(E)) and/or establish a gamma-band-synchronized communication channel selective for the input from the attended stimulus (Figure 3.1(F)). Furthermore, especially in V1 where neural receptive fields are small, attention may reduce lateral interference via cholinergic mechanisms (Figure 3.1(A)).

ATTENTIONAL ENHANCEMENT OF NEURAL POPULATION RESPONSES BY SYNCHRONIZATION

So far we have reviewed the effects of voluntary visual-spatial attention on the responses of single neurons. When competing stimuli are presented far apart, falling on separate neuronal receptive fields, attentional modulation of neuronal spike rates is relatively modest, less than 40% on average (e.g., McAdams & Maunsell, 1999a; Spitzer et al., 1988; Williford & Maunsell, 2006; or equivalent to about a 50% increase in luminance contrast for V4 neurons, Reynolds, Pasternak, & Desimone, 2000) or there is no modulation when the attended stimulus is small and high contrast (e.g., Moran & Desimone, 1985; Reynolds, Pasternak, & Desimone, 2000). This is inconsistent with the fact that behavioral studies have demonstrated robust attention effects on visual detection, classification, and localization even when a single small high-contrast target is presented in the absence of any distractor stimuli (e.g., Guzman-Martinez et al., 2011; Posner, 1980; Posner et al., 1980; Suzuki & Cavanagh, 1997).

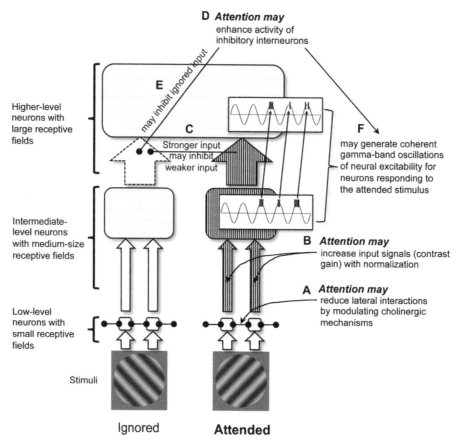

FIGURE 3.1   A schematic diagram of visual processing from low level (bottom) to high level (top), highlighting the different ways in which voluntary visual-spatial attention may exert its influence. The rectangles represent neural receptive fields, with the upward arrows representing feedforward sensory input. The circular buttons represent inhibitory influences. In low-level processing, each small receptive field may capture a portion of a stimulus, where attention may primarily (A) modulate cholinergic mechanisms to reduce lateral interactions and increase spatial resolution. In intermediate-level processing, each mid-size receptive field may capture a whole stimulus, where attention may primarily (B) increase the input signals (contrast gain) with normalization. In mid- to high-level processing, each large receptive field may capture multiple stimuli, entailing within-receptive-field stimulus competition. In this case (C) the enhanced input from the attended stimulus may inhibit the weaker input from the ignored stimulus. Attention may also (D) enhance the activity of inhibitory interneurons. This may (E) directly inhibit the input from the ignored stimulus, and/or (F) generate coherent gamma-band oscillations of excitability across the neurons responding to the attended stimulus (illustrated with phase-aligned sinusoidal curves), making them likely to spike at the peaks of excitability (illustrated with short vertical lines). At the neuronal level, this coherent oscillation may selectively gate attended signals to higher-level processing because coincident excitability facilitates neural communication. At the neural-population level, the coherent oscillation may allow a population of visual neurons to generate coincident action potentials, which are especially effective in driving downstream neurons. (B), (C), and (E) are relevant to the biased-competition model (see text for details).

One possibility is that the attentional enhancement of gamma-band oscillations of neural excitability, potentially establishing synchronized channels to resolve within-receptive-field input competition (see above), might also increase the impact of attended signals at the population level. The impact of neural signals on downstream processing is increased when afferent action potentials are synchronized (e.g., Azouz & Gary, 2000; Salinas & Sejnowski, 2000). As attention enhances the gamma-band rhythm of excitability in the population of visual neurons responding to an attended stimulus,[2]

those neurons would tend to respond in synchrony at the low-inhibition phases of the oscillatory rhythm. Thus, even in conditions where attention effects on neuronal spike rates are modest, attention could enhance the impact of selected signals at the population level by synchronizing stimulus-driven action potentials. Is there evidence in support of this possibility?

Electroencephalography (EEG) provides a method to noninvasively record population electrophysiological activity in humans. One way to evaluate whether attention increases the synchronization of stimulus-evoked neural-population responses is to use periodically flickered stimuli and determine whether attention increases the phase-locking of EEG responses to the selected stimuli.

[2]Except in V1 because attention does not increase gamma-band neural oscillations in V1 (see above).

An advantage of using periodically flickered stimuli is that different flicker frequencies can be assigned to the attended and ignored stimuli. In this way, the neural-population responses to the attended and ignored stimuli can be clearly segregated in the EEG signals based on their corresponding Fourier components, despite the poor spatial resolution of scalp-recorded EEG measures. For example, if a square is flickered at X Hz and an adjacent circle at Y Hz, the Fourier power of EEG at X Hz (and its harmonics) reflects the neural-population response to the square and the Fourier power of EEG at Y Hz (and its harmonics) reflects the neural-population response to the circle. This method is referred to as "frequency tagging" and the oscillatory EEG signals evoked by periodically flickered stimuli are referred to as steady-state visual-evoked potentials (SSVEPs). This method is particularly useful for monitoring the effects of voluntary sustained attention on neural-population responses to attended and ignored stimuli (e.g., Andersen, Müller, & Hillyard, 2009; Di Russo, Spinelli, & Morrone, 2001; Morgan, Hansen, & Hillyard, 1996; Müller et al., 1998). For example, a fundamental question is whether it is possible to sustain visual-spatial attention at two nonadjacent locations without attending to a location in between. By recording the frequency-tagged SSVEPs from a row of stimuli (each flickered at a distinct frequency), Müller, Malinowski, Gruber, and Hillyard (2003) showed that attending to nonadjacent stimuli increased the SSVEP power for those stimuli without affecting the SSVEP power for the in-between stimulus, demonstrating that visual-spatial attention can be sustained at two separate locations.

Crucial for our discussion here is the degree to which stimulus-evoked neural-population responses are synchronized by voluntary visual-spatial attention. The degree of response synchronization in SSVEPs can be estimated by computing inter-trial phase coherence (ITPC). ITPC indexes the degree to which SSVEP phase (relative to the flickered stimulus) is constant across trials (e.g., Delorme & Makeig, 2004; Tallon-Baudry, Bertrand, Delpeuch, & Pernier, 1996). If neuronal responses to a periodically flickered visual stimulus are perfectly synchronized within a population, that is, if each neuron responds at the same delay to each volley of stimulus flicker, the resultant waveform of the population-level field potentials (SSVEPs) should always have a constant phase delay relative to the flickering stimulus. SSVEP phase should then be constant across trials, yielding an ITPC of 1. In contrast, if neuronal responses to the periodic stimulus are not synchronized, that is, if each neuron responds at an independently variable delay to each volley of stimulus flicker, the resultant potentials should have variable phase delays from the flickering stimulus over time. SSVEP phase should then be variable across trials, yielding an ITPC less than 1. Thus, if

attention increases neural response synchronization to the stimulus at the population level, attention should increase ITPC for the attended stimulus.

Indeed, in a prior study we demonstrated that, when competing stimuli were presented in separate visual hemifields (yielding one stimulus per receptive field for the majority of visual neurons), voluntary visual-spatial attention selectively increased ITPC for the attended stimulus (Kim, Grabowecky, Paller, Muthu, & Suzuki, 2007). The results, however, did not conclusively indicate that attention increases neural response synchronization, because attention also increased SSVEP power. That is, attention also increased the amplitude of the stimulus-evoked neural-population responses. The brain generates oscillatory activity across a broad range of frequencies (falling off at higher frequencies), and these intrinsic neural oscillations are randomly phase-shifted relative to the periodic signal from the flickered stimulus. Because the stimulus-evoked oscillatory responses are superimposed on these intrinsic oscillations in SSVEPs, increasing the amplitude of the stimulus-evoked responses necessarily increases ITPC by reducing the relative contribution of random-phased intrinsic oscillations to SSVEPs. Nevertheless, because Kim et al. (2007) computed SSVEP amplitudes after averaging EEG waveforms across trials, their SSVEP amplitudes preferentially reflected the component of oscillatory waveforms that were consistent in phase across trials. It is thus possible that the increased SSVEP amplitudes for the attended stimulus might actually reflect attentional enhancements of neural response synchronization. Furthermore, the SSVEP enhancement with attention was strongest in the high-contrast portion of the contrast-response function, even though SSVEP amplitudes for the ignored stimulus saturated at high contrast for at least one of the two flicker frequencies. This result fits with the idea that SSVEP effects reflected increased synchronization rather than increased spike rates. However, it is also possible that the stimuli were large relative to the relevant receptive fields; in that case, the normalization model of attention would also predict that attention would increase neuronal spike rates especially for high-contrast stimuli.

Another recent study examined the time course of attention effects on SSVEP amplitudes and ITPCs (Kashiwase, Matsumiya, Kuriki, & Shioiri, 2012). To reduce the contribution of response synchronization to the measure of SSVEP amplitudes, SSVEP amplitudes were separately computed for each trial and then averaged across trials. It was found that attention increased ITPCs about 130 ms before it increased SSVEP amplitudes (Figure 3.2), suggesting that attention-induced increases in neural response synchronization drive attention-induced increases in SSVEP amplitudes. Importantly, the time course of behavioral benefits of attention was

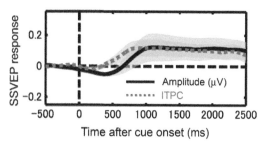

FIGURE 3.2 The time courses of SSVEP amplitude (solid black curve) and ITPC (inter-trial phase coherence; dotted gray curve) for the attended stimulus relative to the onset of a central attention cue (the EEG responses averaged from contralateral-posterior electrodes). The data clearly show that voluntary visual-spatial attention increases ITPC (indicative of neural response synchronization) before it increases SSVEP amplitude. The SSVEP amplitude and ITPC are normalized to the precue response. The shaded areas represent ±1 standard error of the mean. See Kashiwase et al. (2012) for details. *Adapted from Kashiwase, Y., Matsumiya, K., Kuriki, I., & Shioiri, S. (2012).*

more closely associated with the time course of ITPCs than that of SSVEP amplitudes.

These SSVEP results with human observers support the idea that attention can substantially influence visual processing even when small high-contrast stimuli are sparsely presented so that attention effects on individual neurons are expected to be relatively small. Attention can still increase the impact of the selected stimulus on downstream perceptual and cognitive processes by synchronizing the stimulus-evoked neural responses at the population level.

PRESERVING PERCEPTUAL FIDELITY IN SPITE OF STRONG ATTENTIONAL MODULATION OF VISUAL RESPONSES

The attentional modulation of neural responses is crucial for stimulus selection. However, it is also important to prevent the modulation from inducing distortion so as to preserve valid information about stimulus intensity. Although a careful psychophysical study has demonstrated that voluntary visual-spatial attention increases perceived contrast (Liu, Abrams, & Carrasco, 2009), the magnitude of this effect, shifting the perceived intensity of a 32%-contrast stimulus by about ±4%, is much smaller than the amount of attentional modulation of neuronal responses. In reality, a "gray paper appears to us no lighter, the pendulum-beat of a clock no louder, no matter how much we increase the strain of our attention upon them" (Fechner, cited by James, 1890, p. 426). In other words, no amount of attention can noticeably change perceived contrast. It is likely that the visual system has mechanisms to preserve contrast information while allowing attention to

substantially modulate responses of visual neurons for stimulus selection.

Recent neurophysiological and electrophysiological results suggest that stimulus contrast and attentional modulation are separately encoded by the visual system. At the neuronal level, a study examining attention effects on the responses of V1 neurons suggests that stimulus contrast is encoded by the contrast-dependent responses of a group of neurons that are relatively unaffected by attention. At the same time, an attended stimulus is encoded by the difference in responses between the group of neurons that are influenced by attention and those that are unaffected by attention (Pooresmaeili, Poort, Thiele, & Roelfsema, 2010). At the neural-population level, we have used the SSVEP method to provide evidence that contrast information and attentional modulation are encoded by neural populations with different dynamic properties (Kim, Grabowecky, Paller, & Suzuki, 2011). Some visual neurons (including simple cells in V1) respond to periodic stimuli with a frequency-following characteristic, whereas other visual neurons (including complex cells in V1) respond to periodic stimuli with a frequency-doubling characteristic (e.g., Benucci, Frazor, & Carandini, 2007; De Valois, Albrecht, & Thorell, 1982; Hubel & Wiesel, 1968). Roughly speaking, frequency-following neurons strongly respond to onsets of their preferred stimuli whereas frequency-doubling neurons strongly respond to both onsets and offsets of their preferred stimuli. These response characteristics have implications for considering how SSVEP measures might be differentially sensitive to these two types of neurons.

Most SSVEP studies have either used on–off flickered or counter-phase flickered stimuli. Although these stimuli are well suited for frequency tagging of EEG responses, they are unsuitable for distinguishing frequency-following and frequency-doubling neural responses. When the on–off flicker is used, both frequency-following and frequency-doubling neural responses contribute to the 1st harmonic SSVEPs. When counter-phase flicker is used, frequency-following neural responses are primarily averaged out in SSVEPs. By using light–dark flicker (flickered stimuli alternating between brighter and darker relative to a mid-gray background), the experimental design of Kim et al. (2011) made it possible to simultaneously monitor both frequency-following responses, reflected in the 1st harmonic SSVEPs, and frequency-doubling responses, reflected in the 2nd harmonic SSVEPs. Two features of the results were critical. First, frequency-following and frequency-doubling responses had segregated scalp distributions, medial-posterior focus for frequency-following responses (Figure 3.3, upper left) and contralateral-posterior focus for frequency-doubling

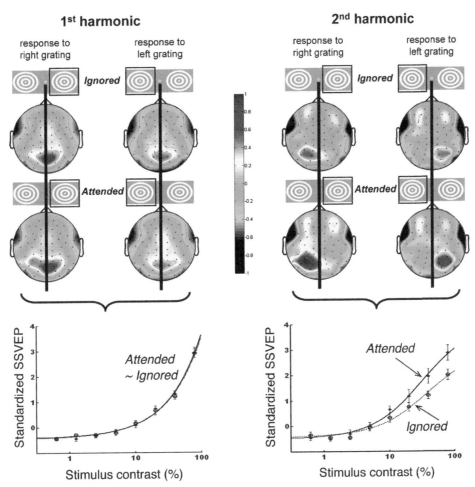

FIGURE 3.3 In this study, dark–light flicker (alternation of dark versus light concentric rings on a mid-gray background) was used so that frequency-following and frequency-doubling visual responses would be segregated in the 1st and 2nd harmonics of SSVEPs, respectively. Voluntary visual-spatial attention clearly increased the contralaterally focused frequency-doubling responses (right column), but it had little effect on the simultaneously recorded centrally focused frequency-following responses (left column). The results suggest that, while frequency-doubling visual processing allows substantial attentional modulation for flexibly highlighting behaviorally relevant signals, frequency-following visual processing at the same time preserves unaltered contrast information irrespective of attention. The error bars represent ±1 standard error of the mean (adjusted for within-participant comparisons). See Kim et al. (2011) for details. *Adapted from Kim, Y.-J., Grabowecky, M., Paller, K. A., & Suzuki, S. (2011).*

responses (Figure 3.3, upper right). Second, whereas frequency-doubling responses were strongly modulated by voluntary visual-spatial attention (especially for high-contrast stimuli) (Figure 3.3, lower right), the simultaneously recorded frequency-following responses were unaffected by attention (regardless of stimulus contrast) (Figure 3.3, lower left). Consequently, it appears that the neural population that collectively exhibits frequency-doubling responses allows strong response modulation by voluntary visual-spatial attention, while at the same time the neural population that collectively exhibits frequency-following responses preserves contrast information irrespective of attention. It is unlikely that these SSVEP results reflect the attention-dependent and attention-independent classes of neurons in V1 (Pooresmaeili et al., 2010), because neural clusters within V1 would

not have produced the substantial scalp segregation of the attention-dependent and attention-independent responses in SSVEPs. Instead, it is likely that the visual system has both neuronal and neural-population mechanisms to separate the encoding of stimulus intensity from attentional modulation of visual signals.

CONCLUSIONS

The design of the ventral visual pathway thought to mediate object identification (e.g., Fang & He, 2005; Goodale & Westwood, 2004; Mishkin et al., 1983) builds on a spatially convergent feedforward architecture where neurons in higher-level visual areas have progressively larger receptive fields. This architecture, required for pooling information across space to encode complex global patterns, necessitates selection mechanisms.

When two (or more) stimuli fall within a high-level visual neuron's receptive field, the input from only one stimulus must be selected while inputs from other stimuli must be inhibited so that the neuron's response indicates whether or not the stimulus of interest is its preferred pattern. This within-receptive-field stimulus selection appears to be mediated by attentional enhancement of fast-spiking inhibitory interneurons. The enhanced activity of inhibitory interneurons might directly inhibit inputs from ignored stimuli, but it might also indirectly facilitate within-receptive-field stimulus selection by generating a gamma-band-synchronized communication channel that tunes the rhythm of the higher-level neuron's excitability to the rhythm of the afferent neurons responding to an attended stimulus. Attentional enhancements of ACh release may further increase the clarity of the attended stimulus by reducing lateral interference, especially in low-level visual areas with small neural receptive fields, where stimulus competition primarily occurs as interference from neighboring neurons.

When a visual scene is sparse and only one stimulus falls within a high-level neuron's receptive field, there is no input competition for the neuron. Accordingly, attention effects at the neuronal level are relatively small, especially when stimuli are high contrast and small (incurring only weak normalization). Nevertheless, behavioral results suggest that strongly attending to one stimulus can make an unexpectedly presented stimulus elsewhere difficult to recognize (or invisible; inattentional blindness, e.g., Mack & Rock, 1998), even if the unexpected stimulus is high contrast, small, and presented far from the attended stimulus so that it falls within the receptive fields of a different population of neurons. Attention-enhanced gamma-band oscillation of neural excitability (relevant to resolving within-receptive-field input competition by establishing synchronized communication channels) may also increase synchronization of neural-population responses to the attended stimulus. This possibility is consistent with recent SSVEP results. Because synchronized spikes are especially effective in driving downstream target neurons, increased synchronization of stimulus-evoked neural responses at the population level would substantially increase the impact of the attended stimulus on higher-level perceptual and cognitive processes.

Attentional selection is clearly necessary for object recognition in the presence of the within-receptive-field stimulus competition that is typical in a cluttered environment, as in most naturalistic situations. However, it is not clear why attentional selection is necessary when, for example, two stimuli are presented in separate visual hemifields, where visual neurons with contralateral receptive fields can in principle separately and simultaneously process both stimuli. One possibility is that selecting one stimulus at a time may be generally desirable for controlling behavior because, for example, attention plays an important role in directing eye movements, and the eyes can fixate only one stimulus at a time (see Awh, Armstrong, & Moore, 2006; Kowler, 2011, for reviews). It might also be beneficial to plan action for one object at a time due to the kinematic constraints of the human body.

In summary, voluntary visual-spatial attention allows us to highlight visual information from a specific location by utilizing a variety of neural mechanisms, by reducing neuronal interference in lower-level visual processing with ACh-related mechanisms, by increasing neuronal responses to attended stimuli by increasing their effective contrast in conjunction with normalization mechanisms, and by enhancing the activity of inhibitory interneurons that may suppress the processing of ignored stimuli and may induce gamma-band synchronization of neural excitability. The latter may facilitate selective transmission of attended signals by establishing a gamma-band-synchronized channel for the attended signals, and may also increase the population-level synchronization of stimulus-evoked neural responses to increase the downstream impact of attended signals. These neuronal and neural-population mechanisms together allow us to flexibly highlight visual information based on location under a variety of conditions, whether the stimulus of interest is dim, bright, small or large, and whether it is in a sparse or cluttered environment.

AFTERTHOUGHTS: ATTENTION VS AWARENESS

The extent to which visual attention and visual awareness reflect separable mechanisms has often been debated. How might our review of the neural mechanisms of voluntary visual-spatial attention contribute to this debate? Evidence suggests that an attended image can become invisible during stimulus competition in spite of any amount of attentional effort one may exert to keep the image visible; typical examples include binocular rivalry, continuous flash suppression, and motion induced blindness (e.g., Bonneh, Cooperman, & Sagi, 2001; Tong, Meng, & Blake, 2006; Tsuchiya & Koch, 2005; Tsuchiya, Koch, Gilroy, & Blake, 2006). These phenomena demonstrate that neither attentionally enhancing effective stimulus contrast, reducing lateral interference in low-level visual processing, generating a selection channel from low- to high-level visual processing by gamma-band synchronizing excitability across neurons responding to the attended stimulus, nor increasing synchronization of stimulus-evoked neural-population responses to the selected stimulus necessarily makes a stimulus consciously visible. In addition, there is no evidence that suggests that any of the attention mechanisms that we have discussed require that the stimulus-evoked neural activity carries the characteristics that generate visual awareness. This is consistent with the fact that some priming effects still require that the location of the prime be attended even if the prime is invisible (e.g., Naccache, Blandin, & Dehaene, 2002; Sumner, Tsai, Yu, & Nachev, 2006).

What might then be the critical neural activity that makes a stimulus consciously visible? Some results suggest that global gamma-band and beta-band oscillations occurring relatively late (~300 ms) after stimulus onset, that broadcast stimulus signals across the neocortex, are important for making the stimulus consciously visible (see Dehaene & Changeux, 2011, for a review). Attention mechanisms do not appear to generate these specific types of oscillatory neural-population activity. For example, visual-spatial attention induces early (50–150 ms) gamma-band oscillations in V4 that are anatomically constrained to neurons that respond to the attended stimulus (Fries et al., 2001). Other results suggest that longer-range lower-frequency synchronization mediates perceptual and cognitive operations that are associated with visual awareness, whereas relatively short-range high-frequency synchronization mediates spatial focusing of attention. For example, mid-frequency gamma-band oscillations appear relevant for stimulus awareness, whereas visual-spatial attention induces high-frequency gamma-band oscillations (Wyart & Tallon-Baudry, 2008). Beta-band rather than gamma-band oscillations in V1 population activity are associated with awareness of visual stimuli (e.g., Wilke, Logothetis, & Leopold, 2006). Furthermore, interactions between attention and working memory, a hallmark of conscious processing, appear to involve gamma-band oscillations that are coupled with slower theta-band oscillations (e.g., Canolty et al., 2006; see Womelsdorf & Fries, 2007; Düzel, Penny, & Burgess, 2010, for reviews).

Although voluntary visual-spatial attention mechanisms do not seem to generate neural activity critical for stimulus awareness, they exert a powerful inhibitory effect on visual signals. Downstream processing of ignored stimuli is substantially curtailed, and inputs from ignored stimuli are virtually "invisible" to higher-level visual neurons when multiple stimuli fall within their receptive fields. Thus, to the extent that awareness of a stimulus requires global sharing of stimulus information (e.g., Dehaene & Changeux, 2011), an ignored stimulus would not reach awareness. This is consistent with the phenomenon of inattentional blindness (Mack & Rock, 1998) and the fact that there is no conclusive empirical evidence of a strongly ignored stimulus reaching awareness (see Cohen, Cavanagh, Chun, & Nakayama, 2012 for a review).

Note that broadly distributed attention is not the same as inattention. That is, when visual-spatial attention is not focused at any specific location, high-level visual neurons with large receptive fields would respond based on how well the entire pattern of stimuli presented within their receptive fields collectively match their preferred patterns. For example, consider a face composed of fruit. When attention is broadly distributed (i.e., when the entire image is attended), a face-tuned neuron would respond but an "apple-tuned" neuron would not. However, when an apple is attended, the apple-tuned neuron would respond but the face-tuned neuron would not. This view is consistent with evidence that people initially perceive the gist of a scene at a glance, and then perceive the details as they begin to focus attention to specific locations (e.g., Hochstein & Ahissar, 2002).

Overall, the available research on neural mechanisms of voluntary visual-spatial attention and visual awareness suggests (1) that we can intentionally select visual signals based on location for downstream processing whether or not we are aware of the signals, and (2) that we can be aware of signals if they come from an attended location and if they additionally produce the type of neural activity that generates visual awareness.

Acknowledgments

This work was supported by National Institutes of Health grant R01 EY021184.

References

Andersen, S. K., Müller, M. M., & Hillyard, S. A. (2009). Color-selective attention need not be mediated by spatial attention. *Journal of Vision, 9*(6), 2, 1–7.

Austin, J. (1918). *Pride and prejudice.* Charles Scribner's Sons.

Awh, E., Armstrong, K. M., & Moore, T. (2006). Visual and oculomotor selection: links, causes and implications for spatial attention. *Trends in Cognitive Sciences, 10,* 124–130.

Azouz, R., & Gary, C. M. (2000). Dynamic spike threshold reveals a mechanism for synaptic coincidence detection in cortical neurons in vivo. *Proceedings of the National Academy of Sciences USA, 97,* 8110–8115.

Benucci, A., Frazor, R. A., & Carandini, M. (2007). Standing waves and traveling waves distinguish two circuits in visual cortex. *Neuron, 55,* 103–117.

Blaser, E., Sperling, G., & Lu, Z. -H. (1999). Measuring the amplification of attention. *Proceedings of the National Academy of Sciences USA, 96,* 11681–11686.

Bonneh, Y. S., Cooperman, A., & Sagi, D. (2001). Motion-induced blindness in normal observers. *Nature, 411,* 798–801.

Bosman, C. A., Schoffelen, J. -M., Brunet, N., Oostenveld, R., Bastos, A. M., Womelsdorf, T., et al. (2012). Attentional stimulus selection through synchronization between monkey visual areas. *Neuron, 75,* 875–888.

Bushnell, M. C., Goldberg, M. E., & Robinson, D. L. (1981). Behavioral enhancement of visual responses in monkey cerebral cortex: I. Modulation in posterior parietal cortex related to selective visual attention. *Journal of Neurophysiology*, *46*, 755–772.

Canolty, R. T., Edwards, E., Dalal, S. S., Soltani, M., Nagarajan, S. S., Kirsch, H. E., et al. (2006). High gamma power is phase-locked to theta oscillations in human neocortex. *Science*, *313*, 1626–1628.

Carrasco, M. (2011). Visual attention: the past 25 years. *Vision Research*, *51*, 1484–1525.

Cavanagh, J. R., Bair, W., & Movshon, J. A. (2002). Nature and interaction of signals from the receptive field center and surround in macaque V1 neurons. *Journal of Neurophysiology*, *88*, 2530–2546.

Cave, K. R., & Bishot, N. P. (1999). Visuospatial attention: beyond a spotlight model. *Psychonomic Bulletin & Review*, *6*, 204–223.

Chalk, M., Herrero, J. L., Gieselmann, M. A., Delicato, L. S., Gotthardt, S., & Thiele, A. (2010). Attention reduces stimulus-driven gamma frequency oscillations and spike field coherence in V1. *Neuron*, *66*, 114–125.

Cheal, M. L., & Lyon, D. R. (1991). Central and peripheral precuing of forced-choice discrimination. *Quarterly Journal of Experimental Psychology: Human Experimental Psychology*, *43A*, 859–880.

Chelazzi, L., Duncan, J., Miller, E. K., & Desimone, R. (1998). Responses of neurons in inferior temporal cortex during memory-guided visual search. *Journal of Neurophysiology*, *80*, 2918–2940.

Cohen, M. A., Cavanagh, P., Chun, M. M., & Nakayama, K. (2012). The attentional requirements of consciousness. *Trends in Cognitive Sciences*, *16*, 411–417.

Colby, C. L., Duhamel, J. R., & Goldberg, M. E. (1996). Visual, presaccadic, and cognitive activation of single neurons in monkey lateral intraparietal area. *Journal of Neurophysiology*, *76*, 2841–2852.

Corbetta, M., & Shulman, G. L. (2002). Control of goal-directed and stimulus-driven attention in the brain. *Nature Reviews Neuroscience*, *3*, 201–215.

De Valois, R. L., Albrecht, D. G., & Thorell, L. G. (1982). Spatial frequency selectivity of cells in macaque visual cortex. *Vision Research*, *22*, 545–559.

Deco, G., & Thiele, A. (2009). Attention—oscillations and neuropharmacology. *European Journal of Neuroscience*, *30*, 347–354.

Dehaene, S., & Changeux, J. -P. (2011). Experimental and theoretical approaches to conscious processing. *Neuron*, *70*, 200–227.

Delorme, A., & Makeig, S. (2004). EEGLAB: an open source toolbox for analysis of single-trial EEG dynamics including independent component analysis. *Journal of Neuroscience Methods*, *134*, 9–21.

Desimone, R., & Duncan, J. (1995). Neural mechanisms of selective visual attention. *Annual Review of Neuroscience*, *18*, 193–222.

Di Russo, F., Spinelli, D., & Morrone, M. C. (2001). Automatic gain control contrast mechanisms are modulated by attention in humans: evidence from visual evoked potentials. *Vision Research*, *41*, 2435–2447.

Doesburg, S. M., Green, J. J., McDonald, J. J., & Ward (2009). From local inhibition to long-range integration: a functional dissociation of alpha-band synchronization across cortical scales in visuospatial attention. *Brain Research*, *1303*, 97–110.

Doesburg, S. M., Roggeveen, A. B., Kitajo, K., & Ward, L. M. (2008). Large-scale gamma-band phase synchronization and selective attention. *Cerebral Cortex*, *18*, 386–396.

Downing, C. J., & Pinker, S. (1985). The spatial structure of visual attention. In M. I. Posner & O. S. M. Marin (Eds.), *Attention and performance, XI*. Hillsdale, NJ: Erlbaum.

Düzel, E., Penny, W. D., & Burgess, N. (2010). Brain oscillations and memory. *Current Opinion in Neurobiology*, *20*, 143–149.

Eriksen, C. W., & Collins, J. F. (1969). Temporal course of selective attention. *Journal of Experimental Psychology*, *80*, 254–261.

Fang, F., & He, S. (2005). Cortical responses to invisible objects in the human dorsal and ventral pathway. *Nature Neuroscience*, *8*, 1380–1385.

Field, D. J., & Hayes, A. (2004). Contour integration and the lateral connections of V1 neurons. In L. M. Chalupa & J. S. Werner (Eds.), *The visual neurosciences*. MIT Press.

Fries, P. (2005). A mechanism for cognitive dynamics: neuronal communication through neuronal coherence. *Trends in Cognitive Sciences*, *9*, 474–480.

Fries, P., Reynolds, J. H., Rorie, A. E., & Desimone, R. (2001). Modulation of oscillatory neuronal synchronization by selective visual attention. *Science*, *291*, 1560–1563.

Funes, M. J., Lupianez, J., & Milliken, B. (2005). The role of spatial attention and other processes on the magnitude and time course of cueing effects. *Cognitive Processing*, *6*, 98–116.

Goodale, M. A., & Westwood, D. A. (2004). An evolving view of duplex vision: separate but interacting cortical pathways for perception and action. *Current Opinion in Neurobiology*, *14*, 203–211.

Gregoriou, G. G., Gotts, S. J., Zhou, H., & Desimone, R. (2009). High-frequency, long-range coupling between prefrontal and visual cortex during attention. *Science*, *324*, 1207–1210.

Guzman-Martinez, E., Grabowecky, M., Palafox, G., & Suzuki, S. (2011). A unique role of endogenous visual-spatial attention in rapid processing of multiple targets. *Journal of Experimental Psychology: Human Perception and Performance*, *37*, 1065–1073.

Hawkins, H. L., Hillyard, S. A., Luck, S. J., Mouloua, M., Downing, C. J., & Woodward, D. P. (1990). Visual attention modulates signal detectability. *Journal of Experimental Psychology: Human Perception and Performance*, *16*, 802–811.

Hess, R. F., Hayes, A., & Field, D. J. (2003). Contour integration and cortical processing. *Journal of Physiology – Paris*, *97*, 105–119.

Hickey, C., McDonald, J. J., & Theeuwes, J. (2006). Electrophysiological evidence of the capture of visual attention. *Journal of Cognitive Neuroscience*, *18*, 604–613.

Hikosaka, O., Miyauchi, S., & Shimojo, S. (1993). Voluntary and stimulus induced attention detected as motion sensation. *Perception*, *22*, 517–526.

Hochstein, S., & Ahissar, M. (2002). View from the top: hierarchies and reverse hierarchies in the visual system. *Neuron*, *36*, 791–804.

Hubel, D. H., & Wiesel, T. N. (1968). Receptive fields and functional architecture of monkey striate cortex. *Journal of Physiology*, *195*, 215–243.

Ito, M., & Gilbert, C. D. (1999). Attention modulates contextual influences in the primary visual cortex of alert monkeys. *Neuron*, *22*, 593–604.

James, W. (1890). *The principles of psychology*, (Vol. 1). Holt and Company.

Jiang, Y., Costello, P., Fang, F., Huang, M., & He, S. (2006). A gender- and sexual orientation-dependent spatial attentional effect of invisible images. *Proceedings of the National Academy of Sciences USA*, *103*, 17048–17052.

Kapadia, M. K., Westheimer, G., & Gilbert, C. D. (1999). Dynamics of spatial summation in primary visual cortex of alert monkeys. *Proceedings of the National Academy of Sciences USA*, *96*, 12073–12078.

Kashiwase, Y., Matsumiya, K., Kuriki, I., & Shioiri, S. (2012). Time courses of attentional modulation in neural amplification and synchronization measured with steady-state visual-evoked potentials. *Journal of Cognitive Neuroscience*, *24*, 1779–1793.

Kastner, S., & Ungerleider, L. G. (2001). The neural basis of biased competition in human visual cortex. *Neuropsychologia*, *39*, 1263–1276.

Kim, Y. J., Grabowecky, M., Paller, K. A., Muthu, K., & Suzuki, S. (2007). Attention induces synchronization-based response gain in steady-state visual evoked potentials. *Nature Neuroscience*, *10*, 117–125.

Kim, Y. -J., Grabowecky, M., Paller, K. A., & Suzuki, S. (2011). Differential roles of frequency-following and frequency-doubling visual responses revealed by evoked neural harmonics. *Journal of Cognitive Neuroscience*, *23*, 1875–1886.

Kowler, E. (2011). Eye movements: the past 25 years. *Vision Research*, *51*, 1457–1483.

Ling, S., & Carrasco, M. (2006). Sustained and transient covert attention enhance the signal via different contrast response functions. *Vision Research, 46,* 1210–1220.

Liu, T., Abrams, J., & Carrasco, M. (2009). Voluntary attention enhances contrast appearance. *Psychological Science, 20,* 354–362.

Luck, S. J., Chelazzi, L., Hillyard, S. A., & Desimone, R. (1997). Neural mechanisms of spatial selective attention in areas V1, V2, and V4 of macaque visual cortex. *Journal of Neurophysiology, 77,* 24–42.

Mack, A., & Rock, I. (1998). *Inattentional blindness.* MIT Press.

McAdams, C. J., & Maunsell, J. H. R. (1999a). Effects of attention on orientation-tuning functions of single neurons in macaque cortical area V4. *Journal of Neuroscience, 19,* 431–441.

McAdams, C. J., & Maunsell, J. H. R. (1999b). Effects of attention on the reliability of individual neurons in monkey visual cortex. *Neuron, 23,* 765–773.

Miller, E. K., Gochin, P. M., & Gross, C. G. (1993). Suppression of visual responses of neurons in inferior temporal cortex of the awake macaque by addition of a second stimulus. *Brain Research, 616,* 25–29.

Mishkin, M., Ungerleider, L. G., & Macko, K. A. (1983). Object vision and spatial vision: two central pathways. *Trends in Neuroscience, 6,* 414–417.

Mitchell, J. F., Sundberg, K. A., & Reynolds, J. A. (2007). Different attention-dependent response modulation across cell classes in macaque visual area V4. *Neuron, 55,* 131–141.

Mitchell, J. F., Sundberg, K. A., & Reynolds, J. A. (2009). Spatial attention decorrelates intrinsic activity fluctuations in macaque area V4. *Neuron, 63,* 879–888.

Moore, T., & Armstrong, K. M. (2003). Selective gating of visual signals by microstimulation of frontal cortex. *Nature, 421,* 370–373.

Moore, T., & Fallah, M. (2004). Microstimulation of the frontal eye field and its effects on covert spatial attention. *Journal of Neurophysiology, 91,* 152–162.

Moran, J., & Desimone, R. (1985). Selective attention gates visual processing in the extrastriate cortex. *Science, 229,* 782–784.

Morgan, S. T., Hansen, J. C., & Hillyard, S. A. (1996). Selective attention to stimulus location modulates the steady-state visual evoked potential. *Proceedings of the National Academy of Sciences USA, 93,* 4770–4774.

Motter, B. C. (1993). Focal attention produces spatially selective processing in visual cortical areas V1, V2, and V4 in the presence of competing stimuli. *Journal of Neurophysiology, 70,* 909–919.

Mountcastle, V. B., Motter, B. C., Steinmentz, M. A., & Sestokas, A. K. (1987). Common and differential effects of attentive fixation on the excitability of parietal and prestriate (V4) cortical visual neurons in the macaque monkey. *Journal of Neuroscience, 7,* 2239–2255.

Müller, M. M., Malinowski, P., Gruber, T., & Hillyard, S. A. (2003). Sustained division of the attentional spotlight. *Nature, 424,* 309–312.

Müller, M. M., Picton, T. W., Valdes-Sosa, P., Riera, J., Teder-Sälejärvi, W. A., & Hillyard, S. A. (1998). Effects of spatial selective attention on the steady-state visual evoked potential in the 20–28 Hz range. *Cognitive Brain Research, 6,* 249–261.

Naccache, L., Blandin, E., & Dehaene, S. (2002). Unconscious masked priming depends on temporal attention. *Psychological Science, 13,* 416–424.

Nakayama, K., & Mackeben, M. (1989). Sustained and transient components of focal visual attention. *Vision Research, 29,* 1631–1647.

Ni, A. M., Ray, S., & Maunsell, J. H. R. (2012). Tuned normalization explains the size of attention modulations. *Neuron, 73,* 803–813.

Orban, G. A. (2008). Higher order visual processing in macaque extrastriate cortex. *Physiological Reviews, 88,* 59–89.

Pastukhov, A., Fischer, L., & Braun, J. (2009). Visual attention is a single, integrated resource. *Vision Research, 49,* 1166–1173.

Pestilli, F., & Carrasco, M. (2005). Attention enhances contrast sensitivity at cued and impairs it at uncued locations. *Vision Research, 45,* 1867–1875.

Pooresmaeili, A., Poort, J., Thiele, A., & Roelfsema, P. R. (2010). Separable codes for attention and luminance contrast in the primary visual cortex. *Journal of Neuroscience, 20,* 12701–12711.

Posner, M. I. (1980). Orienting of attention. *Quarterly Journal of Experimental Psychology, 2,* 3–25.

Posner, M. I., & Cohen, Y. (1984). Components of visual orienting. In H. Bouma & D. G. Bouwhuis (Eds.), *Attention and performance X: control of language processes* (pp. 531–556). Hillsdale, NJ: Erlbanm.

Posner, M. I., Snyder, C. R. R., & Davidson, B. J. (1980). Attention and detection of signals. *Journal of Experimental Psychology: General, 109,* 160–174.

Reynolds, J. H., & Chelazzi, L. (2004). Attentional modulation of visual processing. *Annual Review of Neuroscience, 27,* 611–647.

Reynolds, J. H., Chelazzi, L., & Desimone, R. (1999). Competitive mechanisms subserve attention in macaque areas V2 and V4. *Journal of Neuroscience, 19,* 1736–1753.

Reynolds, J. H., & Desimone, R. (2003). Interacting roles of attention and visual salience in V4. *Neuron, 37,* 853–863.

Reynolds, J. H., & Heeger, D. J. (2009). The normalization model of attention. *Neuron, 61,* 168–185.

Reynolds, J. H., Pasternak, T., & Desimone, R. (2000). Attention increases sensitivity of V4 neurons. *Neuron, 26,* 703–714.

Rolls, E. T., & Tovee, M. J. (1995). The responses of single neurons in the temporal visual cortical areas of the macaque when more than one stimulus is present in the receptive field. *Experimental Brain Research, 103,* 409–420.

Salinas, E., & Sejnowski, T. J. (2000). Impact of correlated synaptic input on output firing rate and variability in simple neuronal models. *Journal of Neuroscience, 20,* 6193–6209.

Sato, T. (1989). Interactions of visual stimuli in the receptive fields of inferior temporal neurons in awake macaques. *Experimental Brain Research, 77,* 23–30.

Sceniak, M. P., Ringach, D. L., Hawken, M. J., & Shapley, R. (1999). Contrast's effect on spatial summation by macaque V1 neurons. *Nature Neuroscience, 2,* 733–739.

Sperling, G., & Melchner, M. J. (1978). The attention operating characteristic: examples from visual search. *Science, 202,* 315–318.

Spitzer, H., Desimone, R., & Moran, J. (1988). Increased attention enhances both behavioral and neural performance. *Science, 240,* 338–340.

Spitzer, H., & Richmond, B. J. (1991). Task difficulty: Ignoring, attending to, and discriminating a visual stimulus yield progressively more activity in inferior temporal neurons. *Experimental Brain Research, 83,* 340–348.

Sumner, P., Tsai, P. C., Yu, K., & Nachev, P. (2006). Attentional modulation of sensorimotor processes in the absence of perceptual awareness. *Proceedings of the National Academy of Sciences USA, 103,* 10520–10525.

Sundberg, K. A., Mitchell, J. F., & Reynolds, J. H. (2009). Spatial attention modulates center-surround interactions in macaque visual area V4. *Neuron, 61,* 952–963.

Suzuki, S. (2001). Attention-dependent brief adaptation to contour orientation: a high-level aftereffect for convexity? *Vision Research, 41,* 3883–3902.

Suzuki, S. (2003). Attentional selection of overlapped shapes: a study using brief aftereffects. *Vision Research, 43,* 549–561.

Suzuki, S. (2005). High-level pattern coding revealed by brief shape aftereffects. In C. Clifford & G. Rhodes (Eds.), *Fitting the mind to the world: Adaptation and aftereffects in high-level vision. Advances in visual cognition series.* (Vol. 2). Oxford University Press.

Suzuki, S., & Cavanagh, P. (1997). Focused attention distorts visual space: an attentional repulsion effect. *Journal of Experimental Psychology: Human Perception and Performance, 23,* 443–463.

Tallon-Baudry, C., Bertrand, O., Delpuech, C., & Pernier, J. (1996). Stimulus specificity of phase-locked and non-phase-locked 40 Hz visual responses in human. *Journal of Neuroscience, 16,* 4240–4249.

Thiele, A., Pooresmaeili, A., Delicato, L. S., Herrero, J. L., & Roelfsema, P. R. (2009). Additive effects of attention and stimulus contrast in primary visual cortex. *Cerebral Cortex, 19,* 2970–2981.

Tiesinga, P., Fellous, J. -M., & Sejnowski, T. J. (2008). Regulation of spike timing in visual cortical circuits. *Nature Reviews Neuroscience, 9,* 97–109.

Tong, F., Meng, M., & Blake, R. (2006). Neural basis of binocular rivalry. *Trends in Cognitive Sciences, 10,* 502–511.

Treue, S. (2004). Perceptual enhancement of contrast by attention. *Trends in Cognitive Science, 8,* 435–437.

Tsuchiya, N., & Koch, C. (2005). Continuous flash suppression reduces negative afterimages. *Nature Neuroscience, 8,* 1096–1101.

Tsuchiya, N., Koch, C., Gilroy, L. A., & Blake, R. (2006). Depth of interocular suppression associated with continuous flash suppression, flash suppression, and binocular rivalry. *Journal of Vision, 6,* 1068–1078.

Wilke, M., Logothetis, N. K., & Leopold, D. A. (2006). Local field potential reflects perceptual suppression in monkey visual cortex. *Proceedings of the National Academy of Sciences USA, 103,* 17507–17512.

Williford, T., & Maunsell, J. H. R. (2006). Effects of spatial attention on contrast response functions in macaque area V4. *Journal of Neurophysiology, 96,* 40–54.

Womelsdorf, T., & Fries, P. (2007). The role of neuronal synchronization in selective attention. *Current Opinion in Neurobiology, 17,* 154–160.

Womelsdorf, T., Schoffelen, J. -M., Oostenveld, R., Singer, W., Desimone, R., Engel, A. K., et al. (2007). Modulation of neuronal interactions through neuronal synchronization. *Science, 316,* 1609–1612.

Wyart, V., & Tallon-Baudry, C. (2008). Neural dissociation between visual awareness and spatial attention. *Journal of Neuroscience, 28,* 2667–2679.

Yantis, S. (1996). Attentional capture in vision. In A. Kramer, M. Coles & G. Logan (Eds.), *Converging operations in the study of selective visual attention* (pp. 45–76). Washington, DC: American Psychological Association.

Yantis, S., & Johnson, D. N. (1990). Mechanisms of attentional priority. *Journal of Experimental Psychology: Human Perception and Performance, 16,* 812–825.

Yeshurun, Y., & Carrasco, M. (1998). Attention improves or impairs visual performance by enhancing spatial resolution. *Nature, 396*(5), 72–75.

Yeshurun, Y., Montagna, B., & Carrasco, M. (2008). On the flexibility of sustained attention and its effects on a texture segmentation task. *Vision Research, 48,* 80–95.

Zoccolan, D., Cox, D. D., & DiCarlo, J. J. (2005). Multiple object response normalization in monkey inferotemporal cortex. *Journal of Neuroscience, 25,* 8150–8164.

Sequential Effects in the Central Cue Posner Paradigm: On-line Bayesian Learning

Antonio Arjona, Carlos M. Gómez

Human Psychobiology Lab, Experimental Psychology Department, University of Seville, Seville, Spain

INTRODUCTION

Attention works through a process of filtering environmental stimuli, assessing which are most relevant, and giving them priority for deeper processing. Currently, there is a tendency to study this phenomenon by appealing to mathematical and probability theory (Bruce & Tsotsos, 2009; Feldman & Friston, 2010; Reynolds & Heeger, 2009). In continuing this line of research, this study aims to shed light on the mechanisms underlying attention allocation induced by spatial cues, and whether the intensity of attention allocation follows a dynamic change as a consequence of previous trial outcome. This dynamic adjustment would be continually influencing decisions in situations of uncertainty.

The attentional mechanisms are continuously providing an assessment of the environment. In other words, there is a continuous estimation of the conditional probabilities of the occurrence of events, based on current perceptions, and prior information the subject has about probabilistic relationships between events (Feldman & Friston, 2010). Thus, the attentional system would try to direct processing resources to the relevant events or stimuli, while trying to predict the occurrence of such events based on our previous experiences, in more formal terms, priors. The "Bayesian brain model" proposed by Friston (2009) would fit this idea of changing the priors probability as a function of the inputs that the agent is receiving from the environment, with the prediction error as the driving force for adaptive changes in synaptic weights. The dynamic change in the synaptic weights would be due to the effects of neuromodulators, based on the prediction error signal (Feldman & Friston, 2010; Friston, 2009; Gómez & Flores, 2011).

In an attempt to clarify and organize the great diversity of theoretical perspectives on the phenomenon of attention, Posner et al. proposed an integrative theory (Posner & Dehaene, 1994; Posner & Petersen, 1990; Posner & Rothbart, 1991) largely based on the so-called Central Cue Posner's Paradigm (CCPP). This sort of paradigm makes it possible to follow on-line the deployment of attention and its effects on the processing of target stimuli (Eimer, 1993; Flores, Digiacomo, Meneres, Trigo, & Gómez, 2009; Gómez et al., 2004; Hopfinger & Mangun, 2000; Mangun & Hillyard, 1991) and the assessment of the validity or invalidity status of a given trial (Gómez, Flores, Digiacomo, Ledesma, & González-Rosa, 2008). This sort of paradigm (Figure 4.1) allows highly reliable testing of the effects caused by the congruence or incongruence between the expected stimulus and the stimulus that actually appears, and the consequences of the outcome value of the actual trial on the processing

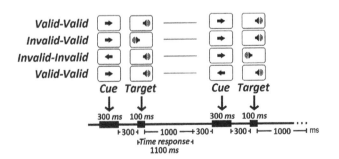

FIGURE 4.1 **Experimental paradigm.** This figure presents the one-trial and two-trial structures for the different types of dyads in the experiment. The temporal sequence of stimulus presentation appears in the lower part of the figure. The central arrow (Cue) was presented in the center of the screen, and the auditory stimulus (Target) was presented monoaurally. The behavioral results in dyads were obtained from the signals in the second trial.

of the next trial (Arjona & Gómez, 2011; Gómez, Flores, Digiacomo, & Vázquez-Marrufo, 2009; Jongen & Smulders, 2007).

Validity and invalidity can be observed in CCPP by an increase in Reaction Times (RTs), and errors in invalid trials with respect to valid trials (Posner, 1980; Posner & Cohen, 1984; Posner, Cohen, & Rafal, 1982; Posner, Nissen, & Ogden, 1978). In the same sense, different studies show that stimuli at attended locations are detected with higher speed and accuracy compared to stimuli presented outside the attentional focus (Jonides, 1981; Miller & Findlay, 1987; Miller & Rabbit, 1989). Furthermore, it has been observed that this effect may be due to the predictive activation of the related sensory area (Flores et al., 2009; Gómez et al., 2004; Hopfinger & Mangun, 2000) and the preparation for issuing a specific motor response (Gómez et al., 2004), as indexed by the contingent negative variation (CNV).

The CNV is characterized as a long-lasting negativity associated with preparation. Therefore the CNV takes place within the period between the warning or spatial directional cue (S1), in the case of CCPP, and the target stimulus (S2). The CNV reflects the expectation created by S1 about the appearance of S2 (Rockstroh, Elbert, Birbaumer, & Lutzenberger, 1982, p. 274; Walter, Cooper, Aldridge, & McCallum, 1964). Furthermore, it is a signal with at least two distinguishable periods: the early period of the signal would be more related to the brain response generated by orientation to S1, and the late phase reflects the preparation for motor response (Gaillard, 1977; Loveless & Sanford, 1974; Rohrbaugh & Gaillard, 1983; Rohrbaugh, Syndulko, & Lindsley, 1976). More recently the late phase of the CNV has also been associated with the preparation of the sensory neural areas prospectively needed for processing expected targets (Brunia & Van Boxtel, 2001; Flores et al., 2009; Gómez et al., 2004).

When spatial cues validly indicate the position of the target, the subject redirects his/her attentional resources to the locations indicated by the cue, and early sensory processing is increased at attended locations with respect to unattended locations, as indexed by P1 and N1 components, in both auditory and visual stimulation (Coull, 1998). A late assessment of the validity or invalidity of the cue occurs at the P3 component level, at which the invalid cue produces an increase in the amplitude of the P3a and P3b components (Eimer, 1993; Gómez et al., 2008; Mangun & Hillyard, 1991). The increase in the P3a to targets in invalid conditions would be related to attentional reorientation, and the increase in P3b to targets in invalid conditions would be related to the updating of the conditional probabilities of the cue–target relationship: p (S2/S1), probability that given a certain cue S1, a target S2 would appear (Digiacomo,

Marco-Pallarés, Flores, & Gómez, 2008; Gómez & Flores, 2011; Gómez et al., 2008; Mangun & Hillyard, 1991). Therefore, the P3 component in CCPP would be related to the cognitive assessment performed by the subject with respect to the validity/invalidity of the current trial (Eimer, 1993; Gómez et al., 2008; Mangun & Hillyard, 1991).

The effects of the assessment of the validity/invalidity of a trial are transferred behaviorally to the next trial in the so-called intertrial validity–invalidity effect: this is a benefit in RTs of valid trials preceded by valid trials (VV) compared to valid trials preceded by invalid trials (IV). On the other hand, there is also a benefit in RTs of invalid trials preceded by invalid trials (II) compared to invalid trials preceded by valid trials (VI). The RTs robustly follow the pattern of VV < IV < II < VI (Arjona & Gómez, 2011; Gómez et al., 2008; Jongen & Smulders, 2007). Furthermore, the anticipation errors follow an inverse pattern to the one previously indicated. The behavioral sequential results in the CCPP suggest that the brain is conducting an ongoing process of updating its neural activity, based on the prediction error computed, which ultimately would change the attentional allocation to the next cue, producing the sequential RTs and anticipations pattern described. An attempt was made to observe whether the CNV following valid or invalid targets indexes these attentional changes; however, a negative result was obtained (Gómez et al., 2008), but very few trials were averaged per subject, producing a low signal to noise ratio. The present experiment tries to overcome this problem by increasing the number of trials and recorded subjects.

In the present study, we will focus on the electrophysiological changes of both (1) the effects caused by the validity or invalidity of the signal in the current trial and (2) the so-called sequential effects or intertrial validity–invalidity effects (Arjona & Gómez, 2011; Gómez et al., 2009; Jongen & Smulders, 2007). This type of effect has been addressed recently, referring to the possible influences that correct or incorrect predictions made in a trial produce on the subsequent trial, in terms of both behavioral and neural level signals. The CNV induced by the first trial cue, the event-related potentials (ERPs) (N1, P2, P3a and P3b) to the targets in the first trial, and the CNV induced by the second trial in the sequence will be analyzed. In the sequential analysis, it is critical to average trials preceded by valid (V-X) or invalid (I-X) trials separately. The ERPs analysis makes it possible to assess (1) the neural preparation induced by the cue (CNV), (2) the process of attentional modulation of perception (N1and P2), (3) the assessment of the validity and invalidity of the present trial (P3a and P3b), and (4) the influence of the evaluation on the processing of the next trial (CNV).

METHODS

Participants

Thirty-four subjects participated in the experiment, but only 29 subjects (16 female and 13 male) between 19 and 35 years of age (mean: 24 years old and SD: 2'87) were fully analyzed (see below). The experiments were conducted with the informed and written consent of each subject, following the rules of the Helsinki Convention. The Ethics Committee of the University of Seville approved the study.

Stimuli and Behavioral Paradigm

The stimulus presentation and response recording were computer-controlled (E-Prime 2.0). Participants were seated 60 cm from a computer screen. The subjects participated in a modified version of the CCPP in which the central cues were arrows appearing in the center of the screen, followed by monoaural auditory stimulation (Figure 4.1). The arrow stimulus was considered the spatial orientation cue, and the monoaural auditory stimulus was the imperative one. The auditory stimuli were delivered to the subject's ears through headphones. Participants were asked to fixate their eyes on a white cross in the center of the screen, and they were instructed to pay attention to the ear indicated by a central arrow, then press the right button as quickly as possible if the auditory stimulus appeared in the right ear, or the left button if the auditory stimulus appeared in the left ear. The response device was the Cedrus model RB-530. The event sequence within a trial was as follows: the central arrow pointer was on for 300 ms, followed by an expectancy period in which a central fixation white cross appeared for 360 ms. Therefore, the total S1–S2 period was 660 ms. The auditory stimulus (1000 Hz) lasted for 100 ms and was randomly presented to the left and right ear with equal probability (0.5). The stimulus had an intensity of 89 db. The window for the response was 1000 ms, followed by a 300 ms period, producing a total intertrial interval of 1300 ms (Figure 4.1).

Each subject was presented with a total of 500 trials divided into five blocks. The central warning stimulus had directional information: in half of the trials it pointed to the right, and in the other half to the left. In 80% of the trials the arrow gave valid information about the target ear (V: valid trials), and in 20% of the trials the arrow pointed to the ear opposite to where the auditory stimulus would appear (I: invalid trials). The cued location (left or right ear) and the trial validity or invalidity were randomly selected. Thus, the experiment presented four types of trials: left valid (200 trials), right valid (200 trials), left invalid (50 trials) and right invalid (50 trials). The subjects had to respond to the monaural auditory stimulus with the index finger of the compatible hand. They were informed that the visual cue had an informative value, indicating with high probability the location of the auditory stimulus. RTs and proportion of correct and incorrect responses (responses to the side opposite the stimulated ear), anticipations (responses of targets faster than 180 ms after the auditory target) and omission responses were computed. The percentage of total errors was computed as the sum of all types of errors. There were 10 training trials.

In the present report, we will focus on the behavioral effects of valid and invalid trials by themselves and when these were preceded by validly or invalidly cued trials. Therefore, apart from the valid and invalid trials, four types of pairs of trials were obtained: Valid trials preceded by Valid trials (VV), Valid trials preceded by Invalid trials (IV), Invalid trials preceded by Invalid trials (II) and Invalid trials preceded by Valid trials (VI). Left and right cue and target presentations were not analyzed because the focus of interest was the validity/ invalidity and the intertrial effects.

EEG Recording, Processing and Analysis

The Electroencephalography (EEG) was recorded from 64 scalp sites in an extended version of the International 10–20 System, using tin electrodes mounted in an electrode cap (electrocap). All the electrodes were connected to the mastoids. Ocular movements Electrooculography (EOG) were recorded from two electrodes at the outer canthus of each eye for horizontal movements, and one electrode under the left eye for vertical movements that was referenced to one electrode above the left eye. Impedance was maintained below 5 Ohms. Data were recorded in DC, and no filtering was applied to them. The amplification gain was 20 (ANT amplifiers). The data were acquired at a sampling rate of 256 Hz, using a commercial AD acquisition and analysis board (eemagine EEG).

EEG recordings were analyzed with the EEGlab (Delorme & Makeig, 2004) and Matlab 2008a (MathWorks Inc., MA, USA) software packages. To eliminate AC power line interference and blink artifacts in the EEG, an independent components analysis (Bell & Sejnowski, 1995; Makeig, Bell, Jung, & Sejnowski, 1996; Makeig, Jung, Ghahremani, Bell, & Sejnowski, 1997) was performed. Criteria for determining these artifactual components were their scalp map distribution, time course, and spectral power. Thus, the eye blink artifact component showed a frontal location, coincided with blinking in the recording of eye movements, and showed low frequency in the power spectrum. These components were discarded, and the EEG signal was reconstructed. The segmented epochs had a duration of 2200 ms. Five subjects out of the 34 recorded were excluded from the analysis, due to the high number of ocular blinks (Electromyography [EMG]), and trend derived contaminations in the EEG.

Artifact corrected recordings were averaged off-line using a rejection protocol based on voltage amplitude. All the epochs for which the EEG exceeded ±90 μV in any channel were automatically discarded for ERP analysis. Moreover, for sequential analysis, the first trial in each block (the experiment had five blocks) had to be rejected because there was no preceding trial. The baseline was the 200–0 ms interval before the cue stimuli. The algebraically-linked mastoids were computed off-line, and used as a reference for analytical purposes. ERPs were obtained for each subject by averaging the EEG, using the switching-on of the target as a trigger.

Two different types of ERPs were obtained: (1) ERPs to targets in valid and invalid trials, and (2) ERPs to the second trial depending on the outcome of the previous trial. V-X refers to the collapsing of the VV and VI conditions, and I-X refers to the collapsing of the IV and II conditions. The latter strategy made it possible to analyze the CNV, after a valid or invalid trial, in order to test the effects of the deployment of attention in a trial depending on the outcome of the previous trial. The same strategy was followed for the VV-X, IV-X, II-X and VI-X three-trial sequence. For all the ERPs obtained, the left and right target stimuli were collapsed, given that the present study is related to main cognitive effects of validity and invalidity, and the expected effects were obtained taking into account the left-right collapsed stimuli.

For the analysis of ERPs, the percentage of averaged trials (500 trials per subject) in the valid condition was 63.64%, and in the invalid condition it was 15.73%. The percentages of trials averaged in sequences of two trials (495 trials per subject) were 68.51% in V-X and 16.76% in I-X sequences. In three-trial sequences (490 trials per subject) the number of analyzed trials was: 52.74% in VV-X, 12.86% in VI-X, 12.86% in IV-X and 3.21% in II-X. The ERPs of the trials in the II-X condition were not analyzed, given the low number of trials obtained.

Statistical Analysis of RTs, Errors and ERPs

RTs and total errors for the VV, IV, II and VI conditions were analyzed by means of analysis of variance (ANOVA) with two factors: First trial (valid and invalid) and Second trial (valid and invalid). The RTs and the errors were computed in the second trial of the sequence. A statistically significant effect of the second trial would mean a simple validity/invalidity effect on the CCPP, while an interaction between the effects of the first and second trial would imply a sequential effect.

In valid and invalid trials, the CNV induced by the cue and the N1, P2, P3a and P3b were analyzed. Repeated-measures ANOVAs were performed on the voltage data in the 64 electrodes for the 29 subjects (for valid

and invalid trials). The ANOVA presented two conditions, trial type (valid and invalid) and the electrodes (64 electrodes). The mean voltage in selected time windows was analyzed independently for different components. The P values were calculated using the Greenhouse–Geisser correction. The very conservative Bonferroni correction for p-values was used to correct statistical significance values for multiple comparisons and represented as a p-map.

Additionally, the amplitude of the CNV after a valid or invalid trial was computed and marked as V-X and I-X, respectively. In the same manner, the CNV were obtained for VV-X, IV-X and VI-X. In both cases, ANOVAS were computed to test possible mean differences in the CNV. For the CNV sequential analysis, the frontal electrodes in which CNV reached the maximum amplitude were selected for analysis (FCz, FC1, FC2, Cz, C1 and C2).

RESULTS

Behavioral Results

The present behavioral results correspond to a reanalysis of 29 subjects from the Arjona and Gómez (2011) study, from which five subjects with a high number of EMGs and trend derived contaminations in the EEG were excluded from the analysis. A more in-depth behavioral analysis can be found in that report.

Reaction Times

A two-factor repeated-measures ANOVA was performed on the means of RTs for the different pairs of trials. The factors considered were *First Trial* (2 levels: Valid and Invalid) and *Second Trial* (2 levels: Valid and Invalid). ANOVAs showed that the *First Trial* factor (F (1, 28) = 4.26, $P < 0.048$), the *Second Trial* factor (F (1, 28) = 58.57, $P < 0.001$) and the effects of the interaction between these two factors (F (1, 28) = 28.50, $P < 0.001$) were statistically significant. The main factor effect of the second trial factor corresponded to the validity–invalidity effect and the interaction of the factor effects corresponded to the intertrial validity–invalidity effects. The RTs in the different sequences of trials appear in Figure 4.2. The fastest condition was VV, followed by IV, II and finally VI.

Errors

A two-factor repeated-measures ANOVA was performed on the percentage of total errors for the different pairs. The factors considered were *First Trial* (2 levels: Valid and Invalid) and *Second Trial* (2 levels: Valid and Invalid). The ANOVA showed that the *First Trial* factor was statistically significant (F (1, 28) = 26.63, $P < 0.001$).

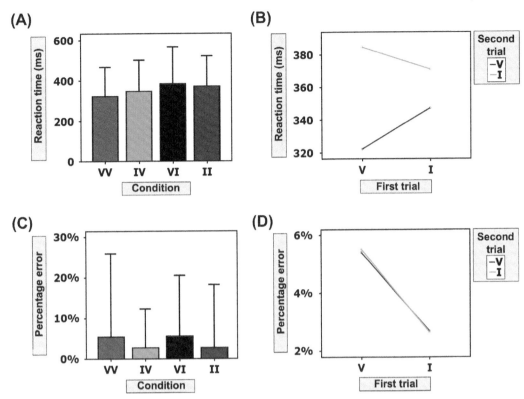

FIGURE 4.2 **RTs and errors in the two trial sequences**. (A) Mean and standard deviation of RTs in the valid-valid (VV), invalid-valid (IV), valid-invalid (VI) and invalid-invalid (II) conditions. Notice that the following RTs pattern was obtained (VV < IV < II < VI). (B) Influence on the RTs of the validity/invalidity in the first trial and the validity/invalidity in the second trial and the interaction effects. (C) Mean and standard deviation of percentage of errors in the valid-valid (VV), invalid-valid (IV), valid-invalid (VI) and invalid-invalid (II) conditions. Notice that the percentage of errors is greater when the previous trial condition was invalid (IV and II). (D) Influence in the percentage of errors of the validity/invalidity in the first trial and the validity/invalidity in the second trial.

The percentages of errors in the different sequences of trials appear in Figure 4.2. The higher number of errors was in the VI condition, followed by VV, IV and finally by the II condition.

Statistical Analysis of ERPs in Valid and Invalid Trials

A sequence of CNV, N1, P2, P3a and P3b components was obtained and statistically analyzed independently for each ERP component (Figure 4.3). The selected time window for each component appears in Figure 4.3. The statistical analysis of ERPs was computed for the one trial mode (valid or invalid) with a two-factor repeated measurement: *Valid/Invalid*, and *Electrodes* (64 electrodes).

Contingent Negative Variation (CNV)

The CNV presented a fronto-central distribution (Figures 4.3 and 4.4). No statistically significant differences were obtained when valid and invalid conditions were compared. The *t*-test comparisons yielded statistically significant differences in fronto-polar electrodes that will not be discussed in the present study, given

that they are probably due to remaining eye and/or blink artifacts.

Auditory Evoked Potential (N1)

The N1 component presented a fronto-central distribution (Figures 4.3 and 4.4) and higher amplitude in the Valid condition than in the Invalid condition. The difference wave presented a centro-parietal distribution. A two-factor repeated-measures ANOVA was performed on the voltage data with 64 electrodes. The mean voltage in the N1 time window was computed for each of the two conditions previously described. The factors considered were the *Type of trial* (2 levels: Valid and Invalid) and the *Electrodes* (64 electrodes). The ANOVA showed that the interaction between *Type of trial* and *Electrodes* was statistically significant (F (4.11, 115.23) = 13.827, $P < 0.001$). The Bonferroni comparisons showed a centro-parietal topography for the statistically significant differences.

P2 Component

The P2 component presented a fronto-central distribution (Figures 4.3 and 4.4) and higher amplitude in the Valid condition than in the Invalid condition. The

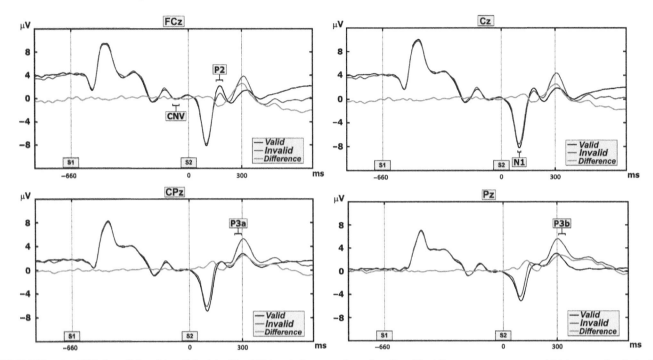

FIGURE 4.3   ERPs in valid and invalid trials. The CNV period was used as a baseline. The N1 component presented higher amplitude in the valid condition than in the invalid condition (Cz electrode). Notice that the P2 component at the FCz electrode presented higher amplitude in the valid condition than in the invalid condition. The P3a and P3b components showed higher amplitude in the invalid condition than in the valid condition (CPz and Pz electrodes respectively).

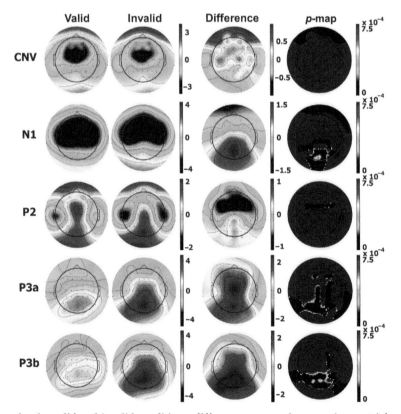

FIGURE 4.4   Voltage maps for the valid and invalid conditions, difference wave and *p*-maps in one-trial sequences. The CNV and N1 component were fronto-centrally distributed. N1 presented a higher amplitude in the valid than in the invalid condition. P2 presented a fronto-posterior topography and higher amplitude in the valid condition than in the invalid condition in frontal electrodes. The P3a and P3b components presented higher amplitude in the invalid condition than in the valid condition, with a central topography for the difference wave in P3a and a posterior topography for the difference wave in the P3b component.

difference wave presented a fronto-central distribution. A two-factor repeated-measures ANOVA was performed on the voltage data with 64 electrodes. The mean voltage in the P2 time window was computed for each of the two conditions previously described. The factors considered were the *Type of trial* (2 levels: Valid and Invalid) and the *Electrodes*. ANOVA showed that the interaction between *Type of trial* and *Electrodes* was statistically significant (F (3.84, 107.52) = 4.58, $p < 0.002$). The Bonferroni comparisons showed a fronto-central topography for the statistically significant differences.

Early Positivity (P3a)

The P3a component presented a central-posterior distribution (Figures 4.3 and 4.4) and higher amplitude in the Invalid condition than in the Valid condition. The difference wave presented a central distribution. A two-factor repeated-measures ANOVA was performed on the voltage data with 64 electrodes. The mean voltage in the P3a time window was computed for each of the two conditions previously described. The factors considered were the *Type of trial* (2 levels: Valid and Invalid) and the *Electrodes*. ANOVA showed that the interaction between *Type of trial* and *Electrodes* was statistically significant (F (4.23, 118.54) = 6.82, $p < 0.001$). Furthermore, the *Type of trial* factor was also statistically significant (F (1, 28) = 16.20, $p < 0.001$). The Bonferroni comparisons showed a central and posterior topography for the statistically significant differences.

The posterior distribution would already be part of the P3b topography.

Late Positivity (P3b)

The P3b component presented a posterior distribution (Figures 4.3 and 4.4) and higher amplitude in the Invalid condition than in the Valid condition. A two-factor repeated-measures ANOVA was performed on the voltage data with 64 electrodes. The mean voltage in the P3b time window was computed for each of the two conditions previously described. The factors considered were the *Type of trial* (2 levels: Valid and Invalid) and the *Electrodes*. ANOVA showed that the interaction between *Type of trial* and *Electrodes* was statistically significant (F (3.62, 97.95) = 8.68, $p < 0.001$). Furthermore, the *Type of trial* factor was also statistically significant (F (1, 27) = 15.26, $p < 0.001$). The Bonferroni comparisons showed a posterior topography for the statistically significant differences.

Contingent Negative Variation (CNV) in the Second Trial of Two-trial Sequences

The CNV showed higher amplitude in the trials preceded by a valid trial than in those preceded by an invalid trial (Figure 4.5). In both cases, and in the difference wave, the topographies presented a fronto-central distribution (Figure 4.6). A two-factor repeated-measures ANOVA was performed on the voltage data for six selected electrodes (FCz, FC1, FC2, Cz, C1 and C2).

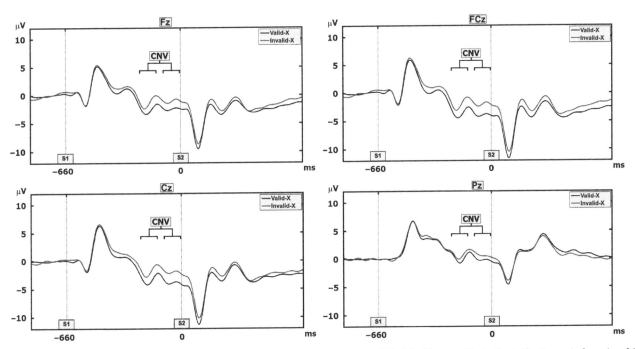

FIGURE 4.5 **The CNV induced by presenting the S1 stimuli after invalid and valid trials**. The graphics indicate the time windows in which early and late CNV were measured. Notice that the previous trial outcome has consistent effects on the amplitude of the CNV induced by the S1 in the current trial, producing a more negative CNV in trials preceded by valid trials (valid-X) than in trials preceded by invalid trials (invalid-X). This effect is greater in fronto-central electrodes (Fz, FCz and Cz), and more reduced in posterior electrodes (Pz).

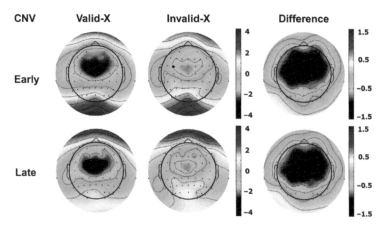

FIGURE 4.6 **Voltage maps of CNV in trials preceded by invalid (I-X) and valid (V-X) trials and the difference wave**. Notice the higher amplitude of the centrally distributed CNV component in trials preceded by valid trials with respect to trials preceded by invalid trials. The difference is consistent in the early and late CNV periods.

These electrodes were selected given the previous CNV topography obtained. The selection of these electrodes was due to the previous information about maximal CNV amplitudes obtained previously. The mean voltage in the CNV time windows (Early: −238/−138 ms and Late: −100/0 ms) was computed for each of the two conditions previously described. The factors considered were: *Validity of previous trial* (2 levels: VX and IX) and *Electrodes*. ANOVA showed statistically significant differences in the Early time window for *Validity of previous trial* ($F (1, 57) = 23.99, p < 0.001$). Statistically significant effects were also obtained in the Late time window for *Validity of previous trial* ($F (1, 57) = 31.28, p < 0.001$).

Contingent negative variation (CNV) in third trial of three-trial sequences

The amplitude of the CNV in the third trial was modulated by the types of previous trials. Figure 4.7 shows the higher amplitude of the CNV in the VV-X sequence compared to the IV-X sequence, and in the IV-X sequence compared to the VI-X sequence. The II-X condition was not included in the analysis because of the very small number of trials obtained for this condition (see the methods section).

A repeated-measures ANOVA was performed on the voltage data from selected electrodes (FCz, FC1, FC2, Cz, C1 and C2) in the third trial for three-trial sequences. The mean voltage in the early and late CNV (Early: −238/−138 ms and Late: −100/0 ms) was analyzed in selected time windows independently for different components under three conditions: Valid-Valid-X (VV-X), Valid-Invalid-X (VI-X) and Invalid-Valid-X (IV-X). The factors considered were: *Type of trial* (3 levels: VVX, VIX and IVX) and *Electrodes*.

ANOVA showed statistically significant differences of CNV amplitude in the early time window for the *Type of trial* factor ($F (1.78, 101.78) = 7.77, p < 0.001$). In order to test

which conditions were different, the different Types of trials were compared. The VV-X vs VI-X ($F (1, 57) = 19.09, p < 0.001$) and the VI-X vs IV-X ($F (1, 57) = 4.35, p < 0.04$) showed statistically significant differences, but the VV-X vs IV-X conditions did not ($F (1, 57) = 2.57, p < 0.114$). For the Late time window, the ANOVA showed statistically significant differences in CNV amplitude for the *Type of trial* factor ($F (1.83, 104.71) = 12.96, p < 0.001$). In order to test which conditions were different, the different Types of trials were compared. The differences between VV-X vs IV-X ($F (1, 57) = 4.75, p < 0.033$), VV-X vs VI-X ($F (1, 57) = 34.56, p < 0.001$) and VI-X vs IV-X ($F (1, 57) = 6.67, p < 0.012$) were statistically significant.

DISCUSSION

The present study tries to assess the effects of predictive attention in a trial with a validly or invalidly cued target, and more importantly, how the assessment of this validity or invalidity is processed in the brain, and the information is transferred to next trial processing. The ERP analysis in the first trial indicated that a CNV was induced after the cue. This change in brain preparation induced an increase in the N1 and P2 components in validly cued targets compared to invalidly cued targets, indicating the attentional facilitation of attended stimuli. However, the P3a and P3b components showed increases in amplitude in the invalid condition compared to the valid condition, indicating an attentional reorientation and assessment of the trial validity, respectively. The trial validity was also observed through a decrease in RTs in the valid condition with respect to the invalid condition. The information on the outcome of the current trial was transferred to the next trial, with the CNV of a trial following a valid trial (V-X) presenting a higher amplitude than the CNV following an

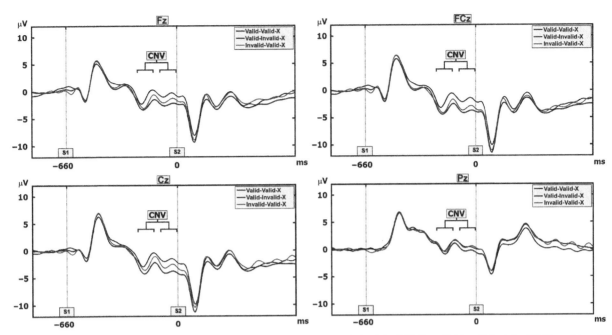

FIGURE 4.7 **The CNV induced by presenting the S1 stimuli after valid-valid trials (VV-X), valid-invalid trials (VI-X) and invalid-valid trials (IV-X).** The displays show the induced CNV in different trial sequences. Notice that the previous trial outcome has consistent effects on the amplitude of the CNV induced by the S1 in the current trial, producing a more negative CNV in trials preceded by two valid trials (VV-X) with respect to trials preceded by the invalid-valid sequence (IV-X), and with the IV-X being more negative than in trials preceded by the valid-invalid sequence (VI-X). This effect is greater in fronto-central electrodes (Fz, FCz, and Cz) and more reduced in posterior electrodes (Pz).

invalid trial (I-X), indicating a dynamic adjustment of attentional deployment as a function of previous trial outcome, which was also reflected as a RTs pattern of VV < IV < II < VI. The three-trial sequences were also explored, and they confirmed the dynamic pattern of attentional adjustment as a function of previous trial outcome. Thus, after two valid trials (VV-X) the CNV presented more amplitude than after an invalid-valid sequence (IV-X), which on its own was also more intense that the valid-invalid sequence (VI-X). All the previous results suggest a continuous updating of the conditional probabilities P (S2/S1), as the assessment of the local history of trial outcomes occurs, following rules which are similar to Bayesian inference.

The CNV is a type of slow wave that appears related to the expectancy and preparation for the arrival of an incoming stimulus (Eimer, 1993; Gómez et al., 2004; Gómez, Flores, & Ledesma, 2007; Gómez, Marco, & Grau, 2003). In our study a CNV develops in the S1–S2 period and is probably caused by the process of activation of task-related sensory areas by the subject before the imminent arrival of the target, but also by motor preparation for the response (Gómez et al., 2004; Tecce, 1972). In a quite similar experiment to the present study, but using Magnetoencephalography (MEG) recordings, Gómez et al. (2004) showed that during the contingent magnetic variation there was a task-specific preparation of the superior temporal gyrus (STG) and the motor cortex contralateral to the directional cue. In the present report,

which remains at a more abstract level, a similar activation pattern can be assumed during the S1–S2 period.

The set of mechanisms underlying the attentional modulation observed in the different studies conducted by the CCPP is an issue that has been thoroughly discussed in recent years, mainly in the visual modality (Eimer, 1993; Gómez et al., 2008; Mangun & Hillyard, 1991; Perchet & García-Larrea, 2000; Perchet, Revol, Fourneret, Mauguière, & Garcia-Larrea, 2001). In the present study, we analyzed intra and intertrial effects: (1) the influence of the validity and invalidity of the cue on target processing in the current trial (N1, P2, P3a and P3b components), and (2) the possible consequences of the previous target processing of the cue in the CNV, and behavioral responses on the subsequent trial.

In the present study, the increase obtained in the valid condition compared to the invalid condition in the N1 and P2 component amplitude can be interpreted as a consequence of this contralateral to the cue sensory cortex preparation. In fact, in the visual modality, the effects of a spatial cue on the attentional modulation of the visual sensory modulation have been extensively studied by analyzing the modulation of the ERPs to valid and invalid cues (Eimer, 1993; Mangun & Hillyard, 1991; Perchet & García-Larrea, 2000; Perchet, Revol, Fourneret, Mauguière, & Garcia-Larrea, 2001). The general result obtained was an increase in visual P1 and N1, and a decrease in P3a and P3b components in validly cued trials with respect to invalid ones. The P1 component is the earliest ERP component modulated by attention, and it is considered to reflect the cost of paying attention to unattended locations (Anllo-Vento, 1995; Coull, 1998; Luck, Heinze, Mangun, & Hillyard, 1990; Mangun & Hillyard, 1991; Mangun, Hillyard, & Luck, 1993; Talsma, Slagter, Nieuwenhuis, Hage, & Kok, 2005). The increase in the N1 component reflects not only the benefit of paying attention to attended locations, but also the starting point of discriminative processes, which are increased at the spatially attended locations. As previously mentioned, the activation of the Extrastriate Cortex Contralateral to the cue, occurring prior to the occurrence of S2, is probably the neural mechanism promoting increased processing at attended locations (Flores et al., 2009; Hopfinger & Mangun, 2000). Therefore, the neural set whose activity has been attentionally biased during the preparatory period could be able to increase the processing level of the attentionally cued stimuli, as indexed by the P1 and N1 components. For the visual (cue)-auditory (target) in CCPP paradigms, the effects of auditory target attentional modulation by visual cues have not been previously studied, although task-related preparation and validity/invalidity RTs results have been obtained during the preparatory period (Chen, Chen, Gao, & Yue, 2012; Gómez et al., 2004). Moreover, when subjects selectively attend to tones in one ear, while tones are presented in both ears, and tones in the unattended ear must be ignored (cocktail party effect), an increase in auditory P1 and N1 components to tones delivered in the attended ear are recorded, indicating an attentional modulation of the Supratemporal Plane (Woldorff et al., 1993; Woldorff & Hillyard, 1991). In addition, the P2 component also presented an increase in the attended ear with respect to the unattended ear. The results obtained in the present experiment of an increased N1 and P2 indicate that endogenous visual cueing is able to modulate the stream of auditory processing in a similar manner to the "cocktail party effect" previously described.

In the present experiment, the validity/invalidity effect on the P300 component turned out to be opposite to the effect on the P1 and N1 components. An increase in the P3a and P3b components was obtained in the invalid condition rather than the valid condition. These results have previously been obtained on visual cues and visual targets CCPP, for both P3a (Digiacomo et al., 2008; Gómez et al., 2008) and P3b components (Digiacomo et al., 2008; Eimer, 1993; Gómez et al., 2008; Mangun & Hillyard, 1991). The present results extend the results previously obtained in the visual modality to the crossmodal visual (cue)-auditory (target) modality, indicating the highly cognitive nature of P3 modulation in CCPP. The increase in the P3a to targets in invalid conditions would be related to attentional reorientation to invalidly predicted targets. The higher amplitude of P3b in invalid with respect to valid trials has been suggested to represent the assessment of the lack of adequacy between

sensory–motor preparation and sensory perception, on the one hand, and the actual action in response to the target stimulus, on the other (Gómez & Flores, 2011; Mangun & Hillyard, 1991). It has been suggested that the most important component of this assessment is the revision of the S1–S2 (cue–target) contingency value (For a review, see Gómez & Flores, 2011).

FMRI studies, by means of comparisons of the BOLD signal between the invalid and valid trials, suggest that important areas for detecting the incongruity between the prepared neural network and the actual target are in the right hemisphere and include the inferior frontal gyrus, the middle and STG, the posterior part of the superior temporal sulcus and the parahippocampal gyrus, and bilateral activation in the intraparietal sulcus (including the right supramarginal gyrus). Moreover, the left thalamus also showed higher activation in invalid targets than in valid targets (Vossel, Thiel, & Fink, 2006). The most ventral part of this distributed network, including the inferior frontal gyrus and the temporal-parietal junction (TPJ), has been proposed to be involved in reorienting the attention to unexpected targets (Corbetta, Patel, & Shulman, 2008). Recently and based on comparisons of the BOLD signal in invalid and valid trials vs neutral trials, a role of the left TPJ has been proposed for changing cue–target contingencies in valid trials, and of both TPJ in invalid trials (Doricchi, Macci, Silvetti, & Macaluso, 2010). The bilateral activation of TPJ in invalidly cued targets would be related to the increased P3b in invalid trials compared to valid trials (Digiacomo et al., 2008; Eimer, 1993; Gómez et al., 2008; Mangun & Hillyard, 1991). To what extent this distributed visuo-visual CCPP network would share neural resources with visuo-auditory types of experiments remains to be tested. The attentional reorientation observed in invalid trials is possibly related to the increased RTs in invalid trials compared to valid trials.

The transfer of information from current trial to next trial has already been demonstrated by behavioral analysis showing the RTs trend of VV < IV < II < VI (Gómez et al., 2008; Jongen & Smulders, 2007), and an anticipation of errors pattern opposite to the RTs trend (Arjona & Gómez, 2011). This pattern of results was also extended to the analysis of triadic sequences of trials (Arjona & Gómez, 2011), in which a similar influence of the local history of validity/invalidity trials affects the more global influence of validity/invalidity in a single trial. The obtained pattern of RTs would be related to the amount of attention deployed in trial $n + 1$ as a function of previous trial outcome (trial n). VV (and VVV) sequences would deploy more attention than IV (and IIV) trials because the previous trial would increase the local credibility of the cue–target contingency; in more formal terms, the conditional probability P (S2/S1) would increase. The lower RTs in the II condition with respect to VI condition would reflect the lower deployment of attention in the second trial if the previous trial was invalid than if previous trial was valid, paying less cost in terms of RTs for attentional deployment in the II condition than in the VI condition.

In this regard, there are several studies showing the contralateral to the cue activation of the indicated sensory cortex (Flores et al., 2009; Gómez et al., 2004; Hopfinger & Mangun, 2000; Mangun & Hillyard, 1991) and the activation of the motor and premotor cortex (Gómez, Vaquero, Vázquez-Marrufo, González-Rosa, & Cardoso, 2005) in the hemisphere opposite to the cue indicated target location, facilitating both the perception and production of the response in the valid trials. All these results fit well with the idea of Bayesian learning, subjects would continuously be making predictions about the place where the target will appear, allowing the generation of a prediction error signal which would modify the a priori probability between the central cue and the target position (Feldman & Friston, 2010; Friston, 2009; Gómez & Flores, 2011).

On the other hand, the so-called biased competition model (Desimone & Duncan, 1995) also supports these results. In this view, the central executive would be responsible for producing this sensory cortex activation in the hemisphere opposite to the side indicated by the key, so that it would take less time to perceive a stimulus that appeared on that side by biasing the activity level (oscillatory and/or tonic activity). In this sense, the dorsolateral fronto-parietal network would be the structure responsible for sending the inputs that activate these sensory cortices (Corbetta et al., 2008; Gómez et al., 2007), while the right inferior frontal gyrus would be one of the areas responsible for perceiving the novelty of the targets in the case of invalid trials (Corbetta et al., 2008; Vossel et al., 2006).

The obtained behavioral results (RTs and error analysis) suggest that in CCPP, the attentional deployment is dynamically changed as a function of previous trial outcome. Consequently, the CNV amplitude on a given trial should be modulated by the validity or invalidity of the previous trial. In fact, in the so-called intertrial validity–invalidity effect, we have observed a more negative CNV in trials preceded by valid trials compared to trials preceded by invalid trials (V-X vs I-X). These results confirm that the subject's expectations about the appearance of the target in the place indicated by the cue are influenced by the previous trial outcome. Valid trials would increase the belief that the next trial will be valid, increasing the expectation created by the cue. In contrast, invalid trials would diminish the credibility of the cue on the following test, reducing its ability to guide the subject's attentional resources. The topographical analysis confirms that there are no substantial differences with respect to

the place of occurrence of the CNV in different types of trial sequences (Figure 4.6). The results were extended to sequences of three trials in which the pattern of amplitude (more negative than) was VV-X > IV-X > VI-X, suggesting that the deployment of attentional resources is dynamically changed.

The CNV is a type of slow wave that appears related to the expectancy and preparation for the arrival of an incoming stimulus (Eimer, 1993; Gómez et al., 2004, 2007, 2003). In our study, the incoming stimulus would be S2. This wave is caused largely by the process of selective attention activated by the subject before the imminent arrival of the target, but also by motor preparation for the response (Tecce, 1972). In the CCPP, the central cue indicates the possible position of the upcoming target, so it generates a CNV, indicating attentional preparation through the fronto-parietal networks, as well as activation of sensory and motor cortices (Fan et al., 2007; Gómez et al., 2004, 2007; Hopfinger & Mangun, 2000). The present results on CNV suggest that subjects would perform a trial-by-trial update of the predictive value assigned to the cue. In this sense, Yu and Dayan (2005) discussed the ability of the CCPP to reflect how subjects are continually updating the probabilities assigned to the possible occurrence of the events around them through Bayesian learning (Feldman & Friston, 2010; Friston, 2009). After an invalid trial, subjects would pay less attention to the cue and be guided more by bottom-up than by top-down prior expectations. The CNV component seems to be a reflection of the activity of supramodal attentional effects based on the activation of fronto-parietal networks and task-specific preparatory activation of the required sensory–motor cortex required for the task (reviewed in Gómez & Flores, 2011). The role of fronto-parietal networks during the CNV would be to modulate the attentional deployment (Corbetta et al., 2008). These results again support the idea that the working dynamic of the human brain would be based on a system similar to Bayesian Statistics (Doya, Ishii, Pouget, & Rao, 2007; Knill & Pouget, 2004).

In summary, our study shows a pattern of evolution of ERPs across trials involving: (1) preparation for next target induced by the visual cue (CNV); (2) attentional modulation of target processing in current trial (N1 and P2 components); (3) attentional reorientation to unexpected targets (P3a); (4) updating of the working memory based on the current trial validity/invalidity status (Duncan-Johnson & Donchin, 1977); and (5) dynamic modulation of attention deployment to next trial as indexed by the CNV and RTs pattern. Based on the latter results, the so-called sequential effects occur, involving the processing of each trial based on the previous trial outcome by modulating the attentional deployment in a dynamic way.

References

Anllo-Vento, L. (1995). Shifting attention in visual space: the effects of peripheral cueing on brain cortical potentials. *International Journal of Neuroscience, 80*, 353–370.

Arjona, A., & Gómez, C. M. (2011). Trial-by-trial changes in *a priori* informational value of external cues and subjective expectancies in human auditory attention. *PLoS One, 6*(6), e21033.

Bell, A. J., & Sejnowski, T. J. (1995). An information-maximization approach to blind separation and blind deconvolution. *Neural Computation, 7*(6), 1129–1159.

Bruce, N. D. B., & Tsotsos, J. K. (2009). Saliency, attention, and visual search: an information theoretic approach. *Journal of Vision, 9*(3), 1–24.

Brunia, C. H., & Van Boxtel, G. J. (2001). Wait and see. *International Journal of Psychophysiology, 43*, 59–75.

Chen, X., Chen, Q., Gao, D., & Yue, Z. (2012). Interaction between endogenous and exogenous orienting in crossmodal attention. *Scandinavian Journal of Psychology.*

Corbetta, M., Patel, G., & Shulman, G. L. (2008). The reorienting system of the human brain: from environment to theory of mind. *Neuron, 58*(3), 306–324.

Coull, J. T. (1998). Neural correlates of attention and arousal: insights from electrophysiology, functional neuroimaging and psychopharmacology. *Progress in Neurobiology, 55*, 343–361.

Delorme, A., & Makeig, S. (2004). EEGLAB: an open source toolbox for analysis of single-trial EEG dynamics. *Journal of Neuroscience Methods, 134*, 9–21.

Desimone, R., & Duncan, J. (1995). Neural mechanisms of selective visual attention. *Annual Review of Neuroscience, 18*, 193–222.

Digiacomo, M. R., Marco-Pallarés, J., Flores, A. B., & Gómez, C. M. (2008). Wavelet analysis of the EEG during the neurocognitive evaluation of invalidly cued targets. *Brain Research, 1234*, 94–103.

Doricchi, F., Macci, E., Silvetti, M., & Macaluso, E. (2010). Neural correlates of the spatial and expectancy components of endogenous and stimulus-driven orienting of attention in the Posner task. *Cerebral Cortex*, July 2010 20, 1574–1585.

Doya, K., Ishii, S., Pouget, A., & Rao, R. P. N. (2007). *Bayesian brain: Probabilistic approaches to neural coding (Computational Neuroscience).*

Duncan-Johnson, C. C., & Donchin, E. (1977). On quantifying surprise: the variation in event-related potentials with subjective probability. *Psychophysiology, 14*, 456–457.

Eimer, M. (1993). Spatial cueing, sensory gating and selective response preparation: an ERP study on visuo-spatial orienting. *Electroencephalography and Clinical Neurophysiology, 88*, 408–420.

Fan, J., Kolster, R., Ghajar, J., Suh, M., Knight, R. T., Sarkar, R., et al. (2007). Response anticipation and response: an event-related potentials and functional magnetic resonance imaging study. *Journal of Neuroscience, 27*, 2272–2282.

Feldman, H., & Friston, K. J. (2010). Attention, uncertainty, and free-energy. *Frontiers in Human Neuroscience, 4*, 215.

Flores, A. B., Digiacomo, M. R., Meneres, S., Trigo, E., & Gómez, C. M. (2009). Development of preparatory activity indexed by the contingent negative variation in children. *Brain and Cognition, 71*, 129–140.

Friston, K. J. (2009). The free-energy principle: a rough guide to the brain? *Trends in Cognitive Sciences, 13*, 279–328.

Gaillard, A. W. K. (1977). The late CNV wave: preparation versus expectancy. *Psychophysiology, 14*, 563–568.

Gómez, C. M., Fernandez, A., Maestú, F., Amo, C., Gonzalez-Rosa, J. J., Vaquero, E., et al. (2004). Task-specific sensory and motor preparatory activation revealed by contingent magnetic variation. *Cognitive Brain Research, 21*, 59–68.

Gómez, C. M., & Flores, A. (2011). A neurophysiological evaluation of a cognitive cycle in humans. *Neuroscience and Biobehavioral Reviews, 35*(3), 452–461.

Gómez, C. M., Flores, A. B., Digiacomo, M. R., Ledesma, A., & González-Rosa, J. J. (2008). P3a and P3b components associated to the neurocognitive evaluation of invalidly cued targets. *Neuroscience Letters, 430*, 181–185.

Gómez, C. M., Flores, A. B., Digiacomo, M. R., & Vázquez-Marrufo, M. (2009). Sequential P3 effects in a Posner's spatial cueing paradigm: trial-by-trial learning of the predictive value of the cue. *Acta Neurobiologiae Experimentalis, 2009*(69), 155–167.

Gómez, C. M., Flores, A., & Ledesma, A. (2007). Fronto-parietal network activation during the contingent negative period. *Brain Research Bulletin, 73*, 40–47.

Gómez, C. M., Marco, J., & Grau, C. (2003). Preparatory visuo-motor cortical network of the contingent negative variation estimated by current density. *Neuroimage, 20*, 216–224.

Gómez, C. M., Vaquero, E., Vázquez-Marrufo, M., González-Rosa, J. J., & Cardoso, M. J. (2005). Alternate-response preparation in a visuo-motor serial task. *Journal of Motor Behavior, 37*(2). Health & Medical Complete p. 127.

Hopfinger, J., & Mangun, G. R. (2000). Shifting visual attention in space: an electrophysiological analysis using high spatial resolution mapping. *Clinical Neurophysiology, 111*, 1241–1257.

Jongen, E. M. M., & Smulders, F. T. Y. (2007). Sequence effects in a spatial cueing task: endogenous orienting is sensitive to orienting in the preceding trial. *Psychological Research, 71*, 516–523.

Jonides, J. (1981). Voluntary versus automatic control over the mind's eye's movement. In J. B. Long & A. D. Baddeley (Eds.), *Attention and performance IX* (pp. 187–203). Hillsdale, NJ: Erlbaum.

Knill, D. C., & Pouget, A. (2004). The Bayesian brain: The role of uncertainty in neural coding and computation. *Trends in Neuroscience, 27*(12), 712–719.

Loveless, N. E., & Sanford, A. J. (1974). Slow potentials correlates of preparatory set. *Biological Psychology, 1*, 303–314.

Luck, S. J., Heinze, H. J., Mangun, G. R., & Hillyard, S. A. (1990). Visual event-related potentials index focused attention within bilateral stimulus arrays. II. Functional dissociation of P1 and N1 components. *Electroencephalography and Clinical Neurophysiology, 75*, 528–542.

Makeig, S., Bell, A. J., Jung, T. P., & Sejnowski, T. J. (1996). Independent component analysis of electroencephalographic data. In D. Touretzky, M. Mozer & M. Hasselmo (Eds.), *Advances in neural information processing systems* (8, pp. 145–151). Cambridge, MA: MIT Press.

Makeig, S., Jung, T. P., Ghahremani, D., Bell, A. J., & Sejnowski, T. J. (1997). Blind separation of auditory event-related brain responses into independent components. *Proceedings of the National Academy of Sciences of the United States of America, 94*, 10979–10984.

Mangun, G. R., & Hillyard, S. A. (1991). Modulations of sensory-evoked brain potentials indicate changes in perceptual processing during visual-spatial priming. *Journal of Experimental Psychology: Human Perception and Performance, 17*, 1057–1074.

Mangun, G. R., Hillyard, S. A., & Luck, S. J. (1993). Electrocortical substrates of visual selective attention. In D. E. Meyer & S. Kornblum (Eds.), *Attention and performance XIV: Synergies in experimental psychology, artificial intelligence, and cognitive neuroscience* (pp. 219–243). Cambridge, MA: MIT Press.

Miller, H. J., & Findlay, J. M. (1987). Sensitivity and criterion effects in the spatial cueing of visual attention. *Perception and Psychophysics, 42*, 383–399.

Miller, H. J., & Rabbit, P. M. A. (1989). Reflexive and voluntary orienting of visual attention: time course of activation and resistance to interruption. *Journal of Experimental Psychology: Human Perception and Performance, 15*, 315–330.

Perchet, C., & García-Larrea, L. (2000). Visuo-spatial attention and motor reaction in children: an electrophysiological study of the "Posner" paradigm. *Psychophysiology, 37*, 231–241.

Perchet, C., Revol, O., Fourneret, P., Mauguière, F., & Garcia-Larrea, L. (2001). Attention shifts and anticipatory mechanisms in hyperactive children: an ERP study using the Posner paradigm. *Biological Psychiatry, 50*, 44–57.

Posner, M. I. (1980). Orienting of attention. *Quarterly Journal of Experimental Psychology, 32*, 3–25.

Posner, M. I., & Cohen, Y. (1984). Components of visual orienting. In H. Bouma & D. G. Bouwhuis (Eds.), *Attention and performance* (pp. 531–556). Hillsdale, NJ: Erlbaum.

Posner, M. I., Cohen, Y., & Rafal, R. D. (1982). Neural systems control of spatial orienting. *Philosophical Transactions of the Royal Society of London, B, 298*, 187–198.

Posner, M. I., & Dehaene, S. (1994). Attentional networks. *Trends in Neurosciences, 17*, 75–79.

Posner, M. I., Nissen, M. J., & Ogden, W. C. (1978). Attended and unattended processing modes: the role of set for spatial location. In J. H. I. Pick & E. Saltzman (Eds.), *Modes of perceiving and processing information* (pp. 137–157). Hillsdale, NJ: Erlbaum.

Posner, M. I., & Petersen, S. E. (1990). The attention system of the human brain. *Annual Review of Neuroscience, 13*, 25–42.

Posner, M. I., & Rothbart, M. K. (1991). Attentional mechanisms and conscious experience. In A. D. Milner & M. D. Rugg (Eds.), *The neuropsychology of consciousness* (pp. 91–112). London: Academic Press.

Reynolds, J. H., & Heeger, D. J. (2009). The normalization model of attention. *Neuron, 61*(2), 168–185.

Rockstroh, B., Elbert, T., Birbaumer, N., & Lutzenberger, W. (1982). *Slow brain potentials and behavior*. Baltimore-Munich: Urban & Schwarzenberg.

Rohrbaugh, J. W., & Gaillard, A. W. K. (1983). Sensory and motor aspects of the contingent negative variation. In A. W. K. Gaillard & W. Ritter (Eds.), *Tutorials in ERP research: Endogenous components* (pp. 269–310). Amsterdam: North-Holland.

Rohrbaugh, J. W., Syndulko, K., & Lindsley, D. B. (1976). Brain wave components of the contingent negative variation in humans. *Science, 191*, 1055–1057.

Talsma, D., Slagter, H. A., Nieuwenhuis, S., Hage, J., & Kok, A. (2005). The orienting of visuospatial attention: an event-related brain potential study. *Cognitive Brain Research, 25*, 117–129.

Tecce, J. J. (1972). Contingent negative variation (CNV) and psychological processes in man. *Psychological Bulletin, 77*, 73–108.

Vossel, S., Thiel, C. M., & Fink, G. R. (2006). Cue validity modulates the neural correlates of covert endogenous orienting of attention in parietal and frontal cortex. *Neuroimage, 32*, 1257–1264.

Walter, W. G., Cooper, R., Aldridge, W. J., & McCallum, W. C. (1964). Contingent negative variation: an electrophysiological sign of sensorimotor association and expectancy in the human brain. *Nature, 203*, 380–384.

Woldorff, M. G., Gallen, C. C., Hampson, S. A., Hillyard, S. A., Pantev, C., Sobel, D., et al. (1993). Modulation of early sensory processing in human auditory cortex during auditory selective attention. *Proceedings of the National Academy of Sciences of the United States of America, 90*, 8722–8726.

Woldorff, M., & Hillyard, S. A. (1991). Modulation of early auditory processing during selective listening to rapidly presented tones. *Electroencephalography and Clinical Neurophysiology, 79*, 170–191.

Yu, A. J., & Dayan, P. (2005). Uncertainty, neuromodulation, and attention. *Neuron, 46*(4), 681–692.

EEG–fMRI Combination for the Study of Visual Perception and Spatial Attention

Francesco Di Russo[1,2], *Sabrina Pitzalis*[1,2]

[1]Department of Human Movement, Social and Health Sciences, University of Rome "Foro Italico", Rome, Italy,
[2]Neuropsychological Unit, Santa Lucia Foundation IRCCS, Rome, Italy

INTRODUCTION

Electroencephalography (EEG) measures electrical brain activity on a millisecond precision and thus permits temporal dynamics of brain function to be analyzed. However, and especially for deeper cerebral structures, attempts to localize the neural sources of the surface electric field are compromised by the "inverse problem" (Friston et al., 2008; Grech et al., 2008; Plonsey, 1963): a given electromagnetic field recorded by scalp EEG can result from an infinite number of different intracranial sources. A priori assumptions can be introduced to limit the number or position of possible field generators. Source estimations are then possible but remain models that are based on strong and not easily verifiable assumptions (Phillips, Rugg, & Friston, 2002). Therefore, the topographical analysis of surface EEG is limited in terms of its localizing capabilities. Conversely, functional magnetic resonance imaging (fMRI) allows an anatomically detailed measurement of neuronal activity including that of deeper cerebral structures, but temporal resolution of fMRI is bound by the time constants of neurovascular coupling. Considering the great temporal resolution of EEG and the excellent spatial resolution of fMRI, the combination of these two techniques is well suited to provide spatiotemporal information superior to either method alone. Through this multimethodological integration, it is now possible to view human brain function in real time.

Although there are several ways to integrate electrophysiological with neuroimaging methods, the most commonly used are the unseeded and seeded models. The unseeded model is the simpler among the two and consists in projecting the coordinates of dipolar source modeled on EEG data alone on an anatomical cortical surface obtained from a template, or from groups of or individual MRI images acquired from the same subjects involved in the EEG experiment. The limit of this "quick and dirty" method is that the spatial resolution is only given by the EEG and therefore it is low because it is based on surface recording and affected by the "inverse problem". When an unseeded model is used, the anatomical MRI images help exclusively to improve the visualization of the EEG-only based localizations.

The seeded model is a more complex and sophisticated method that uses fMRI data to solve the inverse problem. With this method, the locations are fixed (seeded) on fMRI spots found in an fMRI experiment identical to the EEG experiment, with the source orientations optimized to the new locations (seeded model). In visual paradigms, the spatial resolution of the seeded model can be further increased by the combination of standard fMRI data with retinotopy data at the individual level (Pitzalis et al., 2006; Sereno et al., 1995; Tootell et al., 1997). The retinotopic mapping is a demanding and time-consuming tool, which, however, has the great advantage of being able to define the border of the main striate and extrastriate visual areas with a precision comparable to that achieved in invasive single-unit experiments on monkeys. The method can be further improved by the use of a specific functional localizer to define the motion-sensitive regions MT+ (Tootell et al., 1995) and V6 (Pitzalis et al., 2010). The combination of EEG–fMRI data obtained during the same stimulation with the retinotopic mapping enables us to localize the EEG data respective to each single visual area and to specific anatomical regions with a known functional profile, as already done by our group in the past (Di Russo, Martínez, Pitzalis, & Hillyard,

Sereno, 2002; Di Russo, Martínez, Hillyard, 2003; Di Russo et al., 2007, 2005, 2011; Pitzalis, Bozzacchi, et al., 2012; Pitzalis, Strappini, De Gasperis, Bultrini, & Di Russo, 2012). Figure 5.1 shows different results obtained comparing unseeded and *seeded* source models; the colored circles shown in the figure indicate the locations of the dipoles in the *unseeded* model, which for some areas are close to the fMRI spots (as for V1, MT+ and Fusiform region), while for others are quite distant (as for POs and hIPs).

EEG and fMRI might be simultaneously recorded or in separate sessions. The advantage of simultaneous recordings is to measure activity of interest that is not simply reproducible during separate sessions. This is true for studying epilepsy, sleep, resting-state activities, some high-level cognitive tasks or when trial-by-trial correlations are required. However, simultaneous EEG–fMRI recording is not always necessary for studying some passive sensory-evoked or attention-related responses. One has to base this choice on the reproducibility of the task (or stimulus) vs. the possible risk of dealing with largely contaminated EEG data if simultaneously recorded with fMRI. This is in light of the fact that regardless of the theoretical efficacy of artifact correction algorithms for post-processing simultaneously recorded EEG–fMRI data, the outcome of these algorithms is "artificial" and inevitably "worse" than the clear EEG data recorded in a shielded EEG room. So, an important advantage of EEG and fMRI recording in separate sessions is the possibility to record very clean and reliable data in both measures. Finally, simultaneous recording needs time-consuming subject preparation (subject might wait 1 or 2h before starting the experiment). Therefore, a further advantage of separate measures consists of reducing the subject preparation time, a relevant factor in a lab daily schedule.

In this chapter, we describe the advantages in spatial and temporal resolution that can be gained through combining EEG with fMRI methods in the study of visual perception and spatial attention. We focused on EEG–fMRI studies using visual-evoked potentials (VEPs) in passive tasks and event-related potentials (ERPs) in visuospatial attention tasks. We review studies aimed at identifying the sources of VEP and ERP components using focal stimuli located in the four visual quadrants. This stimuli location avoids the activation of widespread regions of retinotopic cortical areas, thereby enhancing the possibility of identifying the exact generator locations.

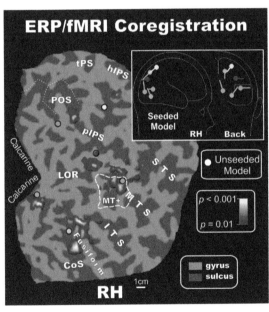

FIGURE 5.1 Combination of the ERP/fMRI attention effects in the right hemisphere for contralateral stimuli in the upper quadrant. Group-averaged contralateral fMRI activations superimposed on the flattened hemisphere (occipital lobe) of the Montreal Neurological Institute (MNI) template. Circles indicate the locations of the dipoles in the unseeded based on the EEG data alone. The pseudocolor scale in the right of the figure indicates the statistical significance of the fMRI activations. Major sulci (dark gray) are labeled as follows: Parieto-occipital sulcus (POS), transverse segment of the parietal sulcus (tPS), intraparietal sulcus (IPS), superior temporal sulcus (STS), middle temporal sulcus (MTS), inferior temporal sulcus (ITS), LOR, Fusiform gyrus (Fusiform), and calcarine fissure (Calcarine). The fundus of the POS is indicated by dashed lines. The dashed outline surrounding MT+ represents the group-averaged location of the motion-sensitive cortex based on separate localizer scans. Inset shows, as an example, the schematic representation of the source locations and orientations in the seeded dipole model. *Data from Di Russo et al., 2011.*

IDENTIFICATION OF THE NEURAL SOURCE OF VEP COMPONENTS

The VEPs are brain waves produced by visual stimuli that can be displayed with different modalities; the most studied one is the pattern-onset modality where visual patterns appear for a short time (from 50 to 400ms) and then disappear. This modality has the great advantage of producing large potentials, however, this kind of stimuli is uncommon in real life because objects usually do not disappear, but might move or vary in local luminance or contrast as when leaves are moved by the wind. A more ecological way to produce VEP is the pattern-reversal modality in which stimuli (e.g., gratings or checkerboard) are continuously present throughout recording, but their pattern continuously reverses in contrast. This modality produces smaller but incredibly systematic potentials in terms of reproducibility. Because of their higher stability in respect to the pattern-onset paradigm, pattern-reversal is often used as an index of neurological dysfunctions of the visual pathways (e.g., Halliday, 1993). Furthermore, to study the visual motion processing, motion-related VEP were extensively used in literature. Among all visual motion-related VEPs tested so far, motion-onset VEPs display the largest amplitudes and the lowest inter- and intrasubject variability (e.g., Kuba, 2006). Motion-onset VEPs are usually produced by moving dots or gratings.

All of these VEP paradigms are defined as transient if the stimulus cadence is slow (one to two stimuli per second) while they are named steady-state if the stimulus is presented at a rate of around 4 Hz or higher. When a repetitive flickering or visual pattern is presented at such a fast rate, a continuous sequence of oscillatory potential changes is elicited in the visual cortex. The steady-state VEP generally appears in scalp recordings as a near-sinusoidal waveform at the frequency of the driving stimulus or its harmonics (reviewed in Di Russo, Teder-Sälejärvi, & Hillyard, 2002).

In literature, the VEP components were labeled in a nonunique way, however, as proposed in several studies of our group, they can be labeled as follows: the C1 (also known as N75 or P85), the P1, the C2, the N1, and the P2. Except for the C1, the successive components are not necessarily generated by a single area. Depending on the stimulation types, they can be separated in subcomponents. A detailed description of their origin is reported below. The very early N70 component found for fast motion stimuli only, will be described in the next section.

The C1 Component

The neural generators of the early components of the VEP have been studied since the original observations of Jeffreys and Axford (1972a). Many studies have obtained evidence that the first major pattern-onset VEP component (C1), with an onset latency between 40 and 70 ms and peak latency between 60 and 100 ms, originates from primary visual cortex (V1, Brodmann's area 17, Calcarine fissure or striate cortex). Evidence that C1 is generated in the striate cortex comes from studies showing that the C1 has a parieto-occipital medial distribution and reverses in polarity for upper vs. lower visual field stimulation (e.g., Butler et al., 1987; Clark, Fan, & Hillyard, 1995; Di Russo, Ragazzoni, & Spagli, 1998; Jeffreys & Axford, 1972a, 1972b; Mangun, 1995). This reversal corresponds to the retinotopic organization of the striate cortex, in which the lower and upper visual hemifields are mapped in the upper and lower banks of the Calcarine fissure, respectively. According to this "cruciform model" (Jeffreys & Axford, 1972a), stimulation above and below the horizontal meridian of the visual field should activate neural populations with geometrically opposite orientations and, hence, elicit surface-recorded evoked potentials of opposite polarity. Such a pattern would not be observed for VEPs generated in other visual areas that lack the special retinotopic organization of the Calcarine cortex, although it cannot be excluded that some degree of polarity shift for upper versus lower field stimuli might be present for neural generators in V2 and V3 as well (Schroeder et al., 1995; Simpson et al., 1995).

The C1 is known to arise from the primary visual area V1. Its localization has been confirmed in many studies

from our (e.g., Di Russo et al., 2011) as well as other (e.g., Clark et al., 1995; Gómez Gonzalez, Clark, Fan, Luck, & Hillyard 1994; Liu, Zhang, Chen, & He, 2009; Zhang, Zhaoping, Zhou, & Fang, 2012) laboratories. Reviewing the extensive VEP literature on this component, it is evident that the C1 has been found in response to many visual stimulation paradigms, such as pattern-onset, pattern-reversal, and motion-onset (Di Russo et al., 2002a, 2005; Pitzalis, Bozzacchi, et al., 2012; Pitzalis, Strappini, et al., 2012). Therefore, the C1 seems to be a general phenomenon related to the activity of area V1, likely reflecting the cortical volley from the lateral geniculate nucleus. Moreover, even though the rapid stimulation rate used in the steady-state VEP does not allow component discrimination, the combined recording of these potentials with fMRI (and retinotopic mapping) allows one to find V1 activity in the early phase of the steady-state VEP second harmonic (Di Russo et al., 2007). The presence of early V1 activity for any visual stimulation confirms its fundamental role along the bottom-up pathway of visual processing.

The P1 Component

P1 is a label to indicate the positive deflection following the C1. The P1 has lateral occipital distribution, contralateral to the stimulated horizontal hemifield and does not change in polarity for the vertical hemifields. Depending on the stimulation used, this activity peaks between 90 and 140 ms. Using pattern-onset VEP, Di Russo et al. (2002) found two subcomponents at 105 and 140 ms (early and late P1) that were localized in areas V3A and V4, respectively. Later on, these data were confirmed by studies using simultaneous EEG–fMRI recording (e.g., Novitskiy et al., 2011). Using pattern-reversal VEP, Di Russo et al. (2005) found a peak at 95 localized in the motion-sensitive area MT+ (or MT complex that encompasses both middle temporal (MT) and medial superior temporal areas; Huk, Dougherty, & Heeger, 2002). Successively, Liu et al. (2009) confirmed the involvement of MT+ at this latency. The motion-sensitive region MT+ is probably activated by pattern-reversal stimuli because such reversal produces a clear motion perception that can be described in terms of motion onset and motion offset-related responses (e.g., Kubova, Kuba, Spekreijse, & Blakemore, 1995). Using motion-onset VEP, the P1 was also localized in MT+ with a peak latency of 120 ms (Pitzalis, Strappini, et al., 2012). Combining steady-state VEP and fMRI, MT+ activity was also found in an early signal phase, successive to that of V1 (Di Russo et al., 2007).

The C2 Component

This component was only seen for pattern-reversal stimuli (Di Russo et al., 2005, 2011) showing a medial occipito-parietal distribution very similar to that of the C1 and (differently from the P1) the C2 change in polarity for the vertical hemifields. This activity peaked at 130 ms and is positive for lower fields and negative for upper fields (the opposite of C1). The C2 was localized in V1 and interpreted as a reentrant feedback activity from extrastriate areas as MT+ (Di Russo et al., 2005, 2011; Liu et al., 2009).

The N1 Component

The N1 is the more complex VEP component because it is produced by multiple areas dependent on the stimulation modality. In pattern-onset VEP, there is both an early anterior N1, peaking at 155 ms and originating in parietal areas, and a later and more posterior activity peaking at 180 ms and originating in visual area V3A (Di Russo et al., 2002; Novitskiy et al., 2011). Pattern-reversal VEP produced three subcomponents at 150, 160, and 180 ms localized in the transverse-parietal sulcus (TPs), V4 and V3A areas, respectively (Di Russo et al., 2005). Motion-onset VEP produced activities at 160 and 180 ms in area V3A and in the lateral occipital regions (LOR), respectively. Using flow-field motion-onset stimuli, an early N1 was localized in motion area V6 at 140 ms and a late N1 in area V3A at 180 ms (Pitzalis, Bozzacchi, et al., 2012).

The P2 Component

The P2 is the less studied component. It peaks between 200 and 250 ms and it was supposed to represent reentrant activity in V1 and V3A areas (Di Russo et al., 2002, 2005). More recently, this component was localized in the intraparietal sulcus (IPs) and in area V6 using motion-onset stimuli (Pitzalis, Bozzacchi, et al., 2012; Pitzalis, Strappini, et al., 2012).

Figure 5.2 shows the comparison between the VEP waveform obtained with pattern-onset, pattern-reversal, and motion-onset stimuli presented in the upper left quadrant. The figure combines the VEP data from Di Russo et al. (2002, 2005) and Pitzalis, Strappini, et al. (2012).

Considering the brain areas involved in visual processing, the aforementioned VEP–fMRI studies indicate that:

- Area V1 is active for any visual stimulation modality with an onset of 50–70 ms. Its first peak of activity is reached at 75–100 ms (C1 component) and, in case of pattern-reversal, it is again active about 50 ms later (C2 component).
- Area MT+ is activated by pattern-reversal and motion-onset stimulations with an onset of 80–100 ms and it reaches the peak activity at 95–130 ms (P1 component). For high speed stimulation, this area showed an earlier response initiating at about 40 ms and peaking at 70 ms (this early activity will be detailed in the next section).

- Area V3A has an early peak activity at 105 ms (onset 95 ms) for pattern-onset VEP (early P1 component) and a later activity (onset 130–150 ms, peak 160–180 ms) for pattern-reversal and motion-onset stimulations (N1p component).
- Area V4/V8 (in the Fusiform gyrus) reaches its peak at 140–180 ms (onset 120–150 ms) for any kind of stimulation (N1 component).
- Parietal regions (IPs and TPs) are active by any stimulation between 155 and 250 ms (onset 130–200 ms). This activity has been labeled as an N1a (anterior N1) component.
- Area V6 was activated early (onset 105 ms, peak 140 ms) by motion-onset flow-field (P140) and later activated at 230–250 m (P2, onset 200–220 m) for both gratings and flow-field motion-onset VEP (the V6 response to flow-field stimulation will be detailed in the next section).

The spatial resolution in the EEG–fMRI coregistration studies from our group was hugely increased by the retinotopic mapping, which was always performed in each

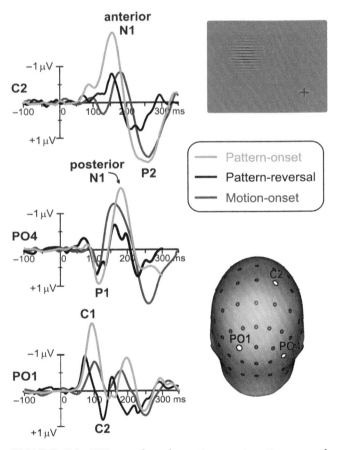

FIGURE 5.2 VEP waveform for pattern-onset, pattern-reversal, and motion-onset stimuli presented in the upper left quadrant. Waveforms show the main VEP component visible on contralateral central and parieto-occipital and medial parieto-occipital electrodes. *Data from Di Russo et al., 2002, 2005; Pitzalis, Strappini, et al., 2012.*

single study to demarcate striate and extrastriate visual areas, but with the more general aim to illustrate the exact relationship between the stimulus-related fMRI activations and the known early visual cortical areas. In each study, retinotopic dorsal (V1, V2, V3, V3A, V6, V7) and ventral (V1, V2, VP, V4v, V4/V8) visual areas were successfully identified by mapping quadrant representations and visual field signs (Sereno et al., 1995). In addition, the classic lateral motion area MT+ was individually mapped by functional localizer (Tootell et al., 1995). The boundaries of all of these visual areas are typically rendered on a flattened version of each participant's reference anatomy. In this way, activations in striate and adjacent extrastriate visual areas could be distinguished despite their close proximity and individual differences in cortical anatomy. Figure 5.3 shows the location of the main cortical visual areas (in colors) mapped with wide-field retinotopic stimuli (Pitzalis et al., 2006) and summarizes the timing of those visual areas found in all VEP–fMRI studies from our group. The location and topography of the cortical areas were based on functional and anatomical magnetic resonance (MR) tests of each subject. The location of the numeric labels indicate the areas found in the aforementioned studies (Di Russo

et al. 2002, 2005; Pitzalis, Bozzacchi, et al., 2012; Pitzalis, Strappini, et al., 2012) and the values indicate the timing their peak activity expressed in ms.

SPATIOTEMPORAL MAPPING OF MOTION PROCESSING

Analysis of visual motion has a crucial biological significance for each species survival, and in humans several brain regions in the primate dorsal visual pathway are specialized for different aspects of visual motion processing. The human dorsal visual stream specialized for visual motion processing begins in V1, extends through several extrastriate areas, and terminates in higher areas of the parietal and temporal lobes. Lateral areas MT+ are classically considered the key motion regions of the dorsal visual stream, being responsive to visual stimuli in motion and showing selectivity for the direction (e.g., Morrone et al., 2000; Smith, Wall, Williams, & Singh, 2006; Tootell et al., 1995) and speed (e.g., Lebranchu et al., 2010; McKeefry, Burton, Vakrou, Barrett, & Morland, 2008; Pitzalis, Strappini, et al., 2012) of movement. In comparison to the lateral temporal cortex, relatively less attention has been devoted to the motion sensitivity of dorsal regions in the medial parieto-occipital cortex. Recent studies from our group have revealed the presence in the human dorsal stream of another key motion region, area V6, located medially in the parieto-occipital sulcus (POS) (Fattori, Pitzalis, & Galletti, 2009; Pitzalis et al., 2006, 2010). As in nonhuman primates, the human V6 is a motion area highly sensitive to coherent motion and flow-fields (Pitzalis et al., 2010, in press), which is probably the most important visual cue for the perception of selfmotion or "egomotion" (i.e., the sensation to be moving in space). While lateral areas MT+ have been widely investigated and their role in motion processing is well grounded, the discovery of the medial motion area V6 is relatively recent and its functional role is still unknown.

VEPs have been extensively used to study motion processing and integrity of the visual system, and in the previous section we have already described the spatiotemporal structure of motion-onset VEP with the support of the fMRI. However, before 2012 there were no studies reporting the electrophysiological correlates of area V6. Moreover, the effect of coherent visual motion has been scarcely investigated by electrophysiological methods (e.g., Kuba, Kubová, Kremlábek, & Langrová, 2007). Further, inconsistent results were found about important questions concerning the response timing of the motion-sensitive areas MT+ and V6 as well as the temporal relationship between these two motion areas and area V1. We addressed these questions in two recent VEP–fMRI studies, which will be reviewed in this section.

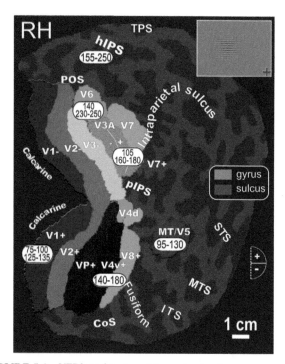

FIGURE 5.3   VEP based timing of the main visual areas represented on flattened right hemisphere (occipital lobe) of the MNI template. Response to stimuli located in the upper left visual quadrant. The boundaries of visual areas defined in the same subject by the retinotopic visual field sign, and by MT+ and V6 mapping. As indicated in the semicircular logos, dashed and solid lines correspond to vertical and horizontal meridians, respectively; the plus and minus symbols refer to upper and lower visual field representations, respectively. Other labels are as in Figure 5.1. *Data from Di Russo et al., 2002, 2005; Pitzalis, Strappini, et al., 2012; Pitzalis, Bozzacchi, et al., 2012.*

In Pitzalis, Strappini, et al. (2012), we localized the main sources of the motion-onset VEPs for high and low speed stimuli by combining high-resolution EEG recordings with neuroimaging data. In doing so, we addressed the question about the response timing of the motion area MT+ respect to that observed in area V1 when slow and fast speed motion stimuli are used.

Some electrophysiological studies have found early activity in MT+, ranging from 35 to 120 ms, which may bypass area V1 (Buchner et al 1997; Ffytche, Guy, & Zeki, 1995; Schoenfeld, Heinze, & Woldorff, 2002). Also, neurophysiological studies on monkeys have found short MT+ latencies to fast stimuli (e.g., Schmolesky et al., 1998). These data should be taken into consideration because the V5 region in nonhuman primates has been shown to have anatomical connections not only from areas V1, V2, V3, V4, and V6 (Galletti et al., 2001) but also directly from subcortical structures that bypass area V1, such as the lateral geniculate (Sincich, Park, Wohlgemuth, & Horton, 2004) and pulvinar (Berman & Wurtz, 2010) nuclei in the thalamus and the superior colliculus (Gross, 1991). In humans, the existence and role of these direct and fast subcortical connections to MT+ are still unclear. However, a few studies on patients with V1 lesions have provided some evidence for the existence of such connections in humans (Ffytche, Guy, & Zeki, 1996). As mentioned above, three electrophysiological studies on healthy subjects (Buchner et al., 1997; Ffytche et al., 1995; Schoenfeld et al., 2002) reported concordant evidence for early parallel inputs into MT+ bypassing V1. However, there are discrepancies among them with respect to the onset and the peak latency of MT+ activity. The study of Pitzalis, Strappini, et al. (2012) tried to clarify these contradictory results concerning the onset and peak latency of MT+ activity measuring its activation timing by combining VEP and fMRI data for both slow and fast-moving stimuli. They found a very early component (N70), which was only present for fast stimuli confirming that motion signals for different speeds may reach the MT+ through different pathways, either through area V1 in the case of slow stimuli or bypassing area V1 in the case of high speed stimuli (Ffytche et al., 1995, 1996).

Additionally, comparing fMRI data for slow vs. fast motion, we found signs of slow-fast motion stimulus topography (i.e., speed-o-topy) along the posterior brain in at least three cortical regions (MT+,V3A, and LOR). Figure 5.4(B) shows slow and fast motion activations (for both upper and lower hemifields) rendered together on the anatomical template Population-Average, Landmark- and Surface-based (PALS). The results support a spatial segregation between the two speeds. The spatial trend is similar in the posterior Intraparietal Sulcus and MT+, where slow and fast motion stimuli activated the antero-dorsal and postero-ventral parts of these regions, respectively. Also, a spatial trend was visible in the LOR,

but only in the superior–inferior direction, with the slow and fast motion activating the more ventral and dorsal portions of this region.

In contrast, area V6 selectively responded to fast speed motion stimuli and independently to the visual quadrant stimulated. It is possible that the high-speed motion stimuli resembled a flickering visual stimulation, which is known to activate area V6 (Pitzalis et al., 2010) and other motion areas.

We also recently addressed another issue concerning the spatiotemporal mapping of motion processing. Specifically, in Pitzalis, Bozzacchi, et al. (2012) we used VEPs, fMRI, and retinotopic brain mapping to find the electrophysiological correlates of V6 and to define its temporal relationship with the activity observed in MT+. We also used wide-field coherent motion stimuli intentionally designed to best activate the area based on the finding in Pitzalis et al. (2010). As expected, we found a V6 strong preference for coherent motion, which is in line with previous fMRI studies (Cardin & Smith, 2010; Helfrich, Becker, & Haarmeier, 2012; Pitzalis et al., 2010, 2013; von Pföstl et al., 2009). Additionally, we found that area V6 is one of the most early stations coding the motion coherence and that its electroencephalographic activity is almost simultaneous with that of MT+. The early timing found of V6 activation (onset latency 105 ms) together with the small temporal gap with the V1 timing (peak latency 75 ms) is in agreement with data on macaque brain, where the existence of a direct connection between V1 and V6 has been proven (Galletti et al., 2001). This result also fits with previous human magnetoencephalography (MEG) studies that found visual activity in POS and V1 in a similar latency range between 60 and 100 ms from stimulus onset (Vanni, Tanskanen, Seppa, Uutela, & Hari, 2001; von Pföstl et al., 2009). We also found a late second activity in V6 in the latency range of the P2, which was also found in our (Di Russo et al., 2011; Pitzalis, Strappini, et al., 2012) and other (Hoffmann & Bach, 2002; Kremlácek, Kuba, Chlubnová, & Kubová, 2004) studies, and it was previously attributed to the processing of complex features of motion (expanding/contracting radial motion) (e.g., Kuba et al., 2007). In Pitzalis, Bozzacchi, et al. (2012), we showed that the analysis of such complex motion signals also occurs much earlier, about 100 ms before (N140), supporting the hypothesis of a V6 involvement in early cortical motion processing. We interpret the late activity in V6 (P230) as a reentrant feedback from other extrastriate visual areas, like V3A, which is strongly connected with V6 in the macaque (Galletti et al., 2001) and is supposed to be involved in extracting form from motion (Vanduffel et al., 2002; Zeki, 1978). Such a type of signal could help V6 to recognize real motion of objects among the plethora of retinal image movements self-evoked by eye and body movements (Galletti, Battaglini, & Fattori, 1990; Galletti & Fattori, 2003).

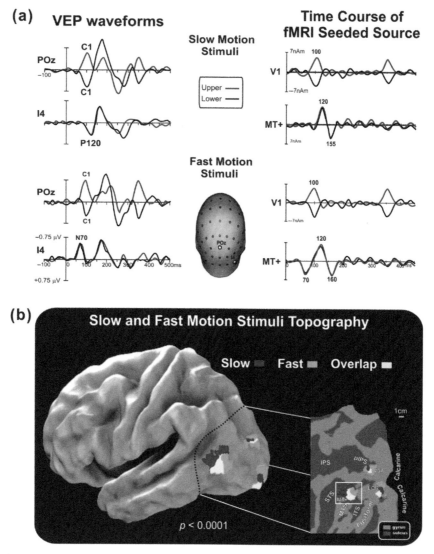

FIGURE 5.4   a) On the left, grand averaged waveforms of motion-onset VEPs for slow and fast motion stimuli presented to the left quadrants for medial parieto-occipital (POz) and contralateral Inion-level (I4) electrodes, of which the location is indicated on the head representation. Shown on the right are the source waveforms of the dipoles seeded to the fMRI activations for the same slow and fast motion stimuli. (b) Group fMRI activations for slow and fast motion stimuli rendered on the semiinflated cortical surface reconstruction of the left hemisphere of the average brain (left section). Results are also shown in a closeup view of the posterior part of the brain rendered on a flat map. Results from upper and lower hemifields are collapsed together. Activations for slow and fast motion conditions are plotted in different colors to represent their topographic specificity. *Data from Pitzalis, Strappini, et al., 2012.*

In Pitzalis, Bozzacchi, et al. (2012), we also provided important data that concerns the spatiotemporal profile of the motion coherency effect on VEPs and the localization of its neural generators. We found a complex sequence of six components located in occipital, parietal, and temporal cortices, including feed-forward and reentrant feedback signals in some specific cortical regions. Specifically, the processing of motion in the cortical network started in V1 (C1 component) approximately 50 ms after stimulus onset (peaking at 75 ms), then was detected in ventral extrastriate areas, likely LOR region (P100) and, almost simultaneously, in MT+ (P130) and V6 (N140). Subsequently, the activity in the

posterior part of the brain was found in V3A (N180) and again in V6 (P230). However, not all of these components were affected by the motion coherence. The earliest VEP components, the C1 and P100, respectively originating from V1 and LOR, i.e., the cortex between dorsal areas V3A and MT+ (Larsson & Heeger, 2006; Smith, Greenlee, Singh, Kraemer, & Hennig, 1998; Tootell & Hadjikhani, 2001) were not modulated by motion coherence. Activities in MT+, V6, and V3A were consistently and differently modulated by motion and its coherence. While both areas V6 (N140 and P230, see above) and MT+ (P130) showed a preference for the coherent motion, though in a different degree, area V3A showed the opposite pattern, being more activated in the random condition (N180).

Our analyses show a rapid sequence of activation from the occipital pole to areas V6 and MT+. These two dorsal motion areas have similar onset latencies (100 and 105 ms), with a delay of about 25 ms with respect to V1 peak. The minimal temporal gap between the two areas supports the view of direct interconnections between V1 and the two motion areas, as found in the macaque brain (Galletti et al., 2001; Shipp & Zeki, 1989). The similar latencies of visual responses in V6 and MT+ also suggest that these areas are anatomically interconnected, as it is the case in the macaque monkey (Galletti et al., 2001).

Overall, our results suggest that motion signals flow in parallel from the occipital pole to the medial and lateral motion areas V6 and MT+. These two areas, in turn, likely exchange information on visual motion. On the functional point of view, it has been suggested that MT+ is involved in the analysis of motion signals (direction and speed of movement) particularly in the central part of the visual field, whereas V6 in both object and selfmotion recognition across the whole visual field (Galletti & Fattori, 2003). In particular, V6 would be involved in "subtracting out" selfmotion signals across the whole visual field (Pitzalis et al., 2010). The small temporal gap between the onset of visual responses in areas MT+ and V6 and the strong interconnection between the two areas observed in monkeys lend support to this view.

IDENTIFICATION OF THE NEURAL SOURCES MODULATED BY SPATIAL ATTENTION

Studies over the past three decades have shown that early ERP components in the 80–250 ms range are enhanced in amplitude by spatially focused attention in the manner of a sensory gain control (Mangun & Hillyard, 1991; Hillyard & Anllo-Vento, 1998; Hillyard, Vogel, & Luck, 1998; Hopf, Heinze, Schoenfeld, & Hillyard, 2009; Hopfinger, Luck, & Hillyard, 2004). In studies of visual-spatial attention that combined ERP recordings with fMRI, it was found that the earliest evoked component (the C1), which has been attributed to V1 generator, was not affected by attention, but all later components attributed to multiple areas of extrastriate visual cortex were enhanced in amplitude (e.g., Martínez, Di Russo, Anllo-Vento, & Hillyard, 2001; Martinez, Di Russo, Anllo-Vento, Sereno, et al., 2001; Di Russo, et al., 2003, 2011).

In apparent contradiction with these results on humans, experiments in monkeys have found that neural activity in V1 may be modulated by attention under certain conditions, in particular, when several competing stimuli are simultaneously present (Ito and Gilbert, 1999; Motter, 1993; Roelfsema, Lamme, & Spekreijse, 1998; Vidyasagar, 1998). Enhanced neural responses in area V1 were typically found to occur at fairly long latencies (80–100 ms or more), well beyond the initial peak of the sensory-evoked response, suggesting that the attentional modulations were carried out via delayed feedback influences from higher visual areas (Vidyasagar, 1999). In support of such a feedback mechanism, Mehta and collaborators (Mehta, Ulbert, & Schroeder, 2000a; Mehta, Ulbert, & Schroeder, 2000b) found that evoked activity in higher tier visual areas (such as V4) was modulated by attention at shorter latencies than that recorded in area V1.

The participation of primary visual cortex during spatial attention tasks is further evidenced by neuroimaging studies in humans (Brefczynski & DeYoe, 1999; Ghandhi et al., 1999; Martínez et al., 1999; Somers, Dale, Seiffert, & Tootell, 1999; Tootell et al., 1998). Using fMRI, these studies found that paying attention to a stimulus resulted in increased neural activity in restricted zones of area V1 (and of higher extrastriate areas as well) that corresponded to the retinotopic projections of the attended locations. Considering the low temporal resolution of the fMRI, however, it was difficult to determine whether these attention-related increases in neural activity in V1 reflected a modulation of early sensory-evoked activity in V1, a delayed modulation of V1 activity produced by feedback from higher areas, or a sustained increase or bias in ongoing neural activity associated with the spatial focusing of attention (Luck, Chelazzi, Hillyard, & Desimone, 1997; Kastner, Pinsk, DeWeerd, Desimone, & Ungerleider, 1999; Ress, Backus, & Heeger, 2000).

The integration of ERP and fMRI measures has been critical in order to exclude alternative explanation of the V1 attention effect. A study by Martinez and colleagues (Martínez et al., 1999) carried out ERP recordings and fMRI sessions (on separate days) while subjects attended to a rapid sequence of stimuli presented to one visual field while ignoring a comparable sequence presented in the opposite field. As in previous studies, the C1 amplitude was found to be unaffected by attention, but its dipolar source was colocalized within a zone of attention-related neural activity in area V1 as shown by the fMRI results. To account for this apparent discrepancy, dipole modeling of the ERP attention effects revealed a delayed response at 150–250 ms attributed to the same Calcarine source as the C1 component (Martínez, Di Russo, Anllo-Vento, et al., 2001; Martinez, Di Russo, Anllo-Vento, Sereno, et al., 2001). Similar delayed attention effects localized to area V1 have been observed in recordings of magnetic field (Aine, Supek, & George, 1995; Noesselt et al., 2002). These results suggested that enhanced long-latency neural activity elicited by attended-location stimuli actually arises from area V1 rather than from neighboring extrastriate areas.

A decisive test of this hypothesis comes from the study of Di Russo et al. (2003), which was performed in the Hillyard laboratory and in the fMRI facilities of the University of California San Diego. This study investigated in detail the retinotopic organization of area V1, with the lower visual field projecting primarily to the upper bank of the Calcarine fissure and the upper visual field primarily to the lower bank. In accordance with this anatomical arrangement, it is expected that stimuli presented to the upper and lower visual fields should elicit scalp potentials of opposite polarity for neural generators in primary cortex, as has been consistently observed for the C1 components (Clark et al., 1995; Di Russo, Martínez, et al., 2002; Jeffreys & Axford, 1972a; Portin, Vanni, Virsu, & Hari, 1999). That experiment investigated whether such a polarity inversion also occurs for long-latency attention effects localized to Calcarine cortex as subjects attend to stimuli presented in the upper or lower visual fields. Converging evidence on the localization of spatial attention effects in both striate and extrastriate areas was obtained by comparing sites of fMRI activation with the calculated positions of dipoles representing the attentional modulations (seeded model).

Results confirmed that the earliest effects of spatial attention on visual processing were manifest in the P1 (onset 70–80 ms) and N1 (onset 130–150 ms) components, which were enlarged in amplitude in response to stimuli at attended locations in the visual field. Dipole modeling of these attention-related amplitude modulations and comparison of the calculated sources with fMRI activations indicated that they arose from multiple sites in extrastriate visual cortex. Also in accordance with previous reports, the initial C1 component (onset at 50–60 ms) was found to be unchanged by attention, and its calculated source location in Calcarine cortex and polarity inversion for upper versus lower field stimuli were consistent with a neural generator in the primary visual cortex (area V1). The major new finding was that the same dipole that fit the C1 component's distribution was also found to account for a longer latency attention effect (at 150–225 ms), which also inverted in polarity for upper vs. lower field stimuli. This inversion, together with the colocalization of the C1/late effect dipole with attention-related fMRI activation in Calcarine cortex, provided solid evidence that neural activity in area V1 is in fact modulated by attention but only after a delay, most likely mediated by feedback projections from higher extrastriate areas.

Most ERP studies of attention have used briefly flashed pattern-onset stimuli and the pattern-reversal was hardly used. The pattern-reversal stimulus importantly differs from the pattern-onset in being continuously present throughout recording and in producing a clear perception of motion during the reversal. As reported in the previous section, Di Russo et al. (2005) combined VEPs with fMRI and brain mapping methods to obtain a comprehensive spatiotemporal picture of the pattern-reversal VEPs and its neural generators. In particular, the results provided strong evidence that both the C1 and C2 components (peaking at 130 ms) arise from activity in area V1. To identify which component and corresponding cortical areas are modulated by spatial attention (especially the C2), Di Russo et al. (2011) recently investigated the effect of spatial attention on the pattern-reversal ERP using a dense electrode array and focal stimulation in each of the visual quadrants. The study was aimed at determining the spatiotemporal profile of attention-related ERP modulations and to localize their neural generators. For this purpose, they used the same combined ERP/fMRI technique and stimulation paradigm previously developed (Di Russo et al., 2005) in the Psychophysiology laboratory of "Foro Italico" university and in the fMRI center of Santa Lucia Foundation in Rome. Cortical sources were identified using dipole modeling based on a realistic head model, taking into account the loci of cortical activation revealed by fMRI while performing the same task. These sources were also localized on flat maps with respect to visual cortical areas identified in individual subjects by wide-field retinotopic mapping (e.g., Pitzalis et al., 2006; Sereno et al., 1995). In addition, two motion-sensitive cortical areas were individually mapped: the classic lateral area MT+ (Tootell et al., 1995), which was previously found to be strongly activated by pattern-reversal stimuli (Di Russo et al., 2005), and a newly defined medial area labeled V6 (e.g., Fattori et al., 2009; Pitzalis et al., 2006, 2010). It was found that attention did not modulate the amplitude of the C1, which was localized to area V1. Over the time range of 80–250 ms, six different ERP components were identified that showed increased amplitudes for stimuli at attended locations. Five of these components were localized to neural generators in extrastriate visual cortex in MT+ (P1), in VP, V4v, V4/V8 (N1b), in V3A (N1c), in the horizontal segment of the intraparietal sulcus (hIPS) (N1a), and in POS that corresponded to the recently described visual area V6 (P2). Attention also modulated the C2 that was localized to V1 as the C1. The conclusion of this study was that spatial attention produces a general amplification of sensory signal strength throughout both dorsal and ventral visual pathways and that both feed-forward and feedback signals are enhanced. Figure 5.5 shows the time-course (dipole moment) of the cerebral sources effected by spatial attention for pattern-onset and pattern-reversal stimulation modality. Sources were fit to the grand averaged ERPs and seeded to the fMRI activations indicated in Figure 5.3. The pattern-reversal mode produces a more complex spatiotemporal pattern of activity including the motion-sensitive areas MT+ and V6. The delayed attentional effect on area V1 is visible in both modalities.

Contrary to the bulk of literature showing no attention effect on the C1, some recent studies have reported that spatial attention can increase the amplitude of the C1 (Fu et al., 2009; Fu, Fedota, Greenwood, Parasuraman, 2010; Kelly, Gomez-Ramirez, & Foxe, 2008), but it may be questioned whether these findings actually represent modulation of the initial feed-forward response in area V1. In the experiment of Kelly et al. (2008), the left and right field stimuli were always aligned along a diagonal, so that the well-known upper vs. lower field polarity inversion seen for the C1 was confounded with a left vs. right field inversion, which could have been produced by a laterally oriented dipole outside of area V1. Moreover, the neural sources that were calculated for the attention-related increase in C1 amplitude (using the LAURA algorithm) were situated 23–24 mm lateral to the midline, at the extreme lateral edge of calcarine cortex. Fu et al. (2009, 2010) also reported attention-related modulation within the C1 latency range (60–90 ms), but this effect appeared to be localized to lateral extrastriate cortex and might have been the result of a sensory interaction between the cue and target stimuli rather than a true attention effect. A recent MEG study (Poghosyan & Ioannides, 2008) reported that spatial attention enhanced an early visual response at 55–90 ms that was localized

to area V1, but this localization was based on averages of only 18 presentations of each visual stimulus type in each visual field per subject. At present, the evidence that attention can influence the initial evoked response in area V1 appears slim indeed.

CONCLUSIONS

Overall, the results described here help to reveal the timing and the neuro-anatomical bases of processes involved in stimulus detection and selection, and to characterize the roles of extrastriate and striate cortex in visuospatial attention.

Regarding visual perception, studies that combined VEP recording with structural and functional MRI and retinotopic mapping of visual cortical areas support the hypothesis that the initial evoked components (C1) arise from neural generators in primary visual cortex while subsequent components (P1, N1 and P2) are generated in multiple extrastriate occipital and parietal cortical areas including V3A, V4/V8, MT+, and V6 with the later two especially involved in the motion processing.

Regarding the effect of visuospatial attention, literature does not show convincing evidence that attended

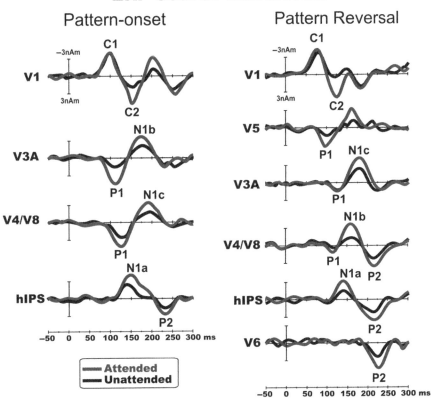

FIGURE 5.5 Source waveforms of the dipoles fit to the grand averaged ERPs and seeded to the indicated fMRI activations. The left and right columns show data from pattern-onset and pattern-reversal stimulation modalities, respectively. *Data from Di Russo et al., 2003, 2011.*

stimuli are preferentially processed during the initial feed-forward response area V1 at 50–80 ms after stimulus onset. However, longer latency activity (peaking at 120–140 ms for pattern-reversal and 150–225 ms for pattern-onset) that was localized to cortical generators in area V1 was enhanced by attention. Beginning at about 80 ms after stimulus, presentation attended-location stimuli elicited enlarged neural responses in multiple extrastriate visual areas in the occipital, parietal, and temporal lobes. The timing of this neural activity modulated by attention was established by electrophysiological recordings of ERPs, and the localization of the underlying generators was reinforced by the mapping of hemodynamic responses in a parallel fMRI experiment. These findings support the hypothesis that a sensory gain-control mechanism selectively amplifies both feed-forward and feedback responses elicited by attended-location stimuli in multiple visual cortical areas of both the dorsal and ventral streams of processing.

References

Aine, C. J., Supek, S., & George, J. S. (1995). Temporal dynamics of visual-evoked neuromagnetic sources: effects of stimulus parameters and selective attention. *International Journal of Neuroscience, 80,* 79–104.

Berman, R. A., & Wurtz, R. H. (2010). Functional identification of a pulvinar path from superior colliculus to cortical area MT. *Journal of Neuroscience, 30,* 6342–6354.

Brefczynski, J. A., & DeYoe, E. A. (1999). A physiological correlate of the 'spotlight' of visual attention. *Nature Neuroscience, 2*(4), 370–374.

Buchner, H., Gobbele, R., Wagner, M., Fuchs, M., Waberski, T. D., & Beckmann, R. (1997). Fast visual evoked potential input into human area V5. *Neuroreport, 8,* 2419–2422.

Butler, S. R., Georgiou, G. A., Glass, A., Hancox, R. J., Hopper, J. M., & Smith, K. R. (1987). Cortical generators of the C1 component of the pattern-onset visual evoked potential. *Electroencephalography and Clinical Neurophysiology, 68,* 256–267.

Cardin, V., & Smith, A. T. (2010). Sensitivity of human visual and vestibular cortical regions to egomotion-compatible visual stimulation. *Cerebral Cortex, 20*(8), 1964–1973.

Clark, V. P., Fan, S., & Hillyard, S. A. (1995). Identification of early visually evoked potential generators by retinotopic and topographic analysis. *Human Brain Mapping, 2,* 170–187.

Di Russo, F., Martínez, A., & Hillyard, S. A. (2003). Source analysis of event-related cortical activity during visuo-spatial attention. *Cerebral Cortex, 13,* 486–499.

Di Russo, F., Martínez, A., Sereno, M. I., PitzalisS, & Hillyard, S. A. (2002a). The cortical sources of the early components of the visual evoked potential. *Human Brain Mapping, 15,* 95–111.

Di Russo, F., Pitzalis, S., Aprile, T., Spitoni, G., Patria, F., Stella, A., et al. (2007). Spatio-temporal analysis of the cortical sources of the steady-state visual evoked potential. *Human Brain Mapping, 28,* 323–334.

Di Russo, F., Pitzalis, S., Spitoni, G., Aprile, T., Patria, F., Spinelli, D., et al. (2005). Identification of the neural sources of the pattern-reversal VEP. *Neuroimage, 24,* 874–886.

Di Russo, F., Ragazzoni, A., & Spagli, P. M. (1998). [Electrophysiological functional exploration of visual cortical area] "Esplorazione funzionale elettrofisiologica delle aree visive della corteccia cerebrale". *Nuova Rivista di Neurobiologia, 8*(5), 139–144.

Di Russo, F., Stella, A., Spitoni, G., Strappini, F., Sdoia, S., Galati, G., et al. (2011). Spatiotemporal brain mapping of spatial attention effects on pattern-reversal ERPs. *Human Brain Mapping, 33*(6), 1334–1351.

Di Russo, F., Teder-Sälejärvi, W. A., & Hillyard, S. A. (2002b). Steady-State VEP and attentional visual processing. In A. Zani & A. M. Proverbio (Eds.), *The cognitive electrophysiology of mind and brain* (pp. 259–274). San Diego, CA: Academic Press.

Fattori, P., Pitzalis, S., & Galletti, C. (2009). The cortical visual area V6 in macaque and human brains. *Journal of Physiology-Paris, 103,* 88–97.

Ffytche, D. H., Guy, C. N., & Zeki, S. (1995). The parallel visual motion inputs into areas V1 and V5 of human cerebral cortex. *Brain, 118,* 1375–1394.

Ffytche, D. H., Guy, C. N., & Zeki, S. (1996). Motion specific responses from a blind hemifield. *Brain, 119,* 1971–1982.

Friston, K., Harrison, L., Daunizeau, J., Kiebel, S., Phillips, C., Trujillo-Barreto, N., et al. (2008). Multiple sparse priors for the M/EEG inverse problem. *Neuroimage, 39*(3), 1104–1120.

Fu, S., Fedota, J. R., Greenwood, P. M., & Parasuraman, R. (2010). Dissociation of visual C1 and P1 components as a function of attentional load: an event-related potential study. *Biological Psychology, 85,* 171–178.

Fu, S., Huang, Y., Luo, Y., Wang, Y., Fedota, J., Greenwood, P. M., et al. (2009). Perceptual load interacts with involuntary attention at early processing stages: event-related potential studies. *Neuroimage, 48,* 191–199.

Galletti, C., Battaglini, P. P., & Fattori, P. (1990). 'Real-motion' cells in area V3A of macaque visual cortex. *Experimental Brain Research, 82,* 67–76.

Galletti, C., & Fattori, P. (2003). Neuronal mechanisms for detection of motion in the field of view. *Neuropsychologia, 41,* 1717–1727.

Galletti, C., Gamberini, M., Kutz, D. F., Fattori, P., Luppino, G., & Matelli, M. (2001). The cortical connections of area V6: an occipito-parietal network processing visual information. *European Journal of Neuroscience, 13,* 1572–1588.

Gandhi, S. P., Heeger, D., & Boynton, G. M. (1999). Spatial attention affects brain activity in human primary visual cortex. *Proceedings of the National Academy of Sciences of the United States of America, 96,* 3314–3319.

Gomez Gonzalez, C. M., Clark, V. P., Fan, S., Luck, S. J., & Hillyard, S. A. (1994). Sources of attention-sensitive visual event-related potentials. *Brain Topography, 7*(1), 41–51.

Grech, R., Cassar, T., Muscat, J., Camilleri, K. P., Fabri, S. G., Zervakis, M., et al. (2008). Review on solving the inverse problem in EEG source analysis. *Journal of NeuroEngineering and Rehabilitation, 7,* 5–25.

Gross, C. G. (1991). Contribution of striate cortex and the superior colliculus to visual function in area MT, the superior temporal polysensory area and the inferior temporal cortex. *Neuropsychologia, 29,* 497–515.

Halliday, A. M. (1993). *Evoked potentials in clinical testing.* Edinburgh: Churchill Livingstone.

Helfrich, R. F., Becker, H. G., & Haarmeier, T. (2012). Processing of coherent visual motion in topographically organized visual areas in human cerebral cortex. *Brain Topography.* http://dx.doi.org/10.1007/s10548-012-0226-1. [Epub ahead of print].

Hillyard, S. A., & Anllo-Vento, L. (1998). Event-related brain potentials in the study of visual selective attention. *Proceedings of the National Academy of Sciences of the United States of America, 95,* 781–787.

Hillyard, S. A., Vogel, E. K., & Luck, S. J. (1998). Sensory gain control (amplification) as a mechanism of selective attention: electrophysiological and neuroimaging evidence. *Philosophical Transactions of the Royal Society of London. Series B, Biological Sciences, 353*(1373), 1257–1267.

Hoffmann, M. B., & Bach, M. (2002). The distinction between eye and object motion is reflected by the motion-onset visual evoked potential. *Experimental Brain Research, 144,* 141–151.

Hopf, J. M., Heinze, H. J., Schoenfeld, M. A., & Hillyard, S. A. (2009). Spatio-temporal analysis of visual attention. In M. S. Gazzaniga (Ed.), *The cognitive neurosciences IV* (pp. 235–250), Cambridge, MA: MIT Press.

Hopfinger, J. B., Luck, S. J., & Hillyard, S. A. (2004). Selective attention: electrophysiological and neuromagnetic studies. In M. S. Gazzaniga (Ed.), *The cognitive neurosciences III* (pp. 561–574). Cambridge, MA: MIT Press.

Huk, A. C., Dougherty, R. F., & Heeger, D. J. (2002). Retinotopy and functional subdivision of human areas MT and MST. *Journal of Neuroscience, 22*, 7195–7205.

Ito, M., & Gilbert, C. D. (1999). Attention modulates contextual influences in the primary visual cortex of alert monkeys. *Neuron, 22*(3), 593–604.

Jeffreys, D. A., & Axford, J. G. (1972a). Source locations of pattern-specific component of human visual evoked potentials. I: component of striate cortical origin. *Experimental Brain Research, 16*(1), 1–21.

Jeffreys, D. A., & Axford, J. G. (1972b). Source locations of pattern-specific component of human visual evoked potentials. II. Component of extrastriate cortical origin. *Experimental Brain Research, 16*(1), 22–40.

Kastner, S., Pinsk, M. A., DeWeerd, P., Desimone, R., & Ungerleider, L. G. (1999). Increased activity in human visual cortex during directed attention in the absence of visual stimulation. *Neuron, 22*, 751–761.

Kelly, S. P., Gomez-Ramirez, M., & Foxe, J. J. (2008). Spatial attention modulates initial afferent activity in human primary visual cortex. *Cerebral Cortex, 18*, 2629–2636.

Kremlácek, J., Kuba, M., Chlubnová, J., & Kubová, Z. (2004). Effect of stimulus localisation on motion-onset VEP. *Vision Research, 44*, 2989–3000.

Kuba, M. (2006). In *Visual evoked potentials and their diagnostic applications* (1st ed.). Hradec Králové: Nucleus HK.

Kuba, M., Kubová, Z., Kremlábek, J., & Langrová, J. (2007). Motion-onset VEPs: characteristics, methods, and diagnostic use. *Vision Research, 47*, 189–202.

Kubova, Z., Kuba, M., Spekreijse, H., & Blakemore, C. (1995). Contrast dependence of motion-onset and pattern-reversal evoked potentials. *Vision Research, 35*, 197–205.

Larsson, J., & Heeger, D. J. (2006). Two retinotopic visual areas in human lateral occipital cortex. *Journal of Neuroscience, 26*, 13128–13142.

Lebranchu, P., Bastin, J., Pelegrini-Issac, M., Lehericy, S., Berthoz, A., & Orban, G. A. (2010). Retinotopic coding of extraretinal pursuit signals in early visual cortex. *Cerebral Cortex, 20*(9), 2172–2187.

Liu, Z., Zhang, N., Chen, W., & He, B. (2009). Mapping the bilateral visual integration by EEG and fMRI. *Neuroimage, 46*(4), 989–997.

Luck, S. J., Chelazzi, L., Hillyard, S. A., & Desimone, R. (1997). Neural mechanisms of spatial selective attention in areas V1, V2, and V4 of macaque visual cortex. *Journal of Neurophysiology, 77*(1), 24–42.

Mangun, G. R. (1995). Neural mechanisms of visual selective attention. *Psychophysiology, 32*(1), 4–18.

Mangun, G. R., & Hillyard, S. A. (1991). Modulations of sensory-evoked brain potentials indicate changes in perceptual processing during visual-spatial priming. *Journal of Experimental Psychology: Human Perception and Performance, 17*, 1057–1074.

Martínez, A., Anllo-Vento, L., Sereno, M. I., Frank, L. R., Buxton, R. B., Dubowitz, D. J., et al. (1999). Involvement of striate and extrastriate visual cortical areas in spatial attention. *Nature Neuroscience, 2*(4), 364–369.

Martínez, A., Di Russo, F., Anllo-Vento, L., & Hillyard, S. A. (2001). Electrophysiological analysis of cortical mechanisms of selective attention to high and low spatial frequencies. *Clinical Neurophysiology, 112*, 1980–1998.

Martinez, A., Di Russo, F., Anllo-Vento, L., Sereno, M. I., Buxton, R. B., & Hillyard, S. A. (2001). Putting spatial attention on the map: timing and localization of stimulus selection processes in striate and extrastriate visual areas. *Vision Research, 41*, 1437–1457.

McKeefry, D. J., Burton, M. P., Vakrou, C., Barrett, B. T., & Morland, A. B. (2008). Induced deficits in speed perception by transcranial magnetic stimulation of human cortical areas V5/MT+ and V3A. *Journal of Neuroscience, 28*, 6848–6857.

Mehta, A. D., Ulbert, I., & Schroeder, C. E. (2000a). Intermodal selective attention in monkeys I: distribution and timing of effects across visual areas. *Cerebral Cortex, 10*, 343–358.

Mehta, A. D., Ulbert, I., & Schroeder, C. E. (2000b). Intermodal selective attention in monkeys II: physiological mechanisms of modulation. *Cerebral Cortex, 10*, 359–370.

Morrone, M. C., Tosetti, M., Montanaro, D., Fiorentini, A., Cioni, G., & Burr, D. C. (2000). A cortical area that responds specifically to optic flow, revealed by fMRI. *Nature Neuroscience, 3*, 1322–1328.

Motter, B. C. (1993). Focal attention produces spatially selective processing in visual cortical areas V1, V2 and V4 in the presence of competing stimuli. *Journal of Neurophysiology, 70*, 909–919.

Noesselt, T., Hillyard, S. A., Woldorff, M. G., Hagner, T., Jaencke, H., Tempelmann, C., et al. (2002). Delayed striate cortical activation during spatial attention. *Neuron, 35*, 575–587.

Novitskiy, N., Ramautar, J. R., Vanderperren, K., De Vos, M., Mennes, M., Mijovic, B., et al. (2011). The BOLD correlates of the visual P1 and N1 in single-trial analysis of simultaneous EEG–fMRI recordings during a spatial detection task. *Neuroimage, 54*(2), 824–835.

Phillips, C., Rugg, M., & Friston, K. (2002). Anatomically informed basis functions for EEG source localization: combining functional and anatomical constraints. *Neuroimage, 16*, 678–695.

Pitzalis, S., Bozzacchi, C., Bultrini, A., Fattori, P., Galletti, C., & Di Russo, F. (2012). Parallel motion signals to the medial and lateral motion areas V6 and MT+. *Neuroimage, 67*, 89–100.

Pitzalis, S., Galletti, C., Huang, R. S., Patria, F., Committeri, G., Galati, G., et al. (2006). Wide-field retinotopy defines human cortical visual area V6. *Journal of Neuroscience, 26*, 7962–7973.

Pitzalis, S., Sdoia, S., Bultrini, A., Committeri, G., Di Russo, F., Fattori, P., et al. (2013). Selectivity to translational egomotion in human brain motion areas. *Plos One, 8*(4): e60241. doi: 10.1371/journal.pone.0060241.

Pitzalis, S., Sereno, M. I., Committeri, G., Fattori, P., Galati, G., Patria, F., et al. (2010). Human V6: the medial motion area. *Cerebral Cortex, 20*(2), 411–424.

Pitzalis, S., Strappini, F., De Gasperis, M., Bultrini, A., & Di Russo, F. (2012). Spatio-temporal brain mapping of motion-onset VEPs combined with fMRI and retinotopic maps. *Plos One, 7*(4), e3577.

Plonsey, R. (1963). Reciprocity applied to volume conductors and the EEG. *IEEE Transactions on Biomedical Engineering, 10*, 9–12.

Poghosyan, V., & Ioannides, A. A. (2008). Attention modulates earliest responses in the primary auditory and visual cortices. *Neuron, 58*, 802–813.

Portin, K., Vanni, S., Virsu, V., & Hari, R. (1999). Stronger occipital cortical activation to lower than upper visual field stimuli. *Experimental Brain Research, 124*, 287–294.

Ress, D., Backus, B. T., & Heeger, D. J. (2000). Activity in primary visual cortex predicts performance in a visual detection task. *Nature Neuroscience, 3*, 940–945.

Roelfsema, P. R., Lamme, V. A. F., & Spekreijse, H. (1998). Object-based attention in the primary visual cortex of the macaque monkey. *Nature, 395*, 376–381.

Schmolesky, M. T., Wang, Y., Hanes, D. P., Thompson, K. G., Leutgeb, S., Schall, J. D., et al. (1998). Signal timing across the macaque visual system. *Journal of Neurophysiology, 79*, 3272–3278.

Schoenfeld, M. A., Heinze, H. J., & Woldorff, M. G. (2002). Unmasking motion-processing activity in human brain area V5/MT mediated by pathways that bypass primary visual cortex. *Neuroimage, 17*, 769–779.

Schroeder, C. E., Steinschneider, M., Javitt, D. C., Tenke, C. E., Givre, S. J., Mehta, A. D., et al. (1995). Localization of ERP generators and identification of underlying neural processes. *Electroencephalography and Clinical Neurophysiology, Supplement, 44*, 55–75.

Sereno, M. I., Dale, A. M., Reppas, J. B., Kwong, K. K., Belliveau, J. W., Brady, T. J., et al. (1995). Borders of multiple visual areas in humans revealed by functional magnetic resonance imaging. *Science, 268,* 889–893.

Shipp, S., & Zeki, S. (1989). The organization of connections between areas V5 and V1 in macaque monkey visual cortex. *European Journal of Neuroscience, 1,* 309–332.

Simpson, G. V., Pflieger, M. E., Foxe, J. J., Ahlfors, S. P., Vaughan, H. G., Jr., Hrabe, J., et al. (1995). Dynamic neuroimaging of brain function. *Journal of Clinical Neurophysiology, 12*(5), 432–449.

Sincich, L. C., Park, K. F., Wohlgemuth, M. J., & Horton, J. C. (2004). Bypassing V1: a direct geniculate input to area MT. *Nature Neuroscience, 7,* 1123–1128.

Smith, A. T., Greenlee, M. W., Singh, K. D., Kraemer, F. M., & Hennig, J. (1998). The processing of first- and second-order motion in human visual cortex assessed by functional magnetic resonance imaging (fMRI). *Journal of Neuroscience, 18,* 3816–3830.

Smith, T., Wall, M. B., Williams, A. L., & Singh, K. D. (2006). Sensitivity to optic flow in human cortical areas MT and MST. *European Journal of Neuroscience, 23,* 561–569.

Somers, D. C., Dale, A. M., Seiffert, A. E., & Tootell, R. B. H. (1999). Functional MRI reveals spatially specific attentional modulation in human primary visual cortex. *Proceedings of the National Academy of Sciences of the United States of America, 96,* 1663–1668.

Tootell, R. B. H., & Hadjikhani, N. (2001). Where is 'dorsal V4' in human visual cortex? Retinotopic, topographic and functional evidence. *Cerebral Cortex, 11,* 298–311.

Tootell, R. B. H., Hadjikhani, N., Hall, E. K., Marrett, S., Vanduffel, W., Vaughan, J. T., et al. (1998). The retinotopy of visual spatial attention. *Neuron, 21*(6), 1409–1422.

Tootell, R. B. H., Mendola, J. D., Hadjikhani, N. K., Ledden, P. J., Liu, A. K., Reppas, J. B., et al. (1997). Functional analysis of V3A and related areas in human visual cortex. *Journal of Neuroscience, 17,* 7076–7078.

Tootell, R. B. H., Reppas, J. B., Kwong, K. K., Malach, R., Born, R. T., Brady, T. J., et al. (1995). Functional analysis of human MT and related visual cortical areas using magnetic resonance imaging. *Journal of Neuroscience, 15,* 3215–3230.

Vanduffel, W., Fize, D., Peuskens, H., Denys, K., Sunaert, S., Todd, J. T., et al. (2002). Extracting 3D from motion: differences in human and monkey intraparietal cortex. *Science, 298*(5592), 413–415.

Vanni, S., Tanskanen, T., Seppa, M., Uutela, K., & Hari, R. (2001). Coinciding early activation of the human primary visual cortex and anteromedial cuneus. *Proceedings of the National Academy of Sciences of the United States of America, 98*(5), 2776–2780.

Vidyasagar, T. R. (1998). Gating of neuronal responses in macaque primary visual cortex by an attentional spotlight. *Neuroreport, 9,* 1947–1952.

Vidyasagar, T. R. (1999). A neuronal model of attentional spotlight: parietal guiding the temporal. *Brain Research Reviews, 30*(1), 66–76.

von Pföstl, V., Stenbacka, L., Vanni, S., Parkkonen, L., Galletti, C., & Fattori, P. (2009). Motion sensitivity of human V6: a magnetoencephalography study. *Neuroimage, 45*(4), 1253–1263.

Zeki, S. M. (1978). The third visual complex of rhesus monkey prestriate cortex. *Journal of Physiology (London), 277,* 245–272.

Zhang, X., Zhaoping, L., Zhou, T., & Fang, F. (2012). Neural activities in V1 create a bottom-up saliency map. *Neuron, 73*(1), 183–192.

6

Source Localization of Visual Stimuli in Peripersonal Space

Katsumi Minakata[1], Wolfgang A. Teder[2]

[1]North Dakota State University, Fargo, ND, USA,
[2]411 14th Street South, Moorhead, MN, USA

INTRODUCTION

The representation of peripersonal space, i.e., the area within direct reach of the extremities, is inherently multisensory in nature. Multisensory integration is different from unisensory processing in that the combined activity of parallel processing is not equivalent to the sum of separately processed unimodal stimuli (Meredith & Stein, 1986; Stein & Meredith, 1993). It has been suggested that different modalities such as vision, audition, and touch are utilized in conjuncture, forming a coherent spatial map representing peripersonal space (Graziano, Hu, & Gross, 1997; Làdavas, Zeloni, & Farnè, 1998).

Neurophysiological evidence was reported by Graziano et al. (1997) and Graziano, Reiss, and Gross (1999) showing bimodal neurons in the ventral premotor (PMv) area of macaque monkeys with overlapping visual and tactile receptive fields which responded to an approaching object moving along a trajectory prone to strike the organism. Similar properties of bimodal audiovisual neurons (Stricanne, Andersen, & Mazzoni, 1996), which can be interpreted as relevant constituents establishing an internal representation of peripersonal space, have been demonstrated.

Corroborating evidence comes from visuotactile neuropsychological studies in human clinical populations examining extinction caused by right-hemisphere lesions (Làdavas et al., 1998). These patients are able to accurately perceive objects when they are individually presented in the left or right hemifield. However, a simultaneous presentation in both hemifields causes a drop in detection rate of contralesionally presented items. Since extinction has also been reliably reported in auditory and tactile modalities, possible mechanisms underlying cross-modal extinction attracted scientific interest (Làdavas et al., 1998) in human stimulus processing based on the work of Graziano et al. (1997) using macaque populations. These authors conducted a complex experiment with five conditions in right-hemisphere lesion patients to assess visuotactile extinction phenomena in peripersonal and extrapersonal space (beyond the reach of extremities). One of their key findings was that bimodal visual-tactile neurons encode combined stimuli within an individual's peri- and extrapersonal space. Specifically, participants failed to detect tactile stimuli under uni- or bimodal stimulation in peripersonal space. However, given extrapersonal (far) stimulus locations, patterns of facilitation and/or recovery from extinction were observed (Làdavas et al., 1998).

Psychophysical and behavioral paradigms have been used to shed further light on spatial patterns related to peripersonal space in healthy, nonclinical human participants. Hari and Jousmäki (1996) used the distance between a visual stimulus projected close to or far from the index finger as an experimental variable and found that reaction times (RTs) were fastest when visual stimuli were presented onto the reacting finger. Furthermore, Dufour and Touzalin (2008) reported improved visual sensitivity in the perihand space, i.e., greater accuracy (fewer errors) in the near-hand field. These authors concluded that bimodal visuotactile cells appear to code peripersonal space centered on body parts.

Lloyd, Azañón, and Poliakoff (2010) used hand presence as the cue for a target in a cuing attention experiment in which participants performed a discrimination task via a foot pedal on the right side of central fixation. The task was to either raise the heel upon presentation of a triangle or raise the toes if the target was a circle while the arms were either in left/right postures congruent with target position or crossed.

The pattern of results indicated that the presence of the hand clearly modulated performance which was consistently faster and more accurate whenever hands and targets were spatially congruent.

Very common approaches for studying peripersonal space in humans are functional magnetic resonance imaging (fMRI) and event-related potentials (ERPs). Based on the fact that the posterior parietal cortex (PPC) and PMv code peripersonal space in human and nonhuman primates, Lloyd, Morrison, and Roberts (2006) employed a fMRI paradigm using painful and nonpainful visual stimuli presented in peripersonal space in conjunction with a rubber hand in close contact to the real hand, which the participants successfully incorporated into their own body representation as long as the position of the artificial hand was anatomically plausible. It was found that the ventral intraparietal area of the PPC (BAs 5, 7) and the inferior parietal lobe (BA 40) exhibited a differential activation pattern to painful vs nonpainful stimuli. This study constitutes the first neuroimaging evidence for specific coding of events in "hand space" in the absence of tactile stimulation of the real hand (Lloyd et al., 2006). There is a large body of research identifying the neural basis for hand-centered encoding of peripersonal space that may also extend onto a prosthetic hand if perceived as one's own (Brozzoli, Gentile, & Ehrsson, 2012).

The ERP technique offers a high temporal resolution and is therefore ideally suited to investigate whether fast-paced laser stimuli projected either onto the hand or onto the desk in front of the participants cause significant amplitude modulations of well-known and robust ERP deflections related to sensory information processing and stimulus classification. A recent study by Qian, Al-Aidroos, West, Abrams, and Pratt (2012) measured visual P2 amplitudes in two separate visual attention experiments using checkerboard reversals and convincingly demonstrated that hand-proximal stimuli benefit from enhanced selective attention during later stages of stimulus processing. Furthermore, these authors were able to show that this effect occurs only for sensory processing at task-relevant locations close to the hands.

In a selective attention experiment, Simon-Dack et al. (2009) used an oddball paradigm to present frequent standard stimuli (85%, single laser dots) and infrequent deviant/target stimuli (15%, paired laser dots) projected onto the index or middle fingers of the left and right hand or, in a different experimental condition, to identical locations with the hands located under the desktop surface. When laser dots were projected onto the fingers, the amplitude of the occipital visual N1 wave was enhanced independent of attentional instruction, suggesting a relatively early, preattentive time course of processing stimuli in peripersonal space. ERP responses to supposedly unattended laser stimuli showed a classic "breakthrough-of-the-unattended" effect, probably due to the fact that the locations of the "Off-hand" laser dots were still too proximal to the hands and, consequently, clearly intruded into the participants' peripersonal space.

These data suggest a refined experimental setup using the surface of the hands rather than discrete fingers and maintenance of a larger spatial separation between laser dots projected onto the hand vs onto the desk surface. With this procedure, it should be possible to investigate whether laser dots projected onto the hand elicit a "pseudotactile" quality as indicated by a more parietal than occipital scalp distribution of modality-specific ERP waveforms. Stimuli in the Off condition (desktop) should fall outside peripersonal space and evoke slower and less accurate behavioral data than responses triggered by laser dots projected onto the hands. This hypothesis coincides with observations made in earlier pilot studies using lasers; it appears that visual stimuli touching the body are very difficult to ignore.

METHOD

Participants

Participants were student volunteers from the North Dakota State University campus. A total of 17 participants (19–24 years, 12 females) reported that they were right-handed and had normal or corrected-to-normal vision. Based on self-report, none of the subjects were color-blind nor did they acknowledge any past history of psychiatric or neurological disease.

Design

A 4-way 2 (laser condition: On vs Off) × 2 (attention: Left vs Right) × 2 (stimulus type: Standards [85%] vs Deviants [15%]) × 2 (stimulus location: Left vs Right) within-subjects factorial design was implemented. Deflections in μV as well as RT and ER were collected as the electrophysiological and behavioral dependent measures, respectively. Partial eta-squared (η_p^2) values are reported as effect-size estimates, i.e., the proportion of the treatment plus error variance that is accounted for by the treatment (Richardson, 2011). As a rule of thumb, a range of 0.01–1.0 (low to high) of partial eta-squared estimates is the variance explained by a given variable of the variance remaining after excluding other sources of variation (Levine & Hullett, 2002).

Stimuli and Apparatus

Stimuli were four small, focused laser points projected onto the fist from an adjustable frame positioned

Experimental setup

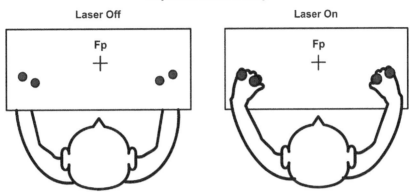

FIGURE 6.1   Description of the experimental setup (see Methods). In two different experimental conditions, the subjects' hands were either on top or under the desk surface. The distance between the hands was 60 cm at an angle of 90°. Fp = fixation point.

above a black desk at which participants were seated (see Figure 6.1).

The red lasers had a luminance of 100 cd/m² (600 nm wavelength) and produced no heat or other physical sensations when they touched the participants. Short bursts of light from the lasers were presented in a fast-paced, random sequence. Standard frequent stimuli were aligned with participants' inner fist on their index finger's knuckle in 100 ms bursts of light. Infrequent "deviant" stimuli occurred 15% of the time and were aligned with participants' outer fist on their little finger's knuckle. Stimuli were presented with an interstimulus interval of 130–360 ms (rectangular distribution). Deviant stimuli never occurred twice in succession.

Procedure

Participants were seated and had their electroencephalogram (EEG) recorded while they performed the experiment. They were instructed to look at a fixation cross on the desk with their hands stretched out in front of them (left/right 45°) (see Figure 6.1). Participants' hands were visible during the On condition and not visible during the Off condition. There were two experimental "laser" conditions: During the On condition, the laser dots were projected onto participants' fists; during the Off condition, participants placed their hands off the table onto their laps, occluded from vision. Further, participants were encouraged to change their body and hand posture as little as possible when they slid their hands beneath the lasers so as to maintain approximate proprioceptive feedback between conditions while performing the task. Participants' fists were also wrapped with medical tape so the reflective surfaces were equal between the conditions. Participants completed 16 blocks, eight of each hand condition. Blocks were 3.5 min each, with a net recording time of 56 min in length. Participants were instructed to attend only to

their left or right hand with attend-left or attend-right blocks interleaved and to ignore all stimuli occurring on or off their unattended hand. The participants' task was to respond to the infrequent deviant (i.e., "target") stimulus occurring in alignment with the attended inner fist location by pressing a foot switch. Participants were instructed to respond only to deviant stimuli aligned with the attended hand.

Behavior

The percentage for correct responses (i.e., hit rate) to target laser bursts was calculated for each of the conditions of the full factorial design (see Figure 6.2). The false alarm rate was derived by calculating the percentage of responses to laser bursts that were not targets. Four 2-way analyses of variance (ANOVAs) were executed on each of the behavioral measures (viz. hit rate, false alarm rate, and RT) for the laser condition (On vs. Off) and attended location (Left vs. Right) factors.

ERP Recordings

The EEG recordings were taken using an Active Two Biosemi Electric System (http://www. biosemi. com; Biosemi, Amsterdam) from 64 scalp locations.

The electrooculogram (EOG) was recorded from six electrodes located at the outer canthi and above and beneath each eye. The EEG sampling frequency was 512 Hz with a pass-band from DC to 150 Hz. The electrode offset was kept below 25 μV. Data were processed using BESA 5.1.8 (Brain Electric Source Analysis, Gräfelfing, Germany) and visually inspected for blinks and eye movements, after which automatic artifact rejection criteria of ±120 μV were applied from −100 to 600 ms poststimulus onset. Remaining trials were averaged per condition with a baseline of −100 to 0 ms. For analysis and display purposes, data were filtered with a zero

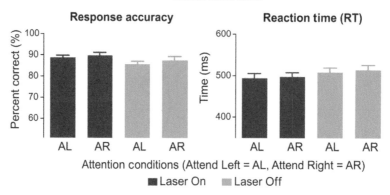

FIGURE 6.2　Behavioral data in terms of response accuracy (percent correct) and reaction time (RT). The bars represent means obtained in two different experimental conditions, and the error bars represent the standard error of the mean (SEM).

phase-shift 35 Hz IV-order Bessel low-pass filter with a fall-off of 24 dB/octave.

ERP Analysis

ANOVAs were run comparing mean amplitudes within specified time windows centered to the peak deflections of interest and referenced to the 100 ms pre-stimulus baseline. Greenhouse-Geisser corrections were applied for violations of sphericity. Partial eta-squared values are reported as a measure of effect size, which indicates the proportion of variance accounted for by the independent variables. The following latency ranges were used for the P1 (115–145 ms), N1 (135–180 ms), P2 (200–235 ms), and P3 (300–450 ms) deflections, which were symmetrical time windows focused on the maximum of each deflection. Mean ERP amplitudes of experimental stimuli were subjected to five-way, within-subjects ANOVAs with the factors laser condition (On, Off), attention (Attended, Unattended), stimulus type (Standard, Deviant), stimulus location (Left, Right), laterality (Left, Right), and anterior–posterior laterality (Centroparietal, Occipital). A P3 is typically only elicited for attended target stimuli. Therefore, we subjected the mean P3 peak amplitudes of attended target stimuli within the latency range of (350–450 ms) to a within-subjects ANOVA with the factors laser condition (On, Off), target location (Left, Right), and electrode cluster (Left, Right). We also analyzed the amplitudes at the onset latency of the P3 due to apparent differences at the initiation of the P3 observed in the grand average. There are several alternatives to determine the onset of the P3 deflection. However, we determined the onset of the P3 deflection by taking the first significant sample as compared to baseline in a series of 10 significant consecutive sample points showing directional monotonicity (for a review, see Hansen & Hillyard, 1980). Finally, we observed that as the P3 was returning to baseline after reaching peak amplitude, there was a longstanding

positivity that appeared to plateau differentially for the On and Off laser conditions with a return to baseline apparently more imminent for the Off condition.

Source Localization

Standardized Low Resolution Brain Electromagnetic Tomography

The grand-average ERP waveforms for each condition were transformed to standardized low resolution brain electromagnetic tomography (sLORETA) current source density (CSD) inverse solution files. This inverse solution algorithm has fewer free parameters than principal and independent component analyses and uses the global field power instead of an average reference as a standard. These files were then visualized to localize the neural generator sources at the study level (see Figures 6.6 and 6.7). Additionally, each participant's ERP waveform was submitted to a nonparametric permutation test that tested each condition at its respective deflection latency (i.e., P1: 115–145; N1: 145–180; P2: 200–235; P3: 300–450 ms) against its baseline.

RESULTS

Behavior

Hit Rate

The condition main effect was statistically significant, $F(1, 16) = 6.84, p = 0.019, \eta_p^2 = 0.30$. Participants were more accurate at responding to the target laser bursts in the On condition ($M = 88.34\%$) relative to the Off condition ($M = 85.54\%$), $p = 0.019$ (see Figure 6.2). There was a significant main effect of attended location, $F(1, 16) = 4.80, p = 0.044, \eta_p^2 = 0.23$. Attended targets in the right hemifield ($M = 88.04\%$) were responded to more accurately than attended targets in the left hemifield ($M = 85.90\%$), $p = 0.044$. The condition × attended location interaction was nonsignificant, $F < 1$.

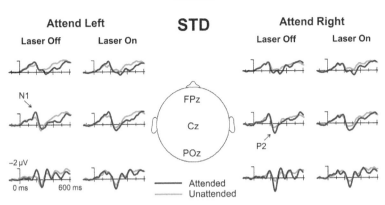

FIGURE 6.3 Grand-averaged event-related potentials (ERPs, referenced to average mastoids) to unattended and attended frequent "standard" (STD) stimuli over three midline sites. Negativity is plotted upwards.

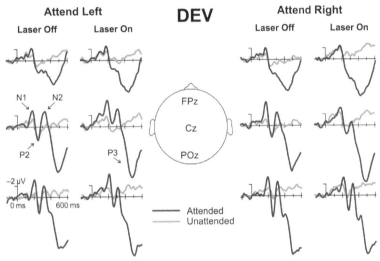

FIGURE 6.4 Grand-averaged event-related potentials (ERPs, referenced to average mastoids) to unattended and attended infrequent "deviant" (DEV) stimuli over three midline sites. Negativity is plotted upwards.

False Alarm Rate

Neither the main effects nor the interaction were statistically significant, $Fs < 3.98$ and $ps > 0.063$.

Reaction Time

The condition main effect was statistically significant, $F (1, 16) = 7.22$, $p = 0.016$, $\eta_p^2 = 0.31$. Participants were faster at responding to the target laser bursts in the On condition ($M = 497.44$ ms) relative to the Off condition ($M = 510.77$ ms), $p = 0.016$. Neither the main effect of attended location nor the condition × attended location interaction was significant, $Fs < 1.25$ and $ps > 0.28$.

Event-Related Potentials

When visual, laser dot stimuli were projected onto the fists of participants, relative to laser dots being projected onto a table, a shift from occipital regions to centroparietal regions occurred in the topographical isopotential maps (see Figure 6.5). In the Off conditions,

attended standard laser stimuli elicited an occipital, contralateral N1 and unattended stimuli elicited a centroparietal, contralateral N1. In the On condition, attended and unattended standard stimuli elicited a centroparietal, contralateral N1 that was more shifted to parietal regions for unattended standard stimuli. The same pattern arose for the deviant laser stimuli (see Figures 6.3 and 6.4).

P1: The anterior–posterior cluster main effect was statistically significant, $F (1, 16) = 15.17$, $p = 0.001$, $\eta_p^2 = 0.47$. No other main effects were statistically significant, $Fs < 1$. The condition × attention × stimulus location and condition × stimulus location × anterior–posterior cluster 3-way interactions were significant, $F (1, 16) = 5.38$, $p = 0.03$, $\eta_p^2 = 0.25$ and $F (1, 16) = 10.01$, $p = 0.0001$, $\eta_p^2 = 0.62$, respectively.

However, the main effect and 3-way interactions were moderated by two significant 4-way interactions. The condition × attention × stimulus location × anterior–posterior cluster and condition × stimulus

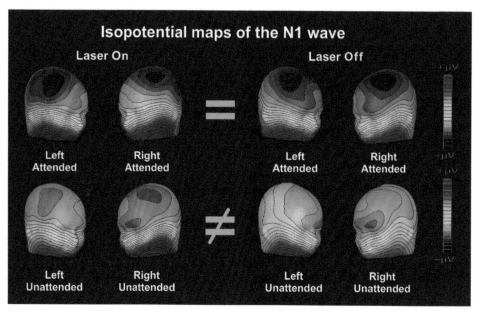

FIGURE 6.5   Isopotential maps of the N1 wave distribution based on grand-average data.

location × anterior–posterior cluster × laterality 4-way interactions were necessary to assess a laterality effect, and they were significant, $F(1,16)=5.95, p=0.03, \eta_p^2=0.27$ and $F(1,16)=10.17, p=0.005, \eta_p^2=0.39$, respectively. For the condition × attention × stimulus location × anterior–posterior cluster interaction, when participants attended to left laser stimuli the P1 mean amplitude was larger in the Off condition $(M=0.14\,\mu V)$ relative to the On condition $(M=-0.23\,\mu V)$, $p=0.003$.

For the condition × stimulus location × anterior–posterior cluster × laterality interaction, the P1 mean amplitude was more positive and contralateral in the occipital cluster for the laser Off condition $(M=0.11\,\mu V)$ when compared to the laser On condition $(M=-0.42\,\mu V)$, $p=0.001$. No other lower- or higher-order interactions were statistically significant, $Fs<3.5$ and $ps<0.10$.

N1: There was a main effect of attention, $F(1,16)=37.08, p=0.005, \eta_p^2=0.40$. The condition × stimulus location, condition × laterality, and stimulus location × laterality 2-way interactions were significant, $F(1,16)=21.09, p=0.001, \eta_p^2=0.57$, $F(1,16)=5.02, p=0.04, \eta_p^2=0.24$, and $F(1,16)=29.54, p=0.0001, \eta_p^2=0.65$, respectively. The condition × attention × stimulus location, condition × stimulus location × anterior–posterior cluster, and condition × attention × laterality 3-way interactions were significant, $F(1,16)=9.48, p=0.007, \eta_p^2=0.37$, $F(1,16)=10.08, p=0.006, \eta_p^2=0.39$, and $F(1,16)=8.30, p=0.01, \eta_p^2=0.34$, respectively.

However, the main effect and lower-order interactions were moderated by the condition × stimulus location × anterior–posterior cluster × laterality 4-way interaction, $F(1,16)=8.21, p=0.01, \eta_p^2=0.34$. In line with the P1 deflection findings, the mean N1 amplitude was more negative and more contralateral in the right parietal cluster for the laser On condition $(M=-2.31\,\mu V)$ when compared to the laser Off condition $(M=-1.05\,\mu V)$, $p=0.001$. No other lower- or higher-order interactions were statistically significant, $Fs<3.5$ and $ps<0.10$.

P2: No main effects were significant, $Fs<3.2$. The condition × laterality, stimulus location × laterality, and anterior–posterior cluster 2-way interactions were significant, $F(1,16)=25.12, p=0.001, \eta_p^2=0.61$, $F(1,16)=40.81, p=0.001, \eta_p^2=0.72$, and $F(1,16)=13.72, p=0.001, \eta_p^2=0.46$, respectively. The condition × attention × laterality, attention × stimulus location × laterality, attention × anterior–posterior cluster × laterality, and stimulus location × anterior–posterior cluster × laterality 3-way interactions were significant, $F(1,16)=38.46, p=0.001, \eta_p^2=0.71$, $F(1,16)=10.11, p=0.006, \eta_p^2=0.39$, $F(1,16)=4.57, p=0.048, \eta_p^2=0.22$, and $F(1,16)=11.97, p=0.003, \eta_p^2=0.43$, respectively.

However, the 3-way interactions were moderated by the significant condition × attention × anterior–posterior cluster × laterality 4-way interaction, $F(1,16)=5.23, p=0.036, \eta_p^2=0.25$. Specifically, when participants attended their left hemifield, a smaller P2 mean amplitude in the ipsilateral (left), parietal cluster was elicited in the On condition $(M=0.17\,\mu V)$ when compared to the Off condition $(M=0.44\,\mu V)$, $p<0.01$. Similarly, when participants attended their left hemifield, a smaller P2 mean amplitude in the contralateral (right), parietal cluster was elicited in the On condition $(M=0.39\,\mu V)$ when compared to the Off condition $(M=0.68\,\mu V)$, $p<0.01$. Thus, the P2 mean amplitude was attenuated for both the left and right parietal areas for when lasers were projected

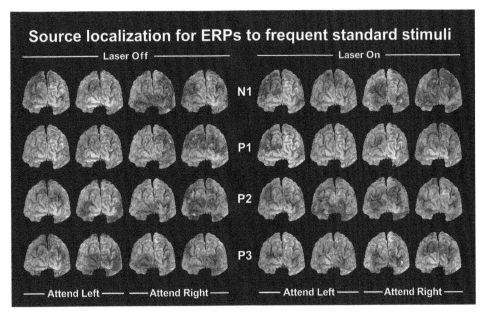

FIGURE 6.6 sLORETA-based three-dimensional distributions of current density for frequent "standard" stimuli for the two experimental conditions laser On vs. Off.

on their hands, relative to when the lasers were projected off their hands onto the table.

When participants attended their right hemifield, a larger P2 mean amplitude in the contralateral (left), occipital cluster was elicited in the On condition ($M = 1.15\,\mu V$) when compared to the Off condition ($M = 0.39\,\mu V$), $p < 0.01$. Similarly, when participants attended their right hemifield, a larger P2 mean amplitude in the contralateral (left), parietal cluster was elicited in the On condition ($M = 0.96\,\mu V$) when compared to the Off condition ($M = 0.37\,\mu V$), $p < 0.01$. Thus, the P2 mean amplitude was larger for both the occipital and parietal areas of their left hemisphere when lasers were projected on their hands, relative to when the lasers were projected off their hands onto the table.

P3: The main effect of anterior–posterior cluster was statistically significant, $F(1, 16) = 5.17, p = 0.037, \eta_p^2 = 0.24$. The target location × laterality and condition × anterior–posterior cluster 2-way interactions were significant, $F(1, 16) = 16.84, p = 0.001, \eta_p^2 = 0.51$ and $F(1, 16) = 16.51, p = 0.001, \eta_p^2 = 0.51$, respectively. However, the 2-way interactions were moderated by the significant condition × target location × anterior–posterior cluster × laterality 4-way interaction, $F(1, 16) = 5.17, p = 0.037, \eta_p^2 = 0.24$. In particular, in the laser On condition, left laser stimuli elicited a contralateral right hemisphere P3 deflection and had a higher mean amplitude in the parietal cluster ($M = 6.73\,\mu V$) relative to the occipital cluster ($M = 4.95\,\mu V$), $p = 0.009$. Similarly, right laser stimuli elicited a contralateral left hemisphere P3 deflection and had a higher mean amplitude in the parietal cluster ($M = 6.95\,\mu V$) relative to the occipital cluster ($M = 5.44\,\mu V$), $p = 0.014$.

Standardized Low Resolution Brain Electromagnetic Tomography

Based on scalp-recorded multichannel data, the sLORETA software was used to compute the three-dimensional distribution of current density (see Figures 6.6 and 6.7). This procedure achieves exact localizations to test point sources but has the property of low spatial resolution on the order of about 5mm (Pascual-Marqui, 2002). This procedure further confirmed and detailed observations based on simple inspection of ERP waveforms and isopotential maps by showing robust differences between the experimental conditions.

The Tables 6.1–6.4 (see Appendix) contain the results of sLORETA-based, statistical nonparametric mapping for statistically significant parts of the P1, N1, P2, and P3. The data were not baseline-corrected; the *p* values were derived by using nonparametric paired *t*-tests.

DISCUSSION

In terms of behavior, it was hypothesized that the hit rate RT would be fastest when laser stimuli were projected onto the hands (On condition) when compared to the hit rate RT when these stimuli were projected onto a surface (Off condition). In addition, the error rate was expected to be smaller in the On condition when compared to the Off condition. It was found that behavioral performance was faster and more accurate in the On condition relative to the Off condition. This evidence was consistent with reports demonstrating faster and more

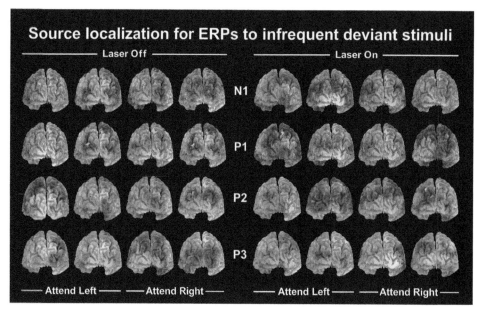

FIGURE 6.7   sLORETA-based three-dimensional distributions of current density for infrequent "deviant" stimuli for the two experimental conditions laser On vs. Off.

accurate behavioral performance when stimuli fall into peripersonal space compared to stimuli outside peripersonal space (Dufour & Touzalin, 2008; Hari & Jousmäki, 1996). It has also been shown that responses of perihand neurons are anchored to the hand itself and represent a combination of proprioceptive, visual, and tactile inputs, and are therefore of multimodal nature (Brozzoli et al., 2012; Graziano et al., 1997).

It was hypothesized that the distribution for the ERP waveforms and topographical isopotential maps for the P1, N1, P2, and P3 deflections would be lateralized for visual stimuli. Indeed, the P1, N1, P2, and P3 deflections did result in lateralized activity in agreement with past visual evoked potential studies (e.g., Witelson, 1976). The lateralization effect found showed a stronger lateralization for the right hemisphere when compared to the left hemisphere lateralization. Again, this is consistent with results that have found a spatial processing specialization for the right hemisphere (Witelson, 1976).

Additionally, it was expected that the deflections of interest would be more occipital in the Off condition and more parietal in the On condition. When the visual stimuli were projected on the participants' fists (i.e., in their peripersonal space), the lateralized occipital activation was shifted to anterior centroparietal regions irrespective of the attention manipulation, as evidenced by the isopotential topographical maps. The sLORETA CSD source localization maps supported this pattern of neural activity (see Figures 6.6 and 6.7).

The P2 deflection was analyzed to determine whether it was sensitive to the peripersonal space manipulation (i.e., On vs. Off conditions). Qian et al. (2012) conducted

a visual evoked potential experiment with the use of checkerboard reversals (centrally or peripherally presented) that participants had to attend to while their hands were either proximal or distal to the screen where the stimuli were presented. It was found that when participants attended to the stimulus that was proximal to their hands, there was a P2 attenuation that was absent when participants attended to the stimulus that was distal to their hands.

The current results are consistent with these findings and indicate that in the On condition P2 mean amplitude was attenuated for both the left and right parietal areas when left-attended lasers were projected on their hands, relative to left-attended lasers that were projected off their hands and onto the table. However, the findings of Qian et al. did not explicitly analyze laterality effects, and the current findings showed that both left and right parietal areas were attenuated for stimuli within peripersonal space. Another dissimilarity to the findings of Qian et al. is that the P2 mean amplitude was larger in the left hemisphere of participants for both occipital and parietal areas when right-attended lasers were projected on their hands, relative to right-attended lasers that were projected off their hands and onto the table. Further, the present findings show a bilateral parietal area effect when participants attend to left hemispace that was not analyzed and obtained in the findings of Qian et al. (2012). Additionally, a unilateral (left; contralateral) occipital and parietal area effect is found when participants attend to right hemispace.

For the sLORETA source localization, in the On conditions, attended and unattended deviant stimuli showed an occipital lobe neural origin. In the On conditions, attended and unattended deviant stimuli showed a centroparietal and frontal lobe neural origin. These results suggest that when visual stimuli are projected within peripersonal space, multisensory and tactile neural regions are recruited when compared to the visual stimuli that are not projected within peripersonal space. In particular, for the On condition, more parietal region generators were found whether or not the visual laser stimuli were attended or unattended. For the Off condition, more occipital region generators were found (see Tables 6.1–6.4, Appendix). The three measure types (i.e., behavioral, ERP, and source localization) suggest that visual stimuli presented within peripersonal space are processed as bimodal (i.e., visuo-haptic) stimuli (by recruiting somatosensory cortices) and are just processed as unimodal (i.e., visual) stimuli when presented outside of an observer's peripersonal space representation.

APPENDIX

TABLE 6.1 Off-Condition, sLORETA-Based, Statistical Nonparametric Mapping of the P1 and N1 Neural Generators

	P1			N1		
Condition	BA	Region	p-value	BA	Region	p-value
OFFAL_LDEV	32	CG	<0.01	24	CG	<0.01
OFFAL_LSTD	6	MFG	<0.01	6	MFG	<0.01
OFFAL_RDEV	19	C	<0.01	34	SG	<0.01
OFFAL_RSTD	40	PostG	<0.01	6	MFG	<0.01
OFFAR_LDEV	9	MFG	<0.01	23	PC	<0.01
OFFAR_LSTD	32	CG	<0.01	6	MFG	<0.01
OFFAR_RDEV	32	MFG	<0.01	24	CG	<0.01
OFFAR_RSTD	6	MFG	<0.01	6	MFG	<0.01

Abbreviations: AC, Anterior Cingulate; AG, Angular Gyrus; BA, Brodmann Area; C, Cuneus; CG, Cingulate Gyrus; IFG, Inferior Frontal Gyrus; IOG, Inferior Occipital Gyrus; IPL, Inferior Parietal Lobule; MFG, Medial Frontal Gyrus; MOG, Middle Occipital Gyrus; MTG, Medial Temporal Gyrus; P, Precuneus; PC, Posterior Cingulate; PG, Precentral Gyrus; PostG, Postcentral Gyrus; SFG, Superior Frontal Gyrus; SG, Subcallosal Gyrus; S-G, Sub-Gyral; SPL, Superior Parietal Lobule; STG, Superior Temporal Gyrus.
Experimental conditions: Laser (Off/On), Attend Left (AL), Attend Right (AR), left (L) and right (R) location, frequent standard stimulus (STD), infrequent deviant stimulus (DEV).

TABLE 6.2 Off-Condition, sLORETA-Based, Statistical Nonparametric Mapping of the P2 and P3 Neural Generators

	P2			P3		
Condition	BA	Region	p-value	BA	Region	p-value
OFFAL_LDEV	32	AC	<0.01	40	IPL	<0.01
OFFAL_LSTD	3	PostG	<0.01	24	CG	<0.01
OFFAL_RDEV	24	CG	<0.01	41	STG	<0.01
OFFAL_RSTD	4	PG	<0.01	6	S-G	<0.01
OFFAR_LDEV	30	PC	<0.01	4	PG	<0.01
OFFAR_LSTD	6	MFG	<0.01	24	CG	<0.01
OFFAR_RDEV	22	STG	<0.01	47	IFG	<0.01
OFFAR_RSTD	37	MTG	<0.01	33	AC	<0.01

For abbreviations see Table 6.1.

TABLE 6.3   On-Condition, sLORETA-Based, Statistical Nonparametric Mapping of the P1 and N1 Neural Generators

	P1			N1		
Condition	BA	Region	p-value	BA	Region	p-value
ONAL_LDEV	6	MFG	<0.01	6	MFG	<0.01
ONAL_LSTD	39	AG	<0.01	39	MTG	<0.01
ONAL_RDEV	18	C	<0.01	18	MOG	<0.01
ONAL_RSTD	19	P	<0.01	6	PG	<0.01
ONAR_LDEV	39	MTG	<0.01	6	PG	<0.01
ONAR_LSTD	24	CG	<0.01	24	CG	<0.01
ONAR_RDEV	40	IPL	<0.01	43	PostG	<0.01
ONAR_RSTD	8	SFG	<0.01	32	AC	<0.01

For abbreviations see Table 6.1.

TABLE 6.4   On-Condition, sLORETA-Based, Statistical Nonparametric Mapping of the P2 and P3 Neural Generators

	P2			P3		
Condition	BA	Region	p-value	BA	Region	p-value
ONAL_LDEV	6	MFG	<0.01	40	PostG	<0.01
ONAL_LSTD	31	CG	<0.01	22	STG	<0.01
ONAL_RDEV	19	C	<0.01	10	MFG	<0.01
ONAL_RSTD	18	IOG	<0.01	31	PC	<0.01
ONAR_LDEV	40	IPL	<0.01	31	CG	<0.01
ONAR_LSTD	39	MTG	<0.01	18	MOG	<0.01
ONAR_RDEV	7	SPL	<0.01	43	PG	<0.01
ONAR_RSTD	24	CG	<0.01	18	C	<0.01

For abbreviations see Table 6.1.

Acknowledgments

The authors thank Enrique Alvarez-Vazquez and Dr Thomas Campbell for technical assistance and Mrs. Christy D. Bright for editing and proofreading. This project was funded by the National Center for Research Resources (NCRR), National Institutes of Health (NIH), P20 RR020151. Its contents are solely the responsibility of the authors and do not necessarily represent the official views of NCRR or NIH.

References

Brozzoli, C., Gentile, G., & Ehrsson, H. H. (2012). That's near my hand! Parietal and premotor coding of hand-centered space contributes to localization and self-attribution of the hand. *The Journal of Neuroscience*, *32*(42), 14573–14582.

Dufour, A., & Touzalin, P. (2008). Improved visual sensitivity in the perihand space. *Experimental Brain Research*, *190*, 91–98.

Graziano, M. S. A., Hu, X. T., & Gross, C. G. (1997). Coding the locations of objects in the dark. *Science*, *277*, 239–241.

Graziano, M. S. A., Reiss, L. A. J., & Gross, C. J. (1999). A neuronal representation of the location of nearby sounds. *Nature*, *397*, 428–430.

Hansen, J. C. & Hillyard, S. A. (1980). Endogenous brain potentials associated with selective auditory attention. *Electroencephalography and Clinical Neurophysiology*, *49*, 277–290.

Hari, R., & Jousmäki, V. (1996). Preference of personal to extrapersonal space in a visuomotor task. *Journal of Cognitive Neuroscience*, *8*, 305–307.

Làdavas, E., Zeloni, G., & Farnè, A. (1998). Visual peripersonal space centred on the face in humans. *Brain*, *121*, 2317–2326.

Levine, T. R., & Hullett, C. R. (2002). Eta squared, partial eta squared and the misreporting of effect size in communication research. *Human Communication Research*, *28*, 612–625.

Lloyd, D., Azañón, E., & Poliakoff, E. (2010). Right hand presence modulates shifts of exogenous visuospatial attention in near perihand space. *Brain and Cognition*, *73*, 102–109.

Lloyd, D., Morrison, I., & Roberts, N. (2006). Role for human posterior parietal cortex in visual processing of aversive objects in peripersonal space. *Journal of Neurophysiology*, *95*, 205–214.

Meredith, M. A., & Stein, B. E. (1986). Visual, auditory, and somatosensory convergence on cells in the superior colliculus results in multisensory integration. *Journal of Neurophysiology*, *56*, 640–662.

Pascual-Marqui, R. D. (2002). Standardized low resolution brain electromagnetic tomography (sLORETA): technical details. *Methods & Findings in Experimental & Clinical Pharmacology*, *24D*, 5–12.

Qian, C., Al-Aidroos, N., West, G., Abrams, R. A., & Pratt, J. (2012). The visual P2 is attenuated for attended objects near the hands. *Cognitive Neuroscience*, *1*, 1–7.

Richardson, J. T. E. (2011). Eta squared and partial eta squared as measures of effect size in educational research. *Educational Research Review*, *6*(2), 135–147.

Simon-Dack, S. L., Cummings, S. E., Reetz, D. J., Alvarez-Vazquez, E., Gu, H., & Teder-Sälejärvi, W. A. (2009). "Touched" by light: event-related potentials (ERPs) to visuo-haptic stimuli in peri-personal space. *Brain Topography*, *21*, 261–268.

Stein, B. E., & Meredith, M. A. (1993). *The merging of the senses*. Cambridge, MA: MIT Press.

Stricanne, B., Andersen, R. A., & Mazzoni, P. (1996). Eye-centered, head-centered, and intermediate coding of remembered sound locations in area lip. *Journal of Neurophysiology*, *76*, 2071–2076.

Witelson, D. F. (1976). Sex and the single hemisphere: specialization of the right hemisphere for spatial processing. *Science*, *193*, 425–427.

7

Involuntary Cross-Modal Spatial Attention Influences Visual Perception

John J. McDonald[1], Jennifer C. Whitman[1], Viola S. Störmer[2],
Steven A. Hillyard[3]

[1]Department of Psychology, Simon Fraser University, Burnaby, BC, Canada, [2]Harvard University, Vision Sciences Laboratory, Cambridge, MA, USA, [3]Department of Neurosciences, University of California San Diego, La Jolla, CA, USA

One of the most firmly established findings in cognitive psychology is that directing attention to a specific location in the visual field results in facilitated responses to subsequent target stimuli at that location (Posner, Snyder, & Davidson, 1980; Wright & Ward, 2008). This spatial cueing effect has been observed in one form or another regardless of the modalities of the cue and target stimuli and regardless of whether attention is directed voluntarily or captured involuntarily by the cue (Prime, McDonald, Green, & Ward, 2008; Spence, McDonald, & Driver, 2004). An enduring controversy has revolved around the question of whether spatial cueing facilitates the early sensory/perceptual processing of target stimuli or has its influence on postperceptual decision and response processes. Psychophysical studies in the visual modality over the past 30 years have provided ample evidence that spatial attention can affect both early sensory and late decision stages of target processing (for reviews, see Carrasco, 2011; Dosher & Lu, 2000; Smith & Ratcliff, 2009). Electrophysiological recordings of event-related brain potentials (ERPs) in spatial cueing tasks have reinforced the view that the processing of targets at attended locations is facilitated at early levels of the visual-cortical pathways (Hopfinger, Luck, & Hillyard, 2004; Luck et al., 1994; reviewed in Mangun & Hillyard, 1991).

CROSS-MODAL CUEING OF ATTENTION ENHANCES PERCEPTUAL SENSITIVITY

The focus of the present chapter is on a series of cross-modal spatial cueing studies that were designed to isolate auditory cueing effects on visual-perceptual processing from decision-level influences. In these studies, psychophysical measures of perceptual processing were combined with ERP recordings to investigate the neural mechanisms by which an auditory cue influences the perception of a subsequent visual target. The first study in this series (McDonald, Teder-Sälejärvi, & Hillyard, 2000) used a signal detection/postcue design in which an auditory cue presented to the left or right side was followed unpredictably by a visual masking stimulus at the same or opposite location as the sound. The task of the participants was to indicate whether or not a weak, threshold-level target preceded the much brighter mask. Since the participant responded only to the information at the location of the mask, which also served as a postcue, this design eliminated the possibility that the auditory cue could have the decision-level effect of reducing the uncertainty of the target's location (Luck et al., 1994).

The results showed that the perceptual sensitivity (d') for detecting the visual target was higher when the target-mask complex was presented at the same location as the preceding auditory cue than when it appeared in the opposite visual field (herein termed valid and invalid trials; Figure 7.1(A)). McDonald and colleagues hypothesized that the auditory cue triggered an automatic shift of attention to its location, which then resulted in enhanced perceptual processing of the subsequent visual stimuli at that location (see also Dufour, 1999; Frassinetti, Bolognini, & Làdavas, 2002). An analogous effect of visual cueing on auditory signal detection was reported by Soto-Faraco, McDonald, and Kingstone (2002), which supports the idea that both sounds and lights activate a common supramodal attentional orienting system that

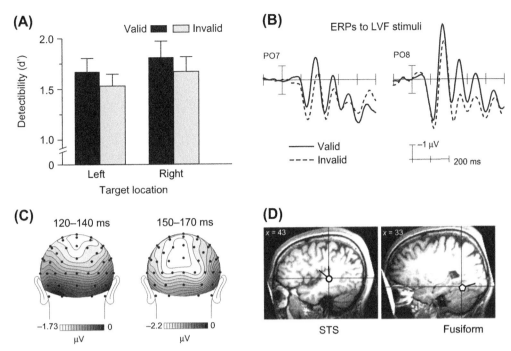

FIGURE 7.1 Cross-modal cueing improves visual perception. (A) Perceptual sensitivity is higher for threshold-level visual targets appearing at the location of a preceding auditory cue than for targets appearing at invalidly cued locations. (B) Grand-averaged ERPs to left-visual-field probes, recorded from electrodes over the left and right occipital scalp (PO7 & PO8). (C) Topographical maps of the valid-minus-invalid differences shown in panel C. (D) Dipolar sources underlying the valid-minus-invalid differences in the 120–170 ms time range. *Source: From McDonald et al. (2000, 2003).*

improves the perceptual quality of stimulus events at the cued location (Farah, Wong, Monheit, & Morrow, 1989).

Recordings of ERPs in this cross-modal cueing paradigm provided confirmatory evidence of a cueing effect on early perceptual processing (McDonald, Teder-Sälejärvi, Di Russo, & Hillyard, 2003). The ERPs elicited by the visual mask presented at the cued and uncued locations began to diverge as early as 100 ms after mask onset (Figure 7.1(B)). The initial phase of this cueing effect on the visual ERP was localized using dipole modeling to the region of the superior temporal cortex, and a subsequent phase beginning 30–40 ms later was localized to the inferior occipito-temporal visual cortex in or near the fusiform gyrus (Figure 7.1(C) and (D)). This spatiotemporal pattern suggested that cross-modal cueing facilitates early visual processing in the ventral visual pathways via a feedback projection from the polymodal region of the superior temporal lobe to the extrastriate visual cortex (see also Macaluso, Frith, & Driver, 2000).

CROSS-MODAL INFLUENCES ON TIME-ORDER PERCEPTION

The signal-detection studies outlined above showed that cross-modal cueing of attention enhances visual perceptual sensitivity. Around the same time, researchers were starting to ask whether the capture of attention

by nonvisual cues would speed up visual perceptual processing and facilitate awareness of competing visual stimuli (Shimojo, Miyauchi, & Hikosaka, 1997). The idea that attended stimuli might be perceived earlier in time than physically identical unattended stimuli has been around for over 100 years (Titchener, 1908). Recent inquiries into this "law of prior entry" have used temporal order judgment (TOJ) tasks in which observers report which of two rapidly presented stimuli occurs first. The general finding has been that when attended and unattended visual stimuli are presented simultaneously, observers report that the attended stimulus appears to occur first (Shore, Spence, & Klein, 2001; Stelmach & Herdman, 1991). Of particular relevance to the hypothesis that spatial attention has supramodal influences, Shimojo and colleagues (Shimojo et al., 1997) found that visual stimuli at attended locations were perceived earlier than at unattended locations even when shifts in attention were induced by spatially nonpredictive auditory or tactile cues.

Not surprisingly, these cueing effects on TOJ have been subjected to the traditional wrangling over whether they represent a true perceptual phenomenon as opposed to a biasing of postperceptual decisions. In the latter view, observers might actually perceive two targets as appearing simultaneously but still report the cued side first because of a decision bias that favors the cued target (Pashler, 1998; Schneider & Bavelier, 2003; Shore et al.,

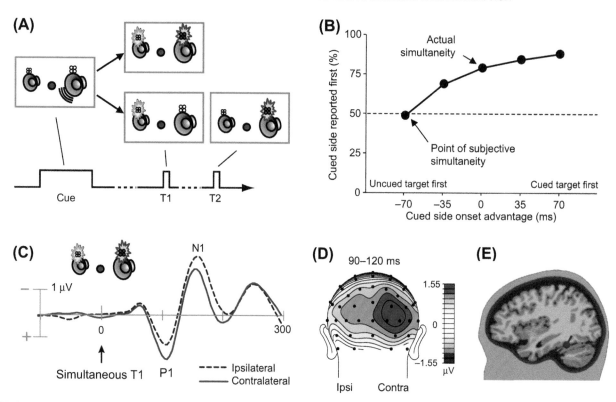

FIGURE 7.2 Cross-modal cueing produces perceptual prior entry. (A) An auditory cue was presented 100–300 ms before a pair of brief visual targets. The targets were presented simultaneously on 50% of trials. (B) Mean percentage of trials in which observers reported seeing the target at the cued location first, as a function of the lead time of the cued-side target (cued-side onset advantage; CSOA). Negative and positive CSOAs indicate the target on the uncued side and the cued side appeared first, respectively. (C) Grand-average ERPs elicited by simultaneous visual targets, recorded from occipital electrodes (PO7/PO8) contralateral and ipsilateral to the cued location. (D) Topographical map of the simultaneous-target ERPs in the time range of the P1. (E) Localization of the dipolar source underlying the contralateral-minus-ipsilateral differences in the time range of the P1. *Source: From McDonald et al. (2005).*

2001). While appropriate experimental designs can mitigate such response bias effects, they are difficult to rule out entirely. ERP recordings bring important evidence to bear on the perceptual vs postperceptual conundrum by revealing whether cueing effects on TOJ are associated with changes in the neural response to targets in the visual cortex. Moreover, cueing effects on the latencies of the target-elicited ERPs can shed light on the question of whether changes in the perceived timing of visual events are encoded by the timing of neural events in the relevant brain pathways or whether perceived timing is represented by some nontemporal aspect of neural activity (Dennett, 1991).

McDonald, Teder-Sälejärvi, Di Russo, and Hillyard (2005) recorded ERPs in a TOJ experiment in which a spatially nonpredictive auditory cue was presented on the left or right side of a video monitor just prior to a bilateral pair of simultaneous or near-simultaneous visual targets (Figure 7.2(A)). As in previous studies, this lateralized cue had a strong effect on the judgments of the temporal order of the two visual targets (Figure 7.2(B)). When the targets actually occurred simultaneously, observers judged the target on the cued side to occur first in 79%

of the trials. In order to achieve perceptual simultaneity, the target on the uncued side had to be presented nearly 70 ms before the target on the cued side.

To study the neural basis of this cross-modal cueing effect on TOJ, McDonald et al. (2005) recorded ERPs to simultaneous visual targets. Contrary to the view that the time course of perceptual experience is based on the timing of target-evoked activity in the visual cortex, there were no latency differences observed between early occipital ERP components recorded contralaterally and ipsilaterally with respect to the side of the auditory cue (Figure 7.2(C)). Instead, cross-modal cueing produced an increased early ERP positivity over the visual cortex contralateral to the cued side without any change in component latencies (Figure 7.2(D)). This positivity began in the latency range of the P1 component (90–120 ms), and its neural generators were localized by dipole modeling to the ventral extrastriate visual cortex (Figure 7.2(E)). This finding suggests that the perceptual prior entry of the target on the cued side is a consequence of a stronger neural response in the contralateral visual cortex induced by cross-modal cueing rather than an actual speeding of neural transmission. How might a stronger neural response lead to earlier perceptual awareness of the cued target? One possibility is that the enhanced response to the cued target causes a perceptual threshold to be reached earlier at a subsequent stage of processing.

These effects of spatially nonpredictive auditory cueing on visual signal detection (McDonald et al., 2000) and TOJ (McDonald et al., 2005) may be interpreted as consequences of the *involuntary* deployment of spatial attention to the location of a sudden sound. While we found that changes in visual ERP amplitude rather than latency were associated with these perceptual effects produced by involuntary orienting, Vibell, Klinge, Zampini, Spence, and Nobre (2007) reported that a small latency change (4 ms) in the visual ERP in association with a much larger visual TOJ effect was produced by the voluntary allocation of attention to the visual modality. This finding raises the possibility that attending voluntarily to the visual modality affects the timing of early visually evoked activity, whereas the involuntary orienting of attention to a location affects only the amplitude of early visual activity. In any case, the finding of early ERP modulations associated with attention-induced TOJ effects provides compelling evidence that cross-modal attention affects early visual-sensory processing and is not solely a consequence of higher-order decision or response biases as proposed by Santangelo and Spence (2008) (see McDonald, Green, Störmer, & Hillyard, 2012 for a more detailed discussion).

CROSS-MODAL CUEING OF ATTENTION ALTERS VISUAL APPEARANCE

The findings outlined in the previous sections indicate that orienting attention reflexively to a sudden sound alters the perception of subsequent visual targets and produces a concomitant boost of target-evoked neural activity in the extrastriate visual cortex. However, none of these studies directly addressed the question of whether orienting attention to sound alters the subjective appearance of visual objects. If an observer were to hear a snap of a twig off to one side, would the colors of visual objects in the vicinity of the sound source appear more colorful than the colors of objects at other locations? Would orienting attention make white objects appear whiter and dark objects appear darker? Psychologists have wondered whether attention alters appearance in such ways for over a century (e.g., Fechner, 1882; Helmholtz, 1866; James, 1890).

Carrasco and colleagues developed a psychophysical paradigm to determine whether attention alters appearance (Carrasco, Ling, & Read, 2004). The paradigm is similar to the TOJ paradigm except that, rather than varying the stimulus onset asynchrony (SOA) between two visual targets and asking participants to judge which one was first, the luminance contrast of two targets is varied and participants are asked to judge which one is higher in contrast. In the original variant of the task, a small, abruptly onsetting black dot was used to summon attention to the left or right just prior to the appearance of two Gabor patches (sinusoidal gratings) at both the left and right locations. When the contrasts of the two Gabor patches were physically similar or identical, observers tended to judge the one on the cued side as being higher in contrast. Based on these and other similar results, Carrasco and colleagues concluded that attention alters the subjective appearance of visual stimuli (for a review, see Carrasco, 2006).

The conclusion that attention altered appearance in these visual-cueing studies met some stiff opposition. One concern was that the apparent boost in contrast was due to sensory interactions between the visual cue and the Gabor patch at the cued location (Schneider, 2006; Schneider & Komlos, 2008). For example, a high-contrast cue such as a black-on-gray abrupt onset might be assimilated with the cued-location Gabor, leading to an attention-independent boost in perceived contrast. Another concern was that the apparent perceptual effect actually reflected a decision- or response-level bias to report the cued Gabor as being higher in contrast (Prinzmetal, Long, & Leonhardt, 2008; Schneider & Komlos, 2008). As was noted earlier, ERPs can be used to help determine whether cue effects are due to changes at early, perceptual stages of processing or at later, decision- or response-level stages.

Störmer, McDonald, and Hillyard (2009) recorded ERPs in a modified version of Carrasco and colleagues' contrast-judgment task to investigate whether orienting attention reflexively to a sound might alter visual appearance. The visual cue was replaced by a spatially nonpredictive noise burst delivered 25° to the left or right of fixation. After a short SOA (150 ms on most trials), two Gabor patches were presented, one at the cued location and one on the opposite side of fixation (Figure 7.3(A)). The subject's specific task was to report the orientation of the Gabor patch that was judged to have higher contrast. The psychophysical findings paralleled those reported by Carrasco et al. (2004). Notably, observers reported the orientation of the cued-location Gabor significantly more often than the uncued-location Gabor (55% vs 45%) when the two Gabors had the same physical contrast (Figure 7.3(B)). This finding indicates that the onset of a salient-but-irrelevant sound boosts the subjective contrast of nearby visual stimuli when the cue–target SOA is in the traditional range of exogenous attention effects. Critically, this cueing effect cannot be attributed to

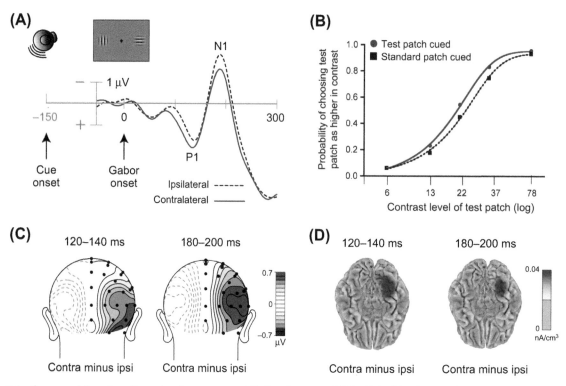

FIGURE 7.3 Cross-modal cueing alters visual appearance. (A) Grand-average ERPs elicited by the equal-contrast Gabor display, recorded from occipital electrodes (PO7/PO8) contralateral and ipsilateral to the side of the auditory cue. ERPs were from short-SOA trials in which the auditory cue preceded the Gabors by 150 ms. (B) Mean probability of reporting the contrast of the test Gabor to be higher than the contrast of the standard Gabor. The contrast of the standard was set at 22%, whereas the contrast of the test varied from trial to trial. The probability of reporting the test Gabor as being higher in contrast was increased when that Gabor appeared at the cued location. (C) Topographical maps of the differences between contralateral and ipsilateral waveforms shown in panel A, in the time ranges of the P1 and N1 peaks. (D) Distributed source activity underlying the contralateral-minus-ipsilateral difference ERP in the time ranges of the P1 and N1 peaks. Source activity was estimated using LAURA and is shown in the contralateral (right) side of the brain only. *Source: From Störmer et al. (2009).*

unimodal sensory interactions such as luminance assimilation because a nonvisual stimulus was used to summon attention.

Störmer et al. (2009) examined the ERPs elicited by the equal-contrast Gabors as a function of cue location to determine whether the lateral noise burst altered visual-perceptual appearance as opposed to a decision or response process. As in the TOJ study outlined in the preceding section, this ERP analysis was premised on the contralateral organization of the visual system and the well-documented lateralized asymmetries of spatial attention effects on the visual ERP (Heinze, Luck, Mangun, & Hillyard, 1990; Luck, Heinze, Mangun, & Hillyard, 1990). Directing attention to one side of such a bilaterally balanced display leads to a larger early positive ERP component at contralateral occipital electrodes than at ipsilateral occipital electrodes (Heinze et al., 1990; Luck et al., 1990; see also McDonald et al., 2005). Based on these earlier findings, Störmer et al. (2009) hypothesized that if the auditory cue captured attention in such a way as to boost visual perceptual processing, the early target-elicited ERP activity over the occipital scalp would be lateralized. Additionally, the authors surmised

that if such attention effects boost perceived contrast, the magnitude of this lateralized ERP activity should correlate with the observers' tendencies to report the cued Gabor as being higher in contrast.

This is exactly what was found. Within 100 ms of target onset, the waveform recorded contralaterally to the cued side became more positive than the waveform recorded ipsilaterally to the cued side, despite the fact that the visual stimuli on the left and right were identical (Figure 7.3(A) and (C)). Importantly, this contralateral positivity was observed only in trials when observers judged the cued-location target to be higher in contrast. Moreover, the tendency to report the cued-location target as being higher in contrast correlated positively with the amplitude of the contralateral ERP positivity measured in the time interval of the P1 component (120–140 ms). Finally, the neural generators of the early contralateral positivity were localized by distributed source analysis to the ventral extrastriate visual cortex (Figure 7.3(D)). Together with the psychophysical findings, these electrophysiological findings provide compelling evidence that cross-modal spatial attention affects visual appearance through modulations at an early sensory–perceptual level rather than by affecting late decision processes.

SALIENT SOUNDS ACTIVATE THE VISUAL CORTEX

Although researchers have pondered the neural mechanisms underlying involuntary cross-modal cue effects for over two decades (e.g., Farah et al., 1989; Macaluso et al., 2000; McDonald et al., 2012; McDonald, Teder-Sälejärvi, & Ward, 2001; Spence & Driver, 1997; Spence et al., 2004; Ward, 1994), little is known about how nonvisual cues come to modulate the processing of subsequent visual targets. Until recently, one outstanding question was whether the nonvisual stimuli used to capture attention in cross-modal cueing paradigms would activate the visual system in the absence of a near-simultaneous visual target. Auditorily evoked occipital activations have been reported in previous functional magnetic resonance imaging (fMRI) studies (e.g., Cate et al., 2009; Wu, Weissman, Roberts, & Woldorff, 2007), but these cross-modal activations were observed in tasks that required the engagement of *voluntary* attention mechanisms.

In addition to modulating the hemodynamic response in the visual cortex, voluntary shifts of spatial attention induced by a symbolic cue have been associated with lateralized ERP components over the posterior scalp in the time interval between the cue and a subsequent target (e.g., Eimer, van Velzen, & Driver, 2002; Eimer, van Velzen, Forster, & Driver, 2003; Green, Teder-Sälejarvi, & McDonald, 2005; Harter, Miller, Price, LaLonde, & Keyes, 1989; Hopf & Mangun, 2000; Nobre, Sebestyen, &

Miniussi, 2000). Interestingly, one such component that has been called the "late attention-directing positivity" (LDAP; occurring 400–800 ms after the onset of a central symbolic cue) appears to originate from the visual cortex and can be observed following nonvisual as well as visual cues (e.g., Eimer et al., 2002; Green et al., 2005). Such findings indicate that orienting attention voluntarily activates the visual cortex even when a nonvisual stimulus is used to initiate the shift of attention. Along these lines, one might expect that orienting attention *involuntarily* to salient, spatially noninformative sounds would also activate the visual cortex, but in a more automatic and fleeting fashion.

Recently, McDonald, Störmer, Martinez, Feng, and Hillyard (2013) sought to determine whether salient but spatially nonpredictive sounds activate the visual cortex and whether such cross-modal activation might be associated with the involuntary cross-modal cue effects on visual perception. They first examined the ERPs elicited by the auditory cue used in the cross-modal contrast-judgment experiment described in the preceding section (Störmer et al., 2009). The analysis focused on long-SOA (630 ms) and no-target trials in which it was possible to record the cue-elicited ERP for several hundreds of milliseconds without an intervening visual stimulus. As expected, the cue elicited the usual auditory ERP components, including the N1 (~100 ms postcue) and P2 (~180 ms postcue) having amplitude maxima over the central scalp. Little ERP activity was seen over the fronto-central scalp following the P2, but a large lateralized ERP positivity emerged over the *occipital* scalp at about 200 ms postcue (Figure 7.4(A)). In the 200–400 ms time range, the ERP recorded over the occipital scalp was significantly more positive contralateral

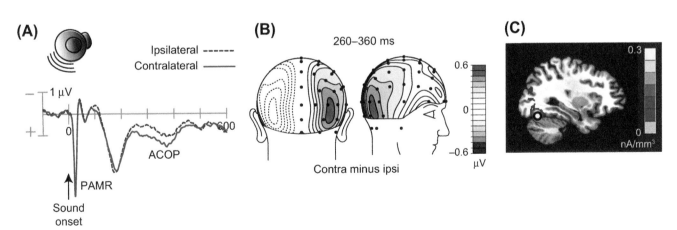

FIGURE 7.4 Salient sounds activate the visual cortex automatically. (A) Grand-average ERPs to a lateral auditory cue in a cross-modal cueing variant of the contrast-judgment task of Carrasco et al. (2004). ERPs were recorded from occipital electrodes (PO7/PO8) contralateral and ipsilateral to the cue's location. A postauricular muscle response (PAMR) occurred immediately following sound onset and was picked up by the reference electrode on the mastoid. An auditorily evoked contralateral occipital positivity (ACOP) occurred 200–400 ms after sound onset. (B) Topographical maps of the difference between contralateral and ipsilateral waveforms shown in panel B, in the time range of the ACOP. (C) Localization of sources underlying the ACOP. The distributed source activity was estimated using LAURA, and the circle represents the location of the best-fitting dipolar source. Both methods placed the neural generators of the ACOP in the ventral occipital cortex. *Source: From McDonald et al. (2013).*

to the cued location than ipsilateral to the cued location. As shown in Figure 7.4(B), the topography of this *auditorily evoked contralateral occipital positivity (ACOP)* resembled other lateralized visual ERP components (e.g. P1, LDAP), and source analyses provided converging evidence that the cortical generator of the ACOP lies within the ventral occipital lobe (Figure 7.4(C)).

As noted in the previous section, participants in this contrast-judgment experiment tended to perceive the cued Gabor as being higher in contrast than the uncued Gabor on the short-SOA trials, even when the physical contrasts of the two Gabors were identical. Critically, this perceptual bias was found to correlate positively with the amplitude of the ACOP: Participants who had larger cue-evoked contralateral positivities over the occipital scalp tended to report seeing the cued Gabor as being higher in contrast on a larger portion of trials. Together with the results of the source analysis, this correlation suggests that the ACOP reflects neural processes within the occipital lobe that are tightly linked to the modulations of visual perception produced by an auditory cue.

In the contrast-judgment experiment, the salient sound that elicited an ACOP (a brief noise burst) was presented in the context of a visual perceptual task. Although the location of the noise burst provided no information about which of the two Gabors would be higher in contrast, the sound did appear at a task-relevant location and did alert observers to the imminent appearance of the task-relevant visual stimuli. Thus, one might assume that the cross-modal activation of the visual system in this experiment was contingent upon an attentional set for task-relevant visual stimuli. Such an assumption would be broadly consistent with several lines of evidence showing that salient *visual* stimuli, such as color singletons and abrupt visual onsets, do not necessarily capture attention if they violate an observer's intention (e.g. Folk, Remington, & Johnston, 1992; Jannati, Gaspar, & McDonald, in press; Yantis & Jonides, 1990). However, McDonald et al. (2013) found that noise bursts elicited ACOPs in purely auditory tasks, even when the noise bursts were temporally and spatially nonpredictive of the auditory target's occurrence and when the auditory target never appeared at the location of the noise burst. These findings suggest that salient-but-irrelevant sounds activate the visual cortex independently of an observer's intentions. That is, salient sounds appear to activate the visual cortex automatically.

CROSS-MODAL CUEING AFFECTS ILLUSORY LINE MOTION

A perceptual phenomenon closely related to the prior-entry effect occurs when a line is flashed and appears to grow from one end to the other. If one end of the line is at a recently cued location and all parts of the line are presented simultaneously, observers asked to judge the direction of line growth typically report that the line grows from the cued end to the uncued end. This effect has been referred to as illusory line motion (ILM) or the "shooting line" illusion (e.g., Hamm & Klein, 2002; Hikosaka, Miyauchi, & Shimojo, 1993; Hikosaka, Miyauchi, & Shimojo, 1996). Tasks eliciting ILM are analogous to TOJ tasks in that the subject is essentially judging which end of the line appears to onset first, and the results from both TOJ and ILM tasks thus suggest that stimuli at attended locations are perceived to occur earlier than stimuli at unattended locations. However, the fact that the ILM task requires a different mode of responding ("does the line grow from the left or the right") from the TOJ task provides evidence that these effects are not limited to a particular task. Moreover, observers note that they actually see the line growing from the cued end, suggesting that the ILM effect is not simply a consequence of response bias.

Hikosaka et al. (1993, 1996) proposed that the effects of attention on both TOJ and ILM were due to an accelerated early visual processing, perhaps beginning with the feed-forward sweep of information through the primary visual cortex. As described in the preceding section on time-order perception, however, the ERP study of McDonald et al. (2005) suggested that the attentional facilitation of TOJ was due to an enhanced amplitude of the early visual cortical ERP to the attended-location stimulus rather than to an acceleration of the timing of the response.

Alternative proposals have attributed the ILM effect to processing that occurs after line presentation. Eagleman and Sejnowski (2003) attributed ILM to *postdiction*— that is, to the integration of successively presented visual events after they have occurred. This postdiction account is based on the finding that the perceived direction of ILM can be reversed if a dot is presented in the initially cued location after the line disappears. A related interpretation attributes ILM to the subject's perception of the cue and subsequent line as a single contiguous object (Downing & Treisman, 1997). This object is perceived to begin as a square (the cue) and after a brief disappearance to grow across the screen to become a horizontal rectangle (the line). This account is a variant of postdiction, because the perception of the cue and the line as a single object can occur only after both the cue and the line have been presented.

The aim of the study reported here was to use ERP recordings to evaluate the early sensory–perceptual vs later postdictive accounts of the ILM effect. Spatially nonpredictive peripheral auditory cues were used to draw attention involuntarily to the left or right side of fixation prior to the onset of a horizontal line target. To determine how ILM is related to real motion, we compared the ERPs elicited by instantaneously presented lines that resulted in ILM to ERPs elicited by actually growing lines that were accurately perceived.

Methods

Thirty-four young adults (21 female) with a mean age of 22.2 years participated for course credit. During testing they were seated in a sound-attenuated chamber facing a 19 inch CRT monitor flanked by two loudspeakers situated 32° of visual angle to the left or right of a central fixation cross. Each trial began with an 80 ms burst of pink noise from the left or right speaker, followed after a random SOA of 100–300 ms (rectangular distribution) by a white, horizontal-line target spanning 17° of visual angle (see Figure 7.5(A)).

Participants completed 20 blocks of 32 trials each, and trials with left or right auditory cues occurred equally often, at random. The target line appeared instantaneously (50% of trials), grew to the left or right in five segments over a period of 50 ms (25% of trials), or grew in two segments over a period of 20 ms (25% of trials). Leftward- and rightward-growing lines occurred equally often, and the direction of line growth was independent of the preceding auditory cue's location. In all cases, the line remained on the display for 500 ms (e.g., 20 ms of growth followed by 480 ms of static display) and was followed by a 2000–2500 ms intertrial interval. The task for 16 of the participants was to indicate by pressing a left or right mouse button the side *from* which the line grew, and for the other 18 participants to indicate the side *toward* which the line grew. They were encouraged to make their "best guesses" when uncertain.

During testing, the electroencephalogram (EEG) was recorded from 63 scalp channels (bandpass 0.1–100 Hz) with a common right-mastoid reference. The horizontal electro-oculogram was also recorded between the left and right outer canthi to monitor eye position. Following artifact rejection, ERPs time-locked to the line-target onset were averaged in 3000 ms epochs that included a 1500 ms prestimulus baseline. ERPs were re-referenced to the average of the left and right mastoids and were digitally low-pass filtered with a −3 dB cutoff at 30 Hz. ERPs were baseline-corrected using a 100 ms prestimulus interval. Of primary interest in this study were the ERPs elicited by the stationary lines. Because the cue–target SOA was short, these ERPs were distorted by overlapping ERPs elicited by the preceding auditory cue. Adjacent response filtering (ADJAR, Woldorff, 1993) was used to estimate and remove the overlapping cue ERP activity from the visual ERPs.

Results and Discussion

As shown in Figure 7.5(B), accuracy in judging the direction of slowly growing lines was very high (mean = 91.1% correct, SD = 10.5), while accuracy in the quickly growing lines was lower (mean = 66.0% correct, SD = 9.3). To determine whether the auditory cue led to ILM, we first examined behavioral responses to the stationary lines. If participants perceived no growth of the stationary lines, they would have indicated the line grew from the cued end on 50% of the trials. That is, they would have guessed the direction of the line growth. This was not the case, however: 76.4% (SD = 10.8) of the participants' responses on these trials were congruent

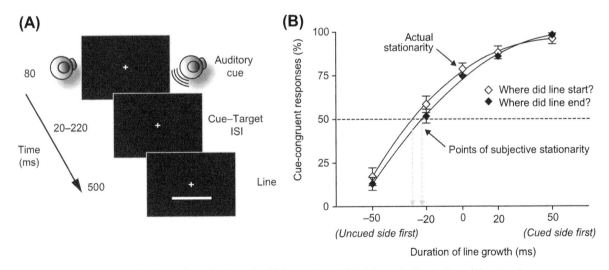

FIGURE 7.5 Methods and psychophysical results from the ILM experiment. (A) Schematic illustration of the stimulus sequence on a stationary-line trial. (B) Mean percentage of trials in which participants reported line motion starting from the cued side (or ending at the uncued side) as a function of the duration of line growth. Positive and negative durations indicate that the line grew from the cued end and from the uncued end, respectively (see text for details). The 0 ms duration indicates that all segments of the line appeared instantaneously. Data were collapsed across left-cue and right-cue trials.

with the cue—that is, participants reported that the line grew away from the cued end or toward the uncued end significantly more often than chance (76.4% vs 50%, $t(33) = 12.58, p < 0.001$). Importantly, the response profiles shown in Figure 7.5(B) were very similar for participants who reported the side where the line started and those who reported where the line ended. This equivalence provides a powerful argument against the ILM effect being primarily a consequence of biased responding toward the side of the cue.

As in TOJ studies of attention-induced prior entry, maximal uncertainty of line growth in the present study occurred not when the line was actually stationary but when the line grew away from the uncued end. In TOJ studies, the lead time of the uncued target that results in maximal uncertainty about the temporal order of the two targets has been labeled the *point of subjective simultaneity*. In the present study, interpolation along the psychophysical curves presented in Figure 7.5(B) shows that the participants were maximally uncertain as to the direction of line growth when the line grew away from the uncued side over the course of 22–29 ms. These points will be referred to as *points of subjective stationarity*.

To investigate the effects of the auditory cue on visual cortical activity, we examined the ERPs elicited by the stationary line at occipital electrodes contralateral and ipsilateral to the side of the auditory cue. Figure 7.6(A) displays the stationary-line ERPs averaged over the 76.4% of trials in which participants judged the line to grow away from the cued end (or toward the uncued end). The ERP waveforms consist of several typical peaks, including the P1 (mean peak latency = 113 ms), N1 (165 ms), P2 (234 ms), N2 (281 ms) and P3 (335 ms). Statistical analyses by analysis of variance of peak latencies at lateral occipital electrode sites PO7 and PO8 showed that only the latencies of P2 and N2 were affected by the cue. Importantly, however, the small latency differences that were observed (3 ms for P2, 5 ms for N2, both $p < 0.05$) were in the opposite direction from that predicted by the sensory-acceleration account of ILM, with longer latencies at the scalp site contralateral to the side of the cue.

It can also be seen in Figure 7.6(A) that the ERP recorded at the site contralateral to the side of the cue showed an enhanced positivity relative to the ipsilateral site beginning at around 100 ms after line onset and extending until around 300 ms. Mean amplitude measures of this contralateral positivity were significant in the latency ranges of P1 (80–120 ms, $p < 0.001$), N1 (140–200 ms, $p < 0.001$), P2 (200–240 ms, $p < 0.002$), and N2 (240–320 ms, $p < 0.02$). Figure 7.6(B) shows the scalp topography of the stationary-line ERP in the time range of the P1 (80–120 ms postline). In this figure, ERPs from left-cue and right-cue trials were combined in such a way as to show ipsilateral and contralateral scalp activity on the left and right sides of the map, respectively. Two

separate P1 maxima are evident, one over each side of the occipital scalp. Consistent with the ERP waveforms, the contralateral maximum was more positive than the ipsilateral maximum.

To isolate the lateralized cueing effect in the P1 time interval, the ERP waveforms recorded at ipsilateral electrodes were subtracted from the ERP waveforms

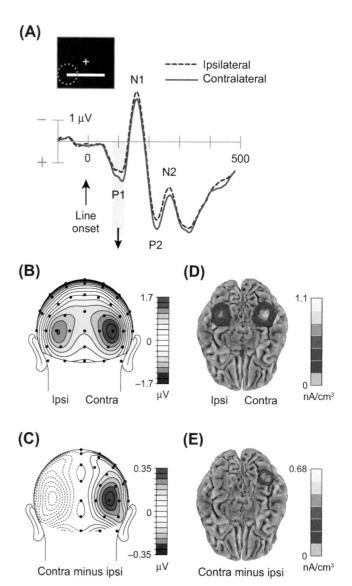

FIGURE 7.6 Grand-averaged ERPs elicited by stationary lines perceived to grow away from the acoustically cued end. (A) ERP waveforms recorded at occipital electrodes (PO7/PO8) contralateral and ipsilateral to the cued end of the line. (B) Topographical maps of the mean ERP amplitudes in the time range of the P1 (80–120 ms). The ERP data were collapsed over the cued side (left, right) and the recording hemisphere (left, right) to show ipsilateral and contralateral ERP distributions on the left and right sides of the maps, respectively. (C) Topographical maps of the contralateral–ipsilateral difference waveforms in the time range of the P1, projected on the right side of the scalp. (D and E) Estimated distributed source activity underlying the ERP waveforms (D) and the contralateral–ipsilateral difference waveforms (E) in the time range of the P1.

recorded at homologous contralateral electrodes (e.g., PO78-contra minus PO78-ipsi) to produce contralateral-minus-ipsilateral difference waves. Figure 7.6(C) shows a mirror-symmetric topographical map of these difference waves, produced by plotting the contralateral–ipsilateral voltage differences on both sides of the head map and zeroing the voltages at the midline electrodes (for similar approaches, see Green, Conder, & McDonald, 2008; Praamstra, Stegeman, Horstink, & Cools, 1996). A posterior positivity is evident in the map, with a lateral-occipital maximum that resembled that of the P1 component itself.

To gain information on the cortical sources giving rise to the P1 component and the enhanced positivity contralateral to the auditory cue in the P1 latency range, we estimated the location of their neural generators using a distributed source analysis approach called CLARA (Classical LORETA Analysis Recursively Applied; BESA 5.3). The CLARA method is an iterative application of weighted LORETA images with a reduced source space in each successive iteration. For the present purposes, two iterations were sufficient to deblur the distributed source activity sufficiently. The resulting CLARA solution revealed P1 source activity on the ventral surface of the occipital lobe, along the fusiform gyrus (Figure 7.6(D)). Consistent with the scalp-recorded P1, greater source activity was seen in the contralateral occipital lobe than in the ipsilateral lobe. The CLARA solution of the isolated contralateral positivity revealed source activity in a nearby region of the occipital lobe (Figure 7.6(E)).

The ERPs elicited by the lines that actually grew from one end to the other were quite different from those elicited by the stationary lines that appeared to grow due to the advance auditory cueing. Whereas the illusory line growth was associated with an enlarged contralateral positivity beginning in the P1 time interval, actual line growth was associated with contralateral–ipsilateral latency differences of both the P1 and N1 components. Figure 7.7(A) shows the ERP to the line that grew from one end to the other over a 50 ms interval, with time zero representing the onset of the first segment of the line. In this case the latencies of the early ERP peaks were substantially shorter over contralateral than over ipsilateral scalp sites (by 17 ms for P1, $p < 0.001$; by 11 ms for N1, $p < 0.001$). This result shows that when a line actually onsets earlier at one end, the initial ERP peaks are elicited more rapidly in the contralateral visual cortex. Thus, if the auditory cue had accelerated the early visual processing of one end of the stationary line, we would have expected a similar finding of earlier P1 and N1 latencies over the hemisphere contralateral to the cue. The fact that no such ERP latency differences were observed implies that the salient auditory cue produces ILM via a different neural mechanism than simple acceleration of early processing.

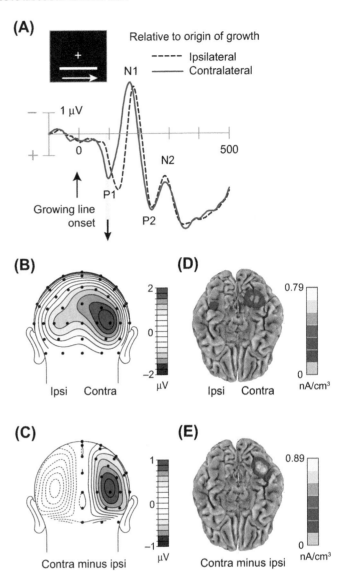

FIGURE 7.7 Grand-average ERPs elicited by slowly growing lines in the ILM experiment. (A) ERPs recorded from electrodes over the occipital scalp (PO7/PO8) contralateral and ipsilateral to the side at which the line motion began. (B–E) Topographical maps and distributed source images, as in Figure 7.6.

To localize the neural generators of the initial ERP activity to slowly growing lines, topographical maps were created for an early phase of the P1 (90–100 ms postline) and for the isolated contralateral-minus-ipsilateral difference waveform in the same time range (Figure 7.7(B) and (C), respectively). During this early phase, the P1 was at maximum over the contralateral scalp and beginning to emerge over the ipsilateral scalp. The contralateral maximum was distributed very similarly to that of the enlarged contralateral P1 to stationary lines that were perceived to grow from the cued end (Figure 7.7(B) vs Figure 7.6(B)). Likewise, the scalp distribution of the contralateral–ipsilateral difference wave in this early P1 interval was nearly identical to that of the enlarged contralateral positivity to the ILM lines (Figure 7.7(C) vs Figure 7.6(C)). CLARA analyses showed distributed source activity in ventral regions of the occipital lobe, near the fusiform gyrus, for both the early P1 and the contralateral–ipsilateral difference waveform in the early P1 time interval (Figure 7.7(D) and (E)). Thus, although different neural mechanisms appear to underlie illusory and actual line growth, these mechanisms appear to involve the same regions of the visual cortex.

The present findings help to settle two debates over cross-modally induced prior entry. First, the finding of equivalent cueing effects on ILM for judgments of "moving toward" and "moving away" from the cued location provides strong support that auditory cueing produces a true perceptual effect and not a response bias. This support is buttressed by the finding of a modulation of early ERP activity originating in the visual cortex. Second, the absence of an ERP latency effect rules out an alternative explanation based on the EEG sampling rate. As reviewed earlier, auditory cues had no effect on the timing of the early ERP components recorded in a TOJ task (McDonald et al., 2005). To account for this finding, Vibell et al. (2007) asserted that a low EEG sampling rate might have caused a type II error. That is, in McDonald et al.'s study, EEG was digitized every 4 ms (250 Hz), and this may have been insufficient to detect a 3–4 ms shift in the early ERP components. In the present ILM study, no latency effect was in evidence despite using Vibell et al.'s preferred 500 Hz sampling rate. Thus, the present findings argue against Vibell et al.'s slow-sampling hypothesis and provide converging support for the conclusion that cross-modally induced prior entry stems from changes in the strength—not timing—of early visual cortical activity.

CONCLUDING REMARKS

The ERP pattern elicited by the stationary line during auditorily induced ILM appears virtually identical to the pattern associated with the cross-modal facilitation of TOJ (Figure 7.2, above) and the cross-modal enhancement of visual contrast (Figure 7.3, above). In each case, a bilaterally symmetrical visual stimulus (a left–right pair of stimuli or a horizontal line) elicited an ERP with enhanced positivity over the hemisphere contralateral to the side of the preceding auditory cue. This positivity had a scalp distribution consistent with a source in the ventral-lateral visual cortex and extended over the interval 100–300 ms after the onset of the visual stimulus. It is not clear how this enhanced positivity is linked with the perceptual modulation of TOJ and ILM, but most likely it reflects an enhanced signal strength of visual inputs from the cued location, resulting in more rapid achievement of a perceptual threshold at a subsequent stage of visual processing. The early onset of the cueing effect (less than 100 ms after the onset of the visual stimulus) shows that it represents an influence on early visual processing and not a purely "postdictive" effect, although such later influences on perceptual responses cannot be ruled out entirely.

Based on these findings, we propose that all of these cross-modally induced changes in visual perception stem from the same physiological process whereby the auditory cue enhances the strength of target-evoked neural responses in the visual cortex starting within 100 ms of target onset. This neural enhancement boosts perceptual contrast and accelerates perceptual awareness in both TOJ and ILM tasks. The cortical sources of these cross-modally induced changes in visual target processing (i.e., the enhanced contralateral positivity) are localized to the same ventral-occipital region as the sources of the cue-elicited ACOP. Moreover, with the cue–target intervals used in these studies (100–300 ms), the timing of the ACOP corresponds with the window of enhancement of the contralateral positivity associated with perceptual facilitation of the visual target. This suggests that the auditory cue sensitizes the extrastriate visual pathways so that a subsequent visual stimulus appearing at the cued location elicits an enhanced response from neurons in those same pathways.

Acknowledgments

This research was supported by grants from the NSERC, CFI, and CRC Programs to JJM and by grants from NSF (BCS-1029084) and NIMH (1P50MH-86385) to SAH.

References

Carrasco, M. (2006). Covert attention increases contrast sensitivity: psychophysical, neurophysiological, and neuroimaging studies. In S. Martinez-Conde, S. L. Macknik, L. M. Martinez, J. M. Alonso & P. U. Tse (Eds.), *Progress in brain research Part 1: Visual perception. Part I. Fundamentals of vision: Low and mid-level processes in perception* (Vol. 154, pp. 33–70). : Elsevier.

Carrasco, M. (2011). Visual attention: the past 25 years. *Vision Research, 51*, 1484–1525.

Carrasco, M., Ling, S., & Read, S. (2004). Attention alters appearance. *Nature Neuroscience, 7*, 308–313.

Cate, A. D., Herron, T., Yund, E. W., Stecker, G. C., Rinne, T., Kang, X., et al. (2009). Auditory attention activates peripheral visual cortex. *PLoS One, 4*, e4645.

Dennett, D. (1991). *Consciousness explained*. The Penguin Press.

Dosher, B. A., & Lu, Z. -L. (2000). Noise exclusion in spatial attention. *Psychological Science, 11*, 139–146.

Downing, P. E., & Treisman, A. M. (1997). The line-motion illusion: attention or impletion? *Journal of Experimental Psychology. Human Perception and Performance, 25*, 768–779.

Dufour, A. (1999). Importance of attentional mechanisms in audiovisual links. *Experimental Brain Research, 126*, 215–222.

Eagleman, D. M., & Sejnowski, T. J. (2003). The line-motion illusion can be reversed by motion signals after the line disappears. *Perception, 32*, 963–968.

Eimer, M., van Velzen, J., & Driver, J. (2002). Cross-modal interactions between audition, touch, and vision in endogenous spatial attention: ERP evidence on preparatory states and sensory modulations. *Journal of Cognitive Neuroscience, 14,* 254–271.

Eimer, M., van Velzen, J., Forster, B., & Driver, J. (2003). Shifts of attention in light and in darkness: an ERP study of supramodal attentional control and crossmodal links in spatial attention. *Cognitive Brain Research, 15,* 308–323.

Farah, M. J., Wong, A. B., Monheit, M. A., & Morrow, L. A. (1989). Parietal lobe mechanisms of spatial attention: modality-specific or supramodal? *Neuropsychologia, 27,* 461–470.

Fechner, G. T. (1882). *Revision der Hauptpunkte der Psychophysik.* Leipzig.

Folk, C. L., Remington, R. W., & Johnston, J. C. (1992). Involuntary covert orienting is contingent on attentional control settings. *Journal of Experimental Psychology: Human Perception and Performance, 18,* 1030–1044.

Frassinetti, F., Bolognini, N., & Làdavas, E. (2002). Enhancement of visual perception by crossmodal visuoauditory interaction. *Experimental Brain Research, 147,* 332–343.

Green, J. J., Conder, J. A., & McDonald, J. J. (2008). Lateralized frontal activity elicited by attention-directing visual and auditory cues. *Psychophysiology, 45,* 579–587.

Green, J. J., Teder-Sälejärvi, W. A., & McDonald, J. J. (2005). Control mechanisms mediating shifts of attention in auditory and visual space: a spatio-temporal ERP analysis. *Experimental Brain Research, 166,* 358–369.

Hamm, J. P., & Klein, R. M. (2002). Does attention follow the motion in the "shooting line" illusion? *Perception and Psychophysics, 64,* 279–291.

Harter, M. R., Miller, S. L., Price, N. J., LaLonde, M. E., & Keyes, A. L. (1989). Neural processes involved in directing attention. *Journal of Cognitive Neuroscience, 1,* 223–237.

Heinze, H. J., Luck, S. J., Mangun, G. R., & Hillyard, S. A. (1990). Visual event-related potentials index focused attention within bilateral stimulus arrays. I. Evidence for early selection. *Electroencephalography and Clinical Neurophysiology, 75,* 511–527.

Helmholtz, H. V. (1866). *Treatise on psychological optics.* Rochester, New York: Optical Society of America.

Hikosaka, O., Miyauchi, S., & Shimojo, S. (1993). Focal visual attention produces illusory temporal order and motion sensation. *Vision Research, 33,* 1219–1240.

Hikosaka, O., Miyauchi, S., & Shimojo, S. (1996). Orienting of spatial attention – its reflexive, compensatory, and voluntary mechanisms. *Cognitive Brain Research, 5,* 1–9.

Hopfinger, J. B., Luck, S. J., & Hillyard, S. A. (2004). Selective attention: electrophysiological and neuromagnetic studies. In M. S. Gazzaniga (Ed.), *The cognitive neurosciences* (Vol. 3, pp. 561–574). Cambridge, MA: MIT Press.

Hopf, J. M., & Mangun, G. R. (2000). Shifting visual attention in space: an electrophysiological analysis using high spatial resolution mapping. *Clinical Neurophysiology, 111,* 1241–1257.

James, W. (1890). *The principles of psychology.* New York: Henry Holt.

Jannati, A., Gaspar, J. M., & McDonald, J. J. (in press). Tracking target and distractor processing in fixed-feature visual search: evidence from human electrophysiology. *Journal of Experimental Psychology: Human Perception and Performance.* 10.1037/a0032251.

Luck, S. J., Heinze, H. J., Mangun, G. R., & Hillyard, S. A. (1990). Visual event-related potentials index focused attention within bilateral stimulus arrays. II: Functional dissociation of P1 and N1 components. *Electroencephalography and Clinical Neurophysiology, 75,* 528–542.

Luck, S. J., Hillyard, S. A., Mouloua, M., Woldorff, M. G., Clark, V. P., & Hawkins, H. L. (1994). Effects of spatial cuing on luminance detectability: psychophysical and electrophysiological evidence for early selection. *Journal of Experimental Psychology: Human Perception and Performance, 20,* 887–904.

Macaluso, E., Frith, C. D., & Driver, J. (2000). Modulation of human visual cortex by crossmodal spatial attention. *Science, 289,* 1206–1208.

Mangun, G. R., & Hillyard, S. A. (1991). Modulations of sensory-evoked brain potentials indicate changes in perceptual processing during visual-spatial priming. *Journal of Experimental Psychology: Human Perception and Performance, 17,* 1057–1074.

McDonald, J. J., Green, J. J., Störmer, V. S., & Hillyard, S. A. (2012). Cross-modal spatial cueing of attention influences visual perception. In M. M. Murray & M. T. Wallace (Eds.), *Frontiers in the neural bases of multisensory processes* (pp. 509–527). Boca Ratan, FL: CRC Press.

McDonald, J. J., Störmer, V. S., Martinez, A., Feng, W., & Hillyard, S. A. (2013). Salient sounds activate human visual cortex automatically. *Journal of Neuroscience, 33,* 9194–9201.

McDonald, J. J., Teder-Sälejärvi, W. A., Di Russo, F., & Hillyard, S. A. (2003). Neural substrates of perceptual enhancement by crossmodal spatial attention. *Journal of Cognitive Neuroscience, 15,* 10–19.

McDonald, J. J., Teder-Sälejärvi, W. A., Di Russo, F., & Hillyard, S. A. (2005). Neural basis of auditory-induced shifts in visual time-order perception. *Nature Neuroscience, 8,* 1197–1202.

McDonald, J. J., Teder-Sälejärvi, W. A., & Hillyard, S. A. (2000). Involuntary orienting to sound improves visual perception. *Nature, 407,* 906–908.

McDonald, J. J., Teder-Sälejärvi, W. A., & Ward, L. M. (2001). Multisensory integration and crossmodal attention effects in the human brain. *Science, 292,* 1791.

Nobre, A. C., Sebestyen, G. N., & Miniussi, C. (2000). The dynamics of shifting visuospatial attention revealed by event-related potentials. *Neuropsychologia, 38,* 964–974.

Pashler, H. E. (1998). *The psychology of attention.* Cambridge: MIT Press.

Posner, M. I., Snyder, C. R., & Davidson, B. J. (1980). Attention and the detection of signals. *Journal of Experimental Psychology: General, 109,* 160–174.

Praamstra, P., Stegeman, D. F., Horstink, M. W. I.M., & Cools, A. R. (1996). Dipole source analysis suggests selective modulation of the supplementary motor area contribution to the readiness potential. *Electroencephalography and Clinical Neurophysiology, 98,* 468–477.

Prime, D. J., McDonald, J. J., Green, J. J., & Ward, L. M. (2008). When crossmodal attention fails. *Canadian Journal of Experimental Psychology, 62,* 192–197.

Prinzmetal, W., Long, V., & Leonhardt, J. (2008). Involuntary attention and brightness contrast. *Perception and Psychophysics, 70,* 1139–1150.

Santangelo, V., & Spence, C. (2008). Crossmodal attentional capture in an unspeeded simultaneity judgement task. *Visual Cognition, 16,* 155–165.

Schneider, K. A. (2006). Does attention alter appearance? *Perception and Psychophysics, 68,* 800–814.

Schneider, K. A., & Bavelier, D. (2003). Components of visual prior entry. *Cognitive Psychology, 47,* 333–366.

Schneider, K. A., & Komlos, M. (2008). Attention biases decisions but does not alter appearance. *Journal of Vision, 8.*

Shimojo, S., Miyauchi, S., & Hikosaka, O. (1997). Visual motion sensation yielded by non-visually driven attention. *Vision Research, 37,* 1575–1580.

Shore, D. I., Spence, C., & Klein, R. M. (2001). Visual prior entry. *Psychological Science, 12,* 205–212.

Smith, P. L., & Ratcliff, R. (2009). An integrated theory of attention and decision making in visual signal detection. *Psychological Review, 116,* 283–317.

Soto-Faraco, S., McDonald, J. J., & Kingstone, A. (2002). Gaze direction: effects on attentional orienting and crossmodal target responses. Poster presented at the annual meeting of the Cognitive Neuroscience Society, San Francisco.

Spence, C., & Driver, J. (1997). Audiovisual links in exogenous covert spatial orienting. *Perception and Psychophysics, 59*, 1–22.

Spence, C., McDonald, J. J., & Driver, J. (2004). Exogenous spatial cuing studies of human crossmodal attention and multisensory integration. In C. Spence & J. Driver (Eds.), *Crossmodal space and crossmodal attention* (pp. 277–320). New York: Oxford University Press.

Stelmach, L. B., & Herdman, C. M. (1991). Directed attention and perception of temporal-order. *Journal of Experimental Psychology: Human Perception and Performance, 17*, 539–550.

Störmer, V. S., McDonald, J. J., & Hillyard, S. A. (2009). Cross-modal cueing of attention alters appearance and early cortical processing of visual stimuli. *Proceedings of the National Academy of Sciences of the United States of America, 106*, 22456–22461.

Titchener, E. N. (1908). *Lectures on the elementary psychology of feeling and attention*. New York: MacMillan.

Vibell, J., Klinge, C., Zampini, M., Spence, C., & Nobre, A. C. (2007). Temporal order is coded temporally in the brain: early event-related potential latency shifts underlying prior entry in a cross-modal temporal order judgment task. *Journal of Cognitive Neuroscience, 19*, 109–120.

Ward, L. M. (1994). Supramodal and modality-specific mechanisms for stimulus-driven shifts of auditory and visual attention. *Canadian Journal of Experimental Psychology, 48*, 242–259.

Woldorff, M. G. (1993). Distortion of ERP averages due to overlap from temporally adjacent ERPs: Analysis and correction. *Psychophysiology, 30*, 98–119.

Wright, R. D., & Ward, L. M. (2008). *Orienting of attention*. New York: Oxford University Press.

Wu, C. T., Weissman, D. H., Roberts, K. C., & Woldorff, M. G. (2007). The neural circuitry underlying the executive control of auditory spatial attention. *Brain Research, 1134*, 187–198.

Yantis, S., & Jonides, J. (1990). Abrupt visual onsets and selective attention: voluntary versus automatic allocation. *Journal of Experimental Psychology: Human Perception and Performance, 16*, 121–134.

FEATURE AND OBJECT ATTENTION

Face invisible – a vase seen instead.
Space divisible
into the haves and have nots
at least in the head.
Attentional fates determined early on by wheres
more than whats though both may matter
for the neural chatter
in a brain laid out to represent the world as it is.
ERPs the electrical whiz kid
that slices and dices time and space whether
readily accessible or somewhere hid
so that cognitive neuroscientists can continue to save face in the competition
about the whys and wherefores of visual cognition.

By Marta Kutas

Object-Category Processing, Perceptual Awareness, and the Role of Attention during Motion-Induced Blindness

Joseph A. Harris[1, 2], David L. Barack[1, 2, 3], Alex R. McMahon[1], Stephen R. Mitroff[1, 2] Marty G. Woldorff[1, 2, 4, 5]

[1]Center for Cognitive Neuroscience, Duke University, Durham, NC, USA, [2]Department of Psychology & Neuroscience, Duke University, Durham, NC, USA, [3]Department of Philosophy, Duke University, Durham, NC, USA, [4]Department of Psychiatry, Duke University, Durham, NC, USA, [5]Department of Neurobiology, Duke University, Durham, NC, USA

INTRODUCTION

The extent of visual processing that occurs outside of awareness is an unresolved issue of broad importance to the field of cognitive neuroscience. Research examining this question is predicated on the notion that any information that is represented in the brain, whether an individual is aware of it or not, holds the potential to affect subsequent behavior in a relevant way. Identifying the information coded in the brain with or without explicit awareness therefore enhances our understanding of what determines or influences behavior.

One method of identifying perceptual processes that occur in the absence of awareness is through the dissociation paradigm, which is comprised of several essential components (Reingold & Merikle, 1988). In vision, for example, once a visual perceptual process of interest is identified, two measures of this process are obtained as a viewer is presented with images invoking this process. An explicit measure is derived from the viewer's behavioral output or report regarding the content of the images, which serves as an index of their level of awareness. A second measure is typically implicit in nature and reflects the processing of the image content of which the viewer may not be aware, as in the case of behavioral priming or neural responses. Through any number of possible manipulations of the presentation parameters

of relevant images (e.g., a manipulation using motion-induced blindness (MIB), for example, as described below), conditions are created in which images are present but not visible to the viewer, which is reflected in a marked decrease of the explicit measure (Kim & Blake, 2005). The implicit measure is then probed in these conditions of reduced awareness vs. those with full awareness. If the implicit measure of the perceptual process is shown to be intact, regardless of the viewer's ability to report relevant image content, then it is inferred that this process is occurring in the absence of awareness (Holender, 1986; Reingold & Merikle, 1988).

Discrimination of object category by the visual system is evident through multiple measures, behavioral and neural, and thus provides explicit and implicit indices that can be used to examine its relationship with visual awareness. A particularly well-studied and readily measured process reflecting such categorical discrimination is face-specific processing. Neural reflections of this process have been most directly observed as enhancements of specific neural responses to face images relative to images of any other object category that are observed in functional modules of the ventral extrastriate and ventral temporal cortices in human and nonhuman primates (Allison et al., 1994; Harries & Perrett, 1991; Perrett, Hietanen, Oram, & Benson, 1992). In normal human observers, for example, face-specific responses have been localized to areas in the fusiform gyrus and lateral occipital cortex using function magnetic resonance imaging (fMRI) measures (Kanwisher, McDermott, & Chun, 1997; Puce, Allison, Gore, & Mccarthy, 1995), and in the occipitotemporal sulcus through intracranial recordings in patients (Puce, McCarthy, Bentin, & Allison, 1997). Using scalp-recorded event-related potential (ERP) measures, face-specific processing has been recorded as a negative-polarity amplitude enhancement over lateral–inferior temporal–occipital regions, peaking at ~170 ms after stimulus onset (Bentin, Allison, Puce, Perez, & McCarthy, 1996), often followed at longer latencies (~300–800 ms) by a smaller amplitude but longer duration negative wave with a very similar scalp distribution (Harris, Wu, & Woldorff, 2011; Philiastides, Ratcliff, & Sajda, 2006). These high temporal resolution electrophysiological measures of this process are especially useful indices of this relatively high-level of object-category discrimination that may not require an explicit report of image content, and thus can serve as an informative implicit measure of this process.

MIB is a relatively recently discovered experimental manipulation that can be used for disrupting visual awareness of target images. In MIB, parafoveally presented static targets are superimposed on a globally moving array of distractors. While maintaining fixation at a specific nontarget spatial position (typically centrally located) and covertly attending to these ever-present static targets, viewers periodically lose and regain awareness of them (Bonneh, Cooperman, & Sagi, 2001). This striking perceptual phenomenon provides a novel and robust manner by which to attenuate visual awareness experimentally and serves as an appealing method by which to examine face-processing in the absence of awareness. To this end, experimenters use MIB to gauge the extent of target-associated processing that occurs in the absence of awareness by probing target-specific processing within and outside of MIB episodes (Kim & Blake, 2005).

A number of behavioral studies have suggested that MIB acts through a high-level or late mechanism to disrupt visual awareness. For example, the formation of negative afterimages, a process likely mediated by a relatively low-level of visual processing, is uninterrupted by MIB (Hofstoetter, Koch, & Kiper, 2004). Similarly, orientation-specific aftereffects persist following exposure to a Gabor patch of a given angle, regardless of whether it was presented during or outside of MIB (Montaser-Kouhsari, Moradi, Zandvakili, & Esteky, 2004; Rajimehr, 2004). Also, higher-level processes of object representation and updating have been demonstrated to occur during MIB. For example, one experiment showed that the sudden physical offset of a perceptually suppressed target "breaks" the blindness episode, making the viewer aware of this transient change. This in turn suggested that changes in the gross physical properties of the target

(i.e., its presence or absence) were being processed during MIB episodes, despite the objects being invisible to the subject (Mitroff & Scholl, 2004). This group also showed that if two previously disparate objects are linked with a connecting line during a blindness episode, they tend to reemerge simultaneously as one object, suggesting that object-based representations can be updated during MIB (Mitroff & Scholl, 2005).

In addition to studies focusing on the visual processes that occur during MIB, research examining the more general dynamics of MIB has supported a mechanism of disruption that acts relatively late in terms of visual processing stages. Specifically, MIB episodes associated with specific static targets are shown to be enhanced (to occur more frequently and for greater durations) when those targets are covertly attended (Carter, Luedeman, Mitroff, & Nakayama, 2009). This is in contrast with a low-level mechanism of disruption, such as that seen in sandwich masking wherein visual mask stimuli occur immediately before and after a target image, which does not appear to be modulated by covert attention (Harris et al., 2011). In addition, the manner in which the visual system accounts for the static target location during blindness episodes is similar to the high-level mechanisms of perceptual filling-in observed for the retinal blindspot or scotomas (Hsu, Yeh, & Kramer, 2006). For example, superimposing a stationary grid over a static target and moving array results in the target being replaced by the stationary pattern, in what amounts to a perceptual filling-in effect based upon context (New & Scholl, 2008). In general, evidence has suggested a rivalrous relationship between the static target and array of moving distractor stimuli that is manifested in the temporal properties of MIB (Carter & Pettigrew, 2003). Although relatively few neural studies of MIB have been performed, this proposed rivalrous relationship has been supported by functional MRI measures that show a competitive relationship between ventral and dorsal visual regions associated with the static target and motion array, respectively, which track the perceptual state of the subject in their respective levels of activity (Donner, Sagi, Bonneh, & Heeger, 2008; Scholvinck & Rees, 2010). Nevertheless, a consensus on the neural mechanisms underlying MIB has yet to be reached.

In the present study, we employed the high temporal resolution measures of face-specific neural processing afforded by electroencephalogram (EEG) to examine the extent and nature of object-category processing that can occur during MIB. In addition, the possible mechanism by which MIB exerts disruption of awareness was investigated. These processes were probed by examining responses associated with the perceptual onset of a static target following a blindness episode. Specifically, two conditions were employed: one in which the disappearance and reappearance of target images was physical in nature (a "static" condition in which a target image actually appeared or disappeared), and the other in which target objects only disappeared and reappeared perceptually due to MIB ("motion condition"). Face-specific neural responses were then tracked across these actual and perceptual onset conditions to gauge the extent of object-category processing in the brain during MIB, the assumption being that a lack of face-specific activity following a perceptual onset (following an MIB episode) would imply that face-processing had been ongoing and intact during the MIB. In addition, activity preceding the perceptual onset of a present image was compared to that preceding the reonset of an image that had actually physically disappeared, to extract an electrophysiological difference between perceptual "reentrance" after an MIB-induced perceptual disappearance and actual perceptual "entrance". This comparison effectively extracts activity reflecting the emergence of awareness of a continually present image of which the viewer was previously unaware, thereby providing insight into the mechanism underlying MIB and, correspondingly, into the neural underpinnings of perceptual awareness.

METHODS

Subjects

Twenty-six neurologically intact subjects with normal or corrected-to-normal vision participated in the study. Before beginning the EEG portion of the study, each subject underwent a behavioral screening procedure to establish a minimal level of susceptibility to the MIB effect (described below). Four subjects were excluded on the basis of inadequate behavioral effects. Two additional subjects were excluded due to excessive eye blink artifacts in the acquired EEG data (trial rejection rate due to blink artifacts greater than 25%). This left 20 subjects with sufficient behavioral effects and viable EEG data for the final analysis (mean age 22.8 ± 2.4 years, eight female, all right-handed). All subjects completed informed consent procedures as approved by the Duke University Institutional Review Board and were paid for the period of time of their participation, even if only for the screening task.

Stimuli and Task

Prior to the EEG session, subjects were screened so as to only include those with a sufficiently robust MIB effect. Subjects were seated with their eyes 70 cm from the center of a 19 inch CRT stimulus presentation monitor with a 60 Hz refresh rate and were asked to covertly attend to a parafoveal static yellow disc (visual angle of 3.37°; eccentricity of 7.46°, located in the upper left quadrant of the screen). This target was superimposed on a full-screen array of blue-cross distractors on a black background, which rotated clockwise as a single surface with its origin at central fixation, at a speed of 15 rounds (360° rotation) per minute (Psychtoolbox, MATLAB). As per the typical MIB task, subjects were asked to press a response button associated with the static target when the target disappeared and to release this button when it reappeared (e.g., Bonneh et al., 2001). If subjects experienced MIB episodes at a rate of at least five disappearances per minute, and of a mean duration of at least 100 ms, they then proceeded to participate in the full experimental session, which differed from the standard MIB task in several ways, as described below.

After applying the EEG cap, the experimental session began. This differed from the screening task in several ways. Static targets were selected randomly and equiprobably from a set of 80 grayscale circular cropped faces and houses, each of the same size and eccentricity as the static targets utilized in the screening task. The background array of distractors was adjusted to be comprised of black crosses over a gray background (rather than blue crosses on a black background), rendering all visual elements in the display grayscale. Two run types were included: a "static" type in which there was no motion of the distractor array, and another in which the distractor array rotated with the same parameters as in the screening task (Figure 8.1), alternating between clockwise and counter-clockwise rotation on each run. Regardless of the run type, subjects were instructed to covertly attend to the location of the static target, and to push a response key as quickly as possible upon the *reappearance* of the target after a disappearance period. Ultimately, this would enable the direct comparison of the brain responses to physical onsets to the responses to strictly perceptual onsets (following MIB), as a means of assessing the preceding processing during MIB. In the case of static runs, the target would physically disappear for a duration that was randomly jittered between 1200 and 1800 ms, and then reappear. Following the button press, a new image (face or house) would be presented at the target location and the sequence would repeat. In the case of the motion condition, the target image only perceptually disappeared (due to MIB) and, following the button press indicating the perceptual reappearance, would switch (after a random period between 800 and 1200 ms) to another selected face or house image that remained onscreen until the subsequent button press. This approach enabled a comparison between actual physical disappearances in which MIB could not occur (during the static condition) and perceptual disappearances in which the target never physically disappeared (during the motion condition). Regardless of the run type, subjects were instructed in an identical manner, namely to press the button upon the reappearance of an image that had previously disappeared.

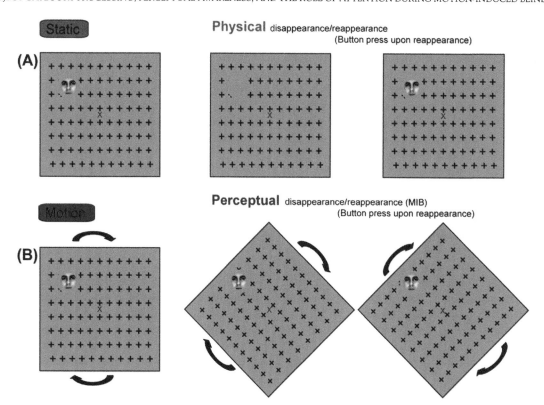

FIGURE 8.1 Stimuli and task: subjects performed the same task for two types of experimental runs. In the static condition (A), randomly selected face and house targets appeared parafoveally (upper left quadrant) for a variable period of time prior to disappearing and then reappearing, at which point subjects were instructed to press a response key as quickly as possible. In the motion condition (B), parafoveal targets superimposed on a coherently rotating array of distractors would perceptually disappear due to MIB (but would never actually physically disappear), with subjects being given the same instructions to press the response key as quickly as possible when observing a reappearance of the target image.

Subjects completed 16 experimental runs, each of which ran for 4 min, with the majority (12) being of the motion run type (in order to obtain comparable numbers of trials across conditions). Button presses were recorded throughout both run types to assess reaction time (RT) in the case of the static condition (relative to the actual reappearance of an actual target), as well as the susceptibility of faces and houses to MIB during the motion condition.

EEG Acquisition and Analysis

EEG data was continuously recorded during static and motion run types from a 64-channel custom cap (Electrocap, Inc., Eaton, OH) with extended scalp coverage, using a right-mastoid reference, a bandpass filter of 0.01–100 Hz, a sampling rate of 500 Hz, and a gain of 1000 (Neuroscan Inc., Charlotte, NC). Eye movements and blinks were monitored and recorded using two horizontal electro-oculogram (EOG) channels referenced to one another and placed on the outer canthi, and two vertical EOG channels placed below the eyes and referenced to frontal electrodes Fp1 and Fp2. Subject behavior was also monitored using a closed circuit video camera.

Following the experimental session, acquired data was analyzed offline using ERPSS, a Linux-based ERP data-analysis software package (University of California at San Diego, La Jolla, CA). Extracted epochs containing eye blinks, eye movements, muscle activity, and slow drift artifacts were rejected offline prior to selective averaging. Artifact-free data were time-locked averaged selectively for the different stimulus types, both to the onset of the stimuli, as well as to button presses indicating the reappearance of images (following physical disappearances in the case of the static condition, and following MIB-induced perceptual disappearances in the motion condition). Averages were low-pass filtered offline using a nine-point running average filter, which attenuates external electrical noise of ~56 Hz frequency content and higher. ERP averages were algebraically rereferenced to the average of all electrodes (common reference) and baseline corrected to the 200 ms preceding stimulus onset in the case of image-locked responses, and to the period of −1000 to −800 ms preceding the button press in the case of response-locked trials. Face-selective effects were extracted by comparing responses to faces to those associated with houses, separately within the static and motion conditions.

In order to examine the extent of face-specific processing that occurred during MIB, ERP activity time-locked to the button presses in response to the reappearance of a face was compared to the corresponding activity associated with the reappearance of a house for the static (physical onset) and motion (perceptual onset) conditions. The extent to which the face-specific effect for these reappearances differed between the static and motion conditions was used to infer the extent of face-specific processing that occurs during MIB. Specifically, in the case of the static condition, a face or house stimulus reappeared after having actually disappeared, meaning that no face-specific processing was possibly occurring during the intervening period. In the case of the motion condition, the targets were always present during the preceding MIB episode, but the extent of face-specific processing during that episode is unknown. Accordingly, if the face-specific ERP responses for the reappearances were identical for perceptual onsets after an MIB as for actual physical onsets, it would suggest that during the preceding MIB no face-specific processing had been ongoing, similar to how there would have been no face-specific processing prior to an actual physical onset because there had been no image present. If however, the extracted face-specific activity surrounding the reappearance button press differed significantly between physical and perceptual onsets of targets, it would not only differentiate the neural processes triggered by those onset events, but it would also differentiate between the ongoing object-related processes preceding those onset events. In particular, if no face-specific activity was observed surrounding a button press in the post-MIB reappearance condition, it would suggest that face-specific processing had been uninterrupted during the preceding MIB, thereby dissociating face-specific processing activity from awareness during the MIB. Finally, to examine more general differences between perceptual and physical onsets, the response-locked data was collapsed across image type (i.e. collapsed across faces and houses), and compared between the static and motion conditions. This comparison was made for assessing whether activity patterns for an image of any type (i.e. not specific to any object category) differed for perceptual vs physical onsets, which would also speak to the mechanisms by which MIB disrupts awareness.

RESULTS

Behavior

In the static condition, whether a disappearing/reappearing stimulus was a face or house had no bearing on the RT of the subjects. Specifically, subjects responded to faces and houses with approximately equal speed, as the mean RT across stimulus type (403 ms for faces and 409 ms for houses) did not differ ($t_{19} = 0.96$, $p = 0.34$). In addition, results showed that MIB was equally effective in diminishing subjects' awareness of faces and houses. In particular, an average of ~10 blindness episodes per stimulus type (mean ± SD: 10.0 ± 4.1 for faces; 9.9 ± 3.5 for houses) per run was observed, with no difference in the mean number of episodes across image type ($t_{19} = 0.13$, $p = 0.90$).

Electrophysiology

Electrophysiological data time-locked to the onset of face and house targets (appearance of a new object in the static condition and a switch to a new object image in the motion condition) showed robust face-specific processing in both the static and motion condition. In both the static and motion conditions, face-specific activity elicited by a new image was characterized by an increased negative-polarity response to faces relative to houses across the poststimulus time window of 150–800 ms over the relevant ventrolateral temporal–occipital scalp area, thus displaying the hallmark face-selective ventrolateral N170 response ($F(1, 19) = 21.6$, $p < 0.001$ for the static condition; $F(1, 19) = 30.2$, $p < 0.0001$ in the motion condition; site TO2; Figure 8.2). This extracted face-specific activity (face minus house) did not differ between the static and motion conditions ($F(1, 19) = 1.0$, $p = 0.33$; Figure 8.2), though some small differences in onset latency and early amplitude, particularly of the raw ERPs to the face and house stimuli, were present. These differences were likely due to the responses in one case (the static condition) being to an image onset following an offset (giving a sharper and earlier deflection) and in the other case (the motion condition) being that of a switch from one image to another (giving less of a raw onset potential). The overall result demonstrates that, despite the various physical differences across the static and motion condition (actual visual offsets occurring in the static but not in the motion condition, as well as constant rotational motion of a distractor array only in the motion condition only), stimulus-locked face-specific processing to actual image onsets was present and equally robust in both conditions, with relatively minor differences.

To investigate the extent of face-specific processing that occurs during MIB, *response-locked face-specific activity* associated with the reappearance of target images was compared across the static and motion condition (Figure 8.3). This peri-response face-specific activity differed significantly between the static and motion conditions during the time period surrounding the button press by the subject indicating reappearance (−150 to +300 ms) ($F(1, 19) = 24.0$, $p < 0.001$; Figure 8.3). This effect was driven by the presence of robust face-specific ERP activity in the static condition ($F(1, 19) = 22.6$, $p < 0.001$)

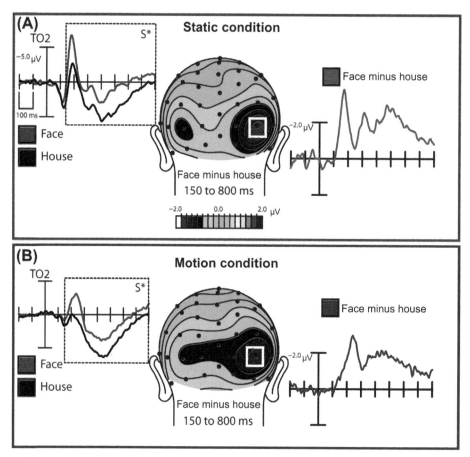

FIGURE 8.2   Face-specific activity to new-image target onsets: face-specific activations were extracted over right temporal–occipital scalp sites in response to new-image target onsets in the static (A) and motion (B) conditions during the poststimulus time window of 150–800 ms. These face-specific responses did not differ across conditions, as shown in a comparison of the face-specific difference waves in the same time window (right side of panel).

and an absence of this activity in the motion condition (F (1, 19) = 0.02, p = 0.90) during the same time period. For the static condition, this button-press-locked response would reflect the convolution of the stimulus-onset-driven face-specific negativity with the response time distribution associated with the button press. If the strictly perceptual onset had actually triggered a comparable face-specific response, a similar activation pattern would be expected in the response-locked averages for the motion condition. Because no discernible face-specific processing was observed for these perceptual onsets, it suggests that face-specific processing had continued uninterrupted during MIB, and that the perceptual onset marked only reentrance of the target into awareness and not the coming online of face-specific processing anew.

Additional analyses collapsing across the face and house object types further examined activity preceding button press responses in the static and motion conditions. This analysis sought to uncover differences in activity preceding the emergence of awareness of an image of any type that had been continuously present (motion condition) to activity preceding the awareness of a physically reappearing image (static condition). This comparison uncovered a significant positive-polarity voltage deflection over parietal scalp sites during the 700 ms preceding a button press in the motion condition, but not in the static condition (F (1, 19) = 47.5, p < 0.0001; Figure 8.4). In the present context, this establishes such activation as distinguishing two types of perceptual reappearances: one in which the object was present but not within awareness, for which this parietal response was present (following MIB), and another in which no object was present and for which no such response was observed.

DISCUSSION

The present results provide electrophysiological evidence that face-specific processing continues relatively intact during MIB, thus supporting the view that MIB disrupts visual awareness through a higher-level mechanism that acts at a relatively late visual processing stage. With

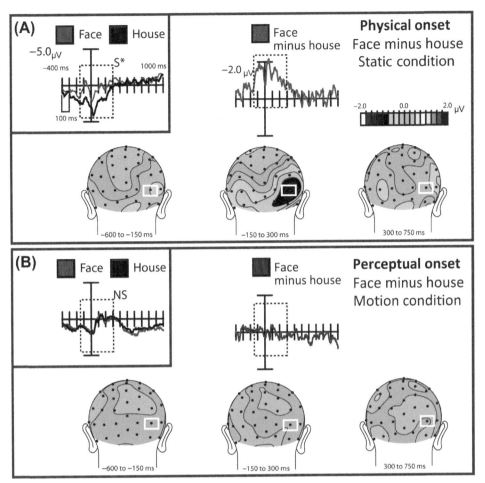

FIGURE 8.3 Response-locked face-specific activations: physical reappearances of faces and houses (static condition) triggered face-specific activations visible in the response-locked averages temporally surrounding the button press (A). In the case of the purely perceptual onsets of faces and houses (motion condition) following MIB episodes, there was no face-specific activation (B). These activations differed significantly across physical and perceptual onsets, during the time window of −150 to 300 ms (surrounding the button press in time).

regard to object-category processing, face-specific neural activity was present in the case of physical onsets, but not in the case of the strictly perceptual onsets that follow MIB episodes. This means that although the disappearance and reappearance of the targets were perceptually similar during the two conditions, the neural processing related to the perceptual appearance and reappearance of targets in the MIB condition was rather unlike that for targets that actually appear or reappear (i.e., in the static condition).

More specifically, the present pattern of results suggests that there was substantial ongoing visual-object processing happening during MIB than during an actual physical absence. In particular, it is clear that in the case of a physical stimulus absence, no face-specific processing could have been happening during that time, given that there was nothing on the screen, and thus the physical reappearance of the stimulus would be expected to trigger a full face-specific response. Thus, by analogy, if there were a complete lack of face-specific processing

during MIB (similar to that seen in the case of a physical absence), a similar face-specific signal would have been expected to occur when the image reentered awareness. The fact that no face-specific activity was actually observed following perceptual reappearance of an image suggests that this activity had been ongoing and intact during MIB. This perseverance of visual neural processing during an MIB despite an absence of awareness is consistent with behavioral MIB studies that suggest that low-level visual perceptual processes intact during MIB. For example, as mentioned earlier, orientation-specific processing (Kouhsari, Moradi, Zand-Vakili, & Esteki, 2002), the formation of negative afterimages (Hofstoetter et al., 2004), the unified nature of an object formed during MIB (Mitroff & Scholl, 2005), and the state of an object following its disappearance during MIB (Mitroff & Scholl, 2004) have all been shown behaviorally to persist during episodes of MIB. The present study, by employing measures of specific neural activity responses, adds

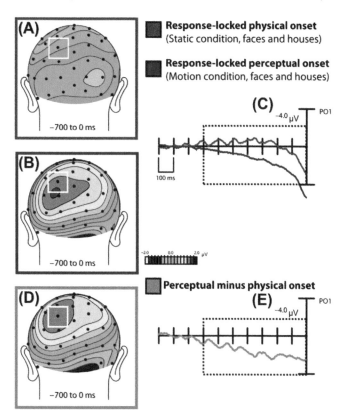

FIGURE 8.4 Perceptual vs physical target onsets: comparisons of physical (A) and perceptual (B) onsets of targets time-locked to the button press, regardless of object category, revealed a positive-polarity voltage deflection over parietal scalp regions during the 700 ms leading up to the button press in the case of perceptual onsets but not physical onsets.

visual object-category discrimination to that list of visual processes that appear to proceed intact during MIB.

The intactness of object-specific processing during MIB is also consistent with some of the proposed mechanisms of MIB. Although a consensus concerning such mechanisms has yet to be reached, one explanation posits that MIB occurs as a result of competing representations of the distractor array and the static target within the visual system (Bonneh et al., 2001). According to this theory, these competing representations are manifested as alternating dominance of the mask display and the static target in terms of what is consciously perceived. This account has been supported neurally by functional imaging studies tracking the relative levels of activity in ventral and dorsal visual regions during and outside of MIB episodes (Donner et al., 2008; Scholvinck & Rees, 2010). In particular, these studies uncovered a pattern of relative levels of activity that seemed to track the subjects' perceptual state, with ventral regions showing higher activity when the static target was within awareness, and dorsal regions showing higher activity during MIB.

The present study speaks to the neural activation patterns that are observed during MIB by measuring the neural correlates of the perceptual events immediately preceding the reemergence of the awareness of an object. Specifically, the perceptual onset, relative to a physical onset, was characterized by a significant increase in parietal activity (during the 700 ms leading to the button press indicating reappearance). This signal could reflect a higher-level process of attentional capture by the continually present target, which would not be observed in the case of a physically absent target, and may mediate its reentrance into visual awareness. This idea of attention breaking an episode of MIB may be distinguished from that put forth in a previous study in which increased endogenous attention to a target enhanced its susceptibility to MIB (Scholvinck & Rees, 2009). In the present case, it may be *exogenous* capture of attention by a present but perceptually suppressed target that appears to facilitate its overcoming of MIB. It makes sense that such an effect would only be seen in the perceptual onset condition, as such attentional switching to the target could underlie its regaining of perceptual dominance in the competitive context of the MIB condition.

Although the neural origin and functional nature of such a parietal scalp signal is not clear as yet, other potentially related effects have implicated a role for parietal processes in the emergence of awareness. For example, disruption of parietal activity has been found to be associated with mediating perceptual switches. When transcranial magnetic stimulation was used to cause transient disruption to left inferior parietal cortex, it facilitated a switch to the subsequent perceptual state, shortened blindness episodes when applied at their onset, and shortened intervals of target awareness when applied with the reemergence of target awareness (Funk & Pettigrew, 2003). The present results thus offer a compelling addition to the body of literature concerning MIB, as well as to that concerning visual processing during the absence of awareness more generally. It must be noted, however, that the interpretation of these results is somewhat constrained by the assumption that the response time distribution in the case of perceptual onsets is reasonably comparable to that of the physical onsets. This assumption is necessary because of the indeterminate nature of the timing of perceptual target onsets in the motion condition, of which the only marker is the button press executed as quickly as possible by the subjects. However, it seems rather unlikely that the total absence of a face-specific effect in the post-MIB case and the presence of a parietal positivity for any object just prior to the button press in that condition could have derived from differences in RT distributions. With regard to face-specific processing, if it were actually present in the motion condition, the RT distribution would have had to be so spread out relative to that of the static condition as to effectively wash out this effect, which seems unlikely. In addition, the observed parietal effect reflecting perceptual onset of a present image is simply not present in the case of static onsets, and cannot be explained by a difference resulting from the convolution of an RT distribution with the same stimulus-locked voltage deflections. Specifically, the parietal difference resulted solely from its presence in the motion condition and complete absence in the static condition. It seems rather unlikely that there was such a variable RT distribution in the motion condition that it could wash out a face-specific ventrolateral-occipital effect in that comparison, while also resulting in an enhanced effect over parietal scalp in another comparison.

CONCLUSIONS

MIB represents a useful tool in disrupting visual awareness while at the same time maintaining low-level visual stimulation. A variety of behavioral studies have suggested that substantial amounts of visual perceptual processing occurs during MIB, and others have proposed high-level mechanisms of competition to account for the effect. The present study adds to the understanding of MIB and visual processing in the absence of awareness in two main ways. First, it shows that although salient images of faces and other objects are susceptible to the effects of MIB, neural activity reflecting object-category discrimination is unaffected as images go in and out of perceptual awareness. Second, it extracts a pattern of parietally distributed activity just prior to the perceptual reappearance of an image (following an MIB episode) that suggests a process of attentional capture by an already present target as it reestablishes its dominance in an MIB setting. Such an attentional process might then constitute a key component of the set of mechanisms mediating MIB.

Acknowledgments

This work was supported by a grant from the National Institutes of Health (R01-MH060415) to M.G.W.

References

Allison, T., Ginter, H., Mccarthy, G., Nobre, A. C., Puce, A., Luby, M., et al. (1994). Face recognition in human extrastriate cortex. *Journal of Neurophysiology, 71*(2), 821–825.

Bentin, S., Allison, T., Puce, A., Perez, E., & McCarthy, G. (1996). Electrophysiological studies of face perception in humans. *Journal of Cognitive Neuroscience, 8*(6), 551–565.

Bonneh, Y. S., Cooperman, A., & Sagi, D. (2001). Motion-induced blindness in normal observers. *Nature, 411*(6839), 798–801.

Carter, O., Luedeman, R., Mitroff, S., & Nakayama, K. (2009). Motion induced blindness: the more you attend the less you see. *Neuroscience Research, 65*. http://dx.doi.org/10.1016/j.neures.2009.09.1573. S17–S17.

Carter, O. L., & Pettigrew, J. D. (2003). A common oscillator for perceptual rivalries? *Perception, 32*(3), 295–305. http://dx.doi.org/10.1068/P3472.

Donner, T. H., Sagi, D., Bonneh, Y. S., & Heeger, D. J. (2008). Opposite neural signatures of motion-induced blindness in human dorsal and ventral visual cortex. *Journal of Neuroscience, 28*(41), 10298–10310. http://dx.doi.org/10.1523/Jneurosci.2371-08.2008.

Funk, A. P., & Pettigrew, J. D. (2003). Does interhemispheric competition mediate motion-induced blindness? A transcranial magnetic stimulation study. *Perception, 32*(11), 1325–1338. http://dx.doi.org/10.1068/P5088.

Harries, M. H., & Perrett, D. I. (1991). Visual processing of faces in temporal cortex – physiological evidence for a modular organization and possible anatomical correlates. *Journal of Cognitive Neuroscience, 3*(1), 9–24.

Harris, J. A., Wu, C. T., & Woldorff, M. G. (2011). Sandwich masking eliminates both visual awareness of faces and face-specific brain activity through a feedforward mechanism. *Journal of Vision, 11*(7). http://dx.doi.org/10.1167/11.7.3. Artn 3.

Hofstoetter, C., Koch, C., & Kiper, D. C. (2004). Motion-induced blindness does not affect the formation of negative afterimages. *Consciousness and Cognition, 13*(4), 691–708. http://dx.doi.org/10.1016/j.concog.2004.06.007.

Holender, D. (1986). Semantic activation without conscious identification in dichotic-listening, parafoveal vision, and visual masking – a survey and appraisal. *Behavioral and Brain Sciences, 9*(1), 1–23.

Hsu, L. C., Yeh, S. L., & Kramer, P. (2006). A common mechanism for perceptual filling-in and motion-induced blindness. *Vision Research, 46*(12), 1973–1981. http://dx.doi.org/10.1016/j.visres.2005.11.004.

Kanwisher, N., McDermott, J., & Chun, M. M. (1997). The fusiform face area: a module in human extrastriate cortex specialized for face perception. *Journal of Neuroscience, 17*(11), 4302–4311.

Kim, C. Y., & Blake, R. (2005). Psychophysical magic: rendering the visible 'invisible'. *Trends in Cognitive Sciences, 9*(8), 381–388. http://dx.doi.org/10.1016/j.tics.2005.06.012.

Kouhsari, L. M., Moradi, F., Zand-Vakili, A., & Esteki, H. (2002). Orientation-selective adaptation in motion-induced blindness. *Perception, 31*, 42–43.

Mitroff, S. R., & Scholl, B. J. (2004). Seeing the disappearance of unseen objects. *Perception, 33*(10), 1267–1273. http://dx.doi.org/10.1068/P5341.

Mitroff, S. R., & Scholl, B. J. (2005). Forming and updating object representations without awareness: evidence from motion-induced blindness. *Vision Research, 45*(8), 961–967. http://dx.doi.org/10.1016/j.visres.2004.09.044.

Montaser-Kouhsari, L., Moradi, F., Zandvakili, A., & Esteky, H. (2004). Orientation-selective adaptation during motion-induced blindness. *Perception, 33*(2), 249–254. http://dx.doi.org/10.1068/P5174.

New, J. J., & Scholl, B. J. (2008). "Perceptual scotomas" – a functional account of motion-induced blindness. *Psychological Science, 19*(7), 653–659.

Perrett, D. I., Hietanen, J. K., Oram, M. W., & Benson, P. J. (1992). Organization and functions of cells responsive to faces in the temporal cortex. *Philosophical Transactions of the Royal Society of London Series B-Biological Sciences, 335*(1273), 23–30.

Philiastides, M. G., Ratcliff, R., & Sajda, P. (2006). Neural representation of task difficulty and decision making during perceptual categorization: a timing diagram. *Journal of Neuroscience, 26*(35), 8965–8975. http://dx.doi.org/10.1523/Jneurosci.1655-06.2006.

Puce, A., Allison, T., Gore, J. C., & Mccarthy, G. (1995). Face-sensitive regions in human extrastriate cortex studied by functional MRI. *Journal of Neurophysiology, 74*(3), 1192–1199.

Puce, A., McCarthy, G., Bentin, S., & Allison, T. (1997). ERP and functional MRI studies of face perception in human ventral visual cortex. *Brain Topography Today, 1147*, 329–333.

Rajimehr, R. (2004). Unconscious orientation processing. *Neuron, 41*(4), 663–673.

Reingold, E. M., & Merikle, P. M. (1988). Using direct and indirect measures to study perception without awareness. *Perception and Psychophysics, 44*(6), 563–575.

Scholvinck, M. L., & Rees, G. (2009). Attentional influences on the dynamics of motion-induced blindness. *Journal of Vision, 9*(1). http://dx.doi.org/10.1167/9.1.38. Artn 38.

Scholvinck, M. L., & Rees, G. (2010). Neural correlates of motion-induced blindness in the human brain. *Journal of Cognitive Neuroscience, 22*(6), 1235–1243.

Feature- and Object-Based Attention: Electrophysiological and Hemodynamic Correlates

Mircea Ariel Schoenfeld[1, 2, 3], *Christian Michael Stoppel*[1]

[1]Department of Neurology, Otto-von-Guericke-University, Magdeburg, Germany,
[2]Leibniz-Institute for Neurobiology, Magdeburg, Germany, [3]Kliniken Schmieder, Allensbach, Germany

INTRODUCTION

Since in everyday life a visual scene is typically analyzed by making eye movements from one spatial location to another, it is not surprising that empirical attention research initially focused on location-based mechanisms of attentional selection. In analogy to the overt eye movements during free vision, Posner and colleagues suggested that visual attention could also be focused covertly in a location-specific manner (Posner, 1980). This notion is captured by the popular metaphor of spatial attention as a spotlight that is directed to a unitary contiguous region of visual space. This spotlight will enhance the processing of all stimuli that fall within its focus, but it has to be shifted across space whenever stimuli at different locations need to be analyzed in more detail. Numerous psychophysical, neurophysiological, and functional neuroimaging studies have provided compelling evidence in favor of the space-based account of attentional selection. This account has been the subject of several recent reviews (Carrasco & Yeshurun, 2009; Hopf, Boehler, Schoenfeld, Heinze, & Tsotsos, 2010; Reynolds & Chelazzi, 2004; Yantis & Serences, 2003). In a nutshell, spatial attention induces a gain enhancement of single neurons/cortical regions whose sensory representation match the attended location (Brefczynski & DeYoe, 1999; Chawla, Rees, & Friston, 1999; Heinze et al., 1994; Hillyard & Mangun, 1987; Luck, Chelazzi, Hillyard, & Desimone, 1997; Moran & Desimone, 1985; Motter, 1993; Spitzer, Desimone, & Moran, 1988), which is accompanied by an improved behavioral performance,

such as increased contrast sensitivity, enhanced spatial resolution, or reduced distractor interference, for stimuli presented at the attended location (Cameron, Tai, & Carrasco, 2002; Hawkins et al., 1990; Lu & Dosher, 1998; Luck, Hillyard, Mouloua, & Hawkins, 1996; Shiu & Pashler, 1995; Yeshurun & Carrasco, 1998). The neural mechanisms underlying these processes are described in Chapter 1 ("Profiling the Spatial Focus of Visual Attention").

Based on many of these psychophysiological and neurophysiological findings, attentional models have argued that space plays a unique role in attentional processing: spatial selection is believed to be an inevitable prerequisite for the processing of featural information, or to accomplish the binding of individual features into holistic objects when stimuli compete for processing resources (Cave & Bichot, 1999; Hillyard & Anllo-Vento, 1998; Treisman & Gelade, 1980). However, individual object attributes (like a stimulus' shape, color or motion) are not only passive recipients of a processing boost due to prior spatial selection, but they might in reverse also be capable of guiding the allocation of spatial attention to potential target objects (Cave, 1999; Wolfe, 1994; Wolfe, Cave, & Franzel, 1989; Wolfe & Horowitz, 2004). This is especially true for situations in which an observer has no prior information about the location of a potential target, but rather must rely on featural information for its detection. Imagine, for example, a situation where you search for a certain person in a crowd. From a computational perspective, it is overly costly to scan every single object that is part of the scenery (here every single person) by focusing onto its spatial location. However, if you possess prior knowledge on the constituent features of the target (e.g., you might know that the person you are looking for is wearing a green sweater), these attributes might aid in guiding your attention and gaze, which ultimately results in an improved detection performance of the target object. This example illustrates that attention cannot only be allocated to particular spatial locations, but also to individual stimulus features. Although the mechanisms of feature-based attention have been investigated less intensively than those underlying spatial selection, recent neurophysiological investigations in primates in conjunction with human neuroimaging studies provided insights into the neural mechanisms underlying feature-based attention. In this chapter, we outline some of the principles underlying feature-based selection processes that have emerged from recent work. We will start by reviewing data from neurophysiological studies in nonhuman primates investigating the effects of feature-based and object-based attention on the processing of distinct stimulus features. This discussion is followed by an outline of functional neuroimaging findings on feature-selective modulations as a result of feature-based and object-based attention. Finally, we will review the results of recent research providing novel insights into the temporal dynamics of feature-based selection processes as revealed by electroencephalographic and magnetoencephalographic recordings in human observers.

NEUROPHYSIOLOGICAL EVIDENCE FOR FEATURE-BASED SELECTION

The first neurophysiological demonstration of feature-selective attentional modulations at a single neuron level emerged more than 25 years ago. In the seminal study by Moran and Desimone (1985), two stimuli were simultaneously presented within the receptive fields of neurons located in macaque regions V4 and IT. One of the stimuli matched the feature selectivity of the particular neurons, while the other was ineffective in driving their response (Moran & Desimone, 1985). When the monkey was required to identify the stimulus corresponding to the neurons' preferred color and orientation, the neurons displayed an increase in their firing rate, while the firing rate was reduced when the nonpreferred stimulus was attended. Although this study clearly showed that a neurons' response is modulated in dependence of the particular features that were attended. Nevertheless, these modulations might also be explained in a space-based selection framework: the behaviorally relevant features only might have guided spatial attention, which finally modulated the neurons' response. While space-based explanations cannot be entirely excluded, these

findings showed that the response of single neurons depends on the similarity between their feature preferences and the features of the attended stimulus. Consistently, numerous subsequent studies reported similar effects for different feature dimensions across multiple visual areas including color-selective modulations in V2, V4, and IT (Luck et al., 1997; Motter, 1994; Reynolds, Chelazzi, & Desimone, 1999), orientation-specific effects in V1, V2, and V4 (McAdams & Maunsell, 1999; Motter, 1993), motion-selective effects in MT (Treue & Maunsell, 1996, 1999), and modulations based on complex objects in V4 and IT (Chelazzi, Duncan, Miller, & Desimone, 1998; Chelazzi, Miller, Duncan, & Desimone, 1993; Chelazzi, Miller, Duncan, & Desimone, 2001). Based on these findings, researchers formulated the biased competition model (Desimone, 1998; Desimone & Duncan, 1995), which asserts that objects presented simultaneously compete for neural representation, and that this competition may be biased in favor of neurons encoding the relevant (attended) information, thus attaining a competitive advantage over neurons that represent the unattended stimulus.

In its initial formulation, the biased competition model mainly referred to competition that is resolved based on spatial mechanisms. More recent studies have shown that neural responses can also be biased in an entirely feature-specific manner, and that these modulations are spatially global, i.e., they occur throughout the entire visual field (Martinez-Trujillo & Treue, 2004; Treue & Martinez Trujillo, 1999). By recording activity from single neurons located in the macaque MT region, Treue and Martinez Trujillo could demonstrate that the response profile of direction-selective neuron scales in a multiplicative manner when attention is directed toward a stimulus' motion direction (Martinez-Trujillo & Treue, 2004; Treue & Martinez Trujillo, 1999). More generally speaking, neurons whose feature preference closely matches the attended feature value (e.g., a specific motion direction) increase their firing rate; while responses of neurons tuned to opposite feature values (e.g., movements opposed to the attended direction) are suppressed. These findings gave rise to the "feature-similarity gain model", which posits that an individual neuron's response depends on the feature similarity between a behaviorally relevant target and the feature preference of that neuron. Importantly, this gain modulation occurs in an entirely location-independent manner. In agreement with the results of Treue and colleagues, other researchers have reported similar feature-selective effects for orientation stimuli in primate area V4 (McAdams & Maunsell, 2000) and for spectral tuning of V4 neurons during natural vision (David, Hayden, Mazer, & Gallant, 2008). In addition, the feature-similarity gain model states that similarity pertains not only to distinct object features, but also to a stimulus' spatial location (feature similarity for location). Accordingly, an additivity of spatial and feature-based modulations has also been observed (Hayden & Gallant, 2005; Martinez-Trujillo & Treue, 2004; Treue & Martinez Trujillo, 1999), but more recent data suggest that both processes might nevertheless rely on distinct mechanisms (Cohen & Maunsell, 2011; Hayden & Gallant, 2005, 2009).

FEATURE-SELECTION AND OBJECT-BASED ATTENTION: NEUROPHYSIOLOGICAL FINDINGS

While psychophysiological evidence for object-based attentional selection dates back to almost half a century ago (Neisser, 1967; Neisser & Becklen, 1975), unequivocal demonstrations on the neurophysiological level did not emerge until the end of the twentieth century. In 1998, Roelfsema, Lamme, and Spekreijse (1998) investigated object-based selection in monkeys using a curve-tracing task, in which one curve had to be attended and an overlapping curve needed to be ignored. With this approach, they demonstrated that the firing of neurons located in area V1, whose receptive fields covered parts of the attended curve, was enhanced, which was not the case for neurons with receptive fields that spatially matched parts of the distracter curve. While this early finding still has been controversial in terms of location-based explanations, later studies were capable to investigate the neurophysiological signs of object-based selection without any location confounds. This was achieved by use of an elegant design developed by Valdes-Sosa and colleagues, which they originally employed to investigate object-based mechanisms of attentional selection in psychophysical experiments (Valdes-Sosa, Bobes, Rodriguez, & Pinilla, 1998; Valdes-Sosa, Cobo, & Pinilla, 1998; Valdes-Sosa, Cobo, & Pinilla, 2000). To exclude space-based attentional selection, Valdes-Sosa and colleagues presented their study participants with a circular aperture in which two populations of dots moved clockwise and counterclockwise, and thus were perceived as two superimposed transparent surfaces. Several studies have adopted this type of stimulus for use in primate neurophysiological experiments. For instance, in a study by Fallah, Stoner, and Reynolds (2007) monkeys were exogenously biased to attend to one of two superimposed transparent surfaces (composed of counter-rotating dots) by a delayed onset of one of the two surfaces. They showed that V4 neurons increase their firing rate when the attended surface's color matched the neurons' color preference, while the firing rate decreased when the color was nonpreferred (Fallah et al., 2007). Similarly, it has been shown that neurons located in primate area V5/MT increase their firing rate when stimuli,

having a task-relevant color and a task-irrelevant motion direction, fall into the neurons' receptive field, even when only the stimulus' color was attended. These data showed that attentional modulations in the extrastriate visual cortex could be observed even when the attended dimension does not match the tuning properties of the recorded neuron. This appears to be accomplished by a cross-featural spread of the attentional enhancement across different object features (Buracas & Albright, 2009; Katzner, Busse, & Treue, 2009; Wannig, Rodriguez, & Freiwald, 2007). These results confirm that the neural processing of task-irrelevant features can be facilitated when they are part of an attended object (an effect termed "same-object advantage").

FUNCTIONAL NEUROIMAGING EVIDENCE FOR FEATURE-BASED SELECTION

In agreement with the aforementioned findings from primate neurophysiology, studies using functional neuroimaging methods in humans also observed feature-selective attentional effects based on a stimulus' color, shape, orientation, or motion direction. Such modulations at neural population levels were identified across multiple subcortical (Schneider, 2011) and cortical regions along the visual hierarchy, including V1 (Huk & Heeger, 2000; Kamitani & Tong, 2005; Liu, Larsson, & Carrasco, 2007), V2 (Kamitani & Tong, 2006; Liu et al., 2007), V3 (Buchel et al., 1998; Chawla et al., 1999; Saenz, Buracas, & Boynton, 2002), V4/V8 (Corbetta, Miezin, Dobmeyer, Shulman, & Petersen, 1990; Liu et al., 2007; Saenz et al., 2002), IT (Corbetta et al., 1990), and human MT (Buchel et al., 1998; Chawla et al., 1999; Corbetta et al., 1990; Huk & Heeger, 2000; O'Craven, Rosen, Kwong, Treisman, & Savoy, 1997; Saenz et al., 2002). Moreover, feature-selective activations even occurred in absence of direct visual stimulation, i.e. in pure anticipation of the to-be presented stimulus, evident as the increased hemodynamic baseline activity in regions that process the expected stimulus attribute (Chawla et al., 1999; Kastner, Pinsk, De Weerd, Desimone, & Ungerleider, 1999; McMains, Fehd, Emmanouil, & Kastner, 2007; Serences & Boynton, 2007; Shibata et al., 2008). While most hemodynamic studies initially targeted the mere functional localization of feature-based modulations for stimuli presented within the focus of attention, subsequent work also demonstrated the global efficacy of feature selection across the visual field (Saenz et al., 2002; Serences & Boynton, 2007).

Thus, the general mechanisms of feature-selection as revealed by single-cell recordings in primates also apply to the modulations at population levels shown by functional neuroimaging in humans. Importantly, most of the conventional hemodynamic investigations addressed feature selectivity by comparing hemodynamic activations across different feature dimensions, e.g., attention to color vs attention to motion. A central hallmark of feature selectivity in primate neurophysiology, however, is the multiplicative scaling of single-neuron responses in dependence of the similarity between a neurons' feature preference and the attended feature value *within* a single feature dimension ("feature-similarity gain"; Martinez-Trujillo & Treue, 2004; Treue & Martinez Trujillo, 1999). Such feature selectivity has recently been addressed by some functional magnetic resonance imaging (fMRI) investigations employing pattern classification methods for data analysis (Jehee, Brady, & Tong, 2011; Kamitani & Tong, 2006; Liu, Hospadaruk, Zhu, & Gardner, 2011; Serences & Boynton, 2007; Serences, Saproo, Scolari, Ho, & Muftuler, 2009). These studies indeed revealed feature-selective activity *within* a feature dimension across multiple stages along the visual hierarchy (Jehee et al., 2011; Kamitani & Tong, 2006; Liu et al., 2011; Serences & Boynton, 2007). These effects, however, were not confined to the cortical regions known to process the physical attributes of the presented stimuli, as demonstrated by neurophysiological studies in primates. Therein, the results from decoding studies do not necessarily imply the existence of feature-selective populations across all regions with above-chance classification accuracy (Serences & Boynton, 2007). Besides factual feature-selective population activity, such a response profile also might entail feed-forward/feedback activity from lower and higher tier visual areas (Sillito, Cudeiro, & Jones, 2006).

While decoding studies require at least some caution with regard to the interpretation of their results due to the above-mentioned neurophysiological constraints, conventional fMRI investigations mostly failed to provide evidence for feature-selective modulations *within* a feature dimension. This lack of direct fMRI evidence for feature selectivity most likely results from methodological limitations, in that the responses of feature-selective neurons to different feature values *within* a feature dimension are probably beyond the spatial and temporal resolution provided by conventional fMRI analysis techniques. To overcome these methodological restrictions, we recently employed a novel task design to assess the influence of feature-selective attention on neural population activity by means of fMRI (Stoppel et al., 2011). The experimental setup was based on a classical feature-based attention task and is illustrated in Figure 9.1(A). During the task, subjects were cued to attend to a certain motion direction (left or right) of a transparent surface (a moving dot field) in a block-wise fashion. During subsequent trials, the motion coherence of the surface was then parametrically manipulated, while the main movement of the dots (left or right) was either directed

into or opposed to the attended direction. This approach allowed investigating the magnitude of hemodynamic activity as a function of direction-selective attention (i.e., feature-selective modulations *within* a feature dimension) under varying noise characteristics (motion coherence) of the stimuli. The magnitudes of these direction-dependent and coherence-dependent modulations across several motion-sensitive regions are depicted in Figure 9.1(B). Note that the activation magnitude of hMT is positively correlated with a stimulus' coherence when its motion direction is attended (mirroring the subjects' behavioral performance). In contrast, when the stimulus moved opposed to the attended direction a reverse relationship was observed (an inverse correlation between motion coherence and activation magnitude). It is important to note that hMT was the only region that exhibited this specific pattern (compare activation patterns between regions shown in Figure 9.1(B)). These data provide evidence for the validity of the feature-similarity gain hypothesis at the level of hMT's entire neural population (Martinez-Trujillo & Treue, 2004), and suggest that feature-based attention improves behavioral performance by modulating direction-selective population activity within area hMT. Recent pattern classification studies (Jehee et al., 2011; Kamitani & Tong, 2006; Liu et al., 2011; Serences & Boynton, 2007) reported attentional modulations of direction-selective responses not only in hMT, but also at multiple stages of the visual processing hierarchy. Future studies will have to investigate the nature of these direction-selective responses in order to link neurophysiological mechanisms to patterns exhibiting above-chance classification accuracy observed across multiple stages along the visual hierarchy in studies using decoding techniques.

FEATURE-SELECTION IN OBJECT-BASED ATTENTION: FUNCTIONAL NEUROIMAGING EVIDENCE

The first fMRI demonstration of a cross-featural enhancement by object-based attention (in terms of a same-object advantage) has been provided by O'Craven, Downing, and Kanwisher (1999). In their study, subjects were presented with superimposed semitransparent pictures of houses and faces, one of which was moving while the other remained stationary. While subjects were cued to attend either to the houses, faces, or the stimulus' motion, increased hemodynamic activations were not restricted to cortical regions selective for the attended object attribute, but also occurred in regions processing the task-irrelevant object feature. Similar as to the early psychophysical and neurophysiological accounts on object-based selection, these results have initially been called into question in terms of space-based explanations.

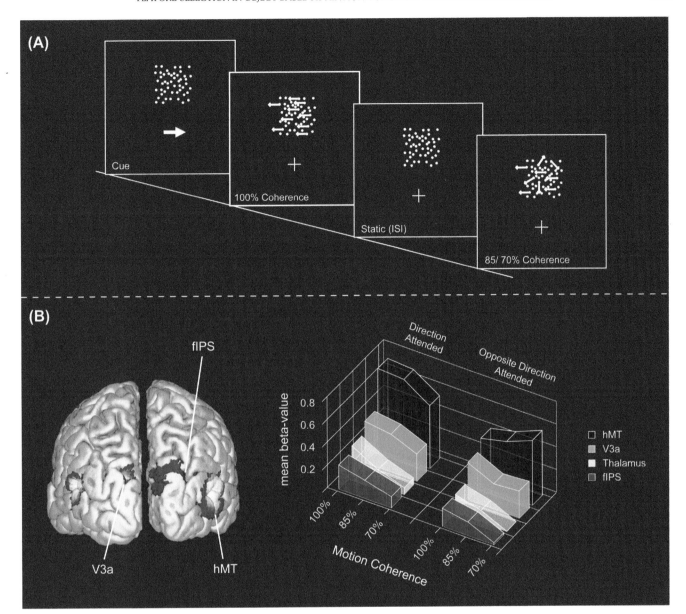

FIGURE 9.1 **(A) Schematic illustration of the experimental design used in the study of** Stoppel et al. (2011). Before each block subjects were cued (arrow pointing to the left or right) to attend to a particular motion direction of a moving transparent surface consisting of 100 white dots. During each trial the dots either moved into or opposed to the attended direction, while their motion coherence was concurrently manipulated (100%, 85% and 70%). On some trials, the movements were of higher speed, and subjects were required to respond to those in the attended direction as targets regardless of their motion coherence. This design allowed comparing the magnitude of hemodynamic activations as a function of direction-selective attention (slow movements into or opposed to the attended direction) under varying noise levels of the stimuli (100%, 85% or 70% coherence). **(B) Attentional modulation of neural activations to visual motion coherence in extrastriate and thalamic regions.** The activation map on the left shows regions exhibiting higher activity during (nontarget) motion trials than during the presentation of stationary dots. On the right, the magnitudes of hemodynamic activations (beta parameter estimates) to each coherence level are depicted for both attention conditions (movements into or opposed to the attended direction). Note that hMT is the only region showing an inverse linear relationship between motion coherence and the magnitude of the signal estimates for attended and unattended conditions. *Adapted from Stoppel et al. (2011).*

However, during the past decade a growing body of functional imaging evidence for object-based selection has accumulated. First, using high-resolution retinotopic mapping, it has been shown that activity in early visual cortex not only is enhanced at the retinotopic coordinates representing the spatial focus of attention, but also at retinotopic locations correspondent to the parts of an object that are not directly (spatially) attended (Muller & Kleinschmidt, 2003; Shomstein & Behrmann, 2006). Moreover, fMRI studies using overlapping transparent surfaces (similar to those employed in neurophysiological research as described above) observed hemodynamic modulations to task-irrelevant object features in terms of a same-object advantage

(Ciaramitaro, Mitchell, Stoner, Reynolds, & Boynton, 2011; Safford, Hussey, Parasuraman, & Thompson, 2010; Schoenfeld et al., 2003). Such a feature spread is not even bound to a certain modality, but rather seems to spread across modalities arguing for the existence of multisensory objects (e.g., enhanced processing of a sound that is perceived as belonging to an attended visual stimulus; Busse, Roberts, Crist, Weissman, & Woldorff, 2005). And finally, recent investigations have shown that the object-based enhancement of task-irrelevant features is not confined to the attended object, but also spreads (globally) to spatially nonattended locations in a similar manner, as it has been observed for simple feature-based selection (Busse et al., 2005; Lustig & Beck, 2012; Sohn, Chong, Papathomas, & Vidnyanszky, 2005).

In summary, consistent evidence for a cross-featural enhancement as a result of object-based selection has independently been provided by psychophysical, neurophysiological, as well as functional neuroimaging research. However, most of the studies discussed so far did not permit inferences about the timing of the underlying processes to be made due to the poor temporal resolution of hemodynamic methods. This is not only true for the object-based enhancement of distinct object features as discussed here, but also applies to the effects driven by mere feature-based selection as outlined in previous paragraphs. This gap should be closed in the following section, which addresses the temporal aspects of feature selection, as provided by noninvasive electroencephalographic and magnetoencephalographic investigations in humans.

THE TIMING OF FEATURE-BASED ATTENTIONAL SELECTION

Noninvasive electrophysiological investigations in humans have shown that event-related electroencephalographic (event-related potentials; ERPs) and magnetoencephalographic (event-related fields; ERFs) responses are modulated by feature-based attention. The general principle behind these studies was to compare the magnitude of ERPs and ERFs elicited by a stimulus whose features were attended to situations when the constituent features of the same stimulus were ignored. The feature-selective modulations observed by this approach were generally evident as broad negative or positive deflections in the evoked responses over centroposterior electrodes in the ERP (the so-called selection negativity or -positivity, SN/SP; for review see Harter & Aine, 1984; Hillyard & Anllo-Vento, 1998). Importantly, based on their precise temporal resolution, these electrophysiological studies not only revealed that the selection of task-relevant features (such as spatial frequency, orientation, color, motion direction,

or shape) is reflected in amplitude modulations per se, but also allowed to assess the timing of these effects on a scale of tens of milliseconds. Numerous studies demonstrated that feature-based selection operates in the time range of the N1 ERP-component, i.e., between 120 and 180 ms after stimulus onset (Anllo-Vento & Hillyard, 1996; Beer & Roder, 2004, 2005; Harter & Aine, 1984; Kenemans, Baas, Mangun, Lijffijt, & Verbaten, 2000; Kenemans, Kok, & Smulders, 1993; Martinez et al., 2001; Motter, 1994; Smid, Jakob, & Heinze, 1999; Torriente, Valdes-Sosa, Ramirez, & Bobes, 1999). The variation in onset latencies between these studies have been suggested to result from differences in the relative discriminability between the attended and unattended features (Hillyard & Anllo-Vento, 1998). Following this logic, feature selection should proceed faster, if a given discrimination process is less demanding. This view has received empirical support by a recent study combining ERP and ERF recordings in human observers (Schoenfeld et al., 2007). The rationale behind this study was, that if attention is directed to entire feature dimensions (e.g., motion vs. color), the selection process should proceed faster than when it involves discrimination between particular feature values belonging to the same dimension (e.g., one motion direction vs. another). The task design employed by Schoenfeld et al. (2007) is illustrated in Figure 9.2(A). Subjects were presented with a squared aperture comprising 100 stationary white dots that, during each trial, either changed their color (either to red or orange) or moved coherently to the right (either fast or slow). By cueing the subjects to discriminate the color change or the motion velocity in a block-wise fashion, the task design aimed to maximize the selective processing of either the stimulus' color or motion. As a result, feature-selective processing could be compared between blocks in which the respective feature dimension was attended (e.g., the dots moved and motion was task relevant) with those in which it was task irrelevant (the dots moved but color was attended). In agreement with previous studies, enlarged amplitudes could be observed for both feature dimensions, when the corresponding dimension was attended compared to when it was ignored (motion-related attentional modulations are shown in Figure 9.2(B), while color-selective effects are depicted in Figure 9.2(C)). Importantly, these attention-related facilitations occurred rapidly, beginning as early as 90–120 ms after stimulus onset (compare original waveforms and see difference waves in Figures 9.2(B) and (C)). These results showed that entire feature dimensions could be selected much earlier (already evident at ~100 poststimulus) than different feature values *within* a single feature dimension (typically starting between 120 and 180 ms after stimulus onset). These data add to the notion that the timing of feature-selective

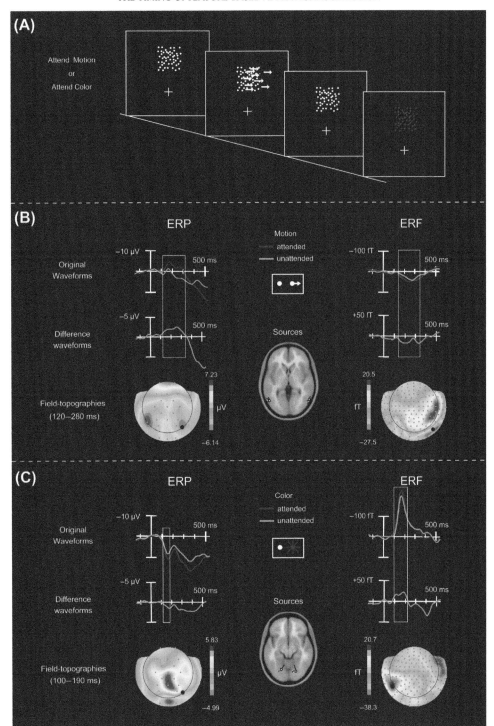

FIGURE 9.2 **(A) Experimental design of the study by** Schoenfeld et al. (2007). Subjects were presented with 100 white dots, that either moved to the right (with high or low velocity) or changed their color (to red or orange) for 300 ms during each trial. Before each block of 16–20 stimuli the subjects were cued either to attend to the stimulus' motion (to identify fast movements) or to its color (to identify an orange color change). This design permitted to compare trials in which a particular feature dimension was attended (e.g., the dots moved and motion was task relevant) with those in which it was unattended (the dots moved but color was task relevant). **The effect of attention on the processing of motion (B) and on the processing of color (C)**. Original ERP and ERF waveforms elicited by the motion and color standards (slow movements/color changes to red) are shown in the upper rows of (B) and (C). Original waveforms from trials in which the particular feature was attended are drawn in red, while those from unattended motion or color trials are depicted in blue. Difference waves (in green—middle rows in (B) and (C)) were obtained by subtracting the waveforms elicited by unattended from attended motion (B) or color (C) trials, respectively. Electrode and sensor locations are indicated by black dots in the corresponding topographical field distributions (lower rows in (B) and (C)). Note that the attentional enhancement of stimulus motion (B) and color (C) both were already evident at ~110 ms in the ERPs (motion and color) and after ~90 ms (color) and ~120 ms (motion) in the ERFs. The estimated source dipoles accounting for the surface topographies of the particular difference waveforms are shown in the middle columns of (B) and (C). The neural generators of the motion-related effect were localized to bilateral middle occipitotemporal cortex, while the color-related modulations were shown to originate from bilateral posterior fusiform/lingual gyrus. *Adapted from Schoenfeld et al. (2007).*

II. FEATURE AND OBJECT ATTENTION

modulations depends on the relative discriminability (i.e., different processing requirements) between the attended and unattended stimulus' features.

While the data discussed so far demonstrated a temporal flexibility of feature-based attentional selection depending on the stimulus-discriminability, other recent work has shown that the temporal dynamics of feature selection also might vary in dependence of other factors. One such aspect is the spatial location at which stimuli are presented with respect to the focus of attention. With this said, it is important to note that a common denominator of the aforementioned studies was that the stimulus material was presented in the attended part of space. However, as outlined above, feature-based selection seems to operate in a spatially global manner. Hence, it is critical to know if the electrophysiological signs of feature-selection show a comparable spatiotemporal pattern when the stimuli are presented outside the focus of spatial attention. Recently, we explicitly addressed this question using combined electroencephalographic and magnetoencephalographic recordings using an experimental design that is illustrated in Figure 9.3(A) (Stoppel et al., 2012). During the task participants attended to the direction of a moving transparent surface located in the left visual field, while task-irrelevant probe stimuli executing brief movements into varying directions were presented in an aperture located in the opposite (spatially unattended) visual field. This allowed the direct comparison of the magnitude of ERPs elicited by the spatially unattended motion probes in dependence of the similarity of their direction of movement to the motion direction of the spatially attended surface. The results demonstrated a feature-selective modulation of the ERPs over central electrodes, whose magnitude varied as a function of the similarity between the motion directions of the spatially attended and unattended stimuli (Figure 9.3(B), left column). A correspondent feature-selective modulation also was observed in the simultaneously recorded ERFs over left occipitotemporal sensors (Figure 9.3(B), right column). Importantly, these parametric modulations reflecting globally enhanced processing of the attended feature were observed to start not before 200 ms poststimulus (see ERP and ERF original waveforms in Figure 9.3(B)). This relative delay in comparison to tasks in which the stimuli were presented at spatially attended locations as outlined above (with modulations arising between 100 and 180 ms after stimulus onset) indicates that the spread of feature-selective modulations from attended to spatially unattended locations is a time-consuming process.

Referring to this relative delay, it is important to note that the stimuli presented at the spatially unattended location were always task irrelevant. Thus, while feature discrimination indeed had to be accomplished in the attended surface, the feature did not serve to guide the deployment of spatial attentional resources, because

the location of the target stimulus was always known. A qualitatively different situation, however, emerges during visual search where the location of the target changes from trial to trial. In such tasks, feature-based attention might guide spatial attention to potential target objects (Cave & Bichot, 1999; Treisman & Sato, 1990; Wolfe, 1994), which raises the question how feature selection is implemented in visual search. Based on guided search theories, feature selection would be expected to precede the indices of location selection during visual search. Hopf, Boelmans, Schoenfeld, Luck, and Heinze (2004) addressed this prediction using a search task in which multiple nontarget items (comprising some target-defining features) could be presented in the visual field containing or being opposed to the factual target (for illustration of the task design see Figure 9.4(A)). This design permitted to dissociate processes related to the selection of task-relevant features from neural responses reflecting the focusing of attention onto the location of the target stimulus (as indexed by the N2pc ERP-component). This, in turn, enabled the authors to investigate the spatiotemporal correlates of feature-based and location-based selection during visual search (Hopf et al., 2004). As visible in Figure 9.4(B), an enhanced response to distractor stimuli containing the target feature was observed in the ERPs and ERFs contralateral to the side of stimulus presentation. Importantly, this feature-selective modulation emerged as early as 140 ms after the onset of the search array, while the N2pc component indicating the focusing of attention onto the location of the target did not arise until 170 ms poststimulus (Figure 9.4(C); the relative timing of both processes is depicted in the right part of Figure 9.4(C)). These data demonstrate that in visual search the processing of task-relevant features precedes the selection of the target location, indicating that feature-based selection can guide spatial attention to the location of the target object. Hence, the data further add to the notion that feature selection is temporally flexible and adapts according to the specific task requirements.

So far, we have outlined the temporal characteristics of feature selection putting aside the effects originating from object-based attentional selection. The timing of such feature-specific effects during object-based selection will be addressed in the following. The first compelling demonstration of object-based effects with electrophysiological methods in humans was provided by Valdes-Sosa and colleagues (Valdes-Sosa, Bobes, et al., 1998). They presented participants with two overlapping counter-rotating dot patterns, which appeared as two perceptually separable but spatially perfectly overlapping transparent surfaces. While observers were required to detect the occurrence of a particular target movement within only one of the two surfaces, brief task-irrelevant lateral displacements could occur within both of them. This allowed to compare the motion-evoked ERPs if the particular

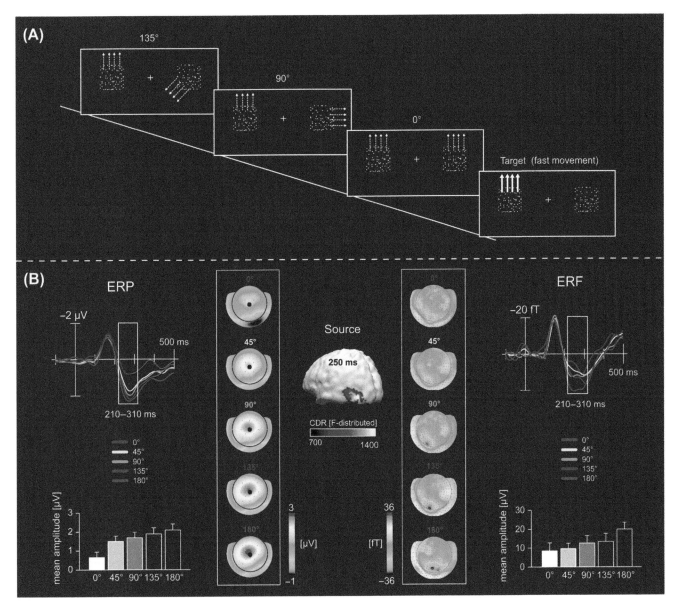

FIGURE 9.3   **(A) Experimental design in the study by** Stoppel et al. (2012). Subjects viewed two squared apertures located in the left and right visual field, each of which was composed of 100 white dots. In the left aperture, all dots moved either coherently up (during even runs) or downward (during odd runs) and were perceived as a transparent surface. The subjects' task was to indicate brief accelerations in the motion speed of this surface by a button-press response. During such target trials and during the intertrial intervals all dots within the right aperture remained stationary. On probe trials, in contrast, all dots in the right aperture performed brief coherent displacements into one of the eight cardinal or ordinal directions, thus deviating from the motion direction of the attended surface by 0°, 45°, 90°, 135° or 180°, respectively. These motion probes were completely task irrelevant and subjects were instructed to ignore them. **(B) Original waveforms and mean amplitudes (210–310 ms poststimulus) of the probe-related ERP (left column) and ERF (right column) responses**. The location of the electrode and sensor are indicated by black dots within the field distribution maps. Note that the ERP and ERF amplitudes varied as a function of the similarity between the probes motion direction and that of the attended surface. The corresponding field distributions show a maximal positivity over midline central electrode sites for the ERPs (left topography maps) and an efflux—influx field transition over left occipitotemporal sensors for the ERFs (right topography maps). The neural source reflecting this parametric modulation was localized to the left middle occipitotemporal cortex (the current source density distribution 250 ms after stimulus onset is shown in the middle of the figure). *Adapted from Stoppel et al. (2012).*

surface was attended or unattended, and thus to investigate how object-based attentional selection modulates the processing of a particular feature. With this elegant design the authors could demonstrate that almost the entire ERP response (up to 700 ms post-onset) was suppressed when the particular surface was ignored. This general finding that object-based selection leads to a competitive advantage in the processing of features that are bound to an attended in comparison to an unattended object has subsequently been extended by other electrophysiological investigations. Using different stimulus material and varying task designs these studies not only replicated the

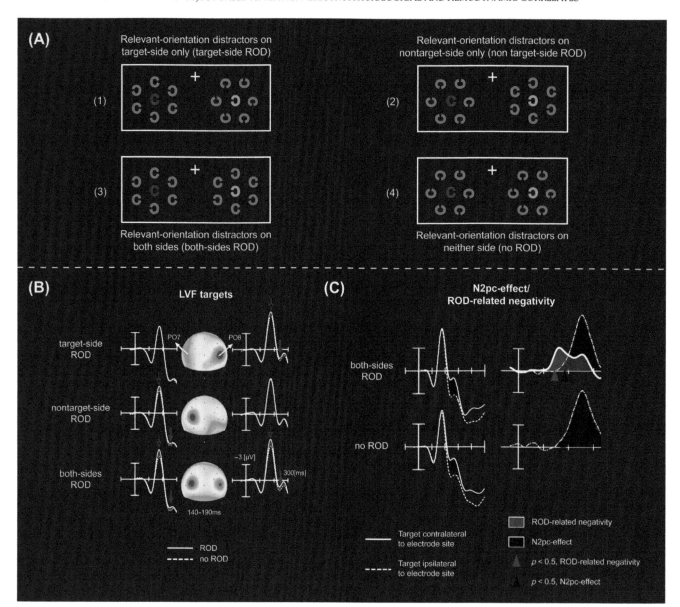

FIGURE 9.4   **(A) Stimuli from the study of** Hopf et al. (2004). Search frames consisted of distinctively colored C's (red or green), one presented to the left and one to the right visual field, which both were surrounded by blue distractors. On each half of the trial blocks, either the red or the green C served as the search target, whose orientation (left or right gap) had to be discriminated by the subjects. In contrast to the search targets, the distractor stimuli could be arranged in that their gap was also oriented to the left and right (relevant orientation distracters, RODs), or it was arranged perpendicular (up and down) to that of the target stimulus (irrelevant orientation distracters). The location of the RODs varied relative to the location of the target item, such that they appeared (1) on the target side only (target-side ROD), (2) on the nontarget side only (nontarget-side ROD), (3) on both sides (both-sides ROD), or (4) on neither side (no ROD). **(B) ERP responses elicited by targets presented to the left visual field (LVF)**. Original waveforms of the different ROD conditions (solid lines) are separately depicted (target-side ROD— top row, nontarget-side ROD—middle row, both-sides ROD—bottom row) each overlaid onto the control condition (no ROD, dashed lines). The correspondent field distributions of the voltage differences between the ROD conditions and the control condition are shown in the middle column. An enhanced negativity in the time range between 140 and 300 ms poststimulus emerged contralateral to the location of the RODs (indicated by red arrows and filled in red between ERP traces). **(C) Target-related effect (N2pc effect) and relative timing of the N2pc and the ROD-related negativity.** Average waveforms elicited by target items contralateral (solid line) and ipsilateral (dashed line) to electrodes PO7/PO8 are depicted on the left. The N2pc effect is highlighted in blue between waveforms. Time courses of the N2pc (contralateral minus ipsilateral targets; broken lines—area under the curve drawn in blue) and the ROD-related negativity (thick solid line—area under the curve drawn in red) are shown on the right. The arrowheads mark the onset latencies of the ROD-related negativity (red) and of the N2pc effect for the both-sides ROD condition (blue). Note that the ROD-related negativity arises ~30–40 ms before the N2pc. *Adapted from Hopf et al. (2004).*

findings by Valdes-Sosa, Cobo, and Pinilla (1998), but also provided data on the timing of feature processing during object-based selection. Therein, it has consistently been shown that the ERPs elicited by features that are bound to attended in comparison to unattended objects display an increased amplitude in the time range of the N1 component, starting around 150–170 ms after stimulus onset (Martinez et al., 2006; Pinilla, Cobo, Torres, & Valdes-Sosa, 2001; Rodriguez & Valdes-Sosa, 2006). The timing of these modulations as a result of object-based selection thus closely resembles the timing of feature-selective effects that are driven by purely feature-based selection as outlined above. Importantly, however, while all studies mentioned so far demonstrated facilitatory effects of object-based selection on the processing of particular features, they did not investigate putative signs of the same-object advantage as evident from psychophysiological, neurophysiological, and functional neuroimaging studies.

This gap has been closed by two recent investigations addressing the neurophysiological mechanisms underlying the same-object advantage by means of noninvasive electrophysiology in humans (Boehler, Schoenfeld, Heinze, & Hopf, 2011; Schoenfeld et al., 2003). Schoenfeld et al. (2003) presented participants with a squared aperture comprising 200 stationary white dots. During each trial, each half of the dots moved into opposite directions (left and right), which thus were perceived as two overlapping transparent surfaces (the task design is illustrated in Figure 9.5(A)). The subjects' task was to attend to one of the two surfaces and to detect the occurrence of a fast movement in the attended direction. In addition to the changes in motion speed, a task-irrelevant color change could occur either within the attended or the unattended surface (Schoenfeld et al., 2003). This design permitted the investigation of the neurophysiological signs of the same-object advantage by comparing trials in which the color change occurred in the attended surface to those in which the color of the unattended surface changed, while in both cases color was completely irrelevant to the task. As shown in Figure 9.5(B), the ERPs and ERFs evoked by a color change was of higher amplitude when it appeared in the attended object in comparison to the unattended object. This neuronal facilitation of an entirely task-irrelevant feature, only by virtue of its belonging to an attended object (i.e., a same-object advantage), did not arise until 220–240 ms after stimulus onset (see original waveforms and difference waves in Figure 9.5(B)). This delay in the processing of a task-irrelevant object feature relative to its direct selection by feature-based attention (starting at 220–240 vs 100–180 ms poststimulus) indicates that the spread of feature-selective modulations toward task-irrelevant object attributes needs time. Hence, both the spread of feature-selective modulations toward spatially unattended locations (Stoppel et al., 2012), as well as between task-relevant and task-irrelevant features of

an object (Schoenfeld et al., 2003) seem to be dynamic time-consuming processes.

The findings that task-irrelevant features are modulated because they are part of an attended object raises two important further questions: (1) Since feature selection is known to proceed globally, does this object-based modulation of task-irrelevant features also spread to unattended locations? and (2) Do the temporal costs for the attentional spread from task-relevant to task-irrelevant object features (as shown by Schoenfeld et al., 2003; also see Figure 9.5) sum up to the costs for spreading from attended to unattended locations (as shown in Stoppel et al., 2012; see Figure 9.3)? Both questions have nicely been addressed by a very recent electroencephalographic investigation (Boehler et al., 2011). In the task employed by Boehler et al. (2011), subjects were presented with two three-dimensional spheres, one of which was located in the left and the other in the right visual field (the task design is illustrated in Figure 9.6(A)). Both spheres were composed of two halves, each of which was drawn in a different color (red, green, blue, or yellow). Before each block, subjects were cued to search for a particular color (e.g., red as shown Figure 9.6(A)), which on each trial appeared in one of the half spheres, either in the left or the right visual field. The other colors were randomly assigned to the remaining half spheres, in that one of the nontarget colors could either appear in both visual fields (and thus was part of the target containing *and* of the irrelevant object—see upper left panel of Figure 9.6(A)), or all four half spheres were assigned a different color (see middle left panel of Figure 9.6(A)). This design allowed us to assess if the ERP response evoked by a particular color of the nontarget sphere was modulated as a function of whether this color was present or absent in the attended sphere. Thereby, the authors could investigate whether the object-based selection of a task-irrelevant feature, when simultaneously presented at an unattended location, leads to a global enhancement of that feature (irrelevant feature effect, IFE). To verify that such an IFE indeed depends on object-based selection of the task-irrelevant feature, the authors included additional control trials into their design, in which the half spheres were cut apart and slightly rotated relative to each other, such that each color now belonged to a separate object (see right panels of Figure 9.6(A)).

The main results of this study are shown in Figure 9.6(B) and (C). As can be seen in the upper row of Figure 9.6(B), trials in which the nontarget color was presented to both visual fields (dashed traces) showed a relative negativity in their ERP amplitudes at electrode sites contralateral to the distracter sphere when compared to trials where the nontarget colors differed between both spheres (solid lines; see right upper panel in Figure 9.6(B)). This amplitude modulation (IFE) did not become significant until 270 ms after stimulus onset. Importantly, such an amplitude difference was

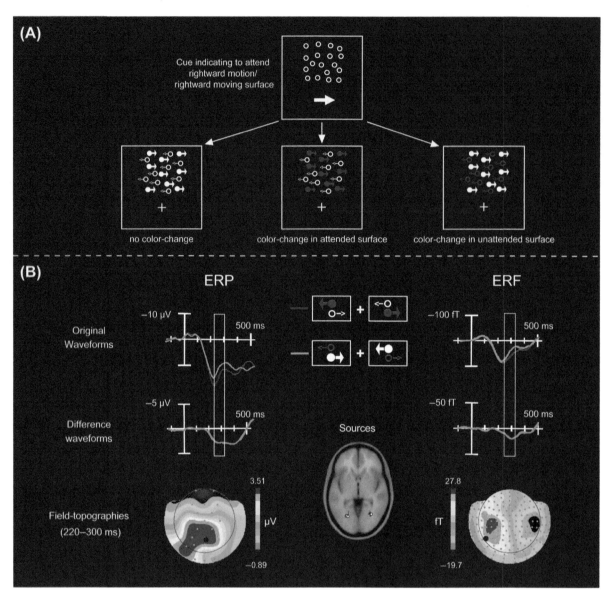

FIGURE 9.5 **(A) Experimental design of the study by** Schoenfeld et al. (2003). Subjects were presented with a squared aperture containing 200 stationary white dots. On each trial, a random half of the dots moved to the left and the other half to the right for 300 ms, and were perceived as two superimposed transparent surfaces. Subjects were cued to attend either to the left-moving or right-moving surface, and to identify occasional targets (fast movements) in the attended surface. On probe trials, either the leftward or rightward moving surface could change its color to red, or both surfaces could remain plain gray. This design allowed comparing responses to trials in which a task-irrelevant color change occurred in the attended surface to responses to the same physical stimulus but where the other surface was attended. **(B) The effect of object-based attention on the processing of task-irrelevant color**. Original waveforms depict the ERP and ERF responses to color changes occurring in the attended (red tracings) or unattended (blue tracings) surface. The difference waveforms formed by subtracting the blue from the red waveforms are shown in green. Note that the object-based attentional enhancement of the irrelevant color emerged not before 220 ms after stimulus onset. The topographical maps represent the field distributions of the difference waveforms for the time range between 220 and 300 ms. The black dots in the topographical maps indicate the locations of the electrode and sensor. The correspondent source dipoles that were estimated to account for the difference waveform topography were localized to bilateral ventral occipital cortex (fusiform/lingual gyrus—shown in between the topography maps). *Adapted from Schoenfeld et al. (2003).*

neither observed for electrodes contralateral to the target sphere (left upper panel in Figure 9.6(B)), nor was any modulation observed in analog comparisons of the waveforms for the separate object condition (see lower row of Figure 9.6(B)). These data clearly demonstrate that the object-based selection of a task-irrelevant

feature proceeds in a spatially global manner. Beyond this finding, the study also provided information concerning the timing of the IFE in relation to modulations reflecting the focusing of spatial attention onto the target object (Figure 9.6(C)). For this purpose, the authors analyzed the timing of the N2pc component, which was

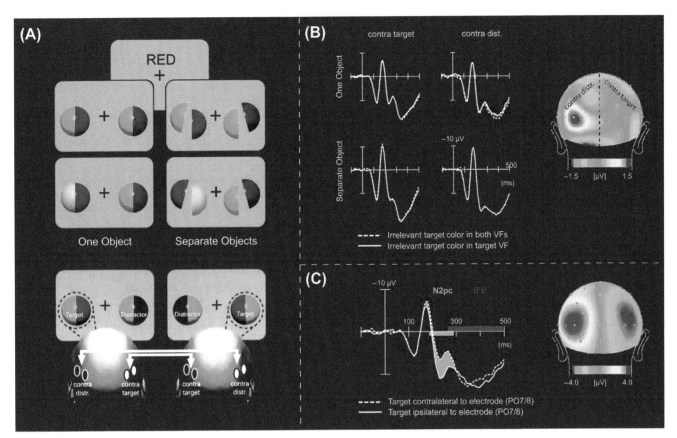

FIGURE 9.6 **Stimulus setup of the study by** Boehler et al. (2011). (A) Example search arrays of the one object condition (left arrays) and of the control condition (right arrays). The upper left panel depicts an array in which the irrelevant color (green) is part of both the target (red/green) and the distractor object (blue/green). The lower left panel shows a trial in which the same distractor object (blue/green) is not accompanied by simultaneous presentation of one of its constituent colors within the target object (red/yellow). Both panels on the right depict the same example search arrays as those on the left, but for the separate object condition, in which the half spheres were cut apart and slightly displaced and rotated. Bottom panels illustrate the data assessment/collapsing performed during analysis. ERP responses to targets and distractors correspond to opposite-hemisphere electrodes (white and black circles). Therefore, activity from electrodes reflecting the distractor (white) and those reflecting the target (black) was collapsed across trials in which the target was presented to the left and to the right visual field (see arrows). (B) ERP waveforms elicited by the whole object (upper row) and separate objects conditions (lower row) at occipital electrodes (P7/8, PO7/8) contralateral to the target (left column) or to the distracter (right column). Note that a relative positivity (filled in red between the ERP traces) was only observed in the whole object condition if the irrelevant color was part of both the target and the distractor object (irrelevant feature effect; IFE). The scalp distribution of this IFE (irrelevant target color in both visual fields minus irrelevant color only in the target) at 400 ms after search frame onset shows a pronounced positivity over lateral occipital electrodes contralateral to the distractor object. **(C) Target-related effect (N2pc effect) and relative timing of the N2pc and the IFE.** Average ERPs elicited by targets contralateral (dashed line) and ipsilateral (solid line) to electrodes PO7/PO8 reveal a classical N2pc effect (filled in blue between traces). The topographical field distribution shows the N2pc (left minus right visual field target difference) at 250 ms after search frame onset. Horizontal bars above and below the x-axis denote the time range in which the N2pc (blue bar) and the IFE (red bar) were significant. Note that the N2pc arises ~80 ms earlier than the IFE, that became significant not until 270 ms after stimulus onset. *Adapted from Boehler et al. (2011).*

derived by comparing ERP responses between trials in which the target appeared contralateral (dashed lines in Figure 9.6(C)) vs ipsilateral (solid lines in Figure 9.6(C)) relative to lateralized posterior electrodes (PO7/PO8). As apparent in Figure 9.6(C), the N2pc arose at about 190 ms poststimulus (time course indicated as blue horizontal bar), which was significantly earlier than the IFE—starting not before 270 ms after stimulus onset (indicated as red horizontal bar). Taken together, the results provided by Boehler and colleagues not only showed that the object-based selection of a task-irrelevant feature is spatially global, but also demonstrated that this

modulation appears after attention has been focused onto the target object. More importantly, however, in conjunction with other findings as outlined above, these results point to a more general framework of the temporal dynamics of feature-based attentional selection.

When features are presented within the focus of attention, they can be readily selected within 100–180 ms after stimulus onset, depending on the relative processing requirements of the task. Therein, selection proceeds faster when it involves entire feature dimensions (~100 ms; Schoenfeld et al., 2007) instead of different feature values of the same dimension (~120–180 ms; for review see Hillyard & Anllo-Vento, 1998). If in contrast, a task-relevant feature is presented at spatially unattended locations, its selection occurs ~50 ms later (~200 ms poststimulus onset; Stoppel et al., 2012), indicating that the spatial spread of feature-based selection takes ~50 ms of time. In addition to these temporal costs for spreading across spatial locations, feature selection also has been shown to require ~40–50 ms to spread from an attended to an unattended feature, which are both part of the same object (arising around 220 ms poststimulus; Schoenfeld et al., 2003). Finally, the data provided by Boehler et al. (2011) showed that attention not only spreads across features within the same object, but also to other spatially unattended objects, that also possess the task-irrelevant feature of the attended object (Boehler et al., 2011). This so-called irrelevant-feature effect appeared at ~270 ms poststimulus, indicating that the temporal costs for the attentional spread from the task-relevant to the task-irrelevant object feature sum up to the costs required for feature-based attention to spread across spatial locations.

GENERAL CONCLUSIONS

Hemodynamic and electrophysiological measures have both proven to be extremely useful in the characterization of neural activity during selective attention in the human brain. The relationship between space-based, feature-based, and object-based attentional mechanisms appears to be highly flexible. Not only the priority of mechanisms can be switched, but the mechanisms can also be combined in order to adapt rapidly to ongoing behavioral demands.

References

Anllo-Vento, L., & Hillyard, S. A. (1996). Selective attention to the color and direction of moving stimuli: electrophysiological correlates of hierarchical feature selection. *Perception and Psychophysics, 58*(2), 191–206.

Beer, A. L., & Roder, B. (2004). Attention to motion enhances processing of both visual and auditory stimuli: an event-related potential study. *Cognitive Brain Research, 18*(2), 205–225.

Beer, A. L., & Roder, B. (2005). Attending to visual or auditory motion affects perception within and across modalities: an event-related potential study. *European Journal of Neuroscience, 21*(4), 1116–1130.

Boehler, C. N., Schoenfeld, M. A., Heinze, H. J., & Hopf, J. M. (2011). Object-based selection of irrelevant features is not confined to the attended object. *Journal of Cognitive Neuroscience, 23*(9), 2231–2239.

Brefczynski, J. A., & DeYoe, E. A. (1999). A physiological correlate of the 'spotlight' of visual attention. *Nature Neuroscience, 2*(4), 370–374.

Buchel, C., Josephs, O., Rees, G., Turner, R., Frith, C. D., & Friston, K. J. (1998). The functional anatomy of attention to visual motion. A functional MRI study. *Brain, 121*(Pt 7), 1281–1294.

Buracas, G. T., & Albright, T. D. (2009). Modulation of neuronal responses during covert search for visual feature conjunctions. *Proceedings of the National Academy of Sciences United States of America, 106*(39), 16853–16858.

Busse, L., Roberts, K. C., Crist, R. E., Weissman, D. H., & Woldorff, M. G. (2005). The spread of attention across modalities and space in a multisensory object. *Proceedings of the National Academy of Sciences United States of America, 102*(51), 18751–18756.

Cameron, E. L., Tai, J. C., & Carrasco, M. (2002). Covert attention affects the psychometric function of contrast sensitivity. *Vision Research, 42*(8), 949–967.

Carrasco, M., & Yeshurun, Y. (2009). Covert attention effects on spatial resolution. *Progress in Brain Research, 176*, 65–86.

Cave, K. R. (1999). The FeatureGate model of visual selection. *Psychological Research, 62*, 182–194.

Cave, K. R., & Bichot, N. P. (1999). Visuospatial attention: beyond a spotlight model. *Psychonomic Bulletin and Review, 6*, 204–223.

Chawla, D., Rees, G., & Friston, K. J. (1999). The physiological basis of attentional modulation in extrastriate visual areas. *Nature Neuroscience, 2*(7), 671–676.

Chelazzi, L., Duncan, J., Miller, E. K., & Desimone, R. (1998). Responses of neurons in inferior temporal cortex during memory-guided visual search. *Journal of Neurophysiology, 80*(6), 2918–2940.

Chelazzi, L., Miller, E. K., Duncan, J., & Desimone, R. (1993). A neural basis for visual search in inferior temporal cortex. *Nature, 363*(6427), 345–347.

Chelazzi, L., Miller, E. K., Duncan, J., & Desimone, R. (2001). Responses of neurons in macaque area V4 during memory-guided visual search. *Cerebral Cortex, 11*(8), 761–772.

Ciaramitaro, V. M., Mitchell, J. F., Stoner, G. R., Reynolds, J. H., & Boynton, G. M. (2011). Object-based attention to one of two superimposed surfaces alters responses in human early visual cortex. *Journal of Neurophysiology, 105*(3), 1258–1265.

Cohen, M. R., & Maunsell, J. H. (2011). Using neuronal populations to study the mechanisms underlying spatial and feature attention. *Neuron, 70*(6), 1192–1204.

Corbetta, M., Miezin, F. M., Dobmeyer, S., Shulman, G. L., & Petersen, S. E. (1990). Attentional modulation of neural processing of shape, color, and velocity in humans. *Science, 248*(4962), 1556–1559.

David, S. V., Hayden, B. Y., Mazer, J. A., & Gallant, J. L. (2008). Attention to stimulus features shifts spectral tuning of V4 neurons during natural vision. *Neuron, 59*(3), 509–521.

Desimone, R. (1998). Visual attention mediated by biased competition in extrastriate visual cortex. *Philosophical Transactions of the Royal Society of London B, Biological Science, 353*(1373), 1245–1255.

Desimone, R., & Duncan, J. (1995). Neural mechanisms of selective visual attention. *Annual Review of Neuroscience, 18*, 193–222.

Fallah, M., Stoner, G. R., & Reynolds, J. H. (2007). Stimulus-specific competitive selection in macaque extrastriate visual area V4. *Proceedings of the National Academy of Sciences United States of America, 104*(10), 4165–4169.

Harter, M. R., & Aine, C. (1984). Brain mechanisms of visual selective attention. In R. Parasuraman & D. R. Davies (Eds.), *Varieties of attention* (pp. 293–321). New York: Academic Press.

Hawkins, H. L., Hillyard, S. A., Luck, S. J., Mouloua, M., Downing, C. J., & Woodward, D. P. (1990). Visual attention modulates signal detectability. *Journal of Experimental Psychology: Human Perception and Performance, 16*(4), 802–811.

Hayden, B. Y., & Gallant, J. L. (2005). Time course of attention reveals different mechanisms for spatial and feature-based attention in area V4. *Neuron, 47*(5), 637–643.

Hayden, B. Y., & Gallant, J. L. (2009). Combined effects of spatial and feature-based attention on responses of V4 neurons. *Vision Research, 49*(10), 1182–1187.

Heinze, H. J., Mangun, G. R., Burchert, W., Hinrichs, H., Scholz, M., Münte, T. F., et al. (1994). Combined spatial and temporal imaging of brain activity during visual selective attention in humans. *Nature, 372*(8), 543–546.

Hillyard, S. A., & Anllo-Vento, L. (1998). Event-related brain potentials in the study of visual selective attention. *Proceedings of the National Academy of Sciences United States of America, 95*(3), 781–787.

Hillyard, S. A., & Mangun, G. R. (1987). Sensory gating as a physiological mechanism for visual selective attention. *Electroencephalography and Clinical Neurophysiology Supplement, 40,* 61–67.

Hopf, J. M., Boehler, C. N., Schoenfeld, M. A., Heinze, H. J., & Tsotsos, J. K. (2010). The spatial profile of the focus of attention in visual search: insights from MEG recordings. *Vision Research, 50*(14), 1312–1320.

Hopf, J. M., Boelmans, K., Schoenfeld, M. A., Luck, S. J., & Heinze, H. J. (2004). Attention to features precedes attention to locations in visual search: evidence from electromagnetic brain responses in humans. *Journal of Neuroscience, 24*(8), 1822–1832.

Huk, A. C., & Heeger, D. J. (2000). Task-related modulation of visual cortex. *Journal of Neurophysiology, 83*(6), 3525–3536.

Jehee, J. F., Brady, D. K., & Tong, F. (2011). Attention improves encoding of task-relevant features in the human visual cortex. *Journal of Neuroscience, 31*(22), 8210–8219.

Kamitani, Y., & Tong, F. (2005). Decoding the visual and subjective contents of the human brain. *National Neuroscience, 8*(5), 679–685.

Kamitani, Y., & Tong, F. (2006). Decoding seen and attended motion directions from activity in the human visual cortex. *Current Biology, 16,* 1096–1102.

Kastner, S., Pinsk, M. A., De Weerd, P., Desimone, R., & Ungerleider, L. G. (1999). Increased activity in human visual cortex during directed attention in the absence of visual stimulation. *Neuron, 22*(4), 751–761.

Katzner, S., Busse, L., & Treue, S. (2009). Attention to the color of a moving stimulus modulates motion-signal processing in macaque area MT: evidence for a unified attentional system. *Frontiers in Systems Neuroscience, 3,* 12.

Kenemans, J. L., Baas, J. M., Mangun, G. R., Lijffijt, M., & Verbaten, M. N. (2000). On the processing of spatial frequencies as revealed by evoked-potential source modeling. *Clinical Neurophysiology, 111*(6), 1113–1123.

Kenemans, J. L., Kok, A., & Smulders, F. T. (1993). Event-related potentials to conjunctions of spatial frequency and orientation as a function of stimulus parameters and response requirements. *Electroencephalography and Clinical Neurophysiology, 88*(1), 51–63.

Liu, T., Hospadaruk, L., Zhu, D. C., & Gardner, J. L. (2011). Feature-specific attentional priority signals in human cortex. *Journal of Neuroscience, 31*(12), 4484–4495.

Liu, T., Larsson, J., & Carrasco, M. (2007). Feature-based attention modulates orientation-selective responses in human visual cortex. *Neuron, 55*(2), 313–323.

Luck, S. J., Chelazzi, L., Hillyard, S. A., & Desimone, R. (1997). Neural mechanisms of spatial selective attention in areas V1, V2, and V4 of macaque visual cortex. *Journal of Neurophysiology, 77*(1), 24–42.

Luck, S. J., Hillyard, S. A., Mouloua, M., & Hawkins, H. L. (1996). Mechanisms of visual-spatial attention: resource allocation or uncertainty reduction? *Journal of Experimental Psychology: Human Perception and Performance, 22*(3), 725–737.

Lu, Z. L., & Dosher, B. A. (1998). External noise distinguishes attention mechanisms. *Vision Research, 38*(9), 1183–1198.

Lustig, A. G., & Beck, D. M. (2012). Task-relevant and task-irrelevant dimensions are modulated independently at a task-irrelevant location. *Journal of Cognitive Neuroscience.*

Martinez-Trujillo, J. C., & Treue, S. (2004). Feature-based attention increases the selectivity of population responses in primate visual cortex. *Current Biology, 14*(9), 744–751.

Martinez, A., DiRusso, F., Anllo-Vento, L., Sereno, M. I., Buxton, R. B., & Hillyard, S. A. (2001). Putting spatial attention on the map: timing and localization of stimulus selection processes in striate and extrastriate visual areas. *Vision Research, 41*(10–11), 1437–1457.

Martinez, A., Teder-Salejarvi, W., Vazquez, M., Molholm, S., Foxe, J. J., Javitt, D. C., et al. (2006). Objects are highlighted by spatial attention. *Journal of Cognitive Neuroscience, 18*(2), 298–310.

McAdams, C. J., & Maunsell, J. H. (1999). Effects of attention on orientation-tuning functions of single neurons in macaque cortical area V4. *Journal of Neuroscience, 19*(1), 431–441.

McAdams, C. J., & Maunsell, J. H. (2000). Attention to both space and feature modulates neuronal responses in macaque area V4. *Journal of Neurophysiology, 83*(3), 1751–1755.

McMains, S. A., Fehd, H. M., Emmanouil, T. A., & Kastner, S. (2007). Mechanisms of feature- and space-based attention: response modulation and baseline increases. *Journal of Neurophysiology, 98*(4), 2110–2121.

Moran, J., & Desimone, R. (1985). Selective attention gates visual processing in the extrastriate cortex. *Science, 229*(4715), 782–784.

Motter, B. C. (1993). Focal attention produces spatially selective processing in visual cortical areas V1, V2, and V4 in the presence of competing stimuli. *Journal of Neurophysiology, 70*(3), 909–919.

Motter, B. C. (1994). Neural correlates of attentive selection for color or luminance in extrastriate area V4. *Journal of Neuroscience, 14*(4), 2178–2189.

Muller, N. G., & Kleinschmidt, A. (2003). Dynamic interaction of object- and space-based attention in retinotopic visual areas. *Journal of Neuroscience, 23*(30), 9812–9816.

Neisser, U. (1967). *Cognitive psychology.* Englewood Cliffs: NJ: Prentice Hall.

Neisser, U., & Becklen, R. (1975). Selective looking: attending to visually specified events. *Cognitive Psychology, 7,* 480–494.

O'Craven, K. M., Downing, P. E., & Kanwisher, N. (1999). fMRI evidence for objects as the units of attentional selection. *Nature, 401*(6753), 584–587.

O'Craven, K. M., Rosen, B. R., Kwong, K. K., Treisman, A., & Savoy, R. L. (1997). Voluntary attention modulates fMRI activity in human MT-MST. *Neuron, 18,* 591–598.

Pinilla, T., Cobo, A., Torres, K., & Valdes-Sosa, M. (2001). Attentional shifts between surfaces: effects on detection and early brain potentials. *Vision Research, 41*(13), 1619–1630.

Posner, M. I. (1980). Orienting of attention. *Quarterly Journal of Experimental Psychology, 32,* 3–25.

Reynolds, J. H., & Chelazzi, L. (2004). Attentional modulation of visual processing. *Annual Review of Neuroscience, 27,* 611–647.

Reynolds, J. H., Chelazzi, L., & Desimone, R. (1999). Competitive mechanisms subserve attention in macaque areas V2 and V4. *Journal of Neuroscience, 19*(5), 1736–1753.

Rodriguez, V., & Valdes-Sosa, M. (2006). Sensory suppression during shifts of attention between surfaces in transparent motion. *Brain Research, 1072*(1), 110–118.

Roelfsema, P. R., Lamme, V. A., & Spekreijse, H. (1998). Object-based attention in the primary visual cortex of the macaque monkey. *Nature, 395*(6700), 376–381.

Saenz, M., Buracas, G. T., & Boynton, G. M. (2002). Global effects of feature-based attention in human visual cortex. *National Neuroscience, 5*(7), 631–632.

Safford, A. S., Hussey, E. A., Parasuraman, R., & Thompson, J. C. (2010). Object-based attentional modulation of biological motion processing: spatiotemporal dynamics using functional magnetic resonance imaging and electroencephalography. *Journal of Neuroscience, 30*(27), 9064–9073.

Schneider, K. A. (2011). Subcortical mechanisms of feature-based attention. *Journal of Neuroscience, 31*(23), 8643–8653.

Schoenfeld, M. A., Hopf, J. M., Martinez, A., Mai, H. M., Sattler, C., Gasde, A., et al. (2007). Spatio-temporal analysis of feature-based attention. *Cerebral Cortex, 17*(10), 2468–2477.

Schoenfeld, M. A., Tempelmann, C., Martinez, A., Hopf, J. M., Sattler, C., Heinze, H. J., et al. (2003). Dynamics of feature binding during object-selective attention. *Proceedings of the National Academy of Sciences United States of America, 100*(20), 11806–11811.

Serences, J. T., & Boynton, G. M. (2007). Feature-based attentional modulations in the absence of direct visual stimulation. *Neuron, 55*(2), 301–312.

Serences, J. T., Saproo, S., Scolari, M., Ho, T., & Muftuler, L. T. (2009). Estimating the influence of attention on population codes in human visual cortex using voxel-based tuning functions. *Neuroimage, 44*(1), 223–231.

Shibata, K., Yamagishi, N., Goda, N., Yoshioka, T., Yamashita, O., Sato, M. A., et al. (2008). The effects of feature attention on prestimulus cortical activity in the human visual system. *Cerebral Cortex, 18*(7), 1664–1675.

Shiu, L. P., & Pashler, H. (1995). Spatial attention and vernier acuity. *Vision Research, 35*(3), 337–343.

Shomstein, S., & Behrmann, M. (2006). Cortical systems mediating visual attention to both objects and spatial locations. *Proceedings of the National Academy of Sciences United States of America, 103*(30), 11387–11392.

Sillito, A. M., Cudeiro, J., & Jones, H. E. (2006). Always returning: feedback and sensory processing in visual cortex and thalamus. *Trends in Neuroscience, 29*(6), 307–316.

Smid, H. G., Jakob, A., & Heinze, H. J. (1999). An event-related brain potential study of visual selective attention to conjunctions of color and shape. *Psychophysiology, 36*(2), 264–279.

Sohn, W., Chong, S. C., Papathomas, T. V., & Vidnyanszky, Z. (2005). Cross-feature spread of global attentional modulation in human area MT+. *Neuroreport, 16*(12), 1389–1393.

Spitzer, H., Desimone, R., & Moran, J. (1988). Increased attention enhances both behavioral and neuronal performance. *Science, 240*(4850), 338–340.

Stoppel, C. M., Boehler, C. N., Strumpf, H., Heinze, H. J., Noesselt, T., Hopf, J. M., et al. (2011). Feature-based attention modulates direction-selective hemodynamic activity within human MT. *Human Brain Mapping, 32*(12), 2183–2192.

Stoppel, C. M., Boehler, C. N., Strumpf, H., Krebs, R. M., Heinze, H. J., Hopf, J. M., et al. (2012). Spatiotemporal dynamics of feature-based attention spread: evidence from combined electroencephalographic and magnetoencephalographic recordings. *Journal of Neuroscience, 32*(28), 9671–9676.

Torriente, I., Valdes-Sosa, M., Ramirez, D., & Bobes, M. A. (1999). Visual evoked potentials related to motion-onset are modulated by attention. *Vision Research, 39*(24), 4122–4139.

Treisman, A. M., & Gelade, G. (1980). A feature-integration theory of attention. *Cognitive Psychology, 12*(1), 97–136.

Treisman, A., & Sato, S. (1990). Conjunction search revisited. *Journal of Experimental Psychology: Human Perception and Performance, 16*(3), 459–478.

Treue, S., & Martinez Trujillo, J. C. (1999). Feature-based attention influences motion processing gain in macaque visual cortex. *Nature, 399*(6736), 575–579.

Treue, S., & Maunsell, J. H. (1996). Attentional modulation of visual motion processing in cortical areas MT and MST. *Nature, 382*(6591), 539–541.

Treue, S., & Maunsell, J. H. (1999). Effects of attention on the processing of motion in macaque middle temporal and medial superior temporal visual cortical areas. *Journal of Neuroscience, 19*(17), 7591–7602.

Valdes-Sosa, M., Bobes, M. A., Rodriguez, V., & Pinilla, T. (1998). Switching attention without shifting the spotlight object-based attentional modulation of brain potentials. *Journal of Cognitive Neuroscience, 10*(1), 137–151.

Valdes-Sosa, M., Cobo, A., & Pinilla, T. (1998). Transparent motion and object-based attention. *Cognition, 66*(2), B13–B23.

Valdes-Sosa, M., Cobo, A., & Pinilla, T. (2000). Attention to object files defined by transparent motion. *Journal of Experimental Psychology: Human Perception and Performance, 26*(2), 488–505.

Wannig, A., Rodriguez, V., & Freiwald, W. A. (2007). Attention to surfaces modulates motion processing in extrastriate area MT. *Neuron, 54*(4), 639–651.

Wolfe, J. M. (1994). Guided search 2.0: a revised model of visual search. *Psychonomic Bulletin and Review, 1*, 202–238.

Wolfe, J. M., Cave, K. R., & Franzel, S. L. (1989). Guided search: an alternative to the feature integration model for visual search. *Journal of Experimental Psychology: Human Perception and Performance, 15*(3), 419–433.

Wolfe, J. M., & Horowitz, T. S. (2004). What attributes guide the deployment of visual attention and how do they do it? *Nature ReviewsNeuroscience, 5*(6), 495–501.

Yantis, S., & Serences, J. T. (2003). Cortical mechanisms of space-based and object-based attentional control. *Current Opinion in Neurobiology, 13*(2), 187–193.

Yeshurun, Y., & Carrasco, M. (1998). Attention improves or impairs visual performance by enhancing spatial resolution. *Nature, 396*(6706), 72–75.

10

Neural Mechanisms of Feature-Based Attention

Matthias M. Müller

Department of Psychology, University of Leipzig, Germany

SELECTION UNITS OF VISUAL ATTENTION AND THE FEATURE SIMILARITY GAIN MODEL

Research on visual attention is one of the most studied fields in psychology and the neurosciences and looks back to many decades. Commencing with behavioral data in the middle of the twentieth century, research was focused on spatial selection, which is not surprising given that the visual system has inherently spatial properties. Systematic studies of spatial attention in the 1970s and 1980s lead to influential theories, such as the spotlight (Posner, 1980), zoom-lens (Eriksen & Collins, 1969; Eriksen & St. James, 1986), or feature integration model (Treisman & Gelade, 1980). Location as a unique selection property was questioned in 1984 when empirical evidence emerged that the visual system can prioritize perceptual processes on the basis of whole objects (Duncan, 1984). And only a few years ago, in 1999, it was shown that selection can also be performed on the basis of features leading to the feature-similarity gain model (Treue, 2001; Treue & Trujillo, 1999). Thus, research on feature-based attention is a very new field with growing interest over the last years. Based on single-cell recordings in monkey visual cortex (see below for the "classical" experiment), the model mainly proposes that:

- Feature-based attention modulates the gain of cortical neurons tuned to the attended feature, anywhere in the visual field (global effect of attention).
- Attentional enhancement by spatial selection employs the same mechanisms as nonspecial, feature-based selection.
- The attention effect of the neural response is additive for different features.

Evidently, long before the feature-similarity gain model was formulated, a number of studies were able to show that attending to a certain feature, such as color or motion, selectively increases the response in cortical areas that process that particular feature, such as motion in human middle temporal complex (MT+) or color in V4 (cf. Anllo-Vento & Hillyard, 1996; Corbetta, Miezin, Dobmeyer, Shulman, & Petersen, 1990; O'Craven, Rosen, Kwong, Treisman, & Savoy, 1997). In all of these previous studies, however, stimulus location was still an important property. In addition, stimuli were transiently presented with no spatial or temporal overlap between a to-be-attended or ignored stimulus. The new dimension that was brought in by the feature-similarity gain model was the fact that particular features such as clouds of moving dots were presented together at one location to investigate the neural responses of feature processing while a competing stimulus was presented as well. As a further side note, it is worth mentioning, that the feature-similarity gain model has its origin in single-cell recordings in monkeys (Treue & Trujillo, 1999) as this is the case with the biased competition approach (Desimone, 1998; Desimone & Duncan, 1995) and, thus, they are fine examples of models with a genuine foundation in the neurosciences. Together, these two models are currently the most influential models of visual attention in cognitive neuroscience and the neurosciences.

What was the initial experiment for the feature-similarity gain model? In the 1999 study, Treue and Martinez-Trujillo recorded the response of cells in MT with a specific motion direction preference that were contralateral to the to-be-ignored visual hemifield. Monkeys attended to a display in which two clouds of dots moved in the preferred and the antidirection in the opposite visual hemifield (Figure 10.1). When the dots in the ignored hemifield moved in the preferred direction of the recorded cells and monkeys attended to that direction in the to-be-attended hemifield, they responded with higher responses compared to when dots in the

Attention to preferred direction   **Attention to null-direction**

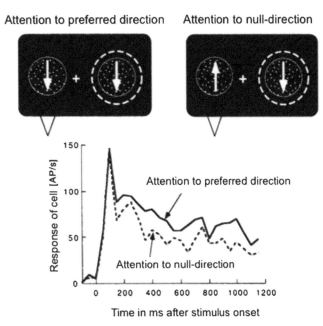

FIGURE 10.1 Schematic representation of stimulation. The monkey attended to the left visual hemifield. Cell responses were recorded at the right visual hemifield. Recorded cell preferred downward motion. The response of the cell at the to-be-ignored location was significantly higher, when dots moved in the preferred direction compared to the null-direction at the attended location in the opposite visual hemifield. *Source: Courtesy of Stefan Treue.*

attended hemifield moved in the antidirection. Thus, the authors demonstrated a global effect of feature-based attention, that is, when the monkey attends to a certain motion direction, all cells with that preferred direction became more activated, regardless at what location the monkey has deployed its attention.

Only 3 years later in 2002, Saenz, Buracas, and Boynton (2002) were able to show the global spread of feature-based attention in the human brain as well. Similar to the monkey experiment, the authors measured the response in human MT+ at the to-be-ignored side with functional magnetic resonance imaging (fMRI). In addition, they were able to show that this global effect is not restricted to motion but can be demonstrated for color in human area V4 as well.

TOP-DOWN SENSORY GAIN OR SHARPENING OF TUNING FUNCTIONS

In a subsequent monkey study, Martinez-Trujillo and Treue (2004) were investigating whether feature-based attention changes the selectivity of neurons. As a result of that study, they reported a multiplicative attentional modulation of the neuron's response and not of a change in the tuning function. Importantly, the strength of that response depended on the similarity of the to-be-attended feature and the preference of the recorded

cells. Cells that preferred the antidirection showed a markedly decreased response. In other words, on the population level—rather than changing the selectivity of neurons—preferred processing of the attended feature was reported to be a mixture of increasing the response of neurons optimally tuned to the feature and a suppression of neuronal activity of the opposite preference (such as the antidirection for cells in MT).

Besides this gain mechanism, David, Hayden, Mazer, and Gallant (2008) reported a change of the tuning function of V4 neurons in feature-based attention. As a consequence, a neuron can change its preferred stimulus and tune it toward the to-be-attended spectral range. Thus, it seems that both mechanisms are available. According to these authors, altering the gain seems a mechanism that is linked to spatial attention, while changing the tuning properties is linked to feature-based attention.

Both mechanisms, a change of the gain of the target as well as changes in the tuning function, are linked to the particular feature of the relevant stimulus and exclusively affect so-called "on-target" neurons. However, just recently it was shown that a third mechanism is possible for better discrimination under top-down control (Scolari, Byers, & Serences, 2012; Scolari & Serences, 2010) and is best observed when subjects were required to perform a difficult discrimination task, i.e., targets and nontargets are very similar. In that particular case, it seems more optimal if attention to a particular feature, such as orientation in the studies by Scolari and colleagues, alters the gain of neurons that have a slightly different tuning function compared to the to-be-attended orientation (off-target gain). In other words, top-down activation of neurons that are tuned away from the target orientation result in an improved fine-grained discrimination between similar features, because their increase in firing rate results in a much better signal-to-noise ratio compared to the gain on on-target neurons (see for more details Scolari & Serences 2010; 2012). Importantly, the authors were able to demonstrate that off-target gain predicted behavioral responses.

THE STEADY STATE VISUAL EVOKED POTENTIAL AS SOLUTION TO OVERCOME LIMITATIONS OF PREVIOUS STUDIES

The limitation of the monkey studies as well as of the above-mentioned fMRI study was the fact that neural responses at the to-be-ignored side were always measured without any competitive stimulus in the same visual hemifield. The different-direction or different-color cloud was always at the attended hemifield. The neural response was measured at the to-be-ignored hemifield with nonoverlapping stimuli. Thus, the

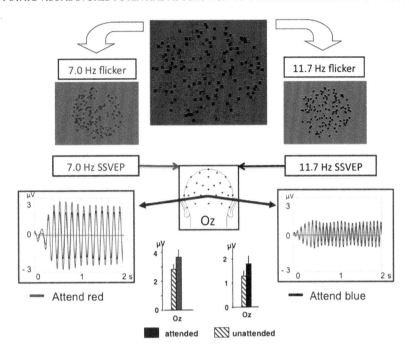

FIGURE 10.2 Schematic representation of stimulus configuration. Red dots were flickering at 7.0 Hz and blue dots at 11.7 Hz, evoking distinguishable SSVEPs. In the depicted example, the red fixation cross instructed observers to attend to the red random dot kinematogram. Change in SSVEP amplitude at electrode Oz for one subject while attending to red (left) or blue (right). The increase in SSVEP amplitude is clearly visible and maintains throughout the stimulation. Bars show the mean (+standard error) across all subjects for electrode Oz when subjects attended (full bars) or ignored (striped bars) the respective color.

question whether feature-based attention enhances the response of the attended feature when stimuli with different features share the same spatial location remained unanswered. To investigate that question, we (Müller et al., 2006) presented our subjects spatially superimposed red and blue random dot kinematograms (RDKs, Figure 10.2) and instructed them to either attend to the blue or red RDK. Feature-based attention would clearly predict that subjects are able to selectively attend to the one or other color to perform a task. A spatial account, however, would come to a different conclusion. In 1982, Treisman stated that "… attention cannot be distributed over a subset of items (e.g., the red ones) when these are spatially scattered among other items in a randomly mixed display" (Treisman, 1982, p. 199). This is simply due to the fact that in such a display the attentional spotlight includes both colors.

When simultaneously presenting two sets of stimuli, it is important to make sure that one can independently measure the neural response of each stimulus set. This is impossible with fMRI, because there is no solution to differentiate the measured response elicited by the red from the one elicited by the blue RDK. In electrophysiological (electroencephalography, EEG) recordings the simultaneous presentation of two stimuli needs some technical "trick" because conventional event-related potential (ERP) stimulation and analysis techniques are also not able to differentiate the neural responses of the two stimuli. The technical trick is to frequency-tag

stimuli at different frequencies. Continuous presentation of flickering visual stimuli elicits the steady state visual evoked potential (SSVEP, Regan, 1989). In EEG recordings, the SSVEP is a sinusoidal brain response that can easily be analyzed in frequency domain because it has the same frequency and its harmonics as the driving stimulus or the driving stimuli in case of more than one flicker stimulus. In previous spatial-based studies, we were showing that attending to a flickering stimulus significantly enhances the SSVEP amplitude compared to when that stimulus had to-be-ignored (cf. Müller & Hübner, 2002; Müller, Malinowski, Gruber, & Hillyard, 2003; Müller, Picton, et al., 1998). Given the attentional modulation of SSVEPs and the possibility to obtain distinguishable neural responses with frequency-tagged stimuli, in our experiment we flickered red and blue RDKs at a frequency of 7 Hz (red) and 11.67 Hz (blue). We found that when subjects attended to the blue RDK, 11.67 Hz SSVEP amplitude was significantly increased compared to when subjects attended the red RDK. Attending the red RDK, in turn, resulted in a significant increase of the 7.0 Hz SSVEP amplitude (Figure 10.2). To assure that subjects were not using flicker frequency as a feature to solve the task, we conducted a behavioral control study and found no behavioral differences when red and blue RDKs flickered at the same compared to different frequencies, clearly indicating that subjects were not using frequency to discriminate between the two RDKs (Müller et al., 2006).

FEATURE-BASED SELECTION AND ITS GLOBAL EFFECT

Results of that study were in the middle of the discussion, whether there is something like feature-based attention or whether it all is based on spatial cues (Shih & Sperling, 1996). Of course, that discussion was not just of academic interest, because some authors seriously questioned a feature-based selection mechanism in general (cf. Moore & Egeth, 1998; Shih & Sperling, 1996; Tsal & Lavie, 1993). To resolve that question, we created a task in which the individual dots of the red and blue RDK randomly changed position to make sure that subjects did not have the possibility to attend to a restricted special location within the RDK (Andersen, Müller, & Hillyard, 2009). Furthermore, tasks were no longer defined by coherent motion events as in our previous study. We used luminance changes instead. We were able to fully replicate the results of our previous study and settled that long lasting controversy.

The question remains: Can we demonstrate the global effect of feature-based attention with our method as well? To this end, we presented superimposed red and blue clouds of dots in the left and right visual hemifield (Figure 10.3). Each cloud flickered at a different frequency and a central cue instructed subjects to attend to a certain color at the left or right visual hemifield (Andersen, Fuchs, & Müller, 2011). Thus, in contrast to all other studies that were conducted up to that moment, we were in the unique position to test the global effect in a full factorial design.

Based on findings in monkeys (Treue & Trujillo, 1999) and human fMRI (Saenz et al., 2002), we expected an increase of SSVEP amplitude that was elicited by the RDK at the to-be-ignored location but shared the same color as the to-be-attended one. In addition, given that the to-be-ignored color at the to-be-attended location shared the same feature location, we expected an increase in amplitude for that RDK as well. This was exactly what we found. SSVEP amplitudes were smallest for the RDK that neither shared the attended color nor location. Greatest amplitudes were found for the RDK that shared both, attended color and location. As depicted in Figure 10.3, and in line with the feature-similarity gain model, we found that SSVEP amplitudes were significantly increased when RDKs either shared the same color at the to-be-ignored location or were sharing the same location compared to when neither of these attributes applied (Andersen et al., 2011). However, as can also be seen in Figure 10.3, the attention effect for the attended color at the attended hemifield is significantly greater compared to the one of the same color but at the to-be-ignored side. As will be outlined below, this is due to the additive effect of location and color. Together, our result with a full factorial design and the research

reported so far convincingly supported central predictions of the feature-similarity gain model.

FEATURE-BASED ATTENTION AND VISUAL SEARCH

But what is feature-based attention good for? An obvious field, which is also one of the central research topics in psychology and the neurosciences, is visual search. Everyday life experience gives a number of examples in which we are confronted with visual search tasks. We want to pick up a friend at the railway station, search for a face in a crowd, or look for our car at a big parking lot. Closely linked to research in visual attention, visual search was dominated by the idea that spatial information is the most important feature. Feature integration theory (FIT) postulated a master map of location as the top-level layer. Visual search is performed in a serial manner, that is, the spotlight of attention moves from location to location (Treisman & Gelade, 1980). Subordinate to that master map of location are feature maps of different feature dimensions, such as color, orientation, or motion. These feature maps are further subdivided into the different characteristics of a particular feature, such as red, green, or yellow for the feature map color. In visual search, different features that define an object are only bound together at the attended location reflected by the finding that search time linearly increases with the amount of objects in the search display (Treisman, 1998; Treisman & Gormican, 1988; Treisman & Sato, 1990).

In contrast to FIT, Wolfe and colleagues (Wolfe, 1994; Wolfe, Cave, & Franzel, 1989; Wolfe & Horowitz, 2004) suggested that visual search can be performed on the basis of parallel perceptual processes. Given that subjects know for what they are looking for, knowledge of the features that define the search item can activate certain feature maps in parallel to facilitate visual search. Thus, search is guided by a priori knowledge of central features. Contrary to spatial-based attention for which anticipatory activation in visual cortex was shown in the absence of any stimulus (Kastner, Pinsk, De Weerd, Desimone, & Ungerleider, 1999), anticipatory or "guided" knowledge of a feature such as a particular color has not been shown to activate feature processing related areas in the absence of the visual stimulus. But what had recently been shown is a spreading effect to locations without any stimulus by means of increased blood oxygenation level-dependent (BOLD) responses in early visual areas in the absence of direct visual stimulation at these locations (Serences & Boynton, 2007).

Interestingly, the guided search and the feature-similarity gain model have another common central assumption. Both models predict that features of the search item

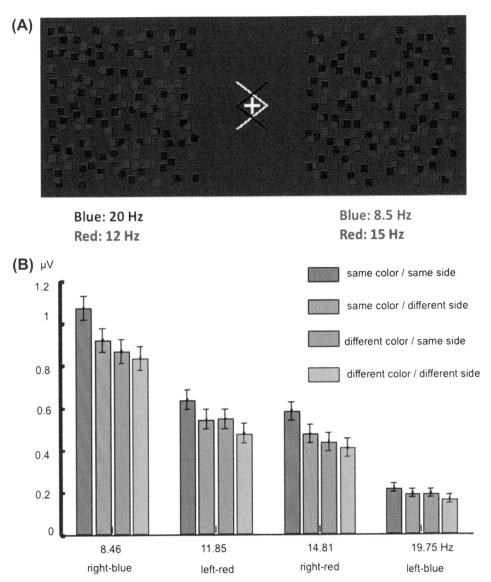

FIGURE 10.3 (A) Schematic illustration of stimulation. Red and blue random dot kinematograms were presented in the left and right visual hemifield. Each random dot kinematogram flickered at a different frequency as indicated at the bottom of the illustration. A central arrowhead cued subjects to which side and color they had to attend to. In the given example: Blue in the left visual hemifield. (B) Grand mean SSVEP amplitudes for each frequency when subjects attended to a color in that hemifield (orange), the attended color was at the unattended hemifield (brown), the hemifield was attended but the color had to-be-ignored (dark green), or the hemifield as well as the color was ignored (bright green). Error bars correspond to 95% within-subjects confidence intervals of the mean.

add-up cumulatively (Wolfe, 1994; Wolfe et al., 1989; Wolfe & Horowitz, 2004). Given that only one stimulus aggregates all features, the to-be-searched object should outstand from other objects in the activation map resulting in much shorter search times, compared to serial search. It is important to mention here, that both models, although they have some common assumption, were independently developed and is not the case that feature-similarity gain has been subsumed by Wolfe's guided search model.

We tested the assumption of additive feature conjunction in a full factorial design experiment, by presenting our subjects with red or blue horizontal or vertical bars (Andersen, Hillyard, & Müller, 2008). As with all of our experiments, each stimulus set was flickering at a different frequency and we instructed subjects to attend to one set of stimulus bars that conjoined color and orientation, e.g., red horizontal bars (Figure 10.4). We expected that SSVEP amplitudes would be increased for all stimuli that share one of the two features (color or orientation) of the attended stimulus and that color and orientation resulted in an additive SSVEP response. That was exactly what we found. As depicted in Figure 10.4, stimuli that shared one of the features of the attended stimulus elicited significantly increased SSVEP amplitudes compared to those stimuli that shared none of the

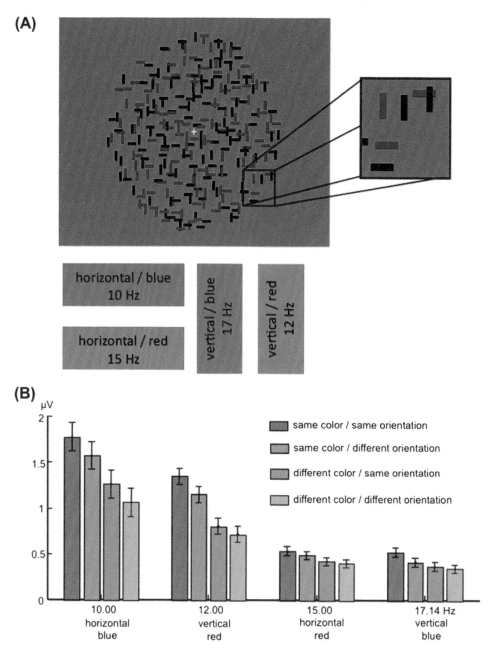

FIGURE 10.4   (A) Schematic illustration of stimulation. Four types of bars were presented and flickered at different frequencies as indicated at the bottom of the illustration. Bars either shared the same orientation or color. Before stimulus onset, subjects were cued to what bar they had to attend to. (B) Same as in Figure 10.3 but for each bar type, respectively.

features. The interaction between color and orientation was not significant, signifying an additive effect of the main factors color and orientation.

We also found an additive effect of color and location in our study in which we tested the global effect of feature-based attention reported above (Andersen et al., 2011). The interaction between color and location was not significant. This fits well with the idea that there is nothing special about space. Location is just another feature of the stimulus (Desimone & Duncan, 1995). However, when we look at behavioral data, we

found that false alarms were clearly limited to the attended location, in other words, subjects were not responding to events at the to-be-ignored location. In the same line, analysis of the P3 amplitude of the ERP that was elicited by coherent motion events showed that an attentional modulation was restricted to the attended location.

Given our ERP results, it seems quite likely that one has to consider two different functional differences between feature-based attention and target processing. Feature-based attention produces a global facilitation of stimuli that share identical features as the to-be-searched one. Full identification of the search target seems to take place at much later stages of stimulus processing and seems to be linked to the attended location. Exactly such an interplay of parallel and serial mechanisms in visual search was reported by Bichot, Rossi, and Desimone (2005). They recorded activity in monkey V4 cells while they performed a visual search task under free viewing conditions. Enhanced and synchronized responses were found whenever a stimulus in the cell's receptive field matched a feature of the search target, speaking for a global and parallel process. In addition, the authors found enhanced neural responses when a stimulus was selected for saccades to foveate that particular stimulus signifying a serial component during visual search.

SUPPRESSION OF NEURAL RESPONSES OF THE UNATTENDED FEATURE FOLLOWS AMPLIFICATION OF THE TO-BE-ATTENDED ONE

But what happens with irrelevant features that are not shared with the search item? Polk, Drake, Jonides, Smith, and Smith (2008) conducted an fMRI experiment in which they used a Stroop task. When subjects attended to the color of the font while they ignored the word, they found enhanced BOLD responses in color areas and decreased responses in word areas. These results indicate that processing of irrelevant features will be suppressed.

In one of our own studies we found a similar result (Andersen & Müller, 2010). As in our first study, we presented our subjects intermingled RDKs of red and blue dots that flickered at different frequencies (Figure 10.2). Unlike our first study, the RDKs started to flicker and after a while we presented a color cue, instructing subjects to shift attention to either red or blue. We found a mixture of amplification of the to-be-attended and suppression of the to-be-ignored color. As depicted in Figure 10.5, the most interesting result was the exact time course of these two processes. After the presentation of the cue, we observed an early amplification that was followed after about 130 ms by an SSVEP amplitude suppression. That pattern is different from what we observed for spatial shifts that resulted in the facilitation of the newly to-be-attended location only (Müller, 2008; Müller, Teder-Sälejärvi, & Hillyard, 1998). This delay in amplitude suppression for the to-be-ignored color clearly speaks against a strictly limited resource model of visual processing. If this were case, one would expect that shifting resources to one stimulus must invariably lead to a suppression of the unattended stimulus. Thus, it seems likely that

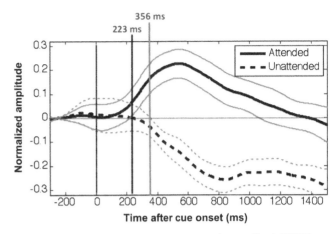

FIGURE 10.5 Grand mean time course of normalized SSVEP amplitudes collapsed over red and blue random dot kinematograms. At time point zero, the cue instructed our subjects to what color they had to shift their attention. Significant amplification of the to-be-attended color SSVEP compared to baseline (before cue onset) was found 223 ms after the cue. Amplification was followed by a suppression of SSVEP amplitude about 130 ms later at 356 ms after the onset of the cue. Gray lines correspond to 95% confidence intervals.

in feature-based attention under conditions of spatial overlap an early sensory gain mechanism triggers competitive interactions as suggested by the biased competition model (Desimone, 1998; Desimone & Duncan, 1995).

A further interesting result was the finding that the time course of behavioral data to coherent motion events as a function of the cue-event time interval followed a measure of sensitivity, i.e., the time course of attended minus unattended stimulus SSVEPs. A still open question is whether suppression of the unattended color globally occurs in the visual field (as is the case for amplification), or whether it is restricted to the location of focused attention. Very preliminary results from an ongoing study at the moment of writing this book chapter indicate that suppression is not global but restricted to the attended location.

FEATURE-BASED VS LOCATION-BASED SELECTION

A further point to deal with in this chapter is the question of when and where feature-based attention modulates poststimulus processing. Furthermore, what are the underlying brain circuits that guide feature-based attention? Are they different from the ones that are linked to spatial attention?

For many years, it was set that processing of features follows spatial processing. Besides the "dogma" of spatial priority in visual processing, a number of ERP studies have shown that the P1 component with a poststimulus latency of about 80–100 ms was only modulated by spatial attention (cf. Hillyard, 1993; Hillyard & Anllo-Vento, 1998; Hillyard, Mangun, Woldorff, & Luck, 1995; Hillyard, Vogel, & Luck, 1998). When subjects were instructed to selectively attend to a certain feature, such as color or motion, the earliest attentional modulation was reported at a latency of about 160–180 ms, the so-called selection negativity (cf. Anllo-Vento & Hillyard, 1996; Anllo-Vento, Luck, & Hillyard, 1998; Hillyard & Münte, 1984; Müller & Keil, 2004).

A certain limitation of the frequency-tagging method can be seen in the fact that poststimulus processing to the onset of the stimulus stream is difficult. The evoked response is a mixture of the ERP to stimulus onset and the build-up of the SSVEP that lasts about 400–500 ms depending on the stimulation frequency. However, once the SSVEP is established, one can concurrently analyze SSVEPs and ERPs by filtering-out the SSVEP from the ERP elicited by events embedded in the stimulation stream (Müller & Hillyard, 2000).

Zhang and Luck (2009) presented subjects a color display, similar to the one that was used by Saenz et al. (2002), i.e., superimposed red and green dots in one visual hemifield to which subjects were instructed to attend to. In the opposite, the to-be-ignored hemifield, they presented short probes that were either in the attended or unattended color. By analyzing ERPs evoked by these probes they found an attentional modulation of the P1 component that had been seen as a purely spatial component. Thus, it seems that in conditions where stimuli compete for processing resources feature-based and location-based mechanisms seem to operate at the same time scale. It has to be mentioned, however, that long before Zhang's and Luck's study, Anllo-Vento et al. (1998) reported an early positivity that started 100 ms after stimulus onset with a source in lateral occipital cortex that was modulated by attention to color. However, in that early study the authors, perhaps erroneously, were not attributing this early effect to the P1. One has to keep in mind that this early study was conducted in times of the spatial priority "dogma" and the feature-similarity gain mechanism had yet to be discovered. Given a similar latency and an almost identical topographical distribution as in the Zhang and Luck study conducted 10 years later, one is tempted to claim that both publications reported the same neural mechanism of early feature-based attentional modulation. Interestingly, in the early study color stimuli in the form of checkerboards were sequentially presented, but at the same location. Perhaps the usage of big colored checkerboards resulted in that early modulation without direct spatial competition. In line with such an early effect in the evoked potential is our consistent finding of attentional SSVEP amplitude modulation in early visual processing areas as depicted in Figure 10.6 (cf. Andersen et al., 2008; Müller et al., 2006).

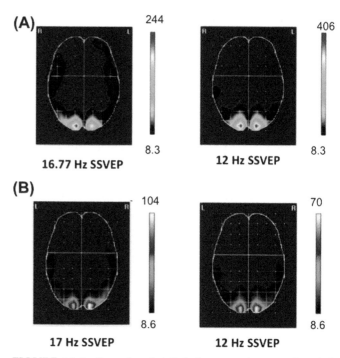

(A)   244   8.3   **16.77 Hz SSVEP**

406   8.3   **12 Hz SSVEP**

(B)   104   8.6   **17 Hz SSVEP**

70   8.6   **12 Hz SSVEP**

FIGURE 10.6 Examples of statistical parametric maps of cortical current density distributions that give rise to the SSVEP amplitude difference between attended and unattended stimuli from two different experiments. (A) SSVEPs elicited by blue or red random dot kinematograms (*Source*: *adapted from* Andersen & Müller, 2010; see Figure 10.1 for stimulus display). (B) SSVEPs elicited by bars as depicted in Figure 10.4 (*Source*: *adapted from* Andersen et al., 2008). Scales represents t^2 values, and the $p < 0.001$ threshold for the attended versus unattended comparison corresponds to 8.3 in (A) and 8.6 in (B).

NEURAL CIRCUITS OF FEATURE-BASED AND SPATIAL ATTENTION

This section deals with the question of whether spatial and feature-based attention are mediated by different or similar neural mechanisms. On the one hand, both selection units seem to serve different purposes to some extend. On the other hand, they have to play together in a number of everyday situations, such as in visual search.

In a delayed match-to-sample task, Hayden and Gallant (2005) recorded from monkey single cells in V4 to extract the time course of spatial and feature-based attention. Spatial attention was manipulated by cueing attention either to the receptive field of V4 cells or to the opposite visual hemifield. At both locations a stream of small pictures was presented and monkeys had to respond to a precue sample stimulus at the attended location. They found different time courses of spatial and feature-based responses. While feature-based attention resulted in a relatively constant response across time, spatial-based attention resulted in a somewhat weaker response at short latencies and a stronger response at longer latencies. From that difference in time course, the authors concluded that the two mechanisms serve different purposes. While feature-based attention is goal driven and seems to be linked to maintaining an internal representation of the match, spatial attention represents a mixture of stimulus- and goal-driven mechanisms that are important to guide saccades. It is commonly accepted that spatial attention is linked to preparation and execution of saccades or bigger eye movements. Very likely, top-down control of spatial attention is performed through the frontal eye field (FEF) and lateral intraparietal area (cf. Gregoriou, Gotts, Zhou, & Desimone, 2009; Herrington & Assad, 2010; Kastner & Ungerleider, 2000; Moore, Armstrong, & Fallah, 2003). Thus, for many years it seemed logical that FEF is tightly linked to the spatial-attention network.

Just recently, experimental evidence was provided that FEF play a role in feature-based attention as well (Zhou & Desimone, 2011). The authors simultaneously recorded from cells in monkey FEF and V4, while the animals performed a visual search task. They reported of feature-based attentional modulation in both areas. Interestingly, the magnitude of the response enhancement was inversely related with the number of saccades required to find the target. However, a closer inspection of the time course of responses revealed shorter feature-based latencies in FEF than the latencies recorded in V4. This suggests that FEF might serve as a top-down control source in feature-based attention. On the other side, latencies of purely shape and color driven responses, i.e. bottom-up information of basic features were much shorter in V4. Together, these results suggest a close link between FEF and V4 in a way that V4 provides sensory information of stimulus features to create an internal template. FEF, on the other hand, creates top-down influences to bias attention in favor of the features of the to-be-detected target that can be used to guide saccades to the location of the target.

In a human fMRI study, Greenberg, Esterman, Wilson, Serences, and Yantis (2010) reported common activation in posterior parietal cortex (PPC) and prefrontal cortex when subjects were instructed to either voluntarily shift between spatial locations or to shift between colors at a fixed location. However, when they tested their data with a multivariate pattern classification, they found differences in the spatiotemporal activation pattern in PPC, suggesting that there are different subsets of neurons tuned to feature- or spatial-based control.

Besides the possible differences in strategic control, the last two studies suggest that feature-based and spatial attention are basically managed in identical fronto-posterior networks but perhaps activate subpopulations of neurons that are tuned to different domains. Along that line, Cohen and Maunsell (2011) also concluded that feature-based and spatial attention act on a common neural mechanism. They recorded from monkey V4 neurons in both hemispheres while monkeys performed either a spatial frequency or orientation task with Gabor patches. Both, feature-based and spatial attention resulted in an enhancement and synchronization of neural responses, thus, they acted on an identical modulation mechanism. However, while feature-based attention acted across both hemispheres, spatial attention was restricted to the hemisphere contralateral to the to-be-attended location. Given that result, it is quite obvious whenever location is important, spatial attention acts locally to increase the neural response in early retinotopically organized areas. However, from where and how the global activation of feature-based attention is guided is currently still unknown. On the basis of the findings from Zhou and Desimone (2011), FEF seem to be one of the likely candidates, but from what we have learned from Greenberg et al. (2010), PPC is a likely candidate as well.

FEATURE-BASED VS OBJECT-BASED SELECTION

Contrary to the comparison of feature-based vs spatial selection, research on a direct comparison of feature- vs object-based attention is sparse. As mentioned above, Duncan's experiments in 1984 demonstrated that spatial selection does not have a unique position in perception. His results showed, although two objects were presented in the attentional spotlight, dual judgments for one object were significantly better compared to when these judgments incorporated two objects. Many years later in 1999, in an elegant fMRI study, O'Craven et al. (1999) demonstrated selective activation in the fusiform face or parahippocampal place area when subjects attended to either a face or a building with spatially superimposed images. Given that both stimuli, faces and buildings, were in the center of the attentional spotlight, a purely spatial account would have predicted that there is no difference in neural activation regardless of what stimulus subjects have to attend to. In contrast to that prediction, O'Craven and colleagues showed selective activation of these areas even when the face or the building needed not to be identified to solve the task. Their finding resulted in the formulation of the "integrated competition account" of object selective attention. At its heart is the prediction that all attributes (features) that constitute an object will be processed regardless of whether or not a particular attribute of the attended object is required to perform the task.

The temporal dynamics of integrated competition were investigated in a combined EEG/magnetoencephalography (MEG) and fMRI study (Schoenfeld et al., 2003). The authors presented two arrays of dots moving in opposite directions. In some of the displays all dots were presented as black circles (i.e., white dots), in other displays one array of dots was presented in red. Subjects were instructed to attend to one direction of motion and to detect short speed changes of motion in the to-be-attended surface. Importantly, subjects were never instructed to attend to the color of the dots. Results showed increased neural activity in color sensitive early visual areas when subjects attended to red dots to detect changes of speed. EEG/MEG analysis of ERPs/ERFs (event related fields) revealed that attentional modulation of color information followed about 50 ms after the modulation caused by attending to the direction of motion. The authors interpreted that result as direct evidence of rapid binding processes of all features that constitute the to-be-attended object, as hypothesized by the integrated competition account.

In a similar vein, Katzner, Busse, and Treue (2009) interpreted their findings by means of extracellular recordings from single cells in MT in monkeys. Monkeys were trained to attend to either motion or color of random dot patterns. They found attentional modulation of MT neurons, regardless of whether monkeys attended to color or motion, supportive for the idea of integrative processing of relevant and irrelevant features that form an object. Wannig, Rodriguez, and Freiwald (2007) reported similar results in favor of integrated object processing in monkey intracranial MT recordings. They presented transparent spatially overlapped rotating surfaces and monkeys were trained to attend to one surface, while ignoring the other. MT neurons responded much stronger to the attended surface compared to the unattended one. Furthermore, that effect was even pronounced when surfaces were presented in different colors.

It is very likely that the amount of supportive findings for the integration account, i.e., all properties (features) of an object will be bound together and processed, were discouraging research on comparing feature- vs object-based selection. Nobre, Rao, and Chelazzi (2006) showed that attending to a particular feature of an object selectively modulates behavioral and ERP responses. The authors used a negative-priming paradigm with objects that were either bidimensional (color and motion) or unidimensional (either color without motion or gray with motion). On the behavioral level they reported a decrease in performance if, for example, a certain color had to be detected that was the to-be-ignored color in the preceding bidimensional stimulus (negative priming for color). A modulatory response of negative priming was additionally mirrored in early (P1 and N1) and later ERP components (P3).

In our yet unpublished study, we presented our subjects with outlined squares that were rotating in steps of 10° of visual angle every 118 ms (Figure 10.7). In addition to the "jumpy" rotation that produced an SSVEP at 8.5 Hz, the squares changed color from red to green or

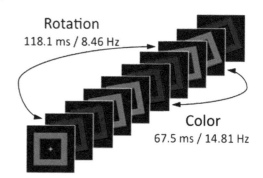

FIGURE 10.7 Schematic representation of stimulation. Rotation elicited an SSVEP at 8.46 Hz, while color changes drove an SSVEP response at 14.81 Hz. Subjects were instructed to attend to either rotation or color changes and to detect target events in the to-be-attended attribute (feature) of the squares.

vice versa at a rate of 33 ms, eliciting an SSVEP at 14.8 Hz (Figure 10.7). As with all of our experiments, colors were isoluminant. Subjects were instructed to attend to either color changes, i.e., rotation was task irrelevant, or attend to rotation, i.e., color changes were task irrelevant, and to detect target events, respectively.

The integrated competition account would predict that SSVEP amplitudes will not be modulated, regardless to what feature subjects had to attend to. However, as depicted in Figure 10.8, we found significant attentional modulation of 8.5 and 14.8 Hz SSVEP amplitudes at posterior electrodes when subjects attended to rotation or color, respectively. Source reconstruction of the respective attention effect (i.e., attended minus unattended) resulted in distinct centers of gravity, with modulated activation in early visual cortex (V1–V3) for color and V5 or human MT complex for motion (Figure 10.8).

Together, although there is more experimental evidence in favor of the integrated processing account, results from the later two human experiments allow questioning of the overall validity of it. At least under certain circumstances, it seems the case that attending to a particular feature of an object resulted in neural responses that clearly indicated preferred processing of that feature, rather than integrated processing of all features. Future research is definitely needed to shed light on the basic neural principles that might differ between object and feature processing and the underlying neural circuits.

SUMMARY

As of today it seems that top-down effects of global feature-based attention and local effects of spatial selection are guided by the same cortical networks, but within these higher order cortical structures subpopulations of cells with domain-specific tuning properties seem to exist. The big difference between the two selection domains is that feature-based attention acts globally,

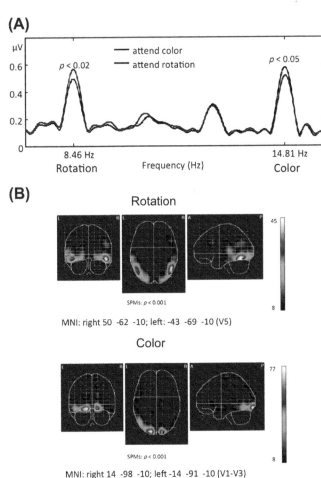

(A)

attend color
attend rotation

$p < 0.02$

$p < 0.05$

8.46 Hz
Rotation

Frequency (Hz)

14.81 Hz
Color

(B)

Rotation

SPMs: $p < 0.001$

MNI: right 50 -62 -10; left: -43 -69 -10 (V5)

Color

SPMs: $p < 0.001$

MNI: right 14 -98 -10; left -14 -91 -10 (V1-V3)

FIGURE 10.8 Spectrum at parietal electrodes and source reconstruction of the attention effect. (A) Stimuli evoked SSVEPs at the respective driving frequency with significant amplitude gains when subjects attended to either rotation or color changes, respectively. Spectra were obtained from individual electrodes out of a parietal area that showed greatest amplitudes averaged across all experimental conditions, respectively. (B) Cortical sources of attention effect (attended minus unattended) for rotation (upper panel) and color (lower panel). Scales represents t^2 values and the $p < 0.001$ corresponds to 8.0. Coordinates of centers of gravity correspond to average probabilistic magnetic resonance imaging atlas (average brain) produced by the Montreal Neurological Institute (MNI; Collins, Neelin, Peter, & Evans, 1994).

while spatial attention is a more local player in visual cortex. Very little is known on the direct comparison between feature- and object-based attention. Although experimental evidence clearly points into the direction that selective processing of a particular attribute (feature) of an object is difficult to demonstrate, given that objects seem to be processes as grouped entities with all features, some results exist that question the generalized validity of that mechanism in the human brain.

As previously mentioned, research on feature-based attention is a relatively new field and many observations are far from being understood. Ongoing and future research will provide more insights into the basic mechanisms and one day in the future we will hopefully gain a

more complete picture as to what extent feature, object, and spatial selection work together hand in hand. What common mechanisms underlie these selection units and where do they differ? A notable paper that is looking for differences and commonalities of these selection units is the recent paper by Kravitz and Behrmann (2011) that used behavioral data to investigate interactions of the three selection units in the organization of visual scenes.

Acknowledgments

The presented work was conducted in close collaboration with Steve Hillyard and Søren Andersen. Søren Andersen did all of the programming and data analysis. Thanks to both of them for support and fruitful discussions that we had and still have. Research was supported by the Deutsche Forschungsgemeinschaft and different grants in the US that were awarded to Steve Hillyard.

References

Andersen, S. K., Fuchs, S., & Müller, M. M. (2011). Effects of feature-selective and spatial attention at different stages of visual processing. *Journal of Cognitive Neuroscience, 23*, 238–246.

Andersen, S. K., Hillyard, S. A., & Müller, M. M. (2008). Attention facilitates multiple stimulus features in parallel in human visual cortex. *Current Biology, 18*, 1006–1009.

Andersen, S. K., & Müller, M. M. (2010). Behavioral performance follows time-course of neural facilitation and suppression during cued shifts of feature-selective attention. *Proceedings of the National Academy of Sciences of the United States of America, 107*, 13878–13882.

Andersen, S. K., Müller, M. M., & Hillyard, S. A. (2009). Color-selective attention need not be mediated by spatial attention. *Journal of Vision, 9*, 1–7.

Anllo-Vento, L., & Hillyard, S. A. (1996). Selective attention to the color and direction of moving stimuli: electrophysiological correlates of hierarchical feature selection. *Perception and Psychophysics, 58*, 191–206.

Anllo-Vento, L., Luck, S. J., & Hillyard, S. A. (1998). Spatio-temporal dynamics of attention to color: evidence from human electrophysiology. *Human Brain Mapping, 6*, 216–238.

Bichot, N. P., Rossi, A. F., & Desimone, R. (2005). Parallel and serial neural mechanisms for visual search in macaque area V4. *Science, 308*, 529–534.

Cohen, M. R., & Maunsell, J. H. (2011). Using neuronal populations to study the mechanisms underlying spatial and feature attention. *Neuron, 70*, 1192–1204.

Collins, D. L., Neelin, P., Peter, T. M., & Evans, A. C. (1994). Automatic 3D registration of MR volumetric data in standardized talairach space. *Journal of Computer Assisted Tomography, 18*, 192–205.

Corbetta, M., Miezin, F. M., Dobmeyer, S., Shulman, G. L., & Petersen, S. E. (1990). Attentional modulation of neural processing of shape, color, and velocity in humans. *Science, 248*, 1556–1559.

David, S. V., Hayden, B. Y., Mazer, J. A., & Gallant, J. L. (2008). Attention to stimulus features shifts spectral tuning of V4 neurons during natural vision. *Neuron, 59*, 509–521.

Desimone, R. (1998). Visual attention mediated by biased competition in extrastriate visual cortex. *Philosophical Transactions of the Royal Society of London – Series B: Biological Sciences, 353*, 1245–1255.

Desimone, R., & Duncan, J. (1995). Neural mechanisms of selective visual attention. *Annual Review of Neuroscience, 18*, 193–222.

Duncan, J. (1984). Selective attention and the organization of visual information. *Journal of Experimental Psychology: General, 113*, 501–517.

Eriksen, C. W., & Collins, J. F. (1969). Temporal course of selective attention. *Journal of Experimental Psychology, 2*, 254–261.

Eriksen, C. W., & St. James, J. D. (1986). Visual attention within and around the field of focal attention. *Perception & Psychophysics, 45*, 225–240.

Greenberg, A. S., Esterman, M., Wilson, D., Serences, J. T., & Yantis, S. (2010). Control of spatial and feature-based attention in frontoparietal cortex. *Journal of Neuroscience, 30*, 14330–14339.

Gregoriou, G. G., Gotts, S. J., Zhou, H., & Desimone, R. (2009). High-frequency, long-range coupling between prefrontal and visual cortex during attention. *Science, 324*, 1207–1210.

Hayden, B. Y., & Gallant, J. L. (2005). Time course of attention reveals different mechanisms for spatial and feature-based attention in area V4. *Neuron, 47*, 637–643.

Herrington, T. M., & Assad, J. A. (2010). Temporal sequence of attentional modulation in the lateral intraparietal area and middle temporal area during rapid covert shifts of attention. *Journal of Neuroscience, 30*, 3287–3296.

Hillyard, S. A. (1993). Electrical and magnetic brain recordings: contributions to cognitive neuroscience. *Current Opinion in Neurobiology, 3*, 217–224.

Hillyard, S. A., & Anllo-Vento, L. (1998). Event-related brain potentials in the study of visual selective attention. *Proceedings of the National Academy of Sciences of the United States of America, 95*, 781–787.

Hillyard, S. A., Mangun, G. R., Woldorff, M. G., & Luck, S. J. (1995). Neural systems mediating selective attention. In M. S. Gazzaniga (Ed.), *The cognitive neurosciences* (pp. 665–681). Cambridge: MIT Press.

Hillyard, S. A., & Münte, T. F. (1984). Selective attention to color and location: an analysis with event-related brain potentials. *Perception & Psychophysics, 36*, 185–198.

Hillyard, S. A., Vogel, E. K., & Luck, S. J. (1998). Sensory gain control (amplification) as a mechanism of selective attention: electrophysiological and neuroimaging evidence. *Philosophical Transactions of the Royal Society of London – Series B: Biological Sciences, 353*, 1257–1270.

Kastner, S., Pinsk, M. A., De Weerd, P., Desimone, R., & Ungerleider, L. G. (1999). Increased activity in human visual cortex during directed attention in the absence of visual stimulation. *Neuron, 22*, 751–761.

Kastner, S., & Ungerleider, L. G. (2000). Mechanisms of visual attention in the human cortex. *Annual Review of Neuroscience, 23*, 315–341.

Katzner, S., Busse, L., & Treue, S. (2009). Attention to the color of a moving stimulus modulates motion-signal processing in macaque area MT: evidence for a unified attentional system. *Frontiers in Systems Neuroscience, 3*, 12. http://dx.doi.org/10.3389/neuro.06.012.2009.

Kravitz, D. J., & Behrmann, M. (2011). Space-, object-, and feature-based attention interact to organize visual scenes. *Attention Perception and Psychophysics, 73*, 2434–2447.

Martinez-Trujillo, J. C., & Treue, S. (2004). Feature-based attention increases the selectivity of population responses in primate visual cortex. *Current Biology, 14*, 744–751.

Moore, T., Armstrong, K. M., & Fallah, M. (2003). Visuomotor origins of covert spatial attention. *Neuron, 40*, 671–683.

Moore, C. M., & Egeth, H. (1998). How does feature-based attention affect visual processing? *Journal of Experimental Psychology: Human Perception and Performance, 24*, 1296–1310.

Müller, M. M. (2008). Location and features of instructive spatial cues do not influence the time course of covert shifts of visual spatial attention. *Biological Psychology, 77*, 292–303.

Müller, M. M., Andersen, S., Trujilllo, H. J., Valdes Sosa, P., Malinowski, P., & Hillyard, S. A. (2006). Feature-selective attention enhances color signals in early visual areas of the human brain. *Proceedings of the National Academy of Sciences of the United States of America, 103*, 14250–14254.

Müller, M. M., & Hillyard, S. A. (2000). Concurrent recording of steady-state and transient event-related potentials as indices of visual spatial selective attention. *Clinical Neurophysiology, 111*, 1544–1552.

Müller, M. M., & Hübner, R. (2002). Can the attentional spotlight be shaped like a doughnut? Evidence from steady state visual evoked potentials. *Psychological Science, 13*, 119–124.

Müller, M. M., & Keil, A. (2004). Neural synchronization and selective color processing in the human brain. *Journal of Cognitive Neuroscience, 16*, 503–522.

Müller, M. M., Malinowski, P., Gruber, T., & Hillyard, S. A. (2003). Sustained division of the attentional spotlight. *Nature, 424*, 309–312.

Müller, M. M., Picton, T. W., Valdes-Sosa, P., Riera, P., Teder-Sälejärvi, W., & Hillyard, S. A. (1998). Effects of spatial selective attention on the steady-state visual evoked potential in the 20–28 Hz range. *Cognitive Brain Research, 6*, 249–261.

Müller, M. M., Teder-Sälejärvi, W., & Hillyard, S. A. (1998). The time course of cortical facilitation during cued shifts of spatial attention. *Nature Neuroscience, 1*, 631–634.

Nobre, A. C., Rao, A., & Chelazzi, L. (2006). Selective attention to specific features within objects: behavioral and electrophysiological evidence. *Journal of Cognitive Neuroscience, 18*, 539–561.

O'Craven, K. M., Rosen, B. R., Kwong, K. K., Treisman, A., & Savoy, R. L. (1997). Voluntary attention modulates fMRI activity in human MT-MST. *Neuron, 18*, 591–598.

Polk, T. A., Drake, R. M., Jonides, J. J., Smith, M. R., & Smith, E. E. (2008). Attention enhances the neural processing of relevant features and suppresses the processing of irrelevant features in humans: a functional magnetic resonance imaging study of the Stroop task. *Journal of Neuroscience, 28*, 13786–13792.

Posner, M. I. (1980). Orienting of attention. *Quarterly Journal of Experimental Psychology, 32*, 3–25.

Regan, D. (1989). *Human brain electrophysiology: Evoked potentials and evoked magnetic fields in science and medicine*. New York: Elsevier.

Saenz, M., Buracas, G. T., & Boynton, G. M. (2002). Global effects of feature-based attention in the human visual cortex. *Nature Neuroscience, 5*, 631–632.

Schoenfeld, M. A., Tempelmann, C., Martinez, A., Hopf, J. -M., Sattler, C., Heinze, H. -J., et al. (2003). Dynamics of feature binding during object-selective attention. *Proceedings of the National Academy of Sciences of the United States of America, 100*, 11806–11811.

Scolari, M., Byers, A., & Serences, J. T. (2012). Optimal deployment of attentional gain during fine discriminations. *Journal of Neuroscience, 32*, 7723–7733.

Scolari, M., & Serences, J. T. (2010). Basing perceptual decisions on the most informative sensory neurons. *Journal of Neurophysiology, 104*, 2266–2273.

Serences, J. T., & Boynton, G. M. (2007). Feature-based attentional modulations in the absence of direct visual stimulation. *Neuron, 55*, 301–312.

Shih, S. I., & Sperling, G. (1996). Is there feature-based attentional selection in visual search. *Journal of Experimental Psychology: Human Perception and Performance, 22*, 758–779.

Treisman, A. (1982). Perceptual grouping and attention in visual search for features and objects. *Journal of Experimental Psychology: Human Perception and Performance, 8*, 194–214.

Treisman, A. (1998). Feature binding, attention and object perception. *Philosophical Transactions of the Royal Society of London – Series B: Biological Sciences, 353*, 1295–1306.

Treisman, A. M., & Gelade, G. (1980). A feature-integration theory of attention. *Cognitive Psychology, 12*, 97–136.

Treisman, A., & Gormican, S. (1988). Feature analysis in early vision: evidence from search asymmetries. *Psychological Review, 95*, 15–48.

Treisman, A., & Sato, S. (1990). Conjunction search revisited. *Journal of Experimental Psychology: Human Perception and Performance, 16*, 459–478.

Treue, S. (2001). Neural correlates of attention in primate visual cortex. *Trends in Neuroscience, 24*, 295–300.

Treue, S., & Trujillo, C. M. (1999). Feature-based attention influences motion processing gain in macaque visual cortex. *Nature, 399,* 575–579.

Tsal, Y., & Lavie, N. (1993). Location dominance in attending to color and shape. *Journal of Experimental Psychology: Human Perception and Performance, 19,* 131–139.

Wannig, A., Rodriguez, V., & Freiwald, W. A. (2007). Attention to surfaces modulates motion processing in extrastriate area MT. *Neuron, 54,* 639–651.

Wolfe, J. M. (1994). Guided search 2.0: a revised model of visual search. *Psychonomic Bulletin and Review, 1,* 202–238.

Wolfe, J. M., Cave, K. R., & Franzel, S. L. (1989). Guided search: an alternative to the feature integration model for visual search. *Journal of Experimental Psychology: Human Perception and Performance, 15,* 419–433.

Wolfe, J. M., & Horowitz, T. S. (2004). What attributes guide the deployment of visual attention and how do they do it? *Nature Reviews Neuroscience, 5,* 495–501.

Zhang, W., & Luck, S. J. (2009). Feature-based attention modulates feedforward visual processing. *Nature Neuroscience, 12,* 24–25.

Zhou, H., & Desimone, R. (2011). Feature-based attention in the frontal eye field and area V4 during visual search. *Neuron, 70,* 1205–1217.

Effects of Preparatory Attention to Nonspatial Features in the Visual Cortex

Sean P. Fannon[1], George R. Mangun[2]

[1]Department of Psychology, Folsom Lake College, Folsom, CA, USA,
[2]Departments of Psychology and Neurology and Center for Mind and Brain, University of California, Davis,
Davis, CA, USA

INTRODUCTION

Covert visual attention to spatial locations or nonspatial features facilitates behavioral and neural responses to attended stimuli (e.g., Corbetta, Miezin, Dobmeyer, Shulman, & Petersen, 1991; Heinze et al., 1994; Hillyard & Munte, 1984; Kingstone, 1992; Posner, 1980; Schoenfeld et al., 2007; Woldorff et al., 1997). In addition to modulating stimulus-evoked responses, a growing number of studies have shown that selective attention can modulate activity in sensory brain regions *before* the onset of an evoking stimulus. Often referred to as "baseline shifts", it is widely presumed that these prestimulus changes in activity represent the top-down signals that bias sensory processing in favor of an attended location or feature (Desimone & Duncan, 1995). Influential models of attention have further proposed that these elevated activity levels play a *causal* role in boosting subsequent neural responses to relevant sensory inputs (e.g., Driver & Frith, 2000; Kastner & Ungerleider, 2000; Reynolds & Heeger, 2009). Some computational (Borgers, Epstein, & Kopell, 2005; Chawla, Lumer, & Friston, 1999, 2000) and physiological studies (e.g., Cossart, Aronov, & Yuste, 2003) have supported the proposal that increased background activity before sensory inputs contributes to the modulation of stimulus-locked transients. If so, this would represent an elegant solution for attentional biasing and possibly provide a convenient way to assess the focus of selective attention in the absence of attended stimuli.

These prestimulus increases in activity have been observed quite consistently in studies manipulating spatial attention. Increased prestimulus activity has been observed in sensory areas that code an attended location in studies using single unit (e.g., Luck, Chelazzi, Hillyard, & Desimone, 1997; Reynolds, Chelazzi, & Desimone, 1999), event-related potential (Harter, Anllo-Vento, & Wood, 1989; Harter & Anllo-Vento, 1991; Hopf & Mangun, 2000; Yamaguchi, Tsuchiya, & Kobayashi, 1994, 1995), and functional magnetic resonance imaging (fMRI) methods (Hopfinger, Buonocore, & Mangun, 2000; Kastner, Pinsk, De Weerd, Desimone, & Ungerleider, 1999). They have even been found to increase in magnitude with the difficulty of an upcoming discrimination, consistent with increased attentional focus to cope with greater task demands (Ress, Backus, & Heeger, 2000).

However, analogous prestimulus activity has been observed far less consistently in studies that direct the subjects' attention to nonspatial features. In those that find the effects, the baseline shifts are not retinotopically specific but rather tend to be specific to the neural populations or cortical regions specialized for processing the attended features. Some studies observe clear increases in activity in relevant sensory neurons or regions (e.g., Chawla, Rees, & Friston, 1999; Chelazzi, Duncan, Miller, & Desimone, 1998; Shulman et al., 1999; Serences & Boynton, 2007; Stokes, Thompson, Nobre, & Duncan, 2009). Others find them inconsistently (e.g., Fannon, Saron, & Mangun, 2007; Haenny, Maunsell, & Schiller, 1988; Ferrara et al., 1994; Wylie, Javitt, & Foxe, 2006) or not at all (Fannon & Mangun, 2008; McMains, Fehd, Emmanouil, & Kastner, 2007; Shulman, d'Avossa, Tansy, & Corbetta, 2002). Reconciling these discrepant results is complicated by the rather wide variability in experimental procedures employed. Nonetheless, resolving this issue is of fundamental importance to our understanding of attention. If baseline shifts in relevant sensory areas are not a consistent property of preparatory attention to nonspatial features, then, despite their consistency in spatial attention, they cannot be regarded as a general mechanism for modulating stimulus-evoked responses, and continued investigation is required to identify the actual mechanisms.

Here we consider some of the various factors that might influence preparatory attention effects in the sensory cortex. Sorting out the conditions under which such activity is observed may help to clarify the mechanisms that underlie the top-down modulation of sensory-evoked responses and to assess the premises underlying prominent models of attention.

CONTROLLING FOR NONSELECTIVE EFFECTS

Studies of selective attention generally compare conditions that vary only in the attribute attended (location, feature, object category, etc.), and efforts are made to ensure that task difficulty, attentional load, and other cognitive and perceptual demands are equated across the various attention conditions. This is done to preclude changes in arousal or nonspecific attention mechanisms from masquerading as effects of selective attention. However, some functional imaging studies reporting effects of selective feature attention have not included adequate controls for these nonselective influences.

In one study of attention to motion (Luks & Simpson, 2004), subjects were presented with a particular type of radial motion and instructed to attend to either the left or right visual field before each block of trials. At the beginning of each trial, the fixation cross changed, cueing subjects to prepare for a series of relevant motion stimuli that were then presented either 1.25 or 9.75 s later. Subjects then had to respond when the particular motion type presented before the block of trials appeared in the attended hemifield during any trial in that block. The authors reported significant increases in activity in a series of posterior brain regions consistent with those previously shown to play a role in motion processing, including MT, following the fixation cross change that signaled the start of each trial. The authors attributed this activity to preparatory motion attention. While the observed activations likely included the effects of selective attention to motion, the activity reported was relative to an inattentive baseline condition and therefore also reflected changes in attention and arousal that were not feature-specific.

Shulman et al. (1999, Experiment 2) also used event-related fMRI to investigate the neural correlates of prestimulus attention to motion. Subjects were cued to the specific direction of motion of the to-be-detected target stimulus at the start of each trial. The authors also

observed increased activity in area MT in response to the cues. However, the increased MT response for direction-specific cues was relative to that evoked by passive cues instructing subjects to do nothing with the upcoming stimulus. Thus, the activity could again reflect nonspecific changes in arousal or other attention mechanisms, instead of or in addition to the attentional preparation for specific directions of motion.

Though the results of studies such as these are informative in other ways, they cannot be used to draw strong conclusions about feature-specific preparatory activity. Hence they also cannot be used to assess the proposition that this preparatory activity is the mechanism by which attention modulates sensory responses to relevant targets, because changes in arousal might mimic a feature-selective baseline shift in these cases.

ELIMINATING SPATIAL ATTENTION

The baseline shifts reported in the study by Luks and Simpson (2004) described above might also have reflected spatially selective preparatory activity, rather than motion-specific preparatory activity. In each trial, subjects were not just attending for a specific type of motion; they were also restricting their attention to a single hemifield. Hence, elevations in activity observed in the visual cortex may have been driven by the allocation of spatial attention.

An earlier study by our group (Giesbrecht, Weissman, Woldorff, & Mangun, 2006) compared the activity elicited by location and color cues in a task that successfully matched the difficulty of the two attentional conditions, thereby eliminating the nonspecific effects of attention or arousal in their comparison. The results showed pre-target activity in visual areas that responded to the color targets following color attention cues, and increased activity in areas that responded to the location targets in response to location cues. However, the location and color targets were presented at different locations within the visual field: The two color targets were spatially superimposed at the fovea, whereas the two location targets were placed in the upper left and right quadrants nearly 6° from fixation. So although subjects were still required to select an object based on color in the color attention condition, their attention was also necessarily directed to a different spatial location than during the location attention condition, and the differences in the locations of cue-related visual activity between the two conditions could therefore reflect the effects of spatial selective attention. Retinotopically specific effects of preparatory spatial attention are, again, a robust finding in the literature.

This interpretation is supported by the findings of an earlier report using some of the same data (Giesbrecht,

Woldorff, Song, & Mangun, 2003). That report included two different target configurations: one in which the color targets were presented foveally as in the 2006 report, and one in which they were presented on the midline above fixation at the same eccentricity as the lateralized location targets. The location of cortical activity elicited by the color cues showed a marked anterior shift for the more eccentric color targets, consistent with a retinotopic shift in the focus of spatial attention to the new target location.

ATTENDING TO FEATURES OR DIMENSIONS

Behavioral studies have demonstrated that prior knowledge of a specific sensory *feature* (e.g., red color or vertical orientation) in an upcoming stimulus can facilitate responses to that stimulus (e.g., Ball & Sekuler, 1980; Humphreys, 1981; Posner & Snyder, 1975). Other studies have cued subjects to a relevant sensory *dimension* (e.g., speed or direction of rotation) along which the feature or features of an upcoming stimulus may vary and must be discriminated or within which a stimulus detection must be made, but they do not specify a particular feature (e.g., 10°/s or clockwise rotation) to expect along that dimension. Functional imaging studies of preparatory attention also differ in this regard, and these differences might account for at least some of the discrepant findings. Studies of visual working memory (WM) suggest that frontal and parietal control regions interact with and activate regions of visual cortex that code the features of the WM representation (e.g., Curtis & D'Esposito, 2003; Xu & Chun, 2006). Perhaps cueing attention to a specific feature activates a neural representation of that feature to serve as an "attentional template" and produces a similar pattern of activity in sensory areas that code the attended feature (e.g., Bundesen, 1990; Duncan & Humphreys, 1989; Desimone & Duncan, 1995). In fact, we recently reported psychophysical evidence for the role of WM in feature-based attention (Bengson & Mangun, 2011). Subjects in this study performed a combined location- and feature-based cueing task. The validity of both feature and location cues was manipulated independently such that we could assess the effectiveness of each for individual subjects. In addition, for each subject we measured operation span as an assessment of WM capacity. We found that subjects' WM capacity predicted the effectiveness of feature-selective attention in the context of combined spatial and feature expectancy. However, cueing an entire *dimension* may be less likely to produce this kind of attentional template than cueing a specific feature, and this may help to account for divergent results among imaging studies of feature-based preparatory attention.

Chawla, Rees, et al. (1999) reported increases in attention-related baseline activity between target events in areas V4 and V5 during color and motion attention blocks, respectively. Subjects viewed 98 s blocks containing events in which radially moving red dots were presented and with green stationary dots displayed continuously during the interstimulus intervals (ISIs). The experimenters used a wide range of ISIs to permit estimation of the neural activity present between events. Subjects were cued at the start of each run to respond to occasional events in which the dots moved more slowly (in motion attention runs) or were a slightly lighter shade of red (in color attention runs). Thus subjects had to attend to a particular feature in order to perform the task effectively.

In their Experiment 1, Shulman et al. (1999) used a task similar to their Experiment 2, described in the preceding section, but in a blocked design that did not allow the dissociation of cue-related activity from target-related activity. This experiment included a condition in which subjects had to detect motion but were not told the direction of the upcoming motion. They referred to this as the neutral cue condition, though in effect it is a cue for the stimulus dimension of coherent motion as opposed to a cue for a particular feature within that dimension (i.e., a specific direction). When direction-specific feature attention cues were compared with this neutral, dimension cue condition, a set of regions including MT+ was shown to be activated in the feature-specific condition more so than in the general dimension condition. While this differential activity could have been generated in response to the cue, the stimulus, or both (the blocked design precludes this dissociation), the pattern of activity was nearly identical to that observed in the direction-specific cue vs passive cue comparison from the event-related design used in Experiment 2, suggesting that it might indeed be generated during the cue period. If this is so, then it likely reflects the subjects' use of information about the direction (a specific feature) of the upcoming stimulus to better prepare for processing that stimulus.

A similar study from the same group (Shulman et al., 2002) cued subjects to specific features, but the task required subjects to discriminate between a standard stimulus and occasional stimuli that differed slightly from a standard. For example, when given a cue for "green", subjects had to press one button for the standard green and another for an occasional target that was a slightly different shade of green. The nonstandard stimulus for a given feature (i.e., green or red color, left or right motion) was always the same for a given subject. While the cues were for specific features, this discrimination task may not have been conducive to activating a specific attentional template the way a detection task might, resulting in an absence of feature-specific baseline shifts.

In an fMRI study by McMains et al. (2007), subjects were cued at the start of each block to attend to either the color or motion dimension of an upcoming train of stimuli at a particular location. The feature of the first subsequent stimulus within the attended dimension then served as the attended feature for the rest of the block. Hence, during the cue-stimulus interval, subjects were not anticipating or attending a specific feature but were preparing for the dimension as a whole. The authors reported no difference between the activity in MT or V4 following these general color and motion dimension cues.

We conducted an event-related fMRI study in which we directly compared the effects of feature and dimension attention cues on preparatory activity in sensory areas in the context of a difficult target detection task (Fannon et al., 2007). It was designed to overcome key limitations of previous such studies (see Figure 11.1). First, we included both feature and dimension cues in the same experiment and within the same runs. Second, we included cues for two separate dimensions (color and motion) to ensure that any effects were selective for the attended attribute and not due to changes in arousal, and also to assess whether any effects of cue specificity (feature vs. dimension) generalized across different dimensions. Finally, we localized color- and motion-sensitive cortical areas in runs separate from the attention runs and

examined the responses evoked by cues and targets in these regions of interest (ROIs) (Figure 11.2). Most studies examining cue-related effects in feature-selective visual areas either localized these areas by a group analysis (Shulman et al., 1999) or did not localize them at all (Chawla, Rees, et al., 1999; Shulman et al., 2002). Wide variability has been demonstrated in the locations of anatomical landmarks across individual brains (e.g., Tamraz & Comair, 2000) and in the locations of functional areas relative to such landmarks and within a stereotactic coordinate system (Aine et al., 1996; Uylings, et al., 2005). Localizing functional regions for individual subjects is therefore preferable because a functional region defined by a group analysis might overlap only partially or not overlap at all with that region in a given subject.

The human color-sensitive region observed in or near the collateral sulcus is often labeled V4 due to its inferred homology with area V4 identified in monkeys (e.g., Zeki, 1990; Zeki & Bartels, 1999; Zeki et al., 1991). However, retinotopic mapping studies suggest that this color-sensitive region does not fall within the fourth retinotopically organized visual area in humans, and has instead been given the tentative alternative label of V8 (Hadjikhani et al., 1998). Our color-sensitive ROIs are consistent with the coordinates of this retinotopically defined V8, and we

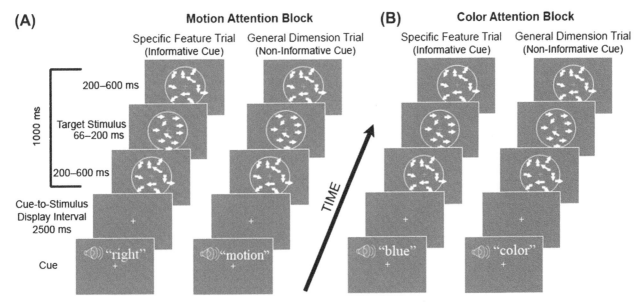

FIGURE 11.1 Schematic illustration of cue and stimulus trials for the motion and color conditions. (A) Stimulus sequences for the motion attention condition showing a specific feature cue trial (left in part A) and a general dimension cue trial (right in part A). Specific feature cues informed the subject of the direction of coherent motion of the upcoming target (if present). In general dimension cue trials, subjects were presented only with the word "motion" indicating that each of the four possible directions of motion was equally likely. The verbal auditory cue was followed 2500 ms later by a 1000 ms display of randomly moving dots. In the midst of this presentation, there could be a motion target, where a portion of the dots briefly moves coherently. During the motion condition, most target displays also contained task-irrelevant color changes. Each trial was followed by an intertrial interval of 1000 ms. (B) Stimulus sequences for the color attention conditions. The left side of part B depicts a specific feature cue trial. The right side of part B shows a general dimension cue trial. Most target displays also contained periods of task-irrelevant coherent motion.

use this revised terminology when referring to our color-sensitive ROIs. Note, however, that these ROIs are in the same location as color-sensitive regions labeled V4 in earlier studies and thus are directly comparable.

The responses to four cue types and their subsequent targets were examined in these functionally defined ROIs. Cues were presented auditorily (to minimize stimulus-driven activity in the visual cortex during the cue period) and consisted of prerecorded spoken words. The cue types were as follows: color dimension (the word "color"), color feature (the name of one of four colors, e.g., "red"), motion dimension (the word "motion"), and motion feature (the name of one of four directions of coherent motion, e.g., "up"). The subjects' task was then to detect brief periods of color or coherent motion, depending on the attentional condition, in a circular display of otherwise randomly moving grayscale dots

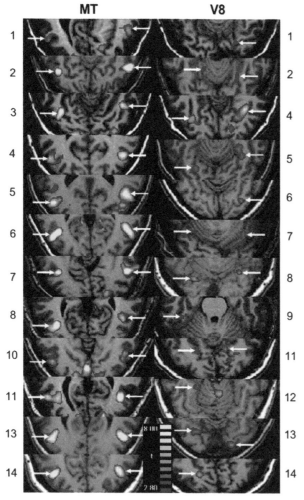

FIGURE 11.2 **Individually defined MT and V8 ROIs.** Arrows indicate the activation(s) from which the ROI(s) for each subject (N = 14) were generated. The left column shows motion area MT and the right shows color area V8.

that appeared 2.5 s after the cue onset and lasted for 1 s. Feature cues were always valid; that is, the color or coherent motion that appeared during the target period was always of the cued color or direction. Cues for specific features and general dimensions were intermixed within runs, but color and motion attention trials were segregated into different runs. "Cue-only" and "null" trials were included to permit individual estimation of cue and target responses (Ollinger, Corbetta, & Shulman, 2001; Ollinger, Shulman, & Corbetta, 2001; Woldorff et al., 2004).

While there were some significant effects of cue specificity (feature vs. dimension) on cue-related activity in sensory areas, their pattern does suggest they can account for discrepancies in the literature with regard to the presence of baseline shifts in nonspatial attention. In MT, feature cues generated larger responses than dimension cues for *both* dimensions (color and motion) (Figure 11.3). Even more surprisingly, in V8 there was no difference between the responses generated by cues for specific colors (color feature cues) and color dimension cues, but cues for specific directions (motion feature cues) elicited a significantly larger response than motion dimension cues, as in MT (Figure 11.4). In MT there was also no difference between color and motion cues generally, though targets elicited a significantly larger response when subjects were detecting coherent motion than when there were detecting color changes.

The results suggest a complex relationship between prestimulus activity and the specificity of nonspatial attention cues. Larger baseline shifts do not necessarily follow cues for specific visual features in their respective feature-selective visual areas. This manipulation thus does not appear to explain discrepancies in the literature. More crucially, the lack of correspondence between the magnitude of baseline shifts and subsequent target-driven responses undermines the proposition that increases in preparatory activity boost subsequent stimulus-driven responses in the sensory cortex, at least at the level of functionally defined visual areas. We observed differences between the responses to attention cue conditions that failed to translate into a difference in the amplitude of subsequent target responses. Conversely, we observed differences in the response to different target conditions despite statistically identical baseline activity associated with the preceding cue types. This dissociation between preparatory and stimulus-driven activity was reinforced by examining the relationship between these responses on a subject-by-subject basis. For a given visual area, we correlated the amplitude of cue-driven responses and target-driven responses for each cue condition across subjects. Of 12 possible correlations (four cue types, plus activity in each dimension collapsed across cue

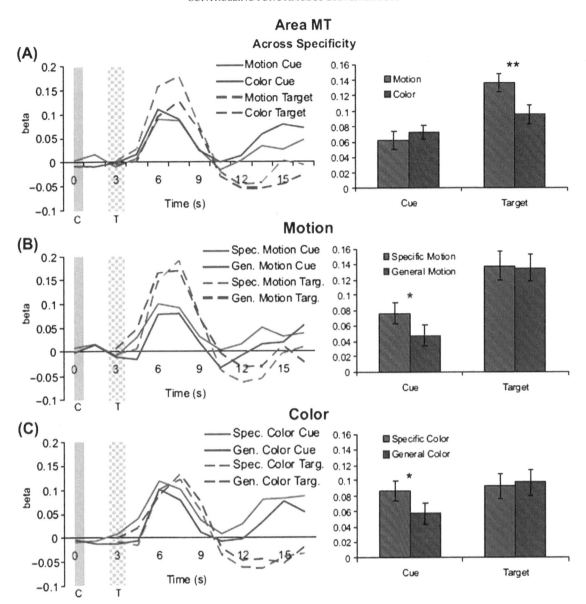

FIGURE 11.3 **Cue and target responses in area MT**. The left column shows BOLD response time course estimates (beta weights) in MT. The solid and checkered gray bars represent the cue (C) and target (T) onsets and offsets, respectively. The right column shows the amplitudes of cue and target responses averaged over the three TRs capturing the peak of the hemodynamic response. All individual cue and target responses are significantly different from the zero baseline. (A) Hemodynamic responses collapsed across specific feature and general dimension trials for motion and color cues and targets in MT. Cue responses for motion and color conditions were not significantly different. Target responses were significantly larger for attention to motion than attention to color (across cue specificity). (B) Hemodynamic responses for specific feature and general dimension motion cues and targets in MT. Specific motion direction cues elicited larger responses than general dimension motion cues, but there was no effect of motion cue specificity on target responses. (C) Hemodynamic responses for specific feature and general dimension color cues and targets in MT.

specificity, for two cortical sensory regions), only four showed significant relationships and these were all negative, meaning that for these areas and cue-target pairs, larger baseline shifts were associated with smaller target responses. This is clearly inconsistent with the view that elevated prestimulus activity in a visual area potentiates larger sensory responses to the attended stimuli in that area.

CONTROLLING FOR STIMULUS-DRIVEN EFFECTS

Another element that varies across imaging studies of feature attention is the presence of irrelevant stimuli during the expectation periods prior to or between relevant targets. Many studies that have reported feature- or dimension-specific baseline shifts

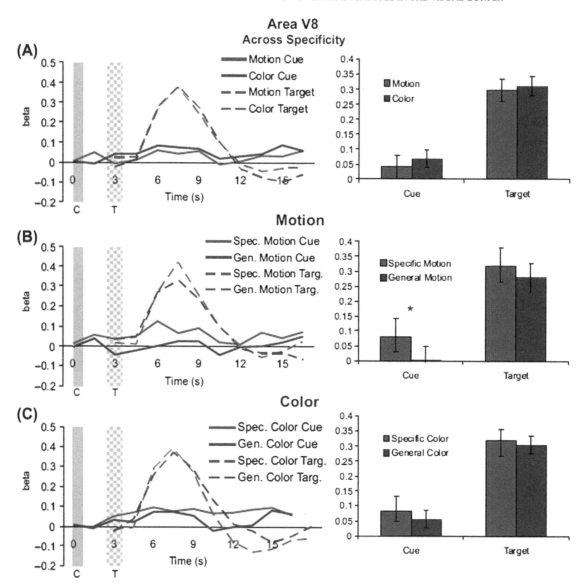

FIGURE 11.4 **Cue and target responses in area V8.** Data presented as in Figure 11.3. Cue responses are all significantly different from the zero baseline except for general dimension motion cues (panel B). (A) Hemodynamic responses collapsed across specific feature and general dimension trials for motion and color cues and targets in V8. Unlike MT, there were no significant differences in the amplitude of target responses with attention. (B) Hemodynamic responses for specific feature and general dimension motion cues and targets in V8. (C) Hemodynamic responses for specific feature and general dimension color cues and targets in V8.

displayed prominent, though task-irrelevant, visual stimuli while subjects were preparing for the next target. For example, in the experiment of Chawla, Rees, et al. (1999) described above, a display of static green dots was present continuously between relevant (red) moving dot targets. Ongoing anticipatory attention to color or motion may have enhanced the sensory response to this irrelevant stimulus in areas that coded the attended feature. Similarly, Shulman et al. (1999) observed cue-related activity in MT in both experiments, and in both experiments an array of static dots was displayed in the same aperture in which the subsequent moving dot stimuli would be presented. This

might also explain the absence of cue-related activity in a subsequent study by the same group (Shulman et al., 2002). In this latter study, as in ours (Fannon et al., 2007), the display was left blank during the cue-target interval.

We explicitly tested the hypothesis that attention-related baseline shifts in feature-sensitive visual areas are a function of the presence of these irrelevant stimuli during the pretarget period (Fannon & Mangun, 2008). Color- and motion-sensitive regions were functionally localized, and subjects were precued to expect specific colors or directions of motion as in our study described above, though instead of manipulating cue specificity by including general dimension cues, the presence of irrelevant pretarget stimuli was varied across runs. During half the runs, there was only a small fixation cross present between target periods (the "pattern-absent" condition) as in our previous study, but during the other half of the runs a static random dot pattern (the "pattern-present" condition, essentially a single frame of the random dot motion stimuli) was displayed throughout the run during the periods between targets, including the cue-target intervals. If attention modulates the response to irrelevant stimuli while subjects anticipate the relevant target stimulus, this modulation should be apparent as a difference in activity following color and motion cues in color- and motion-sensitive visual areas.

First, we should note that the results in the pattern-absent condition exactly replicated those of our previous study (Fannon et al., 2007), in which the display was also blank between targets (apart from the small fixation cross) (Figure 11.5). The replication confirms our conclusion that attention-related baseline shifts in visual areas need not influence the amplitude of subsequent target responses there. In addition, the result also rules out a possible confound. In our previous study, color and motion cues were segregated into separate runs, allowing the possibility that differences in activity level or arousal between runs influenced the relative amplitude of responses to these cue types. In this follow-up study,

color and motion cues were intermixed within each run, eliminating this potential confound. Despite this change, the results were identical.

The crucial new finding, though, came from the comparison of these results (the pattern-absent conditions) with those from the pattern-present runs. Preparatory attention to color and motion did *not* modulate the response to the irrelevant dot pattern and there were still no feature-specific baseline shifts (Figures 11.6 and 11.7). The responses elicited by cues in the pattern-present and pattern-absent runs were virtually identical. These results rule out the attentional modulation of the response to irrelevant pretarget stimuli as a possible explanation for discrepancies among the results of other studies.

MEASURING THE APPROPRIATE NEURAL ACTIVITY

The work discussed so far fails to offer convincing evidence that attention-related baseline shifts in visual areas coding the attended feature constitute the means by which feature attention modulates the sensory response to subsequent targets. Some studies did not sufficiently control for factors unrelated to feature attention, and in studies that did, baseline shifts were observed inconsistently and, crucially, did not predict sensory modulation

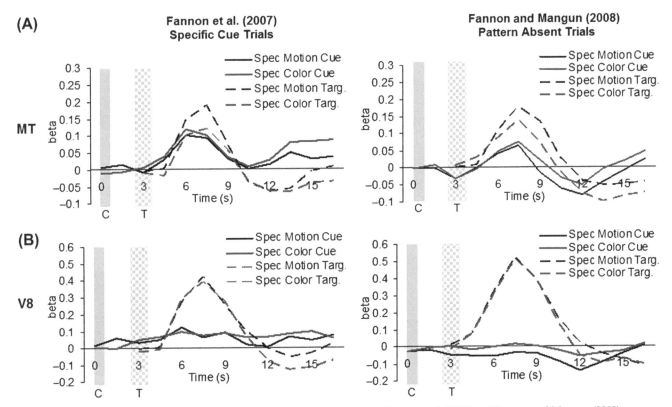

FIGURE 11.5 Close replication of cue and target responses between Fannon et al. (2007) and Fannon and Mangun (2008).

of subsequent targets. However, these were functional imaging studies that measured the effects of preparatory attention and stimulus response modulation within rather large ROIs, represented in some cases by hundreds of voxels. Regions this large necessarily contain individual neurons with a variety of feature preferences. If preparatory attention exerts differential effects across these cells, the changes might not be observable in the hemodynamic response measured across the imaged region.

Feature-based attention has been shown to increase the response in single cells tuned for directions (Martinez-Trujillo & Treue, 2004; Treue & Martinez Trujillo, 1999), colors (Motter, 1994; Spitzer, Desimone, & Moran, 1988), and orientations (Haenny & Schiller, 1988) when the animal is attending for the cell's preferred feature. Importantly, these excitatory effects may be accompanied by response *suppression* in cells tuned for unattended features (Haenny & Schiller, 1988; Martinez-Trujillo & Treue, 2004; Motter, 1994). For example, Martinez-Trujillo and Treue (2004) recorded the responses of MT neurons in response to dot motion in a range of directions, while monkeys attended for a

particular direction of motion at a location well outside the receptive field (RF) of the recorded cell. This produces a pure effect of feature attention, as spatial attention was directed elsewhere. Consistent with the authors' "feature-similarity gain model", under these conditions a given cell's response to its preferred direction of motion was enhanced when the animal was attending to the same motion in the opposite hemifield and suppressed when it was attending to the antipreferred direction. The level of enhancement or suppression varied with the degree of similarity between the cell's preferred direction and the attended direction. Across the population of directionally tuned neurons, then, attention to a given direction would increase the response of some cells and decrease the response to others, potentially resulting in little or no overall change in the activity of the population. Bridwell and Srinivasan (2012) recorded steady-state evoked potentials (SSVEPs) during a task that manipulated the degree to which subjects enhanced or suppressed the processing of nonspatial visual features. They found electrophysiological evidence of both enhancement and suppression. If preparatory feature attention also produces both enhancement and suppression of activity within a

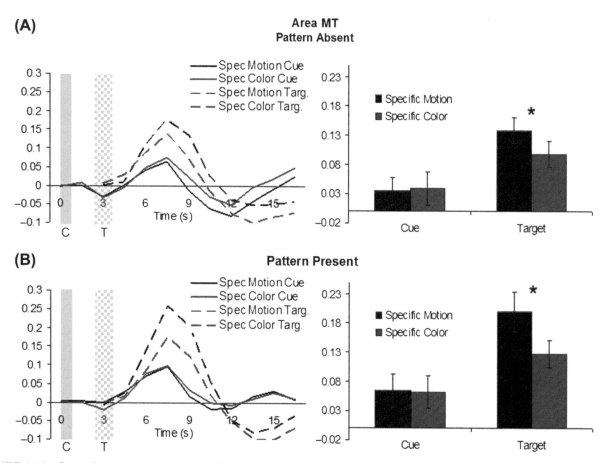

FIGURE 11.6 Cue and target responses in area MT during runs in which the static dot stimulus was absent between targets (pattern absent) and runs in which it was present (pattern present). The presence of the irrelevant stimulus does not interact with preparatory attention to influence the level of baseline activity in MT.

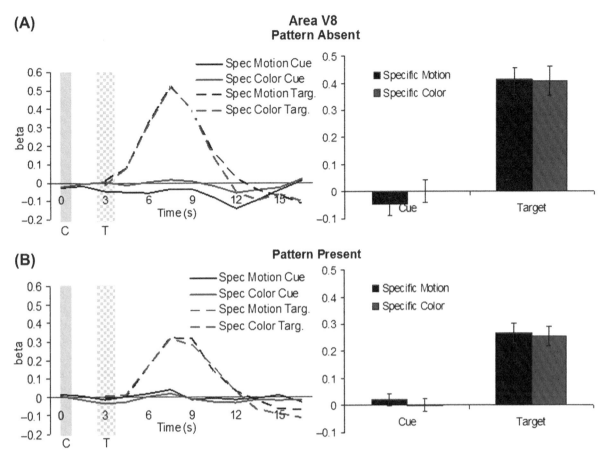

FIGURE 11.7   Data for area V8 presented as in Figure 11.6. Again, the presence of the irrelevant stimulus during the cue-target interval does not influence the amplitude of baseline activity.

visual region, this could make detecting the effects difficult or impossible using standard fMRI methods.

Chelazzi et al. (1998) found evidence consistent with this explanation. In their study, macaques performed a visual search task during which they were shown an object foveally and then were required to make a saccade to the same object when it was presented again, along with one or more distractor stimuli, following a 1500 ms delay. Following Moran and Desimone (1985), the target and distractor stimuli were chosen such that a given cell responded well to one (the "good stimulus"), but not to the others (the "bad stimuli"). Trials were either blocked, with the same cue object repeated over 10–30 trials, or randomized, with each trial presenting a different cue object. Most IT cells showed higher delay activity when a good stimulus was the target to be searched for than when a bad stimulus was the target. The baseline activity was also higher *preceding* a good cue if the animal expected that cue to occur (as in the blocked condition). This finding shows that the baseline shift was not simply a sustained visual response to the cue object, but was instead a function of the animal's knowledge of the relevant stimulus, suggesting that nonspatial baseline shifts occur selectively in individual cells that code the

expected feature or set of features. A later study by the same group found similar results in area V4 (Chelazzi, Miller, Duncan, & Desimone, 2001). While the analyses reported could not distinguish between enhancement of activity for good stimuli and suppression of activity for bad stimuli during the delay period, the results nonetheless reveal preparatory activity in relatively few feature-selective cells within the neural population. Such activity would likely be difficult to detect using standard fMRI methods.

However, other single unit studies have failed to observe such selectivity in the delay period. For example, while recording from individual V4 neurons, Haenny, Maunsell, and Schiller (1988) had macaques perform an orientation match-to-sample task. The animals were cued with one of four orientations, and then were presented with a sequence of target gratings. The animals were then required to release a switch when a target grating matched the cued orientation. Orientation cues were either visual or tactile, and both often elicited increased firing rates in V4 cells during the period before the onset of the first stimulus. A total of 22% of units were selective only for target orientation and not for cue orientation, while 18% were selective only for cue orientation and not target orientation. Most cells were selective for certain orientations of both the cues and stimuli, but these selectivities did not necessarily coincide. For example, a given cell could show an increase in delay period firing after a horizontal cue, but then *decrease* its firing when a horizontal stimulus grating appeared. Thus, the visual response properties of single cells did not necessarily correspond with their selectivity for attended features.

Similarly, Ferrera, Rudolph, and Maunsell (1994) trained monkeys to perform a delayed match-to-sample task where the attribute to be matched was the direction of motion of a field of dynamic random dots undergoing uniform translation. This allowed measurement of the neuronal responses of the test stimuli as a function of stimulus direction (i.e., conventional stimulus selectivity), and also as a function of the sample (or cue) direction. Increased delay period activity relative to baseline was seen in a high percentage of cells in all areas studied (V4, MT, MST and 7a). For all cells, the average delay activity was twice the baseline. However, there was a consistent but weak *negative* correlation between direction selectivity and delay activity. That is, cells that were less sensitive to the direction of motion tended to have higher levels of delay activity. Further, while most cells experienced some change in excitability, as measured by increased or decreased overall levels of activity during the delay, there was no evidence that this activity carried information about the direction of the cue for the vast majority of cells. For example, cells activated by rightward motion did not tend to have higher delay activity after a cue for rightward motion than they did after cues for other motion directions, analogous to the results observed in V4 for attention to orientation (Haenny et al., 1988).

Bisley, Zaksas, Droll, and Pasternak (2004) found little activity in individual MT neurons during the delay period in a motion direction delayed match-to-sample task, but like Ferrera et al. (1994) they found that activity was slightly higher when the sample stimulus was in the antipreferred direction than when it was in a cell's preferred direction. However, in this study the test stimulus was either of two opposite directions or one of four orthogonal directions (up, down, left, or right). The ease with which these test stimuli could be distinguished meant the maintenance of a specific representation of the sample direction was unnecessary to perform the task, and the neural signature of such a representation in the delay period may have been weak as a result.

Conventional fMRI methods have been thought to lack the spatial resolution to distinguish the representations of individual features within the human cortex due to the fact that individual voxels measure the activity of a pool of neurons with a range of feature tuning. The spatial spread of the hemodynamic response, spatial smoothing resulting from image preprocessing, and residual uncorrected head movement further limit spatial resolution. However, while a given voxel contains cells with a range of feature preferences, the distribution of these preferences is unlikely to be perfectly balanced across voxels, leaving each voxel with a weak bias toward a particular feature. As a result, when using multivoxel pattern analysis methods, fMRI studies can reliably detect the object category (e.g., Haxby et al., 2001) and even the specific orientation (Kamitani & Tong, 2005) or direction of motion (Kamitani & Tong, 2006) of the stimulus display. More critically for the current discussion, attention to visual features has also been shown to produce predictable changes in the pattern of responses across voxels using these same analysis techniques (Kamitani & Tong, 2005, 2006).

Perhaps previous studies, including ours, would have found reliable baseline shifts with feature-based attention by analyzing changes in the pattern of activity across voxels in a visual region rather than the overall level of activity within the region. A study by Serences and Boynton (2007) indirectly addressed this question. They used functional magnetic resonance imaging and a pattern classification algorithm to predict the attentional state of human observers as they attended to one of two directions of motion. Following Treue and Martinez Trujillo (1999), subjects attended to a particular direction of motion in one hemifield while the activity in visual cortical areas coding the opposite hemifield was measured. However, Serences and Boynton also included a condition in which there was no stimulus in the unattended hemifield. They found that the pattern of activity in the visual cortex within an *unstimulated* hemisphere was still modulated by the direction of motion to which subjects were attending. That is, feature-based attention induced a systematic modulation of the pattern of activation across an ROI even in the absence of direct stimulation. The same group found similar results for the orientation of gratings coded in the hemisphere ipsilateral to the hemifield in which the remembered stimulus was presented (Ester, Serences, & Awh, 2009). However, these activation patterns were different from the patterns observed when a stimulus was driving the response. Hence, even when analyzing the pattern of activity across a region rather than the overall activity level, there was still a lack of correspondence between the pattern of activity between feature attention with and without visual stimulation.

Although it is tempting to draw a direct comparison between these effects and pretarget baseline shifts, previously reported baseline shifts were observed during the temporal gap between an attention-directing cue and the presentation of the target stimulus or search array. In contrast, observers in the Serences and Boynton (2007) experiment just described were continuously monitoring a stimulus on one side of the visual field, so the spread of feature-based attention may have been driven by hard-wired cross-hemispheric connections between similarly tuned neurons in corresponding visual areas rather than top-down modulation from attentional control regions. A more direct test would be to assess whether the pattern of activity in response to visual feature cues produces a multivoxel pattern of activity similar to that elicited by the cued feature. Stokes et al. (2009) did just this. They used auditory tones to cue subjects to attend to either the letter X or O. Subjects were then required to detect occasional presentations of the attended letter in a slightly smaller font. The authors used multivoxel pattern analysis to identify a swath of LOC bilaterally whose response pattern discriminated between the target shapes (despite similar overall levels of activity elicited by the two shapes). Activity patterns specific to the attended shape were observed throughout the period following the attentional cues. Furthermore, the specificity of this sustained cue-related activity correlated with perceptual performance. While there was dynamic visual noise presented continuously throughout each trial, the results of Fannon and Mangun (2008) described above suggest that this should not have influenced their results. Among functional neuroimaging studies, these results constitute the strongest evidence to date for increases in baseline activity with preparatory attention in feature-specific neural populations. The similar overall activity level elicited by the target types and cue conditions in LOC also highlights the difficulty of detecting such changes using conventional fMRI analysis techniques.

Related studies of visual WM have reported analogous findings. For example, Serences et al. (2009) performed multivoxel pattern analysis on V1 ROIs during the delay period of a delayed match-to-sample task for orientation or color. They found a sustained pattern of activation in V1 that represented only the intentionally remembered feature of a multifeature object, and this pattern was similar to that observed during the discrimination of sensory stimuli. Harrison and Tong (2009) reported similar results.

While the single unit results are inconsistent in this regard, functional neuroimaging studies are beginning to provide evidence that the pattern of activity within the visual cortex, if not the overall level of activity within a region, is associated with preparatory attention to visual features. Though the finding needs replication, at least one study of cued attention and multiple studies of WM showed that the pattern of activity preceding a target stimulus is similar to that generated by the attended or remembered stimulus attribute. This is consistent with models of attention that propose baseline shift bias processing in favor of attended items by boosting their sensory response, though the effect is apparently localized to relatively small neural ensembles rather than later retinotopically or functionally defined visual areas.

ASSESSING SYNCHRONY

Most research on the neural bases of selective attention has focused on changes in firing rate or indirect measures of this activity such as the blood oxygen level dependent (BOLD) response in fMRI. However, a growing body of research documents the capacity for selective attention to also modulate the synchrony of neural activity. Changes in synchrony have the potential to dramatically influence neural computation without necessarily producing changes in overall spike rate or hemodynamic response.

Several electroencephalogram (EEG) studies have documented that attention to spatial locations is associated with retinotopically specific changes in alpha-band activity, even in the absence of visual stimulation. Preparatory decreases of alpha-activity have been observed contralateral to the attended location (Sauseng et al., 2005) and are interpreted to reflect enhanced cortical excitability to facilitate future visual processing at the attended location. In addition, alpha increases have been observed contralateral to the unattended location (Kelly, Lalor, Reilly, & Foxe, 2006; Worden, Foxe, Wang, & Simpson, 2000; Yamagishi et al., 2003), potentially reflecting an active "inhibitory" process suppressing visual input from task-irrelevant locations. Thut, Nietzel, Brandt, and Pascual-Leone (2006) showed that the degree of asymmetry in this prestimulus activity predicts the detection of subsequent targets.

Fries, Reynolds, Rorie, and Desimone (2001) manipulated visual spatial attention in monkeys while recording multiunit and local field potential (LFP) responses with overlapping receptive fields in V4. They observed striking effects of attention on measures of neural synchrony, often in the absence of changes in firing rate, during the stimulus period and, importantly, during the delay period preceding the attended stimulus. Spike-triggered averages, which show oscillatory synchronization between spikes and the LFP recorded from different electrodes, revealed that attention reduced low-frequency (<17 Hz) power by about half during the delay period, without a significant change in overall spike rate. During the stimulus period, this low-frequency synchronization continued to be suppressed and gamma frequency synchronization was enhanced. The authors also calculated spike-field coherence to quantify synchronization between spikes and LFP oscillations as a function of frequency. While the spike-triggered averages did not show gamma frequency modulations of the LFP during the delay period, gamma-band spike-field coherence increased by about 10% during this period. During the stimulus period, low-frequency spike-field coherence was reduced but gamma-band coherence increased. A more recent study (Fries, Womelsdorf, Oostenveld, & Desimone, 2008) found similar results and also observed reduced alpha-band synchronization when attention was directed within the receptive of recorded neurons during the prestimulus period, consistent with the human electrophysiology findings described above. It is unclear why firing rate changes with spatial attention were not observed during the delay period in this study, as they had been observed in similar studies previously (e.g. Luck et al., 1997; Reynolds et al., 1999), but the results indicate that spatial attention might bias visual processing via changes in synchrony, and these can be seen in the prestimulus period.

Bichot, Rossi, and Desimone (2005) observed analogous synchrony changes during a visual search task involving feature-based attention. They examined the responses of V4 neurons and LFPs while monkeys searched displays for a target defined by color, shape, or both. While the animals were searching but had not yet identified a target, neurons showed greater spike activity and greater synchrony in the gamma range whenever a preferred stimulus in their receptive field matched a feature of the target. Measuring human EEG, Muller and Keil (2004) demonstrated larger gamma-band activity in response to stimuli with an attended color. Feature attention thus modulates stimulus-driven gamma synchrony, but what about prestimulus synchrony?

Tallon-Baudry, Bertrand, Henaff, Isnard, and Fischer (2005) recorded gamma oscillations from intracranial electrodes in epilepsy patients in a shape delayed match-to-sample task. In the expectation period before presentation of the sample stimuli, they observed greater gamma oscillations from lateral occipital (LO) cortex, but not fusiform gyrus, in blocks of trials when patients were performing the match task than in blocks where they were performing an unrelated task in which the first stimulus was irrelevant. Surprisingly, the subsequent stimulus-induced gamma activity was *lower* in LO when the stimuli were attended, though it was higher in fusiform gyrus. The results suggest a complex relationship between gamma power and attention that seems to vary by cortical region. Similarly, de Oliveira, Thiele, and Hoffmann (1997) recorded simultaneously from multiple neurons, primarily in MT and MST, while monkeys performed a direction discrimination task. They found that neurons tended to fire synchronously during the expectation period before stimulus presentation, though they observed reductions in synchrony at stimulus onset that scaled with the contrast of the stimuli. However, the temporal correlation did not vary systematically with stimulus direction and therefore did not appear to carry information about the physical stimulus properties.

The findings by Tallon-Baudry et al. and de Oliveria et al. demonstrate synchrony effects of attentive expectation preceding visual stimulation, and other studies have shown that increased synchrony predicts response times and accuracy (Gonzalez Andino et al., 2005; Kaiser, Hertrich, Ackermann, & Lutzenberger, 2006; Linkenkaer-Hansen et al., 2004). However, these studies did not manipulate the visual feature subjects attended and could have reflected nonselective preparatory mechanisms. So while they suggest a role for synchrony in attentive preparation generally, it remains unclear whether these effects can be feature-specific. If preparatory feature-specific attention does influence neural synchrony, however, it might be possible for these changes to bias stimulus processing without revealing themselves in measures that reflect mainly firing rate or postsynaptic activity, and this might account for some of the disparities in the results of such studies.

This might help explain the results of Shibata et al. (2008). They used both magnetoencephalogram (MEG) and fMRI to measure brain responses as subjects were cued to attend to either color or motion. They did not report changes in baseline activity in sensory areas in their fMRI data. However, when they used the MEG data to estimate cortical currents in color- and motion-sensitive areas, localized in individual subjects using fMRI, they observed small feature-specific preparatory attention effects. The effects were transient, rather than sustained, and the time of maximal difference between feature cue conditions varied widely between subjects. These current source estimates would likely be more sensitive to increased synchrony than hemodynamic measures, possibly permitting the detection of smaller effects not visible in the BOLD response.

CONCLUSIONS

Do baseline shifts themselves bias sensory processing? For visual spatial attention, the correspondence between retinotopically specific baseline shifts and subsequent target modulation is quite consistent and in line with a causal role in biasing responses to visual stimuli at the attended locations. However, for preparatory attention to visual features other than location, the answer may depend on the size of the population of neurons one is measuring and possibly whether one considers a change in neural synchrony a baseline shift. Several authors have based their presumption of a causal role for attention-related baseline shifts in sensory modulation, at least in part, on data pooled across rather large functionally or retinotopically defined visual cortical regions observed using fMRI (e.g., Driver & Frith, 2000; Kastner & Ungerleider, 2000). However, at this level of analysis the evidence for baseline shifts affecting stimulus-evoked responses is rather weak, with several well-controlled studies failing to find feature-specific baseline shifts or finding that they do not predict subsequent modulations of sensory processing. But by narrowing the analysis to smaller numbers of neurons or to the pattern of activity within a visual area (and hence reflecting activity in smaller neural ensembles), the evidence becomes more supportive of a general causal role for baseline shifts in biasing sensory processing, especially if one also includes the patterns of delay-period activity in recent functional imaging studies of WM as evidence. Nonetheless, there are discrepancies to be accounted for, particularly among single unit studies of feature-based preparatory attention, though there are, unfortunately, rather few of these. More work is clearly needed to sort out the issue.

But why are location-specific baseline shifts so robust but their feature-specific counterparts so demure? After all, single unit studies suggest that attention to locations and features influences neural responses in similar ways and can do so simultaneously even in the same cells, and with additive effects (e.g., Cohen & Maunsell, 2011), and analogous results have been reported in humans (Saenz, Buracas, & Boynton, 2003). At least for functional neuroimaging and human electrophysiology, the answer may again come down to the spatial resolution of the measurements. Spatial attention appears to increase the gain of all neurons whose receptive fields lie within the attended location. If this boost in gain is preceded by a change in baseline activity of those neurons, then this would be easily discernable within the resolution of standard functional imaging techniques. However, as already discussed, feature attention appears to increase the gain primarily of the neurons that code the attended feature, and it does so globally, across retinotopic regions (Martinez-Trujillo & Treue, 2004; Saenz et al., 2003), and neurons tuned for different features are spatially intermingled. If this feature-specific effect is preceded by a baseline shift (not a settled point), then it would be far more difficult to detect when measuring activity pooled across a large population of cells.

One final point: Even if the proper spatial resolution and means of measurement are achieved such that a consistent relationship between attention-related baseline activity and subsequent sensory modulation can be reliably demonstrated, this would still not entirely settle the matter because causation cannot be inferred from correlation. Attention-related baseline shifts that are perfectly predictive of subsequent sensory modulation could nonetheless be merely a byproduct of—or a reliable epiphenomenon associated with—the mechanism or mechanisms actually mediating the modulation. That is, top-down signals may influence both prestimulus and stimulus-evoked responses in relevant neurons without the former substantially affecting the latter. Establishing a causal role for baseline shifts may require directly manipulating prestimulus activity in the same manner as top-down control signals and then observing a corresponding effect on evoked neural responses and behavior that mirrors those produced by selective attention.

Acknowledgments

Supported by grant MH055714 to G.R.M. and a National Science Foundation Graduate Fellowship to S.P.F.

References

Aine, C. J., Supek, S., George, J. S., Ranken, D., Lewine, J., Sanders, J., et al. (1996). Retinotopic organization of human visual cortex: departures from the classical model. *Cerebral Cortex*, 6(3), 354–361.

Ball, K., & Sekuler, R. (1980). Models of stimulus uncertainty in motion perception. *Psychological Review*, 87(5), 435–469.

Bengson, J. J., & Mangun, G. R. (2011). Individual working memory capacity is uniquely correlated with feature-based attention when combined with spatial attention. *Attention, Perception, and Psychophysics*, 73(1), 86–102. http://dx.doi.org/10.3758/s13414-010-0020-7.

Bichot, N. P., Rossi, A. F., & Desimone, R. (2005). Parallel and serial neural mechanisms for visual search in macaque area V4. *Science*, 308(5721), 529–534. http://dx.doi.org/10.1126/science.1109676.

Bisley, J. W., Zaksas, D., Droll, J. A., & Pasternak, T. (2004). Activity of neurons in cortical area MT during a memory for motion task. *Journal of Neurophysiology*, 91(1), 286–300. http://dx.doi.org/10.1152/jn.00870.2003.

Borgers, C., Epstein, S., & Kopell, N. J. (2005). Background gamma rhythmicity and attention in cortical local circuits: a computational study. *Proceedings of the National Academy of Sciences of the United States of America*, 102(19), 7002–7007. http://dx.doi.org/10.1073/pnas.0502366102.

Bridwell, D. A., & Srinivasan, R. (2012). Distinct attention networks for feature enhancement and suppression in vision. *Psychological Science*, 23(10), 1151–1158. http://dx.doi.org/10.1177/0956797612440099.

Bundesen, C. (1990). A theory of visual attention. *Psychological Review*, 97(4), 523–547.

Chawla, D., Lumer, E. D., & Friston, K. J. (1999). The relationship between synchronization among neuronal populations and their mean activity levels. *Neural Computation*, 11(6), 1389–1411.

Chawla, D., Lumer, E. D., & Friston, K. J. (2000). Relating macroscopic measures of brain activity to fast, dynamic neuronal interactions. *Neural Computation*, 12(12), 2805–2821.

Chawla, D., Rees, G., & Friston, K. J. (1999). The physiological basis of attentional modulation in extrastriate visual areas. *Nature Neuroscience*, 2(7), 671–676. http://dx.doi.org/10.1038/10230.

Chelazzi, L., Duncan, J., Miller, E. K., & Desimone, R. (1998). Responses of neurons in inferior temporal cortex during memory-guided visual search. *Journal of Neurophysiology*, 80(6), 2918–2940.

Chelazzi, L., Miller, E. K., Duncan, J., & Desimone, R. (2001). Responses of neurons in macaque area V4 during memory-guided visual search. *Cerebral Corte*, 11(8), 761–772.

Cohen, M. R., & Maunsell, J. H. (2011). Using neuronal populations to study the mechanisms underlying spatial and feature attention. *Neuron*, 70(6), 1192–1204. http://dx.doi.org/10.1016/j.neuron.2011.04.029.

Corbetta, M., Miezin, F. M., Dobmeyer, S., Shulman, G. L., & Petersen, S. E. (1991). Selective and divided attention during visual discriminations of shape, color, and speed: functional anatomy by positron emission tomography. *Journal of Neuroscience*, 11(8), 2383–2402.

Cossart, R., Aronov, D., & Yuste, R. (2003). Attractor dynamics of network UP states in the neocortex. *Nature, 423*(6937), 283–288. http://dx.doi.org/10.1038/nature01614.

Curtis, C. E., & D'Esposito, M. (2003). Persistent activity in the prefrontal cortex during working memory. *Trends in Cognitive Sciences, 7*(9), 415–423.

de Oliveira, S. C., Thiele, A., & Hoffmann, K. P. (1997). Synchronization of neuronal activity during stimulus expectation in a direction discrimination task. *Journal of Neuroscience, 17*(23), 9248–9260.

Desimone, R., & Duncan, J. (1995). Neural mechanisms of selective visual attention. *Annual Review of Neuroscience, 18*, 193–222.

Driver, J., & Frith, C. (2000). Shifting baselines in attention research. *Nature Reviews Neuroscience, 1*(2), 147–148. http://dx.doi.org/10.1038/35039083.

Duncan, J., & Humphreys, G. W. (1989). Visual search and stimulus similarity. *Psychological Review, 96*(3), 433–458.

Ester, E. F., Serences, J. T., & Awh, E. (2009). Spatially global representations in human primary visual cortex during working memory maintenance. *Journal of Neuroscience, 29*(48), 15258–15265. http://dx.doi.org/10.1523/JNEUROSCI.4388-09.2009.

Fannon, S. P., & Mangun, G. R. (2008). *The effects of irrelevant pre-target stimuli on feature-specific baseline shifts in selective attention.* San Francisco, CA: Cognitive Neuroscience Society. Annual Meeting.

Fannon, S. P., Saron, C. D., & Mangun, G. R. (2007). Baseline shifts do not predict attentional modulation of target processing during feature-based visual attention. *Frontiers in Human Neuroscience, 1,* 7. http://dx.doi.org/10.3389/neuro.09.007.2007.

Ferrera, V. P., Rudolph, K. K., & Maunsell, J. H. (1994). Responses of neurons in the parietal and temporal visual pathways during a motion task. *Journal of Neuroscience, 14*(10), 6171–6186.

Fries, P., Reynolds, J. H., Rorie, A. E., & Desimone, R. (2001). Modulation of oscillatory neuronal synchronization by selective visual attention. *Science, 291*(5508), 1560–1563. http://dx.doi.org/10.1126/science.291.5508.1560.

Fries, P., Womelsdorf, T., Oostenveld, R., & Desimone, R. (2008). The effects of visual stimulation and selective visual attention on rhythmic neuronal synchronization in macaque area V4. *Journal of Neuroscience, 28*(18), 4823–4835. http://dx.doi.org/10.1523/JNEUROSCI.4499-07.2008.

Giesbrecht, B., Weissman, D. H., Woldorff, M. G., & Mangun, G. R. (2006). Pre-target activity in visual cortex predicts behavioral performance on spatial and feature attention tasks. *Brain Research, 1080*(1), 63–72. http://dx.doi.org/10.1016/j.brainres.2005.09.068.

Giesbrecht, B., Woldorff, M. G., Song, A. W., & Mangun, G. R. (2003). Neural mechanisms of top-down control during spatial and feature attention. *Neuroimage, 19*(3), 496–512.

Gonzalez Andino, S. L., Michel, C. M., Thut, G., Landis, T., & Grave de Peralta, R. (2005). Prediction of response speed by anticipatory high-frequency (gamma band) oscillations in the human brain. *Human Brain Mapping, 24*(1), 50–58. http://dx.doi.org/10.1002/hbm.20056.

Hadjikhani, N., Liu, A. K., Dale, A. M., Cavanagh, P., & Tootell, R. B. (1998). Retinotopy and color sensitivity in human visual cortical area V8. *Nature Neuroscience, 1*(3), 235–241.

Haenny, P. E., Maunsell, J. H., & Schiller, P. H. (1988). State dependent activity in monkey visual cortex. II. Retinal and extraretinal factors in V4. *Experimental Brain Research, 69*(2), 245–259.

Haenny, P. E., & Schiller, P. H. (1988). State dependent activity in monkey visual cortex. I. Single cell activity in V1 and V4 on visual tasks. *Experimental Brain Research, 69*(2), 225–244.

Harter, M. R., & Anllo-Vento, L. (1991). Visual-spatial attention: preparation and selection in children and adults. *Electroencephalogr Clin Neurophysiol Suppl. 42*, 183–194.

Harrison, S. A., & Tong, F. (2009) Decoding reveals the contents of visual working memory in early visual areas. *Nature. 458*, 632–635.

Harter, M. R., Anllo-Vento, L., & Wood, F. B. (1989). Event-related potentials, spatial orienting, and reading disabilities. *Psychophysiology, 26*(4), 404–421.

Haxby, J. V., Gobbini, M. I., Furey, M. L., Ishai, A., Schouten, J. L., & Pietrini, P. (2001). Distributed and overlapping representations of faces and objects in ventral temporal cortex. *Science, 293*(5539), 2425–2430. http://dx.doi.org/10.1126/science.1063736.

Heinze, H. J., Mangun, G. R., Burchert, W., Hinrichs, H., Scholz, M., Munte, T. F., et al. (1994). Combined spatial and temporal imaging of brain activity during visual selective attention in humans. *Nature, 372*(6506), 543–546. http://dx.doi.org/10.1038/372543a0.

Hillyard, S. A., & Munte, T. F. (1984). Selective attention to color and location: an analysis with event-related brain potentials. *Perception, & Psychophysics, 36*(2), 185–198.

Hopfinger, J. B., Buonocore, M. H., & Mangun, G. R. (2000). The neural mechanisms of top-down attentional control. *Nature Neuroscience, 3*(3), 284–291.

Hopf, J. M., & Mangun, G. R. (2000). Shifting visual attention in space: an electrophysiological analysis using high spatial resolution mapping. *Clinical Neurophysiology, 111*(7), 1241–1257.

Humphreys, G. W. (1981). Flexibility of attention between stimulus dimensions. *Perception, & Psychophysics, 30*(3), 291–302.

Kaiser, J., Hertrich, I., Ackermann, H., & Lutzenberger, W. (2006). Gamma-band activity over early sensory areas predicts detection of changes in audiovisual speech stimuli. *Neuroimage, 30*(4), 1376–1382. http://dx.doi.org/10.1016/j.neuroimage.2005.10.042.

Kamitani, Y., & Tong, F. (2005). Decoding the visual and subjective contents of the human brain. *Nature Neuroscience, 8*(5), 679–685. http://dx.doi.org/10.1038/nn1444.

Kamitani, Y., & Tong, F. (2006). Decoding seen and attended motion directions from activity in the human visual cortex. *Current Biology, 16*(11), 1096–1102. http://dx.doi.org/10.1016/j.cub.2006.04.003.

Kastner, S., Pinsk, M. A., De Weerd, P., Desimone, R., & Ungerleider, L. G. (1999). Increased activity in human visual cortex during directed attention in the absence of visual stimulation. *Neuron, 22*(4), 751–761.

Kastner, S., & Ungerleider, L. G. (2000). Mechanisms of visual attention in the human cortex. *Annual Review of Neuroscience, 23*, 315–341. http://dx.doi.org/10.1146/annurev.neuro.23.1.315.

Kelly, S. P., Lalor, E. C., Reilly, R. B., & Foxe, J. J. (2006). Increases in alpha oscillatory power reflect an active retinotopic mechanism for distractor suppression during sustained visuospatial attention. *Journal of Neurophysiology, 95*(6), 3844–3851. http://dx.doi.org/10.1152/jn.01234.2005.

Kingstone, A. (1992). Combining Expectancies. *Quarterly Journal of Experimental Psychology Section A. Human Experimental Psychology, 44*(1), 69–104.

Linkenkaer-Hansen, K., Nikulin, V. V., Palva, S., Ilmoniemi, R. J., & Palva, J. M. (2004). Prestimulus oscillations enhance psychophysical performance in humans. *Journal of Neuroscience, 24*(45), 10186–10190. http://dx.doi.org/10.1523/JNEUROSCI.2584-04.2004.

Luck, S. J., Chelazzi, L., Hillyard, S. A., & Desimone, R. (1997). Neural mechanisms of spatial selective attention in areas V1, V2, and V4 of macaque visual cortex. *Journal of Neurophysiology, 77*(1), 24–42.

Luks, T. L., & Simpson, G. V. (2004). Preparatory deployment of attention to motion activates higher-order motion-processing brain regions. *Neuroimage, 22*(4), 1515–1522. http://dx.doi.org/10.1016/j.neuroimage.2004.04.008.

Martinez-Trujillo, J. C., & Treue, S. (2004). Feature-based attention increases the selectivity of population responses in primate visual cortex. *Current Biology, 14*(9), 744–751.

McMains, S. A., Fehd, H. M., Emmanouil, T. A., & Kastner, S. (2007). Mechanisms of feature- and space-based attention: response modulation and baseline increases. *Journal of Neurophysiology, 98*(4), 2110–2121. http://dx.doi.org/10.1152/jn.00538.2007.

Moran, J., & Desimone, R. (1985). Selective attention gates visual processing in the extrastriate cortex. *Science, 229*(4715), 782–784.

Motter, B. C. (1994). Neural correlates of attentive selection for color or luminance in extrastriate area V4. *Journal of Neuroscience, 14*(4), 2178–2189.

Muller, M. M., & Keil, A. (2004). Neuronal synchronization and selective color processing in the human brain. *Journal of Cognitive Neuroscience, 16*(3), 503–522. http://dx.doi.org/10.1162/089892904322926827.

Ollinger, J. M., Corbetta, M., & Shulman, G. L. (2001). Separating processes within a trial in event-related functional MRI. *Neuroimage, 13*(1), 218–229.

Ollinger, J. M., Shulman, G. L., & Corbetta, M. (2001). Separating processes within a trial in event-related functional MRI. *Neuroimage, 13*(1), 210–217.

Posner, M. I. (1980). Orienting of attention. *Quarterly Journal of Experimental Psychology, 32*(1), 3–25.

Posner, M. I., & Snyder, C. R. R. (1975). Facilitation and inhibition in the processing of signals. In P. M. A. Rabbitt & S. Dornic (Eds.), *Attention and performance* (pp. 669–682). New York: Academic Press.

Ress, D., Backus, B. T., & Heeger, D. J. (2000). Activity in primary visual cortex predicts performance in a visual detection task. *Nature Neuroscience, 3*(9), 940–945.

Reynolds, J. H., Chelazzi, L., & Desimone, R. (1999). Competitive mechanisms subserve attention in macaque areas V2 and V4. *Journal of Neuroscience, 19*(5), 1736–1753.

Reynolds, J. H., & Heeger, D. J. (2009). The normalization model of attention. *Neuron, 61*(2), 168–185. http://dx.doi.org/10.1016/j.neuron.2009.01.002.

Saenz, M., Buracas, G. T., & Boynton, G. M. (2003). Global feature-based attention for motion and color. *Vision Research, 43*(6), 629–637.

Sauseng, P., Klimesch, W., Stadler, W., Schabus, M., Doppelmayr, M., Hanslmayr, S., et al. (2005). A shift of visual spatial attention is selectively associated with human EEG alpha activity. *European Journal of Neuroscience, 22*(11), 2917–2926. http://dx.doi.org/10.1111/j.1460-9568.2005.04482.x.

Schoenfeld, M. A., Hopf, J. M., Martinez, A., Mai, H. M., Sattler, C., Gasde, A., et al. (2007). Spatio-temporal analysis of feature-based attention. *Cerebral Cortex, 17*(10), 2468–2477. http://dx.doi.org/10.1093/cercor/bhl154.

Serences, J. T., & Boynton, G. M. (2007). Feature-based attentional modulations in the absence of direct visual stimulation. *Neuron, 55*(2), 301–312. http://dx.doi.org/10.1016/j.neuron.2007.06.015.

Serences, J. T., Ester, E. F., Vogel, E. K. & Awh, E. (2009). Stimulus-Specific Delay Activity in Human Primary Visual Cortex. *Psychological Science, 20*(2), 207–214.

Shibata, K., Yamagishi, N., Goda, N., Yoshioka, T., Yamashita, O., Sato, M. A., et al. (2008). The effects of feature attention on prestimulus cortical activity in the human visual system. *Cerebral Cortex, 18*(7), 1664–1675. http://dx.doi.org/10.1093/cercor/bhm194.

Shulman, G. L., d'Avossa, G., Tansy, A. P., & Corbetta, M. (2002). Two attentional processes in the parietal lobe. *Cerebral Cortex, 12*(11), 1124–1131.

Shulman, G. L., Ollinger, J. M., Akbudak, E., Conturo, T. E., Snyder, A. Z., Petersen, S. E., et al. (1999). Areas involved in encoding and applying directional expectations to moving objects. *Journal of Neuroscience, 19*(21), 9480–9496.

Spitzer, H., Desimone, R., & Moran, J. (1988). Increased attention enhances both behavioral and neuronal performance. *Science, 240*(4850), 338–340.

Stokes, M., Thompson, R., Nobre, A. C., & Duncan, J. (2009). Shape-specific preparatory activity mediates attention to targets in human visual cortex. *Proceedings of the National Academy of Sciences of the United States of America, 106*(46), 19569–19574. http://dx.doi.org/10.1073/pnas.0905306106.

Tallon-Baudry, C., Bertrand, O., Henaff, M. A., Isnard, J., & Fischer, C. (2005). Attention modulates gamma-band oscillations differently in the human lateral occipital cortex and fusiform gyrus. *Cerebral Cortex, 15*(5), 654–662. http://dx.doi.org/10.1093/cercor/bhh167.

Tamraz, J. C., & Comair, Y. G. (2000). *Atlas of regional anatomy of the brain using MRI.* New York: Springer.

Thut, G., Nietzel, A., Brandt, S. A., & Pascual-Leone, A. (2006). Alpha-band electroencephalographic activity over occipital cortex indexes visuospatial attention bias and predicts visual target detection. *Journal of Neuroscience, 26*(37), 9494–9502. http://dx.doi.org/10.1523/JNEUROSCI.0875-06.2006.

Treue, S., & Martinez Trujillo, J. C. (1999). Feature-based attention influences motion processing gain in macaque visual cortex. *Nature, 399*(6736), 575–579.

Uylings, H. B., Rajkowska, G., Sanz-Arigita, E., Amunts, K., & Zilles, K. (2005). Consequences of large interindividual variability for human brain atlases: converging macroscopical imaging and microscopical neuroanatomy. *Anatomy and Embryology, 210*(5–6), 423–431.

Woldorff, M. G., Fox, P. T., Matzke, M., Lancaster, J. L., Veeraswamy, S., Zamarripa, F., et al. (1997). Retinotopic organization of early visual spatial attention effects as revealed by PET and ERPs. *Human Brain Mapping, 5*(4), 280–286.

Woldorff, M. G., Hazlett, C. J., Fichtenholtz, H. M., Weissman, D. H., Dale, A. M., & Song, A. W. (2004). Functional parcellation of attentional control regions of the brain. *Journal of Cognitive Neuroscience, 16*(1), 149–165.

Worden, M. S., Foxe, J. J., Wang, N., & Simpson, G. V. (2000). Anticipatory biasing of visuospatial attention indexed by retinotopically specific alpha-band electroencephalography increases over occipital cortex. *Journal of Neuroscience, 20*(6), RC63.

Wylie, G. R., Javitt, D. C., & Foxe, J. J. (2006). Jumping the gun: is effective preparation contingent upon anticipatory activation in task-relevant neural circuitry? *Cerebral Cortex, 16*(3), 394–404. http://dx.doi.org/10.1093/cercor/bhi118.

Xu, Y., & Chun, M. M. (2006). Dissociable neural mechanisms supporting visual short-term memory for objects. *Nature, 440*(7080), 91–95. http://dx.doi.org/10.1038/nature04262.

Yamagishi, N., Callan, D. E., Goda, N., Anderson, S. J., Yoshida, Y., & Kawato, M. (2003). Attentional modulation of oscillatory activity in human visual cortex. *Neuroimage, 20*(1), 98–113.

Yamaguchi, S., Tsuchiya, H., & Kobayashi, S. (1994). Electroencephalographic activity associated with shifts of visuospatial attention. *Brain, 117*(Pt 3), 553–562.

Yamaguchi, S., Tsuchiya, H., & Kobayashi, S. (1995). Electrophysiologic correlates of visuo-spatial attention shift. *Electroencephalography and Clinical Neurophysiology, 94*(6), 450–461.

Zeki, S. (1990). Parallelism and functional specialization in human visual cortex. *Cold Spring Harbor Laboratory of Quantitative Biology, 55*, 651–661.

Zeki, S., & Bartels, A. (1999). The clinical and functional measurement of cortical (in)activity in the visual brain, with special reference to the two subdivisions (V4 and V4 alpha) of the human colour centre. *Philosophical Transactions of the Royal Society of London. Series B: Biological Sciences, 354*(1387), 1371–1382.

Zeki, S., Watson, J. D., Lueck, C. J., Friston, K. J., Kennard, C., & Frackowiak, R. S. (1991). A direct demonstration of functional specialization in human visual cortex. *Journal of Neuroscience, 11*(3), 641–649.

The Neural Basis of Color Binding to an Attended Object

Marla Zinni, Antígona Martínez, Steven A. Hillyard

Department of Neurosciences, University of California, San Diego, La Jolla, CA, USA

INTRODUCTION

Attention is the cognitive process that allows us to select relevant information from the multitude of signals that the sense organs send to the brain. In some situations, selection is based on the location of the event of interest, while in others a particular nonspatial feature such as color or shape may drive selection. There is increasing evidence that attention may also select entire objects as integrated perceptual units that include all of their constituent features (Scholl, 2001; Chen, 2012). While a substantial amount of research has been conducted to examine the neural mechanisms of space-based attention and a growing amount on feature-based attention, only a few studies have investigated the neural mechanisms of object-based attentional selection (for reviews see Boehler, Schoenfeld, Heinze, & Hopf, 2011; Hopf, Heinze, Schoenfeld, & Hillyard, 2009). Given the importance of object processing to our everyday perceptual experience, understanding the neural basis of object-based attention is of fundamental importance. It has been argued that objects (perceptual groups or units) may be a natural basis for selection because we perceive the world around us as being structured into objects (Vecera & Behrmann, 2001). It is this structure, either based upon grouping by Gestalt principles of visual organization (Wertheimer, 1923/1958) or based upon object familiarity that may serve as the basis for this attentional selection (Vecera & Farah, 1997).

A major unsolved question regarding the neural mechanisms of object-based attention is how the different features of an object, which may be represented in widely dispersed cortical areas, are bound together to form a unified percept. One approach to this "binding problem" comes from Duncan's (1996) "integrated-competition"

model. According to this model, directing attention to one of an object's features produces a competitive advantage for the object in the neural module encoding that feature, which then is transmitted to the modules encoding the other features of the object. The resulting activation of the entire network of specialized modules then underlies the binding of the features into an integrated perceptual object.

An important prediction of the integrated-competition model is that once one feature of an object is selected, attention spreads to its other features such that processing of even behaviorally irrelevant features is facilitated (Duncan, 1996; Duncan, Humphreys, & Ward, 1997). In a seminal study using functional magnetic resonance imaging (fMRI), O'Craven, Downing, and Kanwisher (1999) demonstrated a spread of attention to an object's irrelevant feature, taking advantage of previous findings that specific areas of the brain are differentially activated when either face, house, or moving stimuli are attended. Their visual display consisted of superimposed face and house stimuli, one moving and one stationary, and on different runs attention was directed to either the houses, the faces, or to the moving stimulus. In each brain region studied, the blood oxygen level-dependent (BOLD) signal enhancement was greater when subjects attended to the preferred stimulus for that cortical region than when they attended to a different stimulus in the display. Importantly, however, the task-irrelevant attribute of the attended object was also selected along with the task-relevant attribute that was attended. For example, when participants attended to the object that was moving, a stronger signal was observed in the cortical face-selective region when the faces moved rather than when the houses moved. These results cannot be explained solely by space- or feature-based attentional selection and suggest that object-based attention spreads to cortical areas that process irrelevant attributes of attended objects.

While the study by O'Craven et al. (1999) provided clear evidence for attentional selection of irrelevant features, fMRI measurements do not provide adequate time resolution to determine whether this selection occurs rapidly enough to participate in the binding and perceptual integration of the object. Schoenfeld et al. (2003) investigated the timing of the spread of object-based attention to a task-irrelevant color feature by measuring event-related potentials (ERPs), event-related magnetic fields (ERFs), and the fMRI BOLD response while participants attended to overlapping multifeature objects (surfaces) formed by moving-dot arrays. Participants attended to one of two perceived surfaces formed by superimposed fields of dots moving in opposite directions. Subjects responded to target surfaces moving at a slightly faster velocity. On some trials, dots of one of the surfaces would change color as the motion began. The sensory effect of the color change was revealed by comparing brain responses on trials where the color change occurred on the unattended surface with trials where there was no color change. The effect of attention on processing the irrelevant color was revealed by comparing brain responses to color changes on the attended surface versus color changes on the unattended surface. It was found that the neural responses associated with the task-irrelevant color feature were enhanced when the color belonged to the attended surface. This enhancement occurred within 40–60 ms after the initial sensory color registration. Both the sensory color registration and the attention-related enhancement or irrelevant color processing were localized to the ventral occipital color-selective region of the fusiform gyrus. These findings provided strong evidence in favor of the integrated-competition hypothesis by showing that attending to one of an object's features (direction of movement) resulted in the rapid activation of its irrelevant feature (color) in the neural module specialized for color (Duncan, 1996; Duncan et al., 1997).

While the study of Schoenfeld et al. (2003) demonstrated that enhanced processing of an irrelevant feature occurred rapidly enough to provide a mechanism for the binding and perceptual integration of the multiple features of the attended object, it is unclear whether these effects would generalize beyond the particular features (motion, color) and the rather esoteric object (transparent moving surface) that were used. While motion is an effective cue for object segregation, many of the objects that are processed by the visual system on a daily basis are immobile and are selected on the basis of their shape or form. Accordingly, the three experiments in the present study investigated whether attention spreads to a task-irrelevant color feature of a multifeature object when

the object is defined by its geometric shape instead of its direction of motion. The stimulus displays consisted of superimposed round and rectangular shapes, and subjects attended to either the round or the rectangular shapes on a given run. On some trials, one of the shapes was irrelevantly colored red. Following the analysis techniques of Schoenfeld et al. (2003), we recorded ERPs and calculated (1) the sensory effect of the presence of color in the display and (2) the effect of attention to one shape or the other on the processing of the task-irrelevant color feature. If selection of an irrelevant feature such as color is a general mechanism of perceptual integration, we would expect to find that the processing of the color belonging to the attended shape is rapidly enhanced after the initial sensory registration of color in the V4/V8 region of ventral visual cortex.

MATERIALS AND METHODS

Subjects

Participants were right-handed adults with normal or corrected-to-normal vision and no reported color-blindness or neurological illnesses. Informed consent was obtained from all participants. Paid volunteers between the ages of 19 and 35 years of age ($M = 24.33$ years) served as participants. Thirteen participants were included in Experiment 1 (seven males), 10 participants in Experiment 2 (eight males), and 18 participants (eight males) in Experiment 3.

Stimuli and Task

Overlapping outlines of rectangles and ellipses ($4 \times 4°$ total size) were centrally presented for 161 ms durations on a cathode ray tube (CRT) monitor at an 80 cm viewing distance in a darkened, sound-attenuated and electrically shielded room. A central fixation cross was present throughout each block of stimulus presentations, in which the different overlapping shape stimuli were presented in randomized order.

The stimuli were designed such that subjects would have to attend to the overall shape of the objects and could not distinguish a target on the basis of local features such as intersections between the shapes or the sizes of the shapes (Figure 12.1). Three experiments were conducted in order to balance various aspects of the stimulus properties and further, to provide evidence for replication of the effects across these manipulations. During Experiment 1, the stimulus set consisted of 18 nontarget exemplars that were created by perpendicularly overlapping ellipses and rectangles that were small or large in size. The size of the stimuli was counterbalanced such that an exemplar could have one small and

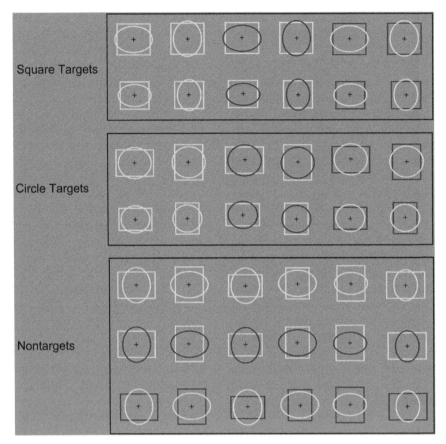

FIGURE 12.1   Stimuli presented in Experiment 1.

one large shape, two large shapes, or two small overlapping shapes. The color of the stimuli (red or gray) was also counterbalanced across trials. Specifically, during one-third of the trials, rectangle stimuli were red, one-third of trials contained red ellipse stimuli, and another third included stimuli in which both shapes were gray. All stimuli were presented on a dark gray background.

The stimuli presented during Experiments 2 and 3 were a subset of those used in Experiment 1 and consisted of only the large ellipses and circles, rectangles, and squares. Unlike Experiment 1 where ellipses and circles were always in the foreground, the foreground/background placement of ellipses and rectangles was counterbalanced in Experiments 2 and 3. In addition, in Experiment 3, the dimensions of the rectangles and ellipses were adjusted to attempt to balance the difficulty of shape discrimination between the two "attention to shape" conditions (attend ellipses or attend rectangles). When combined with the color manipulation, the stimulus sets used during Experiments 2 and 3 consisted of 10 nontarget exemplars, 10 circle target exemplars, and 10 square target exemplars. The percentage of the time each stimulus combination was presented was the same as in Experiment 1 as shown in Table 12.1.

Due to the increased difficulty in discriminating the stimuli, which occurred after adjusting the dimensions

TABLE 12.1   The Frequency With Which Each Stimulus Combination was Presented is Given in Percentages

Stimulus combination	Nontargets	Ellipse target (circle)	Rectangle target (square)
Red ellipses Gray rectangles	26.67%	3.33%	3.33%
Red rectangles Gray ellipses	26.67%	3.33%	3.33%
Gray ellipses Gray rectangles	26.67%	3.33%	3.33%

of the ellipse and rectangle stimuli, the inter-stimulus interval for the third experiment was changed to decrease the pace of the task. As such, inter-stimulus intervals were randomly jittered (between 400–600 ms for Experiments 1 and 2, and between 600–800 ms during Experiment 3).

In all cases, target stimuli consisted of a circle (when ellipses were attended) or square (when rectangles were attended). Circle and square targets were never presented together in the same stimulus. The circle target exemplars and the square target exemplars were created by overlapping circles or squares with either small or large, vertically or horizontally oriented ellipses and rectangles. The shape stimulus combinations were presented in random order with approximately 20% of trials containing a target. Circle and square targets appeared with equal probability, but a response was only required to targets of the attended shape (10% of the trials). The percentage of the time each target stimulus combination was presented is shown in Table 12.1.

Prior to experimental participation, subjective brightness of the red and gray stimuli was equated by minimizing heterochromatic flicker in tests carried out on individual subjects (Wagner & Boynton, 1972). This test was conducted by rapidly alternating the presentation of a filled red square and a filled gray square. The luminance of the red stimulus was held constant. Participants pressed arrows on the keyboard in order to increase or decrease the brightness of the gray square by "adding more white or more black" to the gray patch. When the flicker of the stimulus was perceived to be minimal, participants were to press the Enter key on the keyboard. An average value for the grayscale intensity was established from the average of multiple trials.

At the beginning of each block of stimuli, participants were instructed to attend to either ellipses or rectangles while ignoring the other shape. They were to respond with a button press when the attended shape (ellipse or rectangle) was a target (circle or square). They were explicitly told that the color of the stimuli did not matter and to attend to the entire outline of the attended shape in order to detect the designated target shape.

An initial practice session was given to familiarize participants with the task and to minimize their production of movement related artifacts. This was followed by the experimental session. Each subject was presented with a total of 20 blocks (10 attend ellipse/circle, 10 attend rectangle/square) resulting in 2280 trials in Experiment 1 and 2400 trials in Experiments 2 and 3. The trial number difference is due to the difference in exemplar numbers between stimulus sets. The "attend to ellipse" and "attend to rectangle" block presentation was randomized.

Behavioral data analysis

A response occurring 150–1000 ms after target presentation was scored as correct, a "hit". Responses following nontarget stimuli were scored as false alarms. Hit and false alarm rates were used to calculate d', an estimate of perceptual sensitivity (MacMillan & Creelman, 1991). Mean response times (RT) were calculated for correct trials. For each experiment, sensitivity estimates and response times were entered into two separate 2×3 Analysis of Variance (ANOVA) statistical tests with the factors of attended shape (ellipse or rectangle) and stimulus configuration ("attended red", "unattended red", and "both gray").

Electrophysiological recording and data analysis

The electroencephalogram (EEG) was recorded from 64 scalp electrode sites using a modified 10–20 system montage (Di Russo, Martinez, & Hillyard, 2003). Standard 10–20 sites were FP1, FP2, FZ, F3, F4, F7, F8, CZ, C3, C4, PZ, P3, P4, O1, and O2. Additional electrodes were FPZ, AFZ, AF3, AF4, FCZ, FC1, FC2, FC3, FC4, FC5, FC6, T7, T8, C1, C2, C5, C6, CPZ, CP1, CP2, CP3, CP4, CP5, CP6, P1, P2, TP7, TP8, POZ, PO3, PO4, P5, P6, P7, P8, PO7, PO8, OZ, IZ, I3, I4, I5, I6, SIZ, SI3, SI4, M1, and M2. Eye blinks and movements were monitored by placing electrodes at the right and left external canthi and below the left eye to record horizontal and vertical electro-oculograms (EOGs). Electrodes were referenced to the right mastoid electrode (M1) during recording and were later re-referenced to average of the M1 and M2 electrodes for analysis. Electrode impedances were lowered to 5 kΩ prior to recording. The EEG was digitized at 250 Hz with a gain of 10,000 and was filtered with a bandpass of 0.1–80 Hz. Prior to signal averaging, automated artifact rejection was performed to reject trials containing eye movements, blinks, or amplifier blocking. Two criteria were used to avoid contamination by motor potentials. These were to discard nontarget trials where either (1) the subject produced a false alarm (i.e., subjects pressed the button during a nontarget trial) or (2) when there was a button-press response in the previous trial. For each subject and condition, ERP averages were time-locked to the onset of the overlapping shape stimuli. Prior to data analysis, the averages were digitally low-pass filtered at 25 Hz with a Gaussian finite impulse function to remove high frequency noise and were baseline corrected using the mean amplitude of a 100 ms prestimulus baseline. For all analyses, ERPs to nontarget stimuli of each type were pooled to create grand-average waveforms.

The six experimental conditions that were analyzed are illustrated in Figure 12.2. These six experimental conditions were combined into: (1) "attended red", (2) "unattended red", and (3) "both gray" collapsing over conditions of attention to ellipses and rectangles. ERPs recorded under the various conditions were combined and subtracted to create specific comparisons of interest.

To assess the "sensory effect" of the presence of color, difference waves were calculated by subtracting ERPs elicited by stimuli in which both shapes were gray from ERPs elicited when the unattended shape was colored red (Figure 12.2: ERPs to unattended red (average of 3 and 4) minus ERPs to both gray (average of 5 and 6)). To examine the main effect of interest, "the effect of attention on task-irrelevant color processing", a difference wave was created by subtracting ERPs to "unattended red" stimuli from "attended red" stimuli (Figure 12.2: ERPs to attended red (average of 1 and 2) minus ERPs to unattended red (average of 3 and 4)). Importantly, this comparison was calculated using exactly the same stimuli under different attention conditions. As such, any differences between the two conditions could only be related to the effects of attention and not to physical stimulus differences. Because the analysis was

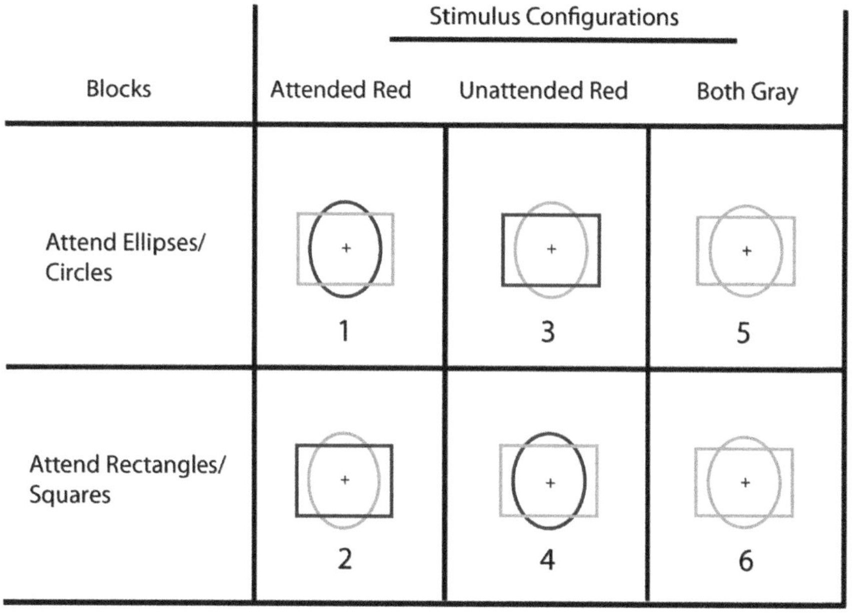

FIGURE 12.2   The six experimental conditions defined by the combination of the stimulus configuration (nontargets only) and the shape attended. Event-related brain potential difference waves were calculated as follows: sensory effect of color = ERPs to unattended red (average of 3 and 4) minus ERPs to both gray (average of 5 and 6); effect of attention on irrelevant color processing = ERPs to attended red (average of 1 and 2) minus ERPs to unattended red (average of 3 and 4).

aimed at investigating whether the task-irrelevant color feature was selected in general, regardless of whether the attended shape is an ellipse or rectangle, ERPs were averaged over the attention to shape variable in this analysis.

For all analyses, difference wave components were quantified as mean amplitudes within specific latency windows around the peak of each identified component. Each effect was measured as the mean voltage over a specific cluster of electrodes at which the component amplitude was maximal. The time window and specific clusters used are listed in the tables given for each experimental ERP effect. All analyses were performed using repeated measures ANOVA and Tukey HSD post-hoc testing unless otherwise indicated.

Source analysis

To estimate the cortical generators of the sensory and attention effects, source localization analyses were performed on the grand-averaged difference waves within the same intervals used for statistical testing. Current density distributions were estimated using a local autoregressive average (LAURA) algorithm (Grave de Peralta Menendez, Gonzalez Andino, Lantz, Michel, & Landis, 2001). LAURA uses a realistic head model with a solution space of 4024 nodes evenly distributed within the gray matter of the Montreal Neurological Institute (MNI) average template brain. It makes no a priori assumptions regarding the number of sources or their locations and can deal with multiple simultaneous active sources

(Michel et al., 2001). LAURA analyses were implemented using the Cartool software (http://brainmapping.unige.ch/cartool). The Talairach coordinates of the current source maxima given by the LAURA algorithm were entered into the Talairach Client (Lancaster et al., 2000) to determine the brain region of the estimated maximal sources. Maps illustrating both the sensory and attention effects and their overlap were created using the AFNI software (Cox, 1996) and were projected onto a structural brain image supplied by MRIcro (Rorden & Brett, 2000).

BEHAVIORAL RESULTS

During Experiment 1, participants were more accurate at discriminating changes in the shape of the ellipses than the rectangles (Mean d' = 3.05 ellipses, Mean d' = 2.26 rectangles) ($F(1, 12)$ = 12.87, $p < 0.01$). Participants were also faster when detecting ellipse targets (circles) than rectangle targets (squares) (Mean RT = 580 ms circles, Mean RT = 613 ms squares) ($F(1, 12)$ = 6.26, $p < 0.05$). The configuration of the stimuli (red attended, red unattended, both gray) did not have significant effects on sensitivity or response time (sensitivity, $F(2, 24)$ = 2.31, $p = 0.12$; response time, $F(2, 24)$ = 0.60, $p = 0.55$). The interaction between attended shape and configuration of the stimuli was not significant for any of the dependent measures (sensitivity, $F(2, 24)$ = 2.17, $p = 0.14$; response time, $F(2, 24)$ = 1.55, $p = 0.23$).

During Experiment 2, there was no significant difference in the ability to discriminate changes in the shape of the ellipses versus the rectangles (Mean d' = 3.36 ellipses, Mean d' = 2.93 rectangles) ($F(1, 9)$ = 1.11, p = 0.32). However, participants were still faster when detecting ellipse targets than rectangle targets (Mean RT = 569 ms circles, Mean RT = 604 ms squares) ($F(1, 9)$ = 12.00, p < 0.01). The configuration of the stimuli (red attended, red unattended, both gray) did not have significant effects on sensitivity or response time (sensitivity, $F(2, 18)$ = 0.39, p = 0.68; response time, $F(2, 18)$ = 1.11, p = 0.35). The interaction between attended shape and configuration of the stimuli was not significant for any of the dependent measures (sensitivity, $F(2, 18)$ = 1.23, p = 0.32; response time, $F(2, 18)$ = 0.21, p = 0.81).

Performance on the task overall was lower during Experiment 3 than during previous versions of the experiment. During this experiment, participants were more accurate at discriminating changes in the shape of the rectangles than the ellipses (Mean d' = 1.96 ellipses, Mean d' = 2.76 rectangles) ($F(1, 17)$ = 13.64, p < 0.01). However, participants were again faster when detecting ellipse targets than rectangle targets (Mean RT = 569 ms ellipses, Mean RT = 581 ms rectangles) ($F(1, 17)$ = 5.73, p < 0.05). The configuration of the stimuli (attended red, unattended red, both gray) did not have significant effects on sensitivity, ($F(2, 34)$ = 2.11, p = 0.14) but did for response time ($F(2, 34)$ = 10.28, p < 0.001). Post-hoc comparisons showed a significant difference between the attended red and both gray configurations (p = 0.01) in which participants were fastest when all of the stimuli were gray. The interaction between attended shape and configuration of the stimuli was not significant for

sensitivity or response time (sensitivity, $F(2, 34)$ = 1.80, p = 0.18; response time, $F(2, 34)$ = 0.27, p = 0.77).

EVENT-RELATED BRAIN POTENTIAL RESULTS

In all experiments, the sensory-evoked ERP waveforms elicited by the shape stimuli were consistent with waveforms typically observed in other visual studies (Hopfinger, Luck, & Hillyard, 2004). In particular, the first prominent component, a laterally distributed occipital-parietal positivity (P1) from 60–140 ms, peaked at about 100 ms. The P1 component was followed by an occipital-parietal negativity (N1), from 140–190 ms, that peaked at about 160 ms, a subsequent positivity (P2) from 180–300 ms, that peaked at 230 ms, and a negativity (N2) from 300–360 ms that peaked at 325 ms.

Sensory Effect of Color

In all three experiments, the sensory effect of color was measured by subtracting the grand-averaged ERPs elicited by stimuli in which both shapes were gray from unattended red stimuli. This sensory effect was first observed as a greater negativity starting at approximately 80–90 ms poststimulus onset (Table 12.2) and was maximal at focal, posterior midline occipital sites.

This "early sensory effect" negativity was accompanied by broad frontal/central positivity during the same time frame and was followed by a negative component

TABLE 12.2 The Sensory Effect of Color

| Time window | Electrodes clustered | ANOVA of the sensory effect | | | Sensory effect | |
		Unatt-Red/Att-Gray μV (SEM)	vs	Att-Gray/Unatt-Gray μV (SEM)	F	p
Experiment 1					$F (1,12)$	
80–127 ms	OZ,IZ	−0.09(0.51)	vs	0.62(0.36)	11.24	<0.01
80–127 ms	AFZ,FZ,FCZ,CZ,CPZ	−1.40(0.37)	vs	−2.09(0.28)	8.65	<0.05
160–219 ms	OZ,IZ,POZ,PZ	−0.23(0.48)	vs	1.35(0.57)	33.11	<0.0001
Experiment 2					$F (1,9)$	
96–127 ms	OZ,IZ	1.92(0.83)	vs	2.68(0.90)	5.41	<0.05
96–127 ms	AFZ,FZ,FCZ,CZ,CPZ	−2.01(0.52)	vs	−2.76(0.50)	7.98	<0.05
160–219 ms	OZ,IZ,POZ,PZ	−0.57(0.86)	vs	0.56(0.84)	27.51	0.001
Experiment 3					$F (1,17)$	
80–127 ms	OZ,IZ	0.32(0.54)	vs	1.32(0.50)	45.38	<0.0001
80–127 ms	AFZ,FZ,FCZ,CZ,CPZ	−1.95(0.38)	vs	−2.52(0.39)	13.34	<0.01
160–219 ms	OZ,IZ,POZ,PZ	−0.58(0.59)	vs	0.55(0.61)	29.50	<0.0001

Att, attended; Unatt, unattended; SEM, standard error of the mean; vs, versus.
Mean voltage amplitude given in μV.

starting at approximately 120–130 ms (the "late sensory effect"). This medial-occipital negativity extended more laterally than the earlier sensory component. The early and late sensory effects obtained in Experiment 1 are shown in Figure 12.3(A) and (B). Very similar patterns of the "early" and "late" sensory effects were also observed in the other two experiments (Figure 12.4(A) and (B)).

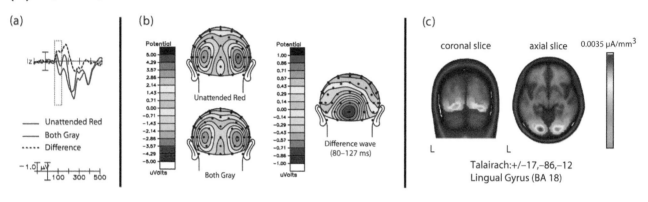

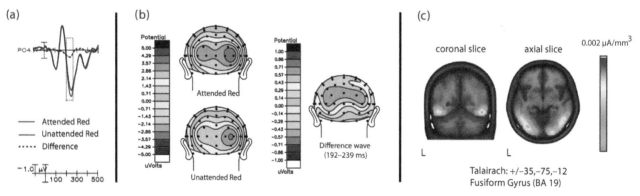

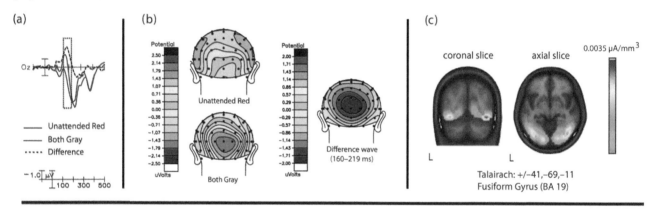

FIGURE 12.3   Data from Experiment 1. Grand-average ERPs (nontarget trials) associated with the early sensory effect are plotted for a midline occipital electrode location in the left column ((A)(a)). The ERPs elicited when red occurred on the unattended shape, when both shapes were gray, and the unattended red minus gray difference wave indexing the sensory effect are shown. ERPs associated with the late sensory effect are plotted from a midline occipital electrode location ((B)(a)). ERPs associated with the effect of attention on the processing of task-irrelevant color from a right parietal-occipital electrode location are shown in the lower left column ((C)(a)). The ERPs elicited when red occurred on the attended shape, when red occurred on the unattended shape, and the "attended red" minus "unattended red" difference wave indexing the attention effects are shown. Dotted line boxes indicate the time windows used for statistical testing. The scalp topography of the conditions and difference waves are shown for each comparison of interest (column (b)). The LAURA source activity estimates for each comparison are displayed in column c.

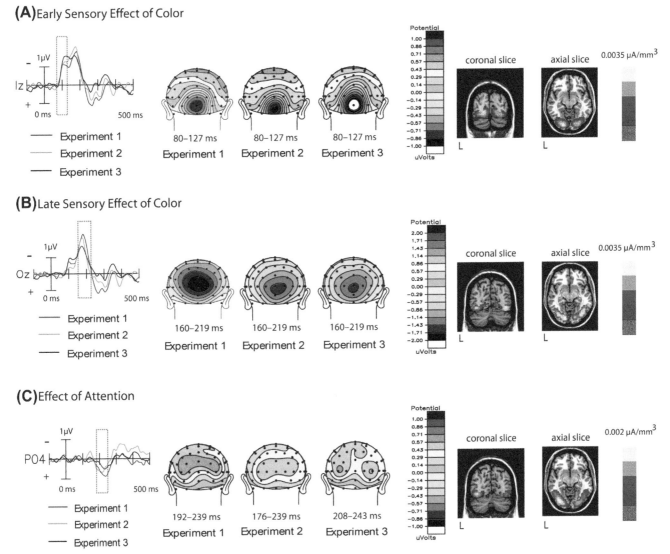

FIGURE 12.4 The ERP difference waveforms for each of the comparisons of interest and for each experiment are shown in the left column. The associated scalp topography for each effect and for each experiment is shown in the center column. The LAURA source activity estimates for each effect, collapsed across experiments, is shown in the right column.

LAURA source analyses were performed on the grand-averaged difference waveforms for the early (115 ms peak) and late sensory (175 ms peak) effects. Source estimates are presented in Table 12.3. The sensory effect of color included bilateral source estimates throughout the lingual and fusiform gyri, for both the early and late sensory effects (Figure 12.3(A) and (B), right column c).

Effect of Attention on Task-Irrelevant Color Processing

The attention effect difference wave in each experiment was isolated by subtracting ERP waveforms on trials in which the red shape was unattended and from trials in which the red shape was attended. Importantly, this comparison was calculated using the same stimuli under different attention conditions. As such, any differences between the two conditions should only be related to the effects of attention.

A significant bilateral occipital positivity was observed beginning at around 170–180 ms in all three experiments (Table 12.4, Figures 12.3(C) and 12.4(C)). In all cases, this difference is the result of a greater positive voltage when the shape containing red was attended versus when it was unattended (Figure 12.3(C)). There was no hemispheric difference in this effect in any of the studies.

LAURA source analyses were also performed on the grand-averaged difference waveforms for the attention effect (225 ms peak), for all experiments. Current source maxima for each of the experiments are given in Table 12.3. The source estimates for the effect of attention showed

TABLE 12.3   Talairach Coordinates and Corresponding Brain Regions of the Current Source Maxima as Modeled by LAURA for the Components in the Sensory and Attention Difference Waveforms

ERP component	x (mm)	y (mm)	z (mm)	Brain region
Experiment 1				
Sensory difference (80–127 ms)	±17	−86	−12	Left lingual gyrus (BA 18)
Sensory difference (160–219 ms)	±41	−69	−11	Right fusiform gyrus (BA 19)
Attention difference (192–239 ms)	±35	−75	−12	Left fusiform gyrus (BA 19)
Experiment 2				
Sensory difference (96–127 ms)	±17	−86	−12	Left lingual gyrus (BA 18)
Sensory difference (160–219 ms)	±35	−75	−12	Left fusiform gyrus (BA 19)
Attention difference (176–239 ms)	±29	−80	−12	Left fusiform gyrus (BA 19)
Experiment 3				
Sensory difference (80–127 ms)	±17	−86	−12	Left lingual gyrus (BA 18)
Sensory difference (160–219 ms)	±17	−86	−12	Left lingual gyrus (BA 18)
Attention difference (208–243 ms)	±35	−75	−12	Left fusiform gyrus (BA 19)

BA = Broadmann's Area.

a lateral occipital distribution that was maximal in the fusiform gyrus (Figure 12.3(C), right column (c)).

Common Neural Sources for the "Sensory" and "Attention" Effects

Altogether, the combined source analysis findings point to common sources in ventral occipital cortex associated with processing of the sensory and attention effects. Because the scalp topographies were similar between the late sensory and attention effects, estimated sources were examined between these two effects collapsed across all experiments (Figure 12.5). Common sources in ventral occipital cortex were observed between cortical localizations of the late sensory effect of color and the effect of shape-selective attention on irrelevant color processing.

ERPs to Target Stimuli

Attended target stimuli in all three experiments elicited a P300 wave indicating that these stimuli were processed in a manner that is consistent with previously reported results obtained in other paradigms in

which infrequent, task-relevant stimuli were presented (for a review see Polich, 2007). Both circle and square targets elicited this widely distributed component that peaked between 500 and 600 ms with a maximum voltage at central-parietal electrode sites (Figure 12.6). In all three experiments, the amplitude of the P300 difference component was larger for attended than unattended targets in both the circle target and square target trials (*circle target*: Experiment 1, $F(1, 12) = 85.23$, $p < 0.0001$; Experiment 2, $F(1, 9) = 53.78$, $p < 0.0001$; Experiment 3, $F(1, 17) = 39.28$, $p < 0.0001$) (*square target*: Experiment 1, $F(1, 12) = 31.77$, $p < 0.0001$; Experiment 2, $F(1, 9) = 35.56$, $p < 0.001$; Experiment 3, $F(1, 17) = 39.28$, $p < 0.0001$). Further, there was no significant mean amplitude difference between the circle target and square target P300 difference wave components for any of the experiments (Experiment 1, $F(1, 12) = 3.07$, $p = 0.11$; Experiment 2, $F(1,9) = 1.91, p = 0.20$; Experiment 3, $F(1, 17) = 1.96, p = 0.18$).

DISCUSSION

An important unanswered question in cognitive neuroscience concerns the mechanism by which the brain binds the multiple features of an object into a unitary, coherent percept. Object-based theories of attention posit that paying attention to one feature of an object results in selection of the entire object as a unit, including its features that are not relevant to the current task. In this study we used ERPs to define the time course of this irrelevant feature processing in a task where subjects attended to shape while color appeared at random as the irrelevant feature. The goal was to obtain information about how attention enhances feature-specific signals in their specialized modules and integrates the task-relevant and irrelevant features into a unified perceptual object.

Recent studies have used moving-dot fields to investigate the neural basis of feature binding and the question of whether attention spreads through all the features of the attended object (Schoenfeld et al., 2003) such that all of its features, both task-relevant and irrelevant, are bound together into an integrated percept. One goal of the present study was to assess whether the attention effects seen in previous studies would generalize to more ecologically valid stimuli consisting of features processed in the ventral stream that included structure, such as edges and corners. Specifically, the temporal dynamics of color binding were investigated for objects defined by geometric shape. In three separate experiments, the timing of the binding of shape and color was determined by comparing two main effects of interest: (1) The sensory effect of color; and (2) The effect of attention to shape on the processing of a task-irrelevant color. The sensory effect of color was defined as the neural activity

TABLE 12.4   The Effect of Attention on Task-Irrelevant Color Processing: Collapsed over Attended Shape

Time window	Electrodes clustered	ANOVA of the attention effect			Attention effect		Hemisphere × attention effect	
		Att-Red/Unatt-Gray μV (SEM)	vs	Att-Gray/Unatt-Red μV (SEM)	F	p	F	p
Experiment 1					$F\,(1,12)$		$F\,(1,12)$	
192–239 ms	P2,P4,P6	2.60(0.49)	vs	2.10(0.42)	6.98	<0.05	0.63	<0.44
	PO4,PO8							
	O2,P1,P3							
	P5,PO3	2.28(0.64)		1.70(0.49)				
	PO7,O1							
Experiment 2					$F(1,9)$		$F(1,9)$	
176–239 ms	P2,P4,P6	0.35(0.66)	vs	−0.09(0.77)	7.18	<0.05	0.08	<0.79
	PO4,PO8							
	O2,P1,P3	1.03(0.77)		0.62(0.90)				
	P5,PO3							
	PO7,O1							
Experiment 3					$F\,(1,17)$		$F\,(1,17)$	
208–243 ms	P2,P4,P6	2.18(0.72)	vs	1.72(0.71)	15.32	<0.01	0.32	<0.58
	PO4,PO8							
	O2,P1,P3	3.01(0.79)		2.51(0.78)				
	P5,PO3							
	PO7,O1							

Att, attended; Unatt, unattended; SEM, standard error of the mean; vs, versus.
Mean voltage amplitude given in μV.

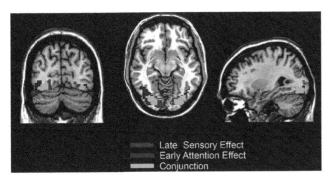

FIGURE 12.5   LAURA source estimates for the "late sensory" effect and the "attention" effect indicating the common source estimates in green.

associated with color processing driven by the physical color difference of the stimuli presented in the display. The effect of attention on the sensory effect of color, the "attention effect", was defined as the neural activity elicited when attention to shape resulted in selection of the task-irrelevant color feature.

The presence of color in the display was first evident as a negative deflection in the ERP difference wave starting at approximately 80 ms over medial-occipital electrode sites. This "early sensory effect" was localized to lateral extrastriate sources in the lingual and fusiform gyri, areas known to be involved in color processing (Clark et al., 1997; Corbetta, Miezin, Dobmeyer, Shulman, & Petersen, 1991). The early effect of color processing was followed by a late sensory effect, a medial-occipital negativity, which onset at approximately 120 ms and extended more laterally than the earlier sensory component.

The effect of attention on task-irrelevant color processing was determined by the comparison of the ERPs elicited by the presence of the color red on the attended versus the unattended shape and was observed as a positivity with an onset of approximately 170 ms. This component had estimated sources in ventral occipital cortex coinciding with the sources estimated for the sensory effects. These results suggest that attention can operate in an object-based manner, selecting not only one object over another, but also, multiple features of an attended object. These findings support the integrated-competition model (Desimone & Duncan, 1995; Duncan et al., 1997) which predicts that selection of an object

Attended and Unattended Target Trials

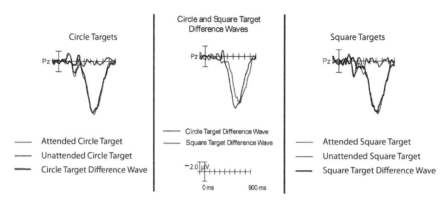

FIGURE 12.6 Grand-average ERPs for circle and square targets from Experiment 1, plotted from a midline parietal electrode location. Waveforms for attended and unattended circle targets and their difference waveforms are presented in the left column. Attended and unattended square targets and their difference waveforms are presented in the right column. Circle and square target difference waves are plotted together in the center column.

in a visual scene containing several objects occurs as a result of enhanced activity in all of the feature modules coding the properties of the selected object, both task-relevant and irrelevant. It is worth noting that in the current study, we did not have a direct behavioral measure of feature binding. While the current findings suggest that the enhancement of the response to the attended, colored object is correlated with the process of binding of the shape and color features, in future studies it would be worthwhile to measure binding more directly. Such a measure could be implemented, for example, by collecting behavioral evidence of feature binding through the use of a priming paradigm in which previous exposure to a specific feature grouping may affect response time to future presentations of that grouping.

As suggested by Schoenfeld et al. (2003), we hypothesized that the binding of the color and shape would occur at some point in time between the onset of the processing of color in the visual system (the sensory effects at 80 and 120 ms), and the attention effect (170 ms). Thus, the time required for the binding of color and shape can be estimated by subtracting the sensory effect from the attention effect. If the late sensory effect and the attention effect are compared due to their similar topographies, this subtraction provides an average estimate of 50 ms for the binding of color and shape (Figure 12.7), on par with the results of Schoenfeld and colleagues.

The current study supports the hypothesis that attention selects objects as wholes for further processing as predicted by biased competition theory (Desimone & Duncan, 1995) and in particular, its integrated-competition hypothesis (Duncan, 1996; Duncan et al., 1997). The integrated-competition hypothesis proposes that the competition between two objects for representation may be resolved by top-down goal

directed behavior (e.g., selection of one or another shape). This theory predicts that there should be widespread selection of the features of the attended object. Thus, for instance, in the current shape study, it would be predicted that once the attended shape became dominant in cortical areas where shape is processed, this facilitation would then spread to the cortical areas that process the other features of the object (e.g., color processing areas if the attended object was colored).

The predictions of the integrated-competition hypothesis are consistent with the effects found in the current study. Differential processing of the task-irrelevant color feature was indicated based upon the "attention effect" seen when color was a part of the attended object vs the unattended object. This provides evidence that the instruction to attend to one object results in the dominance of that object, and as such, these findings strongly suggest that color was also selected when it was a part of that attended object. Furthermore, this "attention effect" difference wave component was localized to occipital brain areas associated with the processing of color (i.e., the fusiform gyrus). The source estimates for this "attention effect" were similar to the source estimates for the "sensory effects" indicating that there was differential processing of color based on whether it was a part of the attended object.

Interestingly, this "attention effect" was not observed as a simple enhancement of the "sensory effects" at either 80 ms or 120 ms, and instead, was observed later in time at approximately 170 ms. While the timing of the "attention effect" provides an upper bound on the estimate of the time required to enhance the processing of the color feature with attention, it does not appear that the amplification of the processing of color with attention occurs during the early period of color processing. Rather, the source estimates suggest a model

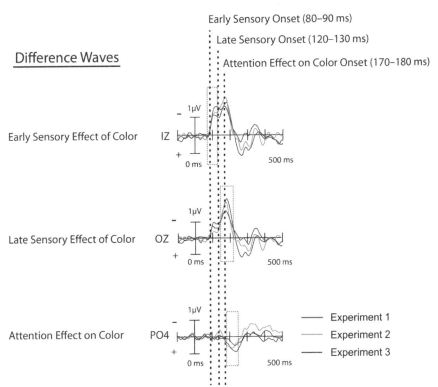

FIGURE 12.7 The ERP difference waveforms for the main comparisons of interest are plotted for each experiment. The timing of the onset of each of these comparisons of interest is indicated by the dotted vertical lines. The binding of color and shape occurred at some point in time between the onset of the processing of color in the visual system (the sensory effects, 80 and 120 ms), and the attention effect (170 ms). Thus, the time required for the binding of color and shape can be estimated by subtracting the sensory effect from the attention effect. If the late sensory effect and the attention effect are compared due to their similar topographies and source estimates, this subtraction provides an average estimate of 50 ms for the binding of color and shape.

that involves a later re-activation of the cortical areas involved in color processing.

Other theories that address feature binding, such as feature integration theory (Treisman, 1993; Treisman, 1998; Treisman & Gelade, 1980) most likely do not account for the data presented here because the objects that competed for attention had considerable overlap in spatial extent. Feature integration theory relies upon a spatial focus of attention to select one object versus another in order to allow for a binding of the features of the selected object. Thus, due to the spatial overlap of the objects, the selection of color most likely could not be based upon a linking of color and the task-relevant attended feature (shape) at a given attended location. Because the shapes were overlapping and might be considered to contain spatial differences in depth, a location-based binding mechanism that utilizes information about the plane on which a given object is presented cannot be ruled out. Such a model would suggest that competition between the two objects for "ownership" of the color feature could be resolved by selecting one plane over another, thus binding the shape and color features through co-location in three-dimensional space.

While this study provides additional evidence for integrated competition, it does not directly address the

neural mechanisms by which selective activation spreads from one cortical area to another. It may be the case that top-down attentional goal signals derived from the frontal and parietal cortices specifically lead to enhancement of the features of the objects (see Yantis & Serences, 2003 for a review). In this model, "a top-down signal that originates in the prefrontal cortex and reflects current behavioral goals arrives at the superior parietal lobule, which responds by transiently increasing its activity. The transient switch signal is received both by extrastriate neural populations and by the intraparietal sulcus and perhaps other structures, which then continuously maintain the new attentive state by providing a constant biasing signal to extrastriate cortical regions" (Yantis & Serences, 2003). An extended alternative that addresses the mechanism more specifically could be the "binding-by-synchrony" hypothesis, which proposes that synchronous oscillations in the gamma range (30–60 Hz) allow for the perceptual binding of various features or segments of an object to occur by synchronizing activity in separate neural populations (Gray & Singer, 1989). This hypothesis provides a temporal means of binding all of the features of an object. In the case of our two overlapping shape objects, such a model may suggest that attention to one object over another would trigger synchrony in the neural populations that code for all the features of the attended object. Further research is critical for advancing and supporting a better understanding of these proposed mechanisms.

CONCLUSIONS

The reported findings suggest that attention can occur in an object-based manner, spreading to all features of the selected object. Furthermore, the effect of attention on a task-irrelevant color feature can be generalized to different objects and is associated with an ERP component that occurs later in time than the initial sensory registration of color. When attending to stimulus shape, the binding of a task-irrelevant color feature takes approximately 50 ms to occur after the sensory registration of color in the display. The source of the selection of the task-irrelevant features of an object occurs in similar cortical regions to those associated with the processing of that feature. This provides evidence of biased competition in favor of all features of the attended object across cortical areas.

Acknowledgments

The authors thank Ricardo Gil da Costa and Raja Parasuraman for valuable comments and discussion and Matthew M. Marlow for technical assistance. The Cartool software was programmed by D. Brunet, and supported by the Center for Biomedical Imaging of Geneva and Lausanne. Portions of this work were submitted in partial fulfillment of the requirements for the doctoral degree of the first author. This work was supported by the National Institute of Mental Health Grant P50MH86385 and the National Science Foundation Grant BCS-1029084.

References

Boehler, C. N., Schoenfeld, M. A., Heinze, H. J., & Hopf, J. M. (2011). Object-based selection of irrelevant features in not confined to the attended object. *Journal of Cognitive Neuroscience, 23*(9), 2231–2239.

Chen, Z. (2012). Object-based attention: a tutorial review. *Attention, Perception, and Psychophysics, 74*, 784–802.

Clark, V. P., Parasuraman, R., Keil, K., Kulansky, R., Fannon, S., Maisog, J. M., et al. (1997). Selective attention to face identity and color studied with fMRI. *Human Brain Mapping, 5*(4), 293–297.

Corbetta, M., Miezin, F. M., Dobmeyer, S., Shulman, G. L., & Petersen, S. E. (1991). Selective and divided attention during visual discriminations of shape, color, and speed: functional anatomy by positron emission tomography. *Journal of Neuroscience, 11*(8), 2383–2402.

Cox, R. W. (1996). AFNI: software for analysis and visualization of functional magnetic resonance neuroimages. *Computers and Biomedical Research, 29*(3), 162–173.

Desimone, R., & Duncan, J. (1995). Neural mechanisms of selective visual attention. *Annual Review of Neuroscience, 18*, 193–222.

Di Russo, F., Martinez, A., & Hillyard, S. A. (2003). Source analysis of event-related cortical activity during visuo-spatial attention. *Cerebral Cortex, 13*(5), 486–499.

Duncan, J. (1996). Cooperating brain systems in selective perception and action. In T. Inui & J. L. McClelland (Eds.), *Attention and performance XVI* (pp. 549–578). Cambridge, MA: MIT Press.

Duncan, J., Humphreys, G., & Ward, R. (1997). Competitive brain activity in visual attention. *Current Opinion in Neurobiology, 7*(2), 255–261.

Grave de Peralta Menendez, R., Gonzalez Andino, S., Lantz, G., Michel, C. M., & Landis, T. (2001). Noninvasive localization of electromagnetic epileptic activity. I. Method descriptions and simulations. *Brain Topography, 14*(2), 131–137.

Gray, C. M., & Singer, W. (1989). Stimulus-specific neuronal oscillations in orientation columns of cat visual cortex. *Proceedings of the National Academy of Sciences of the United States of America, 86*(5), 1698–1702.

Hopf, J. M., Heinze, H. J., Schoenfeld, M. A., & Hillyard, S. A. (2009). Spatiotemporal analysis of visual attention. In M. S. Gazzaniga (Ed.), *The cognitive neurosciences* (4th ed. pp. 235–250). Cambridge, MA: MIT Press.

Hopfinger, J. B., Luck, S. J., & Hillyard, S. A. (2004). Selective attention: electrophysiological and neuromagnetic studies. In M. S. Gazzaniga (Ed.), *The cognitive neurosciences* (3rd ed. pp. 561–574). Cambridge, MA: MIT Press.

Lancaster, J. L., Woldorff, M. G., Parsons, L. M., Liotti, M., Freitas, C. S., Rainey, L., et al. (2000). Automated Talairach atlas labels for functional brain mapping. *Human Brain Mapping, 10*(3), 120–131.

MacMillan, N. A., & Creelman, C. D. (1991). *Detection theory: A user's guide*. New York: Cambridge University Press.

Michel, C. M., Thut, G., Morand, S., Khateb, A., Pegna, A. J., Grave de Peralta, R., et al. (2001). Electric source imaging of human brain functions. *Brain Research Reviews, 36*(2–3), 108–118.

O'Craven, K. M., Downing, P. E., & Kanwisher, N. (1999). fMRI evidence for objects as the units of attentional selection. *Nature, 401*, 584–587.

Polich, J. (2007). Updating P300: an integrative theory of P3a and P3b. *Clinical Neurophysiology, 18*, 2128–2148.

Rorden, C., & Brett, M. (2000). Stereotaxic display of brain lesions. *Behavioral Neurology, 12*, 191–200.

Schoenfeld, M. A., Tempelmann, C., Martinez, A., Hopf, J. M., Sattler, C., Heinze, H. J., et al. (2003). Dynamics of feature binding during object-selective attention. *Proceedings of the National Academy of Sciences of the United States of America, 100*, 11806–11811.

Scholl, B. J. (2001). Objects and attention: the state of the art. *Cognition, 80*, 1–46.

Treisman, A. (1993). Representing visual objects. In D. Meyer & S. Kornblum (Eds.), *Attention and performance XIV* (pp. 163–175). Cambridge, MA: MIT Press.

Treisman, A. (1998). Feature binding, attention and object perception. *Philosophical Transactions of the Royal Society of London: Series B, Biological Sciences, 353*, 1295–1306.

Treisman, A., & Gelade, G. (1980). A feature-integration theory of attention. *Cognitive Psychology, 12*(1), 97–136.

Vecera, S. P., & Behrmann, M. (2001). Attention and unit formation: a biased competition account of object based attention. In T. F. Shipley & P. J. Kellman (Eds.), *From fragments to objects – segmentation and grouping in vision* (pp. 145–180). New York: Elsevier.

Vecera, S. P., & Farah, M. J. (1997). Is visual image segmentation a bottom-up or an interactive process? *Perception and Psychophysics, 59*, 1280–1296.

Wagner, G., & Boynton, R. (1972). Comparison of four methods of heterochromatic photometry. *Journal of the Optical Society of America, 62*(12), 1508–1515.

Wertheimer, M. (1923/1958). Principles of perceptual organization. In D. C. Beardslee & M. Wertheimer (Eds.), *Readings in perception* (pp. 115–135). Princeton, NJ: Van Nostrand. Original work published in 1923.

Yantis, S., & Serences, J. T. (2003). Cortical mechanisms of space-based and object-based attentional control. *Current Opinion in Neurobiology, 13*(2), 187–193.

Switching Attention between the Local and Global Levels in Visual Objects

Mitchell Valdes-Sosa[1], Jorge Iglesias[1], Rosario Torres[2], Nelson Trujillo-Barreto[3]

[1]Cognitive Neurosciences Department, Cuban Center for Neuroscience, Havana, Cuba, [2]Neurodevelopment Department, Cuban Center for Neuroscience, Havana, Cuba, [3]Neuroinformatics Department, Cuban Center for Neuroscience, Havana, Cuba

INTRODUCTION

Steve Hillyard's pioneering work on the neural basis of selective attention helped establish the nascent field of cognitive neuroscience. The experimental strategies that he and his colleagues introduced for event related potential (ERP) research on selective attention continue to shed light on the inner workings of the mind. These strategies have been used to study attentional selection in auditory (Hillyard, Hink, Schwent, & Picton, 1973; Hillyard, Squires, Bauer, & Lindsay, 1971; Hink & Hillyard, 1976; Picton, Hillyard, Galambos, & Schiff, 1971; Schwent & Hillyard, 1975), somatosensory (Desmedt, Huy, & Bourguet, 1983; Desmedt & Robertson, 1977; Michie, Bearparic, Crawford, & Glue, 1987), and visual space (Anllo-Vento & Hillyard, 1996; Clark & Hillyard, 1996; Hillyard & Anllo-Vento, 1998; Luck, Chelazzi, Hillyard, & Desimone, 1997). They have been also applied to examine attentional selection between visual objects (Martinez et al., 2006; Valdes-Sosa, Bobes, Rodriguez, & Pinilla, 1998), of diverse locations inside one object (Martinez, Ramanathan, Foxe, Javitt, & Hillyard, 2007), or of visual features (Andersen, Hillyard, & Muller, 2008). However (for reasons discussed below), these strategies have not been fully applied to analyze the different ways we can look at the same object, as when we selectively attend either the global aspects or the local details of compound objects.

This chapter focuses on attention to different hierarchal levels (i.e., global/local) that coexist within multipart visual objects. We first review some basic principles for studies on the neural basis of selective attention that Steve helped establish. Then we examine why these principals have not been fully adhered to in previous work on attention to compound objects. Later, we define a novel stimulation

method that enables sounder psychophysical and ERP studies of attention within compound letters. Finally, we illustrate the potential of this approach for understanding psychopathology by looking at comparisons of autistic and typical observers using the new paradigm. Our ultimate goal is to understand how we can look at exactly the same object, and yet see distinct things at different times.

SELECTIVE ATTENTION WHEN FACED BY TWO STREAMS OF STIMULI

By 1979, after much tinkering and heated debate in different labs over the world (e.g., Eason, Harter, & White, 1969; Näätänen, 1975; Näätänen, Gaillard, & Mäntysalo, 1978), Hillyard and Picton (1979) were able to distill some basic principles for studying the neural basis of selective attention, initially applied to ERP studies but also valid for other neuroimaging techniques (see the recent review by Luck & Kappenman, 2012). We list below our version of these principles as follows: P1, two streams of information should be presented concurrently on different channels (e.g., the two ears); P2, attention should be directed by turn to both (by means of a discrimination or detection task) in order to compare responses to exactly the same stimuli when attended and when ignored; P3, the stimuli and discrimination task in the two channels should be very similar so that any difference in neural response to the two channels cannot be attributed to differences in global brain states such as arousal; P4, the order of the stimuli should be randomized so participants cannot predict the channel on which each upcoming stimulus was to be presented, thus precluding differential preparatory neural activity; P5, the pace of stimulation should be fast enough, and the subject's task sufficiently difficult, to avoid spillover of surplus attention from the attended to the unattended channel (this idea has resurfaced in the perceptual load theory of Lavie, 1995); and P6, the timing of stimuli should be asynchronous (and with variable interstimulus intervals, (ISI)), to enable the unmixing of overlapping responses to the closely paced stimuli, hence producing independent estimates of each channel's response.

In the visual modality, these principles have been usually incarnated in the fast presentation of two streams of visual objects that replace each other at different locations. Each stream includes many distracters (standards) with a few target (deviant) stimuli, with both types of stimuli sufficiently similar as to make their discrimination challenging, whereas, the difference between streams (channels) should be large. This has been dubbed the Hillyard sustained attention paradigm (Luck & Kappenman, 2012). Many studies have shown that visual spatial attention modulates very early components such as the posterior P1 and N1 (whose neural sources probably lie in visual extra-striate cortices) and the frontal N1, but does not affect the C1 component that originates in striate cortex. These findings have been interpreted as reflecting sensory gating (Anllo-Vento, Schoenfeld, & Hillyard, 2004), and offers support for early selection theories of attention. The application of the principles outlined above, assure us that the measured effects are due to selective attention, and not to unselective or nonspecific effects such as changes in alertness, or differential preparation for processing between the two channels.

A related tradition, using similar fast streams of targets interspersed amidst distracters also emerged in experimental psychology (Broadbent & Broadbent, 1990). This was named rapid visual presentation. However, this technique is perhaps better named rapid serial object substitution (rsoS) since visual objects are continuously created and destroyed in the stream. In this chapter we will use the latter term to contrast it with rapid object transformation (rsoT), in which the visual stream consists of multiple mutations of the same object that do not destroy its spatio-temporal continuity (Valdés Sosa et al., 2003). An important finding with the original rsoS is that when two targets (T1 and T2) are close together in time (about <0.5 s), correct recognition of T1 interferes with recognition of T2. This effect is known as the "attentional blink"((AB); Raymond, Shapiro, & Arnell, 1992; see the recent reviews of the AB by Dux & Marois, 2009; MacLean & Arnell, 2012). Since T2 recognition accuracy is restored by ignoring T1, low order sensory interference (i.e., masking) cannot explain the AB (Duncan, Ward, & Shapiro, 1994; Raymond et al., 1992).

One can strip down the rsoS (and rsoT) from the typical version with multiple distracters to a minimal version that only conserves the two targets (each followed by a visual mask). This is known as the "skeletal" rsoS/rsoT

(MacLean & Arnell, 2012) or the attentional dwell-time paradigm (Duncan et al., 1994), which elicits an AB with similar duration as the one elicited in the "canonical" design. ERPs have been recorded in AB experiments (Luck, Vogel, & Shapiro, 1996), and dual rsoS streams (Chennu, Craston, Wyble, & Bowman, 2008; Śmigasiewicz & Möller, 2011) placed at different visual locations have been used as well, making the connection between the psychological and electrophysiological literature more evident.

Despite their empirical and theoretical connections, crosstalk between skeletal and typical rsoS/rsoT paradigms and ERP designs is still patchy. The connections need to be spelled out in more detail. For example, in principle, it should be possible to predict behavior in the canonical rsoS/rsoT from performance or ERPs in the skeletal design (e.g., McLaughlin, Shore, & Klein, 2001), or to make equivalent predictions in the opposite direction. One should be able to predict the impact of distracters on target identification in the typical rsoS/rsoT design from ERP data, since they provide an unobtrusive index of distracter processing (demanding a behavioral response to a distracter turns it into another target!).

ATTENTION TO THE HIERARCHICAL LEVELS OF COMPOUND OBJECT

Visual scenes and objects can be perceived at different hierarchical levels, moving from the most global down to the narrowest detail. For example, faces have eyes and noses, and eyes have eyelashes. People can selectively attend to these hierarchical levels but have difficulty when trying to apprehend more than one echelon at a time. This failure to consciously perceive different levels at the same time has been assessed with hierarchical stimuli in which a global letter is constructed from smaller letters (Figure 13.1(A)), also known as compound letters (Kinchla, 1974, 1977; Navon, 1977). These figures have the experimental advantage that they equate the complexity and familiarity of the patterns to be identified at both levels.

Most observers are usually faster and more accurate in identifying the global letter than the local forms (Navon, 1977, 2003). Moreover, trying to identify letters at both levels (divided attention) elicits larger interference for the local parts than vice versa (Kim, Ivry, & Robertson, 1999; Modigliani, Brenstein, & Govorkov, 2001). In addition, if the identity of the global and local letters is different in a figure, naming the letter at any level becomes slower. Incongruent global letters interfere more with the naming of local letters than in the opposite direction. All this suggests global precedence, in other words, global information is processed easier and faster than the local details. However, subsequent studies have shown

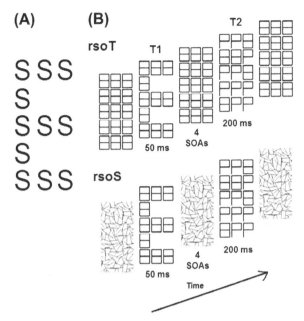

FIGURE 13.1 (A) A compound figure (a.k.a. Navon pattern). In this case the letters defined at the two levels are incongruent. (B) Trial structure in rapid serial object transformation, rsoT (above), and rapid serial object substitution, rsoS (below). The example is a global/local transition. Four different SOAs were used (see Figure 13.2).

that global precedence is not universal, depending on several stimulus factors (Kimchi, 1992). The global precedence effect could be partly a consequence of a competitive advantage for the global level respect to attention. Attempts to indirectly measure this discrepancy in timing were first made with traditional compound stimuli, and tend to support this hypothesis (Filoteo, Friedrich, & Stricker, 2001; Rinehart, Bradshaw, Moss, Brereton, & Tonge, 2000; Robertson, 1996). The time needed to shift attention between different compound letters has been recently assessed with other approaches.

One relevant phenomenon is same-level priming. When asked to identify target letters, subjects are faster if the level at which they were presented is unchanged on successive trials (Hübner, 1997; Lamb, London, Pond, & Whitt, 1998; Lamb & Yund, 1996; Robertson, 1996; Ward, 1982). Since the compound letters change over trials and target letter identity is unpredictable, this facilitation could be attentional in nature. These priming effects can last up to 3 s and seem to be equally strong for both levels (Kim et al., 1999; Lamb & Yund, 1996; Lamb, Yund, & Pond, 1999; Robertson, Egly, Lamb, & Kerth, 1993; Robertson, Lamb, & Knight, 1988). However, a more detailed chronometry of the attentional effects involved would be desirable, which has prompted several studies to look at the AB for compound letters with rsoS designs.

Compound letters have been employed in the canonical rsoS paradigm (Crewther, Lawson, & Crewther, 2007; Lawson et al., 1998; Lawson, Crewther, Junghans, Crewther, & Kiely, 2005). In these studies, unusually long

ABs have been reported, lasting from 1.5 to 2 s. Puzzlingly, there was no advantage for targets at the same level relative to when they appeared at different levels. Compound letters have also been used in a skeletal version of rsoS (two targets followed by noise masks; Srivastava, Kumar, & Srinivasan, 2010). In this case, attentional shifts were faster when both targets appeared at the same hierarchical level. In one of these experiments, local/global and global/local shifts were equivalent in duration, and in another the local/global shift was longer. Both of these findings do not fit with the global dominance hypothesis. Finally, in an interesting design by Kotchoubey, Wascher, and Verleger (1997), participants had to identify which of two target letters was presented at a cued level, but when a different third letter was found, they had to switch and identify the targets at the originally uncued level. However, again responses were slower for the local/global shifts than the global/local shifts.

Several articles describe electrophysiological correlates of directing attention to different levels within compound letters. Some have found larger negativity N2 time window at posterior sites when attention is directed toward local instead of toward global targets (Han, Fan, Chen, & Zhuo, 1997; Han, He, Yund, & Woods, 2001; Heinze & Münte, 1993; Machinskaya, Krupskaya, & Kurgansky, 2010). It is not clear if this effect is related to an increased number of potential targets (many for local vs. only one for global), a factor directly related to N2pc amplitude, or to neural processes more specific to the local level. Some of these authors have also found a larger P1 waveform when attending to the local level (Han et al., 2001; Machinskaya et al., 2010). Interestingly, letter-identity incongruity between levels enhances the amplitude of the N2 waveform (Han et al., 1997, 2001). When the figures were lateralized to one hemifield, larger N2 amplitudes were found when attending to local targets in the left hemisphere and in the right hemisphere when attending to global targets (Schatz & Erlandson, 2003; Volberg & Hübner, 2004). In contrast, in the experiment described above, Kotchoubey et al. (1997) obtained larger- and shorter-latency P1 and N2 components to compound letters when attention was directed to the global level. Furthermore, local/global attentional shifts were associated with a longer P600 latency than global/local shifts.

RAPID VISUAL OBJECT TRANSFORMATION AS A RESEARCH TOOL

We believe that there are two basic problems with many of the experiments reviewed in the previous section that have led to inconsistent results. The first, inherent to rsoS, is that each additional stimulus that pops up in the visual stream must overwrite or destroy the previous one. This means we are looking at a sequence of different objects, which hampers examination of attentional shifts within the same entity (see Valdés Sosa et al., 2003). Furthermore, previous research has established that "new" objects (abruptly emerging within a visual scene) will capture attention automatically (Yantis & Jonides, 1984). This stimulus-by-stimulus resetting of attentional priorities also hampers the study of within-object shifts of attention. The second problem originates with the traditional definition of compound letters. The local and global levels are always presented simultaneously. In fact with traditional stimuli it is impossible to present them separately. This not only limits the options available for psychophysical measurements, it also makes it difficult to unlock the neural responses elicited by the two levels.

To elaborate on this last idea, consider the global and local figures as two channels selectable by attention. Therefore, they should be studied following the principles P1–P6 outlined in a previous section. However in rsoS designs, several of these principles are impossible or difficult to uphold (see Table 13.1). Since the local and global levels are presented at the same time, it is not possible to obtain distinct ERPs to each type of information. To extract ERP or functional magnetic resonance imaging (fMRI) activity selectively associated to different events, we must be able to independently control the timing of each type of stimulus (Dale & Buckner, 1997; Serences, 2004; Woldorff, 1993). Also with abrupt presentation of traditional compound letters, it is not possible to task attention at specific and independent times for each level, which is what is required to directly time attentional shifts.

Therefore, the effects of attention on neural responses specifically associated with a single level (in isolation from the other) have not been studied, as when attended and unattended ERPs from the same visual location (or from the same ear) are compared. We can only contrast the ERPs elicited by the same stimuli after we have tried to weigh attention toward one—and then the other—level. This has the unfortunate consequence that any ERP change is ambiguous, because it could result either from attention being drawn toward one level, or because it is being drawn away from the other. The two alternatives cannot be distinguished in an experiment. In fact, if these two options produce outcomes of opposite polarity, then the net effect would be weak or could even cancel.

To solve these problems we have applied rapid serial object transformation to compound letters (see Table 13.1). In rsoT, instead of the sequential disappearance of "old" and appearance of "new" objects, we use successive transformations of a durable visual entity. This allows the direct timing of attentional shifts between and within objects without contamination from attentional resets due to the abrupt creation of new objects in the scene. Several studies have shown that with rsoT, the AB produced by discrimination of mutations of the same object is smaller than the one produced for different objects (Kellie & Shapiro, 2004; Raymond et al., 1992; Valdés Sosa et al., 2003). In our approach to Navon patterns (Lopez, Torres, & Valdés-Sosa, 2002), participants were presented with a grid of patterns shaped like "8" digits (Figure 13.1(B)), each similar to the seven segment LED numerical displays. Subsequently, either complete "8" patterns were erased briefly, unmasking a global letter, or parts within the individual "8" patterns were eliminated, thus unmasking local letters. Reinstating the original grid served to limit the availability of the letters, without the need to introduce a different and new stimulus as a visual mask (as used in Hübner, 2000; Navon, 1977).

This allows us to dissociate in time the presentation of local and global aspects of the same object (Figure 13.1(B)). One can then unambiguously attract attention to one of the levels of the object at selected time instants. Note that the overall grid (despite its mutations) provides a stable scaffold to which the global and local levels can be anchored. As we show below, rsoT of compound letters

TABLE 13.1 Comparison Between the Classical Navon Paradigm and the rsoT Approach Based on the Principles for Experimentation on Selective Attention Established by Steve Hillyard

	Principle	Previous work using Navon paradigm with rsoS	Our work with rsoT
P1	Two concurrent separate channels (i.e., global and local)	Theoretically yes, practically no	Yes
P2	Attention first to one and then the other over time	Yes	Yes
P3	Equivalent stimuli and task difficulty	Roughly yes (i.e. same letters), but big differences persist	Can be made more equivalent but some differences persist
P4	Random presentation: make which channel upcoming stimulus unpredictable	Impossible	Possible
P5	Fast stimulus pace and large task difficulty to avoid spillover of surplus attention from attended to unattended channel	Yes, but not completely verifiable	Yes, completely verifiable
P6	Asynchronous presentation	Impossible	Possible

permits us to answer new psychophysical questions (such as the direct timing of attentional shifts within levels of the same object), on top of unlocking the neural responses elicited by global and local aspects of the same figure (see Table 13.1). If the baseline grid of "8s" is replaced by a visual noise mask, we have a more traditional rsoS as used in previous work (Figure 13.1(B)), in which different objects are replaced in the visual stream.

DIRECT TIMING OF BETWEEN-LEVEL ATTENTIONAL SHIFTS IN COMPOUND FIGURES

Previous work has suggested that the time to shift attention from the local to the global level of a compound figure could be longer than a shift in the other direction. However, as explained above the direct timing of attentional shifts within the same object cannot be achieved with conventional compound letters. By uncoupling the presentation of these levels with rsoT, we can solve this problem using the same logic developed to directly time attentional shifts between different locations in visual space (Posner, 1980), or between different objects at the

same or separate locations (Chun & Potter, 1995; Raymond et al., 1992; Raymond, Shapiro, & Arnell, 1995; Shapiro, Driver, Ward, & Sorensen, 1997).

In a first experiment using a skeletal version of rsoT (Lopez et al., 2002), a first target letter (T1) was presented at one level and, after a varying stimulus onset asynchrony (SOA), another target letter (T2) was presented either at the same or a different level (Figure 13.1(B)). Both targets were sandwiched between the baseline grid. Pilot runs (in 20 independent participants) allowed us to fix the target durations needed to achieve 85% correct identification: about 50 ms for global- and about 200 ms for local-letters, Four types of transitions were presented (global/global, local/local, local/global, global/local), each in a separate and precued block (100 trials in a block, 25 per SOA), with their order counterbalanced across participants. The identity of T1 and T2 letters (either "E", "S", "H", "U", or "P") were randomly selected on each trial without repetition.

The identification of the second letter (T2) was also highly accurate for same-level trials for all SOAs down to 200 ms, indicating little interference in identifying two target letters at the same hierarchical level (Figure 13.2(A)). In contrast, interference was found for global/local shifts of

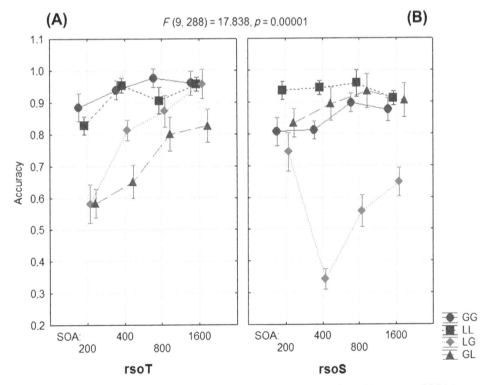

FIGURE 13.2 T2 recognition accuracy (proportion correct) in rsoT and rsoS as a function of transition type and SOA (measured in milliseconds). Only trials in which T1 was correctly identified were considered. In this and subsequent figures the mean and standard error are plotted. (A) In rsoT, transition type (F (3, 48) = 12.3, $p < 0.01$), SOA (F (3, 48) = 32.9, $p < 0.01$) and their interaction (F (9, 144) = 8.4, $p < 0.01$) all had significant effects on T2 identification accuracy. Recognition of T1 did not differ between transition types and SOAs in this design and was highly accurate in all cases (mean > 85%). (B) In rsoS, transition type (F (3, 48) = 30.9, $p < 0.01$), SOA (F (3, 48) = 26.8, $p < 0.01$), and their interaction (F (9, 144) = 19.7, $p < 0.01$) all had significant effects on T2 identification accuracy. Recognition of T1 was also accurate across participants (mean > 85%). *Source: Panel A was modified from Lopez et al. (2002) with permission.*

attention at short SOAs (at 200 ms accuracy dropped about 30%), with a slow recovery that reached the accuracy of same-level trials at about 800 ms. Interestingly, for global/local shifts the impairment in T2 recognition was equally severe at 200 ms, but much longer lasting. In this case, the effects lasted up to1600 ms (Figure 13.2(A)). To summarize: in typical observers, the interference for T2 was very small when both transformations occurred at the same level of the hierarchical figure; it was larger for local/global shifts; and it was much larger for global/local shifts.

Another group of subjects was tested with the same stimuli but in an rsoS design created by replacing the baseline grid of "8s" by visual noise (Figure 13.2(B)). Letter durations were also the same as before. As expected, T2 identification was highly accurate for same-level trials. However, in contrast with rsoT, global/global shifts exhibited a slight (about 10%), but significant drop in performance at the shortest SOAs (200 and 400 ms; (F (3, 16) = 14.9, $p < 0.01$)). The most striking finding was that T2 identification accuracy in different-level trials presented a pattern divergent from the results from the rsoT design (Figure 13.1(B)). Here, global/local shifts presented only a small, albeit significant, drop (about 10%) in accuracy at the shortest SOA. Surprisingly the local/global shifts exhibited a very large impairment for T2 recognition.

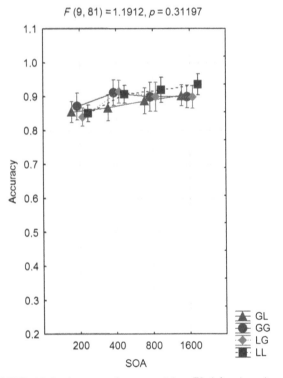

F (9, 81) = 1.1912, p = 0.31197

FIGURE 13.3 Accuracy for recognizing T2 (after ignoring T1) in a rsoT paradigm. All four transition types used are plotted as a function of SOA. A small decrease in accuracy was observed only at the smallest SOA, which resulted in significant effect of SOA accuracy (F (3, 27) = 3.4, $p < 0.04$). However, neither transition type, nor its interaction with SOA, were significant.

Although accuracy was high at the 200 ms SOA possibly a lag-zero effect (Arnell, Howe, Joanisse, & Klein, 2006), for longer SOAs T2 recognition was more inaccurate up to the longest 1600 ms with large drop t 400 ms (falling to 45% accuracy). This is similar to the findings of Srivastava et al. (2010; experiment 2) who also used rsoS.

Are these interference effects attentional in nature? Using the criteria developed in the AB literature in our skeletal rsoT design (Lopez et al., 2002), we asked participants to ignore T1, while focusing attention on—and reporting—only T2, target identification was very accurate (>90%) for all SOAs and all types of trials (Figure 13.3). A slight (4%) drop in accuracy was observed only for the smallest delay. Thus low-level sensory effects (i.e., masking) probably plays a small role (limited to very short SOAs) in the between-level interference effects found in the skeletal rsoT (a similar test for the rsoS task is required).

We believe that our rsoT design allows us to dissect, control, and measure for the first time the covert shifts of attention between levels that are triggered by traditional Navon patterns. Uncovering the local and global letters embedded in the baseline grid at separate moments allows the direct timing of attentional dwell-times (Duncan et al., 1994). The advantage for same-level shifts of attention in rsoT is congruent with the same-level priming previously reported (Robertson et al., 1993), and establishes that it may emerge as fast as 200 ms after attention latches onto one echelon. The greater ease for local/global than for global/local shifts is compatible with (and may partially explain) global precedence. We believe that in rsoT the baseline grid provides a scaffold that unambiguously defines the local and global levels while conserving object continuity. Thus when a traditional compound letter is observed, attention shifts within the object, not to another object. In rsoS by contrast, no scaffold is available in the noise mask, and object continuity is destroyed from one letter to the other. This could help explain why the rsoS data presented here, and that described in previous studies does not comply with the global dominance hypothesis. Note that rsoS plot for local/global shifts resembles the typical AB curves with lag-one sparing, in other words preserved accuracy at the shortest T1–T2 SOA (MacLean & Arnell, 2012). The reason for this effect is not completely clear and requires further exploration (Dux & Marois, 2009).

SUSTAINED ATTENTION TO THE LEVELS OF A COMPOUND FIGURE

Although the sparse design of the skeletal rsoS/rsoT allows direct and detailed timing of attentional shifts, the large number of distracters in the canonical paradigm is better tailored for ERP experiments using the Hillyard sustained-attention method. In this section we turn to typical designs, in which participants in each block either focused attention at one level, or divided attention between the two levels. Based on a comparison of the results from the skeletal rsoT and rsoS in the previous section, we predicted more errors in target identification during the divided-attention blocks, with evidence for global dominance emerging from the former but not in the latter design.

Ten subjects participated in the experiment. Compound letters similar to those described by Lopez et al. (2002) were used. "E" and "P" were selected as targets and "S", "H", and "U" as distracters. Global and local letter durations were first titrated for each subject to achieve 80% identification accuracy. A total of 90 blocks of 20 letters were presented, each separated from the next by either the baseline grid (rsoT) or the noise mask (rsoS). On each block two targets were presented, separated from each other by three to six distracters. In a third of the blocks, targets were presented at only the local level at which participants were asked to focus attention. In another third of the trials, the global level was selected. In the remaining third of the blocks, one local and one global target were presented, and participants were asked to divide attention equally between the two levels. The identity and level of the letters were selected in a pseudo-random order, and subjects identified the targets on a keyboard after each block finished. The ISIs were selected from a uniform distribution from 500 to 800 ms (see Figure 13.4). The variable ISI was necessary for subsequent ERP recordings. Note that the perceptual and memory load created by the targets was equivalent in all blocks.

Figure 13.5 shows mean recognition accuracy as a function of target level for each type of block in the two paradigms. Although in both designs there is a significant cost for dividing attention ($F (1, 9) = 12.5, p < 0.006$), the pattern of effects across blocks differs substantially between rsoT and rsoS as predicted. This was reflected in a significant paradigm X level interaction ($F (1, 9) = 10.2, p < 0.01$). In rsoT, there is a global advantage for the focused attention blocks, and the divided attention cost is more pronounced for the local level. In rsoS, there was

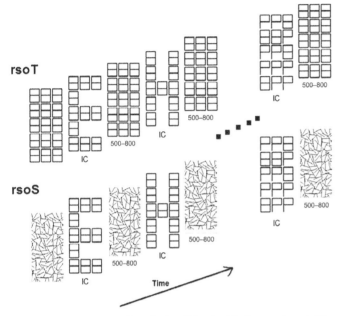

FIGURE 13.4 Examples of stimuli in the block experiment. The first two letters are global (first a target and then a distracter). There were 20 letters in each block. The third letter shown is a target at the local level. The upper sequence is rsoT, whereas the lower is rsoS. IC indicates durations calibrated for each subject to achieve about 85% accuracy.

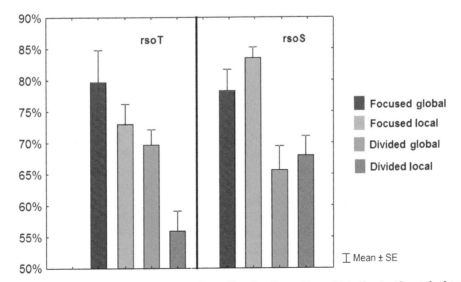

FIGURE 13.5 Mean error rate as a function of block type in the rsoT and rsoS paradigms. Note the significant dual-task cost (see main text), which significant in both rsoT ($F (1, 9) = 9.54, p < 0.013$) and rsoS ($F (1, 9) = 13.4, p < 0.0053$). Whereas the divided attention cost was equivalent for both levels in rsoS, it was more pronounced for the local than the global level ($t(9) = 3.45, p < 0.007$).

a significant cost for divided attention but no effect due to level was found. In other words, clear evidence for global dominance was found in rsoT but not rsoS.

ATTENTIONAL MODULATION OF THE ERPs ELICITED BY DIFFERENT LEVELS OF A COMPOUND FIGURE

Next we used the ability of rsoT to unlock the moments in which global and local letters are presented, in order to segregate neural responses to each level. A canonical rsoT block design was used, similar to that employed in the previous section. Importantly, the intervals between stimuli were randomly jittered, which allows optimal separation of ERP recordings to each type of letter (global vs. local). Here we summarize a more extended report (Iglesisas, Trujillo-Barreto, & Valdes-Sosa, submitted for publication).

The stimuli used were identical to those used in the previously described experiment. Four blocks of stimuli were used. In each block, 120 stimuli (60 global and 60 local), were presented in a random order, separated by baseline period intervals ranging between 600 and 800 ms. Four targets were presented in each block at randomly selected levels. Presentation time for both global and local stimuli were titrated to about 80% recognition accuracy in each individual. The stimuli sequence within each block was randomized. In two of the four blocks, participants were instructed to attend only to the global stimuli (Attend-Global blocks) and in the other two they were instructed to attend only to the local targets (Attend-Local blocks). Block order was counterbalanced across the 17 healthy participants.

Electrodes were placed in 58 active derivations referenced to the nose. In addition eye movements were monitored. Electroencephalogram segments of 800 ms were defined, starting 100 ms before each stimulus. Trials with artifacts or excessive activity in electro-oculogram were rejected, and surviving segments for each condition (on the average about 190 trials) were analyzed separately. Since the temporal overlap of ERPs in fast paced rsoS/rsoT designs usually produces unstable prestimulus baselines, we estimated the average ERPs of each condition in all individuals with a novel methodology (Trujillo-Barreto, Iglesias, & Valdes-Sosa, submitted for publication) dubbed "form-free unmixing for ERPs" (FUN for ERPs), with the same purpose as the previously described adjacent response filter method (ADJAR) (Woldorff, 1993). FUN for ERPs allows robust and efficient extraction of overlapped responses during rapid stimulation paradigms, avoiding "a priori" assumptions about the shape of the underlying ERPs. A permutation method (Galán, Biscay, Rodríguez, Pérez-Abalo, & Rodriguez, 1997) with cluster-mass correction (Maris & Oostenveld, 2007),

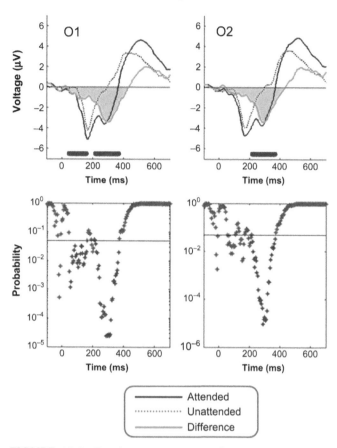

FIGURE 13.6 Grand average responses elicited by global stimuli at selected electrodes O1 and O2. In each panel the upper graphs show the response to attended stimuli (red solid line) and unattended (blue dashed line). The curves below each panel represent the results of comparing both attended and unattended waveforms by means of a permutation test. The red horizontal line shows the probability of $p = 0.05$ (corrected for multiple comparisons). The red bars (above) and dots (below) represent latencies where the test was significant after cluster-mass correction.

was used to estimate the statistical significance of the ERP amplitude elicited by distracter letters when they were attended and when they where unattended.

The ERPs elicited by global stimuli were largest over the occipito-temporal scalp region. As shown in Figure 13.6, two early negative peaks were clearly evident in the attended stimuli, with respective latencies of 170 and 275 ms. This early activity was followed by a positive peak with latency of 485 ms. The amplitude of all components was attenuated when attention was directed away from the global level toward the local level. Interestingly, a significant attenuation of both negative peaks was observed with permutation method that began about 85 ms after stimulus presentation (see Figure 13.6).

Figure 13.7 exhibits the ERPs elicited by local stimuli in both attended and unattended conditions. Attended local letters also evoked ERPs that were also largest over the occipital–temporal scalp (with two negative peaks, latencies of 170 and 275 ms, and a positive peak with

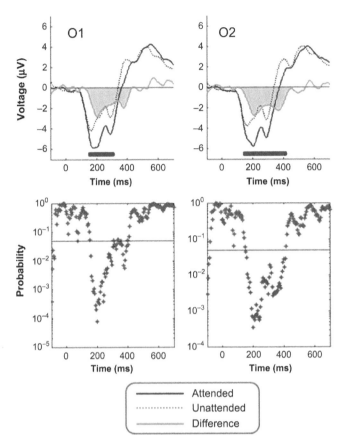

FIGURE 13.7 Grand average responses elicited by local stimuli at selected electrodes O1 and O2. Conventions the same as in Figure 13.6.

latency of 505 ms). Unattended local letters produced smaller ERPs than attended ones. The earliest amplitude difference began at about 175 ms after stimulus onset. This implies that the effects of attention were evident about 100 ms later for the global-as compared to the local-letters in this rsoT experiment.

Note that this is the first report of separate estimates for different letters in a compound figure. The data show that attention modulates early negative ERPs located over the occipital–temporal scalp consistent with early selection. The faster onset of attentional effects for global—than for local—letters is consistent with the global dominance hypothesis, and the corresponding latency difference is of the same magnitude as the traditionally reported global reaction-time advantage (Navon, 1977).

APPLICATIONS OF RAPID OBJECT TRANSFORMATION IN THE STUDY OF AUTISM

As mentioned before, typical observers are faster and more accurate in identifying the global-than the local-letters within traditional compound letters.

Furthermore, when conflicting information is presented at the two levels, interference from the global to the local letters is stronger than in the opposite direction. However, in autistic viewers, recognition of the local letters interferes robustly with identification of the global letter (O'Riordan, Plaisted, Driver, & Baron-Cohen, 2001; Plaisted, Saksida, Alcantara, & Weisblatt, 2003; Rinehart et al., 2000). There are several studies suggesting that autistic individuals are actually faster than typical observers when asked to identify an object embedded in a larger complex pattern (Jolliffe & Baron-Cohen, 1997; Shah & Frith, 1983), which is striking given that cognitive deficits (not advantages) are usually associated with autism (Happé, 1999; Happé & Frith, 2006). Efficient processing of global figures by autistic participants is possible nevertheless when local details can be ignored, a finding that rules out a gross deficiency in their global perception (Plaisted, Swettenham, & Rees, 1999; Posner, 1980).

Current theories of autism have tried to explain this phenomenon by proposing an attentional bias toward local processing (Happé, 1999; Happé & Frith, 2006; Wang, Mottron, Peng, Berthiaume, & Dawson, 2007). If this bias exists, it should translate into slower local/global attentional shifts than found in typical observers. This comparison has been performed twice with an adaptation of the skeletal rsoT procedure first described by Lopez et al. (2002). We first describe our own study, and then summarize findings from an independent study (White, O'Reilly, & Frith, 2009).

We examined nine individuals with autism, conforming to DSM-IV criteria for autism and mental retardation as confirmed by a trained psychiatrist. To control factors such as educational level, verbal, and nonverbal abilities, a control subject with mild mental retardation matched in age (10–26 years), sex (eight male, one female), and nonverbal IQ (Raven's Colored or Standard Progressive Matrices), was recruited for each participant with autism. The autistic and mentally retarded participants were screened beforehand to check that they could identify the letters used as stimuli and perform the task. All of the participants had normal or corrected to normal vision.

A briefer version of the skeletal rsoT procedure described above was designed for clinical populations. Only the 400 ms SOA and accuracy at this interval was used as a surrogate measure for attentional shift duration. One block (consisting of 50 trials) of each transition type was tested and participants were asked to report both T1 and T2. A comparison of T2 recognition accuracy in global/local relative to local/global trials is shown in Figure 13.8(A).

The pattern of performance for the mentally retarded participants was very similar to the majority of typical observers. T2 recognition was larger for local/global

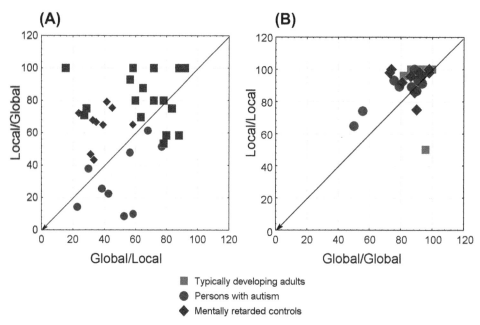

FIGURE 13.8　Scatter-plot of T2 recognition accuracy in autistic, mentally retarded, and typical observers. The diagonal line represents identical performance for the two types of trial. (A) Different level trials (global–local and local–global). Here, autistic participants exhibited a better performance in global/local attentional transitions, as opposed to typical subjects and mentally retarded controls, who performed better in local/global transitions. (B) Same-level trials (global–global and local–local), where no significant differences were found between groups. Only trials were T1 was corrected were included in the figures.

shifts of attention than for global/local shifts, hence all of the mentally retarded and typical viewers fell above the diagonal in Figure 13.8(A). In contrast, almost all autistic observers presented the opposite pattern with poorer local/global than global/local attentional shifts (thereby located under the diagonal in Figure 13.8(A)). Mean T2 recognition accuracy was larger for global/local shifts ($F (1, 16) = 10.4, p < 0.006$) in autistic observers. In the mentally retarded controls mean scores were more accurate for local/global shifts ($F (1, 16) = 17.3, p < 0.0007$). The shift direction interacted significantly with the diagnostic group (mentally retarded vs autistic) in a mixed analysis of variance ($F (1, 16) = 27.27, p < 0.0001$). T2 recognition in same-level shifts did not differ significantly between the autistic and mentally retarded individuals. Therefore our rsoT method confirms that autistic observers do have a bias of attention toward the local level (Filoteo et al., 2001; Robertson, 1996) and allows its precise quantification.

In a study with a much larger sample, White et al. (2009) examined 49 high-functioning 7–12 year olds with autism, of which 12 presented macrocephaly. These children were compared to 25 typical children with the same skeletal rsoT (using only the 400 ms SOA) described above. White et al. (2009) found that children with autism who also had macrocephaly showed a greater processing cost when switching from local to global, than both the children with autism without macrocephaly and the control children. They also found that macrocephaly in the context of normal development was not associated

with this difficulty. They argued that macrocephaly in autism could be associated with abnormal neural connectivity. Overall both studies coincide in showing that in cases of autism, the costs for switching from global to local are increased with respect to controls. This local attentional bias could influence the daily lives of these individuals and be related to the severity of their symptoms. In this sense, correlations between various aspects of visual attention and scores on diagnostic scales have been described (Billington, Baron-Cohen, & Bor, 2007; Kawakubo et al., 2007).

CONCLUSIONS

In this chapter we present a novel experimental approach, rsoT, which allows dissociation of the onset of global and local target letters with the same compound figure. This allowed direct timing of attentional shifts within the same visual object. Shifts of attention to successive targets within the same level were very fast. Typical participants took longer in shifting attention from the global to the local level than from the local to the global level. In contrast to previous work (reviewed above) with the rsoS paradigm, our results are consistent with the well-established literature on global precedence (which suggests more attraction of attention to the global than to the local level) and same-level priming. When we exchange in our stimuli the background/mask pattern that is interspersed between letters from a grid of "8s" for random lines (noise) the design changes from rsoT (same object undergoing mutations) into rsoS (objects appear and disappear). Under these conditions, global/local shifts become faster and local/global much slower, a pattern inverse to our rsoT design but similar to previous reports using this paradigm.

We also show that psychophysically, in rsoT the global and the local aspects of the same stimulus can be considered analogous to the two channels created by spatially separated auditory or visual sources, with significant costs for divided attention relative to focused attention. By exploiting the unlocking of global and local letter onsets in rsoT, we were able to isolate the neural responses to the two levels. Thus all the principles laid down by Steve Hillyard for studies of selective attention (Table 13.1) can be satisfied. We are now using the same rsoT paradigm for fMRI studies, including a multivariate pattern analysis study to examine the coding of global and local letters.

In addition to its contribution to research on basic mechanisms of visual attention, our rsoT method using compound letters is potentially useful for studying attention in neuropsychiatric disorders. In the two studies of children with autism, we review that the typical pattern of longer local/global than global/local attentional shifts was reversed. This potentially offers an explanation for the tendency of autistic participants to focus on details, and perceive global aspects with difficulty. The method could also be applied to characterize attention in other syndromes with atypical processing of compound letters, such as Williams syndrome, Parkinson's disease, Down syndrome, Alzheimer's disease, and schizophrenia.

References

Andersen, S. K., Hillyard, S. A., & Muller, M. M. (2008). Attention facilitates multiple stimulus features in parallel in human visual cortex. *Current Biology, 18*, 1006–1009.

Anllo-Vento, L., & Hillyard, S. A. (1996). Selective attention to the color and direction of moving stimuli: electrophysiological correlates of hierarchical feature selection. *Perception and Psychophysics, 58*, 191–206.

Anllo-Vento, L., Schoenfeld, M. A., & Hillyard, S. A. (2004). Cortical mechanisms of visual attention: electrophysiological and neuroimaging studies. In M. I. Posner (Ed.), *Cognitive neuroscience of attention* (pp. 180–193). Guilford Press.

Arnell, K. M., Howe, A. E., Joanisse, M. F., & Klein, R. M. (2006). Relationships between attentional blink magnitude, RSVP target accuracy, and performance on other cognitive tasks. *Memory and Cognition, 34*, 1472–1483.

Billington, J., Baron-Cohen, S., & Bor, D. (2007). Systemizing influences attentional processes during the Navon task: an fMRI study. *Neuropsychologia, 46*, 511–520.

Broadbent, D., & Broadbent, M. H. P. (1990). Human attention: the exclusion of distracting information as a function of real and apparent separation of relevant and irrelevant events. *Proceedings of the Royal Society of London. Series B: Biological Sciences, 242*, 11–16.

Chennu, S., Craston, P., Wyble, B., & Bowman, H. (2008). Transient attentional enhancement during the attentional blink: ERP correlates of the ST² model. *From associations to rules: Connectionist models of behavior and cognition* (Vol. 17).

Chun, M. M., & Potter, M. C. (1995). A two-stage model for multiple target detection in rapid serial visual presentation. *Journal of Experimental Psychology: Human Perception and Performance, 21*, 109–127.

Clark, V., & Hillyard, S. A. (1996). Spatial selective attention affects early extrastriate but not striate components of the visual evoked potential. *Journal of Cognitive Neuroscience, 8*, 387–402.

Crewther, D. P., Lawson, M. L., & Crewther, S. G. (2007). Global and local attention in the attentional blink. *Journal of Vision, 7*.

Dale, A. M., & Buckner, R. L. (1997). Selective averaging of rapidly presented individual trials using fMRI. *Human Brain Mapping, 5*, 329–340.

Desmedt, J. E., Huy, N. T., & Bourguet, M. (1983). The cognitive P40, N60 and P100 components of somatosensory evoked potentials and the earliest electrical signs of sensory processing in man. *Electroencephalography and Clinical Neurophysiology, 56*, 272–282.

Desmedt, J. E., & Robertson, D. (1977). Differential enhancement of early and late components of the cerebral somatosensory evoked potentials during forced-paced cognitive tasks in man. *The Journal of Physiology, 271*, 761–782.

Duncan, J., Ward, R., & Shapiro, K. (1994). Direct measurement of attentional dwell time in human vision. *Nature, 369*, 313–315.

Dux, P. E., & Marois, R. (2009). The attentional blink: a review of data and theory. *Attention, Perception, and Psychophysics, 71*, 1683–1700.

Eason, R. G., Harter, M. R., & White, C. T. (1969). Effects of attention and arousal on visually evoked cortical potentials and reaction time in man. *Physiology and Behavior, 4*, 283–289.

Filoteo, J. V., Friedrich, F. J., & Stricker, J. L. (2001). Shifting attention to different levels within global–local stimuli: a study of normal participants and a patient with temporal–parietal lobe damage. *Cognitive Neuropsychology, 18*, 227–239.

Galán, L., Biscay, R., Rodríguez, J. L., Pérez-Abalo, M. C., & Rodríguez, R. (1997). Testing topographic differences between event related brain potentials by using non-parametric combinations of permutation tests. [published erratum appears in Electroencephalography and Clinical Neurophysiology (Nov 1998), *107*(5), 380–381], *Electroencephalography and Clinical Neurophysiology, 102*, 240–247.

Grice, R. G., Canham, L., & Boroughs, J. (1983). Forest before trees? It depends where you look. *Perception and Psychophysics, 33*, 121–128.

Han, S., Fan, S., Chen, L., & Zhuo, Y. (1997). On the different processing of wholes and parts: a psychophysiological analysis. *Journal of Cognitive Neuroscience, 9*, 687–698.

Han, S., He, X., Yund, E. W., & Woods, D. L. (2001). Attentional selection in the processing of hierarchical patterns: an ERP study. *Biological Psychology, 56*, 113–130.

Happé, F. (1999). Autism: cognitive deficit or cognitive style? *Trends in Cognitive Science, 3*, 212–222.

Happé, F., & Frith, U. (2006). The weak coherence account: detail-focused cognitive style in autism spectrum disorders. *Journal of Autism and Developmental Disorders, 36*, 5–25.

Heinze, H. J., & Münte, T. F. (1993). Electrophysiological correlates of hierarchical stimulus processing: dissociation between onset and later stages of global and local target processing. *Neuropsychologia, 31*(8), 841–852.

Hillyard, S. A., & Anllo-Vento, L. (1998). Event-related brain potentials in the study of visual selective attention. *Proceedings of the National Academy of Sciences, 95*, 781–787.

Hillyard, S. A., Hink, R. F., Schwent, V. L., & Picton, T. W. (1973). Electrical signs of selective attention in the human brain. *Science, 182*, 177–180.

Hillyard, S. A., & Picton, T. W. (1979). Event-related brain potentials and selective information processing in man. In J. Desmedt (Ed.), *Progress in Clinical Neurophysiology Cognitive Components in Cerebral Event-Related Potentials and Selective Attention*, Vol. 6. Basel: Karger, pp. 1–50.

Hillyard, S. A., Squires, K. C., Bauer, J. W., & Lindsay, P. H. (1971). Evoked potential correlates of auditory signal detection. *Science, 172*, 1357–1360.

Hink, R. F., & Hillyard, S. A. (1976). Auditory evoked potentials during selective listening to dichotic speech messages. *Perception and Psychophysics, 20*, 236–242.

Hübner, R. (1997). The effect of spatial frequency on global precedence and hemispheric differences. *Perception & Psychophysics, 59*, 187–201.

Hübner, R. (2000). Attention shifting between global and local target levels: the persistence of level-repetition effects. *Visual Cognition, 7*, 456–484.

Iglesisas, J., Trujillo-Barreto, N., & Valdes-Sosa, M. (submitted for publication). Separation of event-related response to the global and local levels of compound letters: effects of selective attention.

Jolliffe, T., & Baron-Cohen, S. (1997). Are people with autism and Asperger syndrome faster than normal on the Embedded Figures Test? *Journal of Child Psychology and Psychiatry, 38*, 527–534.

Kawakubo, Y., Kasai, K., Okazaki, S., Hosokawa-Kakurai, M., Watanabe, K., Kuwabara, H., et al. (2007). Electrophysiological abnormalities of spatial attention in adults with autism during the gap overlap task. *Clinical Neurophysiology, 118*, 1464–1471.

Kellie, F. J., & Shapiro, K. L. (2004). Object file continuity predicts attentional blink magnitude. *Attention, Perception, and Psychophysics, 66*, 692–712.

Kimchi, R. (1992). Primacy of wholistic processing and global/local paradigm: a critical review. *Psychological Bulletin, 112*, 24.

Kim, N., Ivry, R. B., & Robertson, L. C. (1999). Sequential priming in hierarchically organized figures: effects of target level and target resolution. *Journal of Experimental Psychology: Human Perception and Performance, 25*, 715–729.

Kinchla, R. A. (1974). Detecting target elements in multielement arrays: a confusability model. *Attention, Perception, and Psychophysics, 15*, 149–158.

Kinchla, R. A. (1977). The role of structural redundancy in the perception of visual targets. *Attention, Perception, and Psychophysics, 22*, 19–30.

Kotchoubey, B., Wascher, E., & Verleger, R. (1997). Shifting attention between global features and small details: an event-related potential study. *Biological Psychology, 46*, 25–50.

Lamb, M. R., & Yund, E. W. (1996). Spatial frequency and attention: effects of level-, target-, and location-repetition on the processing of global and local forms. *Perception & Psychophysics, 58*, 363–373.

Lamb, M. R., London, B., Pond, H. M., & Whitt, K. A. (1998). Automatic and controlled processes in the analysis of hierarchical structure. *Psychological Science, 9*, 14–19.

Lamb, M. R., Yund, E. W., & Pond, H. M. (1999). Is attentional selection to different levels of hierarchical structure based on spatial frequency? *Journal of Experimental Psychology: General, 128*, 88.

Lavie, N. (1995). Perceptual load as a necessary condition for selective attention. *Journal of Experimental Psychology: Human Perception and Performance, 21*, 451.

Lawson, M. L., Crewther, D. P., Duke, C. C., Henry, L., Kiely, P. M., West, S. J., et al. (1998). Attentional blink in global versus local attentional modes. *Australian and New Zealand Journal of Ophthalmology, 26*, S88–S90.

Lawson, M. L., Crewther, S. G., Junghans, B. M., Crewther, D. P., & Kiely, P. M. (2005). Changes in ocular accommodation when shifting between global and local attention. *Clinical and Experimental Optometry, 88*, 28–32.

Luck, S. J., & Kappenman, E. S. (Eds.), (2012). *Oxford Handbook of Event-Related Potential Components*. New York: Oxford University Press.

Lopez, K., Torres, R., & Valdés-Sosa, M. (2002). Medición directa del tiempo de tránsito atencional entre distintos niveles de figuras jerárquicas: observadores normales y autistas. *Revista CENIC Ciencias Biológicas, 33*, 111–117.

Luck, S. J., Chelazzi, L., Hillyard, S. A., & Desimone, R. (1997). Neural mechanisms of spatial selective attention in areas V1, V2, and V4 of macaque visual cortex. *Journal of Neurophysiology, 77*, 24–42.

Luck, S. J., Vogel, E. K., & Shapiro, K. L. (1996). Word meanings can be accessed but not reported during the attentional blink. *Nature, 383*, 616–618.

Machinskaya, R. I., Krupskaya, E. V., & Kurgansky, A. V. (2010). Functional brain organization of global and local visual perception: analysis of event-related potentials. *Human Physiology, 36*, 518–534.

Maris, E., & Oostenveld, R. (2007). Nonparametric statistical testing of EEG and MEG data. *Journal of Neuroscience Methods, 164*, 177–190.

MacLean, M. H., & Arnell, K. M. (2012). A conceptual and methodological framework for measuring and modulating the attentional blink. *Attention, Perception, & Psychophysics, 74*, 1080–1097.

Martinez, A., Ramanathan, D. S., Foxe, J. J., Javitt, D. C., & Hillyard, S. A. (2007). The role of spatial attention in the selection of real and illusory objects. *The Journal of Neuroscience, 27*, 7963–7973.

Martinez, A., Teder-Salejarvi, W., Vazquez, M., Molholm, S., Foxe, J. J., Javitt, D. C., et al. (2006). Objects are highlighted by spatial attention. *Journal of Cognitive Neuroscience, 18*, 298–310.

McLaughlin, E. N., Shore, D. I., & Klein, R. M. (2001). The attentional blink is immune to masking-induced data limits. *The Quarterly Journal of Experimental Psychology: Section A, 54*, 169–196.

Michie, P. T., Bearparic, H. M., Crawford, J. M., & Glue, L. C. (1987). The effects of spatial selective attention on the somatosensory event-related potential. *Psychophysiology, 24*(4), 449–463.

Modigliani, V., Brenstein, D., & Govorkov, S. (2001). Attention and size in a global/local task. *Acta Psychologica, 108*, 35–51.

Näätänen, R. (1975). Selective attention and evoked potentials in humans—a critical review. *Biological Psychology, 2*, 237–307.

Näätänen, R., Gaillard, A. W., & Mäntysalo, S. (1978). Early selective-attention effect on evoked potential reinterpreted. *Acta Psychologica, 42*, 313–329.

Navon, D. (1977). Forest before trees: the precedence of global features in visual perception. *Cognitive Psychology, 9*, 353–383.

Navon, D. (2003). What does a compound letter tell the psychologist's mind? *Acta Psychologica, 114*, 273–309.

O'Riordan, M., Plaisted, K., Driver, J., & Baron-Cohen, S. (2001). Superior visual search in autism. *Journal of Experimental Psychology: Human Perception and Performance, 27*, 719–730.

Picton, T. W., Hillyard, S. A., Galambos, R., & Schiff, M. (1971). Human auditory attention: a central or peripheral process? *Science, 173*, 351–353.

Plaisted, K., Saksida, L., Alcantara, J., & Weisblatt, E. (2003). Towards an understanding of the mechanisms of weak central coherent effects: experiments in visual configural learning and auditory perception. *Philosophical Transactions of the Royal Society of London, Series B, Biological Science, 358*, 375–386.

Plaisted, K., Swettenham, J., & Rees, L. (1999). Children with autism show local precedence in a divided attention task and global precedence in a selective attention task. *Journal of Child Psychology and Psychiatry, 40*, 733–742.

Posner, M. I. (1980). Orienting of attention. *Quarterly Journal of Experimental Psychology, 32*, 3–25.

Raymond, J. E., Shapiro, K. L., & Arnell, K. M. (1992). Temporary suppression of visual processing in an RSVP task: an attentional blink? *Journal of Experimental Psychology: Human Perception and Performance, 18*, 849–860.

Raymond, J. E., Shapiro, K. L., & Arnell, K. M. (1995). Similarity determines the attentional blink. *Journal of Experimental Psychology: Human Perception and Performance, 21*, 653–662.

Rinehart, N. J., Bradshaw, J. L., Moss, S. A., Brereton, A. V., & Tonge, B. J. (2000). Atypical interference of local detail on global processing in high-functioning autism and Asperger's disorder. *Journal of Child Psychology and Psychiatry, 41*, 769–778.

Robertson, L. C. (1996). Attentional persistence for features of hierarchical patterns. *Journal of Experimental Psychology: General, 125*, 227–249.

Robertson, L. C., Egly, R., Lamb, M. R., & Kerth, L. (1993). Spatial attention and cuing to global and local levels of hierarchical structure. *Journal of Experimental Psychology: Human Perception and Performance, 19*, 471.

Robertson, L. C., Lamb, M. R., & Knight, R. T. (1988). Effects of lesions of temporal–parietal junction on perceptual and attentional processing in humans. *The Journal of Neuroscience, 8*, 3757–3769.

Schatz, J., & Erlandson, F. (2003). Level-repetition effects in hierarchical stimulus processing: timing and location of cortical activity. *International Journal of Psychophysiology, 47*, 255–269.

Schwent, V. L., & Hillyard, S. A. (1975). Evoked potential correlates of selective attention with multi-channel auditory inputs. *Electroencephalography and Clinical Neurophysiology, 38*, 131–138.

Serences, J. T. (2004). A comparison of methods for characterizing the event-related BOLD timeseries in rapid fMRI. *Neuroimage, 21*, 1690–1700.

Shah, A., & Frith, U. (1983). An islet of ability in autistic children: a research note. *Journal of Child Psychology and Psychiatry, 24*, 613–620.

Shapiro, K. L., Driver, J., Ward, R., & Sorensen, R. (1997). Priming from the attentional blink: a failure to extract visual tokens but not visual types. *Psychological Science, 8*, 357–371.

Śmigasiewicz, K., & Möller, F. (2011). Mechanisms underlying the left visual-field advantage in the dual stream RSVP task: evidence from N2pc, P3, and distractor-evoked VEPs. *Psychophysiology, 48*, 1096–1106.

Srivastava, P., Kumar, D., & Srinivasan, N. (2010). Time course of visual attention across perceptual levels and objects. *Acta Psychologica, 135*, 335–342.

Trujillo-Barreto, N., Iglesias, J., & Valdes-Sosa, M. (submitted for publication). FUN for ERPs: form-free unmixing of overlapped event related potentials.

Valdés Sosa, M., Bobes, M. A., Rodríguez, V., Acosta, Y., Pérez, A., Iglesias, J., et al. (2003). The influence of scene organization on attention: psychophysics and electrophysiology. In J. Duncan & N. Kanwisher (Eds.), *Attention and performance XX* (pp. 321–344). Oxford, UK: Oxford University Press.

Valdes-Sosa, M., Bobes, M. A., Rodriguez, V., & Pinilla, T. (1998). Switching attention without shifting the spotlight: object-based attentional modulation of brain potentials. *Journal of Cognitive Neuroscience, 10*, 137–151.

Volberg, G., & Hübner, R. (2004). On the role of response conflicts and stimulus position for hemispheric differences in global/local processing: an ERP study. *Neuropsychologia, 42*, 1805–1813.

Wang, L., Mottron, L., Peng, D., Berthiaume, C., & Dawson, M. (2007). Local bias and local-to-global interference without global deficit: a robust finding in autism under various conditions of attention, exposure time, and visual angle. *Cognitive Neuropsychology, 24*, 550–574.

Ward, L. M. (1982). Determinants of attention to local and global features of visual forms. *Journal of Experimental Psychology: Human Perception and Performance, 8*, 562–581.

White, S., O'Reilly, H., & Frith, U. (2009). Big heads, small details and autism. *Neuropsychologia, 47*, 1274–1281.

Woldorff, M. G. (1993). Distortion of ERP averages due to overlap from temporally adjacent ERPs: analysis and correction. *Psychophysiology, 30*, 98–119.

Yantis, S., & Jonides, J. (1984). Abrupt visual onset and selective attention: evidence from visual search. *Journal of Experimental Psychology: Human Perception and Performance, 10*, 601–621.

Contour Integration: Sensory, Perceptual, and Attention-Based ERP Components

Michael A. Pitts[1], Antígona Martínez[2, 3]

[1]Department of Psychology, Reed College, Portland, OR, USA, [2]Department of Neurosciences, School of Medicine, University of California San Diego, La Jolla, CA, USA, [3]Nathan Kline Institute for Psychiatric Research, Orangeburg, NY, USA

INTRODUCTION

Contour integration refers to the visual process that groups together local edge elements to form larger boundaries between surfaces and objects. Based on the Gestalt principle of good continuation, contour integration marks an important intermediate step between lower-level edge detection and higher-level object perception. The ability to link together spatially separate contours to perceive the boundaries of objects is especially useful in real-world settings which commonly involve clutter and occlusion. While much research in this area has employed single-unit recordings in non–human primates (Bauer & Heinze, 2002; Gilbert, Ito, Kapadia, & Westheimer, 2000; Ito & Gilbert, 1999; Kapadia, Ito, Gilbert, & Westheimer, 1995; Li & Gilbert, 2002; Li, Piech, & Gilbert, 2006; Li, Piech, & Gilbert, 2008), functional neuroimaging in humans (Altmann, Bulthoff, & Kourtzi, 2003; Cardin, Friston, & Zeki, 2011; Kourtzi, Tolias, Altmann, Augath, & Logothetis, 2003; Schira, Fahle, Donner, Kraft, & Brandt, 2004), and psychophysical and computational modeling approaches (for a review see Wagemans et al., 2012), the present chapter focuses on event-related potential (ERP) signatures of contour integration.

In neurophysiological studies of contour integration, the stimuli employed are typically variants of those created by Field, Hayes, and Hess (1993) (for a review see Hess & Field, 1999). Within arrays of randomly oriented line segments, the orientations of a subset of line segments are arranged to form larger contours (Figure 14.1). Neural responses elicited by displays containing contours, referred to here as "contour" stimuli (Figure 14.1(A)), are contrasted with neural responses elicited by displays made up entirely of randomly oriented line segments, referred to here as "random" stimuli (Figure 14.1(B)). At first glance, this contrast may seem to violate the so-called "Hillyard principle" which states that when manipulating attention or perception, it is best to compare ERPs elicited by physically identical stimuli (Luck, 2005). The comparison between ERPs elicited by contour-present stimuli and contour-absent stimuli, however, is a necessary first step in assessing purely sensory-driven contour integration processes. The ERP *difference* that results from this contrast can then be compared across various conditions in which attention and perception are manipulated.

Previous ERP studies of contour integration have consistently reported a large negative amplitude shift (>5 μV) at posterior electrode sites for contour compared to random stimuli that begin at ~150 ms (post stimulus-onset) and last until ~300 ms (Casco, Campana, Han, & Guzzon, 2009; Machilsen, Novitskiy, Vancleef, & Wagemans, 2011; Mathes & Fahle, 2007; Mathes, Trenner, & Fahle, 2006). A recent magnetoencephalography study reported an analogous contour-specific effect in event-related magnetic field strength over the posterior scalp (Tanskanen, Saarinen, Parkkonen, & Hari, 2008). The contour-specific ERP component, which we refer to as the "contour integration negativity" (or "CIN"), has been found to vary in latency and amplitude depending on the difficulty of the contour detection task, generally occurring later in time and at reduced amplitudes for more difficult-to-detect contours (Machilsen et al., 2011; Mathes et al., 2006).

For tasks that require overt contour discrimination, the contrast between contour and random stimuli is likely to include not only sensory-driven effects, but also

(A) Contour Stimulus **(B)** Random Stimulus

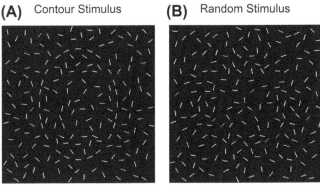

FIGURE 14.1 Examples of stimuli used in contour integration experiments. For contour stimuli (A) the orientations of a subset of line elements are arranged such that a contour is perceived to continue across neighboring lines based on the Gestalt principle of good continuation. For random stimuli (B) the same line segments are present but all are oriented randomly.

postperceptual processes that are only present when the contours are consciously detected. These postperceptual processes include the selection of target candidates for further processing, the comparison of the current contour pattern to a target pattern held in memory, the decision to respond or not, and the preparation and execution of a behavioral response. In other words, it is possible that the CIN reported in previous studies consists of a combination of multiple subcomponents, parts of which reflect contour integration per se, and parts of which reflect selective attention and postperceptual processes related to the subject's task. If so, it should be possible to distinguish which subcomponents of the purported CIN reflect sensory, perceptual, or postperceptual processes, and to determine which of these are modifiable by attention and task demands. The remainder of this chapter describes a series of five experiments aimed at decomposing the CIN via manipulations of stimuli and task, with the overall goal of improving our understanding of the neural processes underlying contour integration.

EXPERIMENT 1: IDENTIFYING THE CIN

Methods and Rationale

As a first step, we sought to replicate the basic finding of a negative amplitude deflection over the posterior scalp at ~150–300 ms for contour vs random stimuli (i.e., the CIN), characterize the scalp topography of the CIN, and test whether its amplitude varies for open vs closed shapes. In this initial study, we created random stimuli and three types of contour stimuli each embedded within a background of randomly oriented line segments: (1) a single vertical contour that could appear in the left or right visual field, (2) a large closed square, and (3) a

(A) Single contour left **(B)** Single contour right

(C) Closed square **(D)** Open square

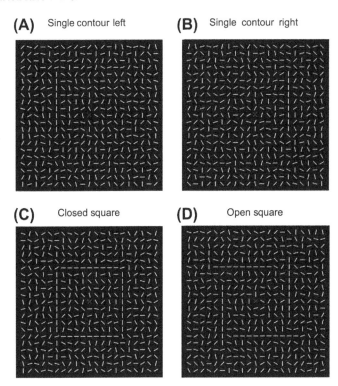

FIGURE 14.2 Example stimuli from experiment 1. The four categories of stimuli consisted of single contours (A, B) appearing at positions slightly above (as shown) or below the horizontal meridian, closed squares (C) of two different sizes (as shown and one notch larger), open squares (D) of two varieties (as shown and a mirror image thereof), and random stimuli (not shown).

large square-like pattern with openings at each corner (see Figure 14.2). The stimulus sequence was randomized and each type of stimulus was 25% probable. For the random stimuli, each 20×20 grid of line segments was created by selecting a random orientation, from $0°$ to $180°$ in $15°$ steps, for the first line segment (e.g., in the bottom left corner of the grid) and then pseudorandomly choosing the orientation of each subsequent line while keeping track of its neighboring line's orientation to prevent accidental collinearity between neighboring lines. For the contour stimuli, we specified the desired orientation of line segments at designated positions on the grid. For all experiments described in this chapter, the stimuli were created with Presentation software (Neurobehavioral Systems, Albany, CA) or a combination of Processing (http://processing.org/) and the Gnu image manipulation program (http://www.gimp.org/). Previous studies have created similar stimuli in Matlab (The Mathworks, Natick, MA) using the grouping elements rendering toolbox (Demeyer & Machilsen, 2012).

Stimuli were presented in a "pattern-change" manner as opposed to an on–off (luminance change) manner. In other words, the arrays of line segments were always visible and ERPs were elicited by line orientation changes rather than array onsets. During the interstimulus

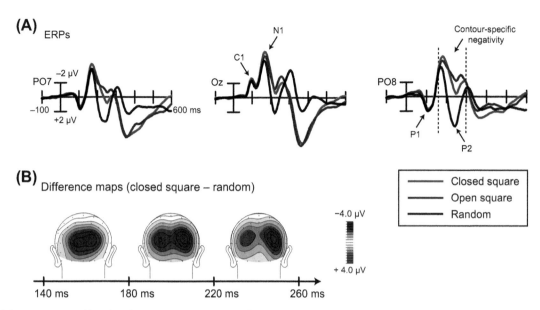

FIGURE 14.3   ERPs elicited by closed square, open square, and random stimuli for three posterior electrode sites (A) the negative voltage deflection for contour stimuli began at ~150 ms and persisted until ~300 ms, overlapping the N1 and P2 peaks (dotted lines indicate range in top right panel). Voltage differences (B) formed by the subtraction of ERPs elicited by squares minus random stimuli plotted over the posterior scalp from 140 to 260 ms.

intervals (ISIs), the line segments were always oriented randomly. The ISI arrays (700–900 ms) briefly switched (for 150 ms) to arrays containing contour patterns or to different random arrays before switching back to an ISI array. These back-to-back changes of line orientations created the perception of apparent rotation of the individual line elements. The decision to present stimuli in this manner as opposed to on–off arrays was motivated by the goal to maximize ERPs specific to contour integration while minimizing the contribution of low-level edge detection. Importantly, to control for local orientation effects, during any particular sequence of stimuli, no two arrays were identical. The orientations of each random control stimulus, each ISI-stimulus, and each stimulus in which contour patterns were embedded were all uniquely generated (thousands of distinct stimuli were created for each subject).

To maintain consistency with previous studies, subjects were trained to perform an overt contour detection task. During four separate blocks of trials (counterbalanced across subjects, $N = 10$), one of the four types of stimuli (single line, closed square, open square, or random) was designated as the target for which subjects were instructed to press a response key upon detection. To isolate the CIN, ERPs elicited by contour stimuli were contrasted with ERPs elicited by random stimuli, excluding blocks in which the stimulus served as the target.

Results and Discussion

ERPs elicited by closed squares, open squares, and random stimuli at three posterior electrode sites are shown

in Figure 14.3(A). In the first 150 ms poststimulus, a typical sequence of visual ERP components (C1, P1, N1) was evident for all stimuli. Amplitudes of the ERPs elicited by contour-present stimuli first diverged from those elicited by random stimuli at around the latency of the N1 (~150 ms). This negative amplitude shift persisted until ~300 ms and was highly similar in timing and general scalp topography to the previously reported contour-specific negativity (e.g., Mathes et al., 2006). Note however that the voltage distribution of the CIN (contour minus random difference maps; Figure 14.3(B)) varied over time and appeared to consist of at least two separate topographies, the first having a central occipital focus and the second showing bilateral occipital–parietal foci with a right hemisphere bias. Also, the amplitude of the CIN was initially greater for closed vs. open squares but this pattern flipped at subsequent latencies (~220 ms), further suggesting the existence of two separable processes.

To investigate the contralaterality of the CIN, ERPs elicited by the single vertical contours were compared to the random stimuli separately for contours appearing in the left and right hemi fields (Figure 14.4). The CIN was evident for these stimuli, albeit at slightly delayed latencies (onset ~200 ms). The CIN was highly contralateral with little or no difference in amplitude between contour and random stimuli at ipsilateral scalp sites. Interestingly, the CIN over the right posterior scalp (elicited by the left hemi field contour) was slightly larger and more focused than the CIN over the left posterior scalp (elicited by the right hemi field contour). This result may suggest a contribution of right hemisphere areas to the detection of contours in both visual fields.

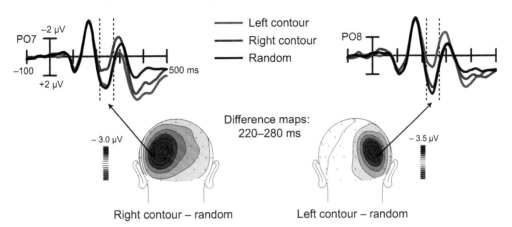

FIGURE 14.4   ERPs elicited by single contours presented to the left or right visual field were compared to those elicited by the random stimuli at left (PO7) and right (PO8) posterior electrode sites. The contour-specific negativity was evident at electrode sites contralateral to the location of the contour. Dotted lines indicate the time windows shown in the difference maps.

To summarize, this experiment replicated the finding of a large (3–6 μV), long-lasting (~150 ms) CIN using our particular stimuli and presentation sequences. It also demonstrated the contralateral nature of the CIN for contours appearing to the left or right of fixation. The shift in scalp topography over time from a central occipital to a bilateral occipital–parietal distribution, as well as the amplitude flip over time for the open and closed shape stimuli, suggests that more than one visual process may contribute to the CIN. The next step was to manipulate the stimuli and the task more systematically in order to directly assess the subcomponents of the CIN.

EXPERIMENT 2: DISTINGUISHING THE CIN FROM THE SELECTION NEGATIVITY

Methods and Rationale

The goal of experiment 2 was to distinguish the CIN from the selection negativity (SN). The SN, originally reported by Harter and Aine (1984), has been characterized as a negative amplitude deflection over the posterior scalp from ~200 to 400 ms elicited by stimuli that contain attended compared to unattended nonspatial features such as a particular color or shape (Hillyard & Anllo-Vento, 1998). For example, Anllo-Vento, Luck, and Hillyard (1998) reported robust SNs for blue checkerboard stimuli when subjects were attending to blue vs. red in order to detect infrequent blue target checkerboards (and similarly for red checkerboards when red was attended). The SN is thought to reflect the selection of a stimulus for further processing in order to determine whether it is a target or not (Hillyard & Anllo-Vento, 1998). Thus, target stimuli and nontarget stimuli that share features with the target elicit robust SNs while stimuli that are less similar to the target elicit weaker or no SNs.

Applying this logic to contour integration, we presented subjects with four types of contour stimuli that consisted of 1, 2, 4, or 5 concentric square-shaped contours (Figure 14.5(A)). On separate blocks, either the 1- or 5-contour stimulus was designated as the target. We expected to observe the largest SNs for the targets in each block and the next largest SNs for stimuli with similar numbers of contours, e.g., the 4 contour stimulus when the target had 5 contours and the 2 contour stimulus when the target had 1 contour. Stimuli that were least similar to the target were expected to show the smallest SNs. Because contour integration is thought to be a low-level sensory-driven process, we expected the CIN to vary in amplitude according to the number of contours (larger for more contours) regardless of which stimulus was the target.

In order to control the overall size of the different contour patterns and to prevent subjects from developing strategies to attend to specific regions of the array, we created size-variants of each type of stimulus so that the location of the inner and outer edges of the contour patterns was balanced across all stimuli. For this experiment, as well as each subsequent experiment described in this chapter, we extended the stimulus duration to 300 ms in order to extend the latency of the stimulus-offset response (the visual ERP elicited by the lines' orientations changing to the next random ISI-stimulus). ISI duration varied between 600 and 800 ms, each type of stimulus was equiprobable (20%), and the order of target blocks was counterbalanced across subjects ($N = 6$). All other methodological details were identical to experiment 1.

Results and Discussion

ERPs elicited by each type of stimulus are plotted separately for blocks in which the 1 contour stimulus was the target and blocks in which the 5 contour stimulus

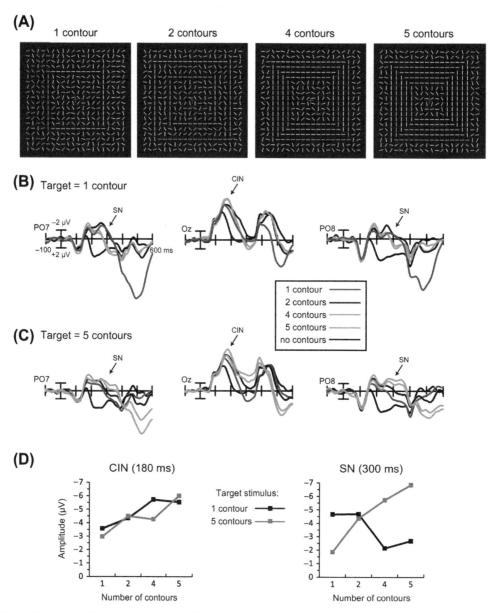

FIGURE 14.5 Example stimuli (A) from experiment 2. ERPs elicited by each stimulus type are displayed separately for trials in which the 1 contour (B) or 5 contour (C) stimulus was the target. The CIN varied in amplitude according to the number of contours, regardless of the target. The SN varied in amplitude according to the target. This pattern of results is summarized (D) by plotting difference amplitudes (contour—random) as a function of number of contours at electrodes Oz and POz for the CIN and SN, respectively.

was the target (Figure 14.5(B) and (C)). The early phase of the broad negative deflection beginning 160 ms post-stimulus was larger for stimuli containing more contours regardless of the target. However, after about 240 ms, negative amplitudes varied according to which stimulus had been designated as the target. Specifically, when the 1 contour stimulus was the target, the 1 contour and 2 contour stimuli produced the most negative ERPs during this latter phase (Figure 14.5(B)); when the 5 contour stimulus was the target, the 5-contour and 4 contour stimuli led to the most negative ERPs (Figure 14.5(C)). The overall pattern of results is summarized in Figure 14.5(D), which

shows that during early time intervals (e.g., 180 ms) difference wave amplitudes (contour minus random) increased as a function of number-of-contours, whereas at later time intervals (e.g., 300 ms), amplitude varied according to target similarity.

This pattern of differential amplitude modulation as a function of number-of-contours vs. behavioral relevance suggests that the early phase of the posterior negativity may be more closely related to contour integration (CIN) while the latter phase reflects selective attention (SN) processes related to target discrimination. Additionally, the scalp topographies of the two phases of the negativity formed by subtracting the random stimulus ERPs from the contour ERPs showed a biphasic pattern similar to experiment 1, i.e., an early central occipital focus followed by bilateral occipital–parietal foci.

In experiments 1 and 2, the contours were always task-relevant and spatially attended. Next, we aimed to manipulate spatial attention and task relevance to determine whether contour integration can occur outside the focus of attention or in situations in which the contours are irrelevant to the task.

EXPERIMENT 3: MODULATION OF CIN AMPLITUDE BY SPATIAL ATTENTION AND TASK RELEVANCE

Methods and Rationale

In experiment 3, we manipulated spatial attention and task relevance in a 2×2 design. In order to assess the effects of spatial attention on contour integration, we split the display into two separate arrays of line segments, each consisting of 10×10 elements, and positioned the arrays to the left and right of fixation (Figure 14.6(A)). During separate blocks of trials, subjects were instructed to attend to either the left or right array and ignore the other array in order to discriminate infrequent target shapes (diamonds: 10% probability) from more frequent standard shapes (squares: 40% probability) and nonshape stimuli (random: 50% probability). The shapes were equally likely to appear in either the left or right array. To assess the effects of task relevance, we overlaid each array with a large red cross and on half of the trials, instead of discriminating shapes, subjects performed a target detection task on the red cross while ignoring the lines segments. On each trial, in synchrony with the line orientation changes, one of the arms of each red cross was slightly reduced in length. Occasionally (10% of trials distributed across the three stimulus types), a cross arm was reduced to a shorter length, and subjects were instructed to press a response key when they detected these larger, infrequent, cross-arm reductions. Thus, contour stimuli could either be spatially attended and task relevant, spatially attended but task irrelevant, spatially unattended but task relevant, or spatially unattended and task irrelevant.

In all four conditions, the stimulus sequence was randomized and stimulus probabilities were identical. Trials including target stimuli were excluded from further analysis. The order in which subjects performed the two tasks (detect diamonds/detect red-cross arm reductions) as well as instructions to attend left or right were counterbalanced across subjects ($N = 16$). All other parameters, including stimulus timing, were identical to experiment 2.

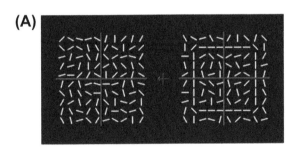

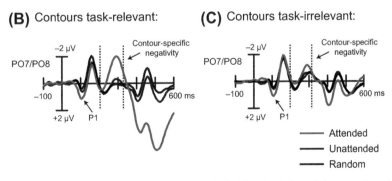

(B) Contours task-relevant:

(C) Contours task-irrelevant:

FIGURE 14.6 Example stimulus (A) from experiment 3. Subjects attended either the left or right array in order to detect diamond-shaped contours (task relevant condition) or reductions in length of the red cross-arms (task irrelevant condition). ERPs (B, C) elicited by square-shaped contours (red & blue) and random stimuli (black) were collapsed over electrode locations contralateral to the contours. The contour-specific negativity was evident for spatially attended contours (red) regardless of task-relevance. Spatially unattended contours (blue) did not elicit significant contour-specific negativities.

The key comparisons were between ERPs recorded at scalp locations contralateral to the square-shaped contours for trials in which spatial attention was present (i.e., focused on the side in which a contour appeared) vs. absent (focused on the opposite side). This same comparison was made for blocks in which the contours were task relevant (subjects responded to diamond targets) vs irrelevant (subjects responded to red cross arm reductions).

Results and Discussion

ERPs recorded at electrodes contralateral to the contours were collapsed across the left/right visual fields, and analyzed according to whether the contours were spatially attended or task relevant. As expected, stimuli containing spatially attended contours elicited enhanced P1 amplitudes compared to ERPs elicited by the same stimuli when unattended. Additionally, spatially attended, task-relevant contours produced robust CIN/SN components (200–320 ms) compared to random stimuli (Figure 14.6(B)). A reduced yet statistically significant negativity was evident between 200 and 300 ms when the eliciting contour stimuli were spatially attended but task irrelevant (Figure 14.6(C)). Spatially unattended yet task-relevant contours, on the other hand, produced a small but insignificant negativity between 260 and 300 ms compared to the random stimuli. ERPs elicited by spatially unattended and task-irrelevant contours did not differ from those elicited by random stimuli.

Based on these results, contour integration appears to require spatial attention given that the CIN and SN components were present for spatially attended contours and absent for spatially unattended contours. In addition, the amplitudes of these posterior negativities were strongly modulated according to task-relevance in the spatially attended condition. A smaller, but still significant negative amplitude shift was evident when the contours were spatially attended but task-irrelevant, suggesting that as long as spatial attention is present contour integration may proceed even if the contours are irrelevant to the task.

This latter finding implies that provided the appropriate setting, i.e., the contours fall within the spotlight of spatial attention, contour integration can occur automatically without any additional top-down amplification or task-based selection processes. To directly test this, it was necessary to ensure that no other processes were contributing to this contour-specific negativity. Notably, in all of the experiments discussed so far, the contours were consciously perceived. In the next experiment, we sought to intentionally hide the contours from subject's conscious awareness via attentional distraction in order to directly assess whether contour integration can proceed automatically.

EXPERIMENT 4: CONTOUR INTEGRATION WITHOUT CONSCIOUS PERCEPTION

Methods and Rationale

To manipulate and measure conscious perception of the contours, we employed an inattentional blindness paradigm, similar to those used by Mack and Rock (1998) and Simons and Chabris (1999). In this type of paradigm, subjects are initially uninformed about a critical stimulus (e.g., a man in a gorilla costume, or in this case a large square) that appears unexpectedly while they perform a distractor task. After being exposed to the critical stimulus in condition 1, subjects are queried as to whether they noticed it. This questioning then acts as a cue such that when subjects are exposed to the same stimulus in condition 2, even while still performing the distractor task, they almost always perceive it. Finally, in condition 3, subjects are instructed to ignore the distractor stimuli and explicitly detect the critical stimulus.

To adapt the inattentional blindness paradigm to an ERP experiment on contour integration, the line segments were presented in the center of the display and were surrounded by a red ring of discs (Figure 14.7(A)). Each time the line segments changed orientation, the surrounding ring rotated clockwise or counterclockwise. The goal was to have subjects diffuse their attention broadly to the surrounding ring of discs in order to complete a difficult target detection task (occasionally one of the discs would dim slightly), and thereby create a situation in which subjects might be inattentionally blind to the square-shaped contours within the task-irrelevant array of line segments.

The key to this version of the inattention paradigm is the subtle difference between condition 1 and condition 2. In both cases, subjects performed the same distractor task on the surrounding ring of discs, i.e., the contours were task-irrelevant in both conditions. The only difference was that subjects who did not notice the contours in condition 1 noticed them in condition 2, due to the intervening questionnaire. Condition 3, in which the task switched to overt contour detection served as a control and was essentially identical to the tasks used in experiments 1 and 2. Thus, this experiment allowed us to compare ERPs elicited by contour vs random stimuli under three conditions in which the contours were: (1) not perceived, (2) perceived but task-irrelevant, and (3) perceived and task-relevant.

Full details of the methods and results of this experiment have been published elsewhere (Pitts, Martinez, & Hillyard, 2012). Briefly, for each of the three conditions, 240 square-shaped contours were presented (40%) along with 300 random stimuli (50%) and 60 diamond-shaped contours (10%). The diamond stimuli served as the targets

(A) Square pattern ────── Random array ──────

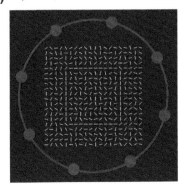 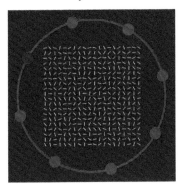

(B) Condition 1: contours not perceived

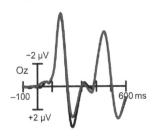

(C) Condition 2: contours perceived but task-irrelevant

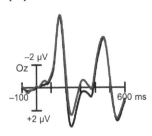

(D) Condition 3: contours perceived and task-relevant

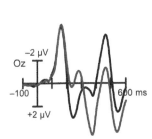

FIGURE 14.7 Example stimuli (A) from experiment 4. ERPs (red = square; black = random) and difference maps (square minus random) for subjects who failed to notice the contours in condition 1 (B–D). The CIN was evident in all conditions, even when subjects were not consciously aware of the contours (B). The CIN was followed by a subsequent negativity (VAN) whenever subjects noticed the contours (C and D). These two components were followed by the SN and a series of P3 components only when the contours were task-relevant (D).

during the contour detection task in the third condition. Following both the first and second conditions, subjects were queried as to whether they noticed any patterns within the array of line segments and asked to describe what they perceived. Regardless of their response to this initial question, they were shown six types of contour patterns: the square, the diamond, and four foil patterns (that never appeared during the experiment) and were asked to rate their confidence in having seen these patterns during the previous round. Based on a combination of responses to these two questions (excluding a few subjects who fell for the foils), 53% of subjects (20 out of 38) failed to perceive the square-shaped contours in condition 1 even after having been exposed to them 240 times. All subjects reported perceiving the contour patterns in condition 2, suggesting that the intervening questions had successfully cued subjects to notice the contours.

Results and Discussion

For each condition, we compared ERPs elicited by the square contour stimuli and the random stimuli. Figure 14.7(B)–(D) shows ERPs and difference topographies for each condition separately. Note that only data from subjects who were inattentionally blind to the contours in condition 1 are plotted here (for the full set of results, see Pitts et al., 2012). During condition 1, even when subjects did not consciously perceive the contour patterns, we observed a significant CIN component over the central occipital scalp from ~220 to 260 ms. When these same subjects later noticed the contours in condition 2, the CIN was followed by a bilateral occipital–parietal negativity from ~300 to 340 ms. This second negativity resembles a component which has previously been linked with conscious perception (see discussion below) and is often referred to as the visual awareness negativity (VAN) (Railo, Koivisto, & Revonsuo, 2011). When the task was altered in condition 3 and the contours became task-relevant, these two posterior negativities (CIN & VAN) shifted to earlier latencies (~180–220 ms and ~220–260 ms, respectively) and were followed by an SN component at ~260–300 ms as well as subsequent P3-like components (~340–380; ~380–420).

This pattern of results, along with the findings from experiment 3, suggests that contour integration can occur automatically and nonconsciously as long as the contours are spatially attended. This process of contour integration is indexed by a central-occipital negativity, designated as the CIN component, that begins anywhere between ~150 and ~250 ms following stimulus onset, depending on the specific task demands. In addition to helping us further characterize the temporal flexibility of the CIN, this experiment suggested a third subcomponent of the large-amplitude, long-duration, posterior negativity observed in our previous experiments. This third subcomponent was temporally situated between the CIN and the SN in condition 3 (contours perceived and task relevant), it appeared after the CIN in condition 2 (contours perceived but task irrelevant), and it was absent in condition 1 (contours not perceived). Hence, this intermediate negativity appeared whenever subjects consciously perceived the contours and was distinguishable from the sensory-based CIN and task-based SN components. Our working hypothesis is that this third subcomponent may index the establishment of the percept itself, thus we refer to this component as the VAN.

Previous studies that have manipulated visual awareness using different methods, such as backward masking and the attentional blink, reported a similar bilateral occipital–parietal negativity at around 200–300 ms (VAN) that distinguishes aware from unaware conditions (Koivisto, Revonsuo, & Lehtonen, 2006; Sergent, Baillet, & Dehaene, 2005; for a review see Railo et al., 2011). An alternative explanation is that the apparent VAN observed these experiments, as well as in condition 2 of this experiment, is actually a small, temporally variable SN. For example, in condition 2 subjects may have shifted their attention to the contours immediately after evaluating the distractor ring for the presence of a target. These attentional shifts may have been marked by SNs, but because of intertrial and intersubject timing variability in searching the distractor ring, the average SN would appear smaller in amplitude and broader in duration compared to condition 3, in which the primary task was contour detection. Nonetheless, in agreement with the VAN interpretation, we observed a frontally distributed selection positivity (SP) that appeared only in condition 3 (contours perceived and task relevant) and not in condition 2 (perceived but task irrelevant). The SP typically precedes the SN by ~20–50 ms and is thought to index similar selective attention processes as the SN (Hillyard & Anllo-Vento, 1998). If the putative VAN in condition 2 is actually an SN, we would expect to see an SP here as well, but instead there were no signs of an SP in condition 2. While the possible identification of an ERP component that indexes conscious perception is intriguing, more work is necessary to fully evaluate whether this midlatency occipital–parietal negativity is really an index of visual awareness that is distinguishable from attention and task-based components such as the SN (e.g., see Verleger, 2010).

EXPERIMENT 5: MODULATION OF CIN LATENCY BY TASK RELEVANCE

Methods and Rationale

To further explore how the latency of the CIN varies according to the task, we conducted a follow-up study to experiment 4 using the same red-ring distractor task but varied the stimuli to include 1, 3, or 5 contours. Each contour stimulus along with a random stimulus was equiprobable (22.5%). A stimulus containing 2 contours (10% probable) served as the target for the contour detection task. Dim red circle targets appeared in 10% of trials distributed across the stimulus types, and all target trials were excluded from analysis. In this experiment, subjects were informed of the presence of contours at the beginning of the experiment, and the tasks (contour detection vs. dim red circle detection) were counterbalanced across subjects ($N = 19$). All other parameters were identical to experiment 4.

Results and Discussion

As in experiment 4, we observed a dramatic latency shift of the CIN according to task relevance (Figure 14.8). Specifically, the onset latency of the CIN was ~140 ms when the contours were task-relevant and ~210 ms when the same contours were task-irrelevant. This negative amplitude shift for contour-present vs. contour-absent stimuli does not appear to be a modulation of the N1 or P2, as it can overlap either peak depending on the task while retaining a consistent scalp topography, i.e., a central-occipital focus. These findings suggest that automatic processes such as contour integration do not follow a rigid time course but, instead, maintain a high degree of temporal flexibility. This flexibility may allow for processing adjustments according to task demands.

GENERAL DISCUSSION

In order to determine the neural basis of contour integration, the present series of experiments suggest that it is critical to distinguish between sensory (CIN), perceptual (VAN), and attention-based (SN) processes. In experiment 1 we replicated the basic finding of a large amplitude, long latency negativity over the posterior scalp for contour-present vs. contour-absent stimuli. In experiment 2,

by parametrically manipulating the number of contours in the stimulus as well as the relationship between each stimulus and the target, we distinguished the CIN from the subsequent SN component. In experiment 3, we determined that spatial attention is necessary for contour integration, while task relevance can modulate but not eliminate the CIN. Experiment 4 revealed that contour integration can occur in the absence of awareness (during inattentional blindness), while also suggesting a third subcomponent intermediate in time to the CIN and SN (the VAN). Finally, experiment 5 confirmed the substantial temporal flexibility of the CIN according to the task.

One of the most interesting and potentially fruitful avenues for research in this area will be to determine how these ERP results correspond to the findings from single-unit recordings and from functional magnetic resonance imaging (fMRI). While it is currently not possible to precisely localize the neuroanatomical sources of ERP components, the scalp topographies along with source estimates (using the LORETA algorithm; Pitts et al., 2012) suggest an early visual cortex generator for the CIN, along with lateral occipital complex (LOC) generators for the subsequent negativities (VAN and SN). If the CIN is generated in V1/V2, its relatively late onset (~150–200 ms) could suggest that this component reflects delayed feedback to anatomically "early" visual areas. Since ERPs are most likely reflections of input to an area rather than output from an area (Kappenman & Luck, 2012), the CIN might reflect feedback from the LOC to V1/V2, while the VAN and SN may index subsequent higher-level processing once contour integration has been carried out and this information is transferred back to the LOC. While feedback and recurrence have been suggested as possible neural correlates of awareness (e.g., Lamme, 2006), the present results suggest that delayed feedback may not be sufficient for awareness, as the CIN component was evident even during inattentional blindness.

With regards to future ERP studies, it will be interesting to see how far the temporal variability of the CIN can be pushed. In the studies reported here, we observed the CIN to onset as early as ~140 ms and as late as ~220 ms,

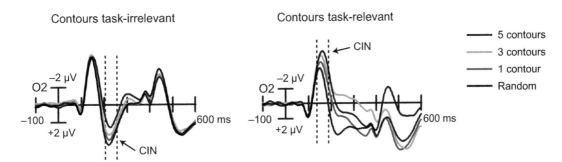

FIGURE 14.8 In a follow-up to experiment 4, subjects were presented 1-, 3-, or 5-contour stimuli while they performed a task on a ring surrounding the line segment arrays making the contours task-irrelevant, or while they performed a contour detection task. The amplitude of the CIN shown here at occipital electrode O2 was modulated by the number of contours in the stimulus, while the latency of the CIN varied according to task relevance.

thus overlapping the N1 and/or P2 components. Might it be possible to configure the stimuli, task, and perceptual training such that the CIN onsets even earlier, possibly overlapping the P1 or C1 peaks, or even later during the N2 peak? The way these line segment arrays are designed permits seemingly infinite options for systematic manipulations of contour salience. The contours can be embedded within dense arrays of randomly oriented distractors (as was the case in our studies here), the distractors could be oriented similarly to create a homogenous background leading to enhanced contrast for the contours, or the contours and/or distractor segments could be made more or less dense to manipulate crowding and thereby alter contour salience. Such studies would help determine the role of surround inhibition in contour integration and more thoroughly assess the automaticity vs. attention-demanding characteristics of contour integration processes.

Another avenue for future research will be to determine how the neural mechanisms supporting texture segregation and contour integration are related. Interestingly, single-unit, fMRI, and ERP studies of texture segregation have reported similar patterns of results to those of contour integration, namely V1 single-cell modulations, increases in LOC activity, and posterior negativities for texture-present stimuli vs. texture-absent stimuli, respectively (Bach & Meigen, 1992, 1997; Kastner, De Weerd, & Ungerleider, 2000; Lamme, 1995). In the ERP literature, this component has been dubbed the texture segregation visual evoked potential (tsVEP). Stimuli used in texture segregation experiments are often created using the same types of multielement line segment arrays as those used in contour integration experiments (e.g., Scholte, Jolij, Fahrenfort, & Lamme, 2008). However, instead of comparing neural responses elicited by stimuli containing collinear segments vs. randomly oriented segments, contrasts are made between stimuli containing patches of similarly oriented line segments within a background of orthogonally oriented segments to stimuli containing only homogenously oriented segments. Notably, texture segregation experiments have reported at least two temporally distinct phases of activity, the first of which appears to be automatic while the latter can be modulated by attention and awareness (Heinrich, Andres, & Bach, 2007; Roelfsema, Tolboom, & Khayat, 2007; Scholte, Witteveen, Spekreijse, & Lamme, 2006). It may be fruitful to directly compare the CIN to the tsVEP within the same study while manipulating attention, perception, or task-relevance.

CONCLUSION

The study of the neural processes supporting contour integration is still in its infancy and much remains to be discovered. The purpose of the series of ERP experiments described in this chapter was to determine whether a distinct ERP component reflecting contour integration (CIN) can be isolated from other related components (e.g., VAN and SN), and to assess the roles of attention and task-relevance on this visual process. The pattern of results reported here may help inform not only future ERP experiments, but also single-unit and fMRI studies, especially with regards to experimental design. It will be increasingly important to encourage collaborative efforts employing various neurophysiological and neuroimaging techniques in order to further our understanding of this important midlevel visual process.

Acknowledgments

The authors thank Jennifer Padwal for her careful and enthusiastic assistance in collecting and analyzing data for a number of experiments described in this chapter. This work was supported in part by the Kavli Institute for Brain and Mind (KIBM Innovative Research Award 2010–2011), the National Institutes of Health (2 R01 EY016984-35 and 1P50MH86385), and the National Science Foundation (BCS-1029084).

References

Altmann, C. F., Bulthoff, H. H., & Kourtzi, Z. (2003). Perceptual organization of local elements into global shapes in the human visual cortex. *Current Biology*, 13(4), 342–349.

Anllo-Vento, L., Luck, S. J., & Hillyard, S. A. (1998). Spatio-temporal dynamics of attention to color: evidence from human electrophysiology. *Human Brain Mapping*, 6(4), 216–238.

Bach, M., & Meigen, T. (1992). Electrophysiological correlates of texture segregation in the human visual evoked potential. *Vision Research*, 32(3), 417–424.

Bach, M., & Meigen, T. (1997). Similar electrophysiological correlates of texture segregation induced by luminance, orientation, motion and stereo. *Vision Research*, 37(11), 1409–1414.

Bauer, R., & Heinze, S. (2002). Contour integration in striate cortex. Classic cell responses or cooperative selection? *Experimental Brain Research*, 147(2), 145–152.

Cardin, V., Friston, K. J., & Zeki, S. (2011). Top-down modulations in the visual form pathway revealed with dynamic causal modeling. *Cerebral Cortex*, 21(3), 550–562.

Casco, C., Campana, G., Han, S., & Guzzon, D. (2009). Psychophysical and electrophysiological evidence of independent facilitation by collinearity and similarity in texture grouping and segmentation. *Vision Research*, 49(6), 583–593.

Demeyer, M., & Machilsen, B. (2012). The construction of perceptual grouping displays using GERT. *Behavior Research Methods*, 44(2), 439–446.

Field, D. J., Hayes, A., & Hess, R. F. (1993). Contour integration by the human visual-system – evidence for a local association field. *Vision Research*, 33(2), 173–193.

Gilbert, C., Ito, M., Kapadia, M., & Westheimer, G. (2000). Interactions between attention, context and learning in primary visual cortex. *Vision Research*, 40(10–12), 1217–1226.

Harter, M., & Aine, C. (1984). Brain mechanisms of visual selective attention. In P. Parasuraman & D. Davis (Eds.), *Varieties of attention* (pp. 293–321). New York: Academic Press.

Heinrich, S. P., Andres, M., & Bach, M. (2007). Attention and visual texture segregation. *Journal of Vision*, 7(6), 6.

Hess, R., & Field, D. (1999). Integration of contours: new insights. *Trends in Cognitive Sciences*, 3(12), 480–486.

Hillyard, S. A., & Anllo-Vento, L. (1998). Event-related brain potentials in the study of visual selective attention. *Proceedings of the National Academy of Sciences of the United States of America, 95*(3), 781–787.

Ito, M., & Gilbert, C. D. (1999). Attention modulates contextual influences in the primary visual cortex of alert monkeys. *Neuron, 22*(3), 593–604.

Kapadia, M. K., Ito, M., Gilbert, C. D., & Westheimer, G. (1995). Improvement in visual sensitivity by changes in local context: parallel studies in human observers and in V1 of alert monkeys. *Neuron, 15*(4), 843–856.

Kappenman, E. S., & Luck, S. J. (2012). ERP components: the ups and downs of brainwave recordings. In S. J. Luck & E. S. Kappenman (Eds.), *The Oxford handbook of event-related potential components.* New York: Oxford University Press.

Kastner, S., De Weerd, P., & Ungerleider, L. G. (2000). Texture segregation in the human visual cortex: a functional MRI study. *Journal of Neurophysiology, 83*(4), 2453–2457.

Koivisto, M., Revonsuo, A., & Lehtonen, M. (2006). Independence of visual awareness from the scope of attention: an electrophysiological study. *Cerebral Cortex, 16*(3), 415–424.

Kourtzi, Z., Tolias, A. S., Altmann, C. F., Augath, M., & Logothetis, N. K. (2003). Integration of local features into global shapes: monkey and human FMRI studies. *Neuron, 37*(2), 333–346.

Lamme, V. A. (1995). The neurophysiology of figure-ground segregation in primary visual cortex. *Journal of Neuroscience, 15*(2), 1605–1615.

Lamme, V. A. (2006). Towards a true neural stance on consciousness. *Trends in Cognitive Sciences, 10*(11), 494–501.

Li, W., & Gilbert, C. D. (2002). Global contour saliency and local colinear interactions. *Journal of Neurophysiology, 88*(5), 2846–2856.

Li, W., Piech, V., & Gilbert, C. D. (2006). Contour saliency in primary visual cortex. *Neuron, 50*(6), 951–962.

Li, W., Piech, V., & Gilbert, C. D. (2008). Learning to link visual contours. *Neuron, 57*(3), 442–451.

Luck, S. J. (2005). *An introduction to the event-related potential technique.* Cambridge, MA: MIT Press.

Machilsen, B., Novitskiy, N., Vancleef, K., & Wagemans, J. (2011). Context modulates the ERP signature of contour integration. *PLos One, 6*(9).

Mack, A., & Rock, I. (1998). *Inattentional Blindness.* Cambridge, MA: MIT Press.

Mathes, B., & Fahle, M. (2007). The electrophysiological correlate of contour integration is similar for color and luminance mechanisms. *Psychophysiology, 44*(2), 305–322.

Mathes, B., Trenner, D., & Fahle, M. (2006). The electrophysiological correlate of contour integration is modulated by task demands. *Brain Research, 1114*(1), 98–112.

Pitts, M. A., Martinez, A., & Hillyard, S. A. (2012). Visual processing of contour patterns under conditions of inattentional blindness. *Journal of Cognitive Neuroscience, 24*(2), 287–303.

Railo, H., Koivisto, M., & Revonsuo, A. (2011). Tracking the processes behind conscious perception: a review of event-related potential correlates of visual consciousness. *Consciousness and Cognition, 20*(3), 972–983.

Roelfsema, P. R., Tolboom, M., & Khayat, P. S. (2007). Different processing phases for features, figures, and selective attention in the primary visual cortex. *Neuron, 56*(5), 785–792.

Schira, M. M., Fahle, M., Donner, T. H., Kraft, A., & Brandt, S. A. (2004). Differential contribution of early visual areas to the perceptual process of contour processing. *Journal of Neurophysiology, 91*(4), 1716–1721.

Scholte, H. S., Jolij, J., Fahrenfort, J. J., & Lamme, V. A. (2008). Feedforward and recurrent processing in scene segmentation: electroencephalography and functional magnetic resonance imaging. *Journal of Cognitive Neuroscience, 20*(11), 2097–2109.

Scholte, H. S., Witteveen, S. C., Spekreijse, H., & Lamme, V. A. (2006). The influence of inattention on the neural correlates of scene segmentation. *Brain Research, 1076*(1), 106–115.

Sergent, C., Baillet, S., & Dehaene, S. (2005). Timing of the brain events underlying access to consciousness during the attentional blink. *Nature Neuroscience, 8*(10), 1391–1400.

Simons, D. J., & Chabris, C. F. (1999). Gorillas in our midst: sustained inattentional blindness for dynamic events. *Perception, 28*(9), 1059–1074.

Tanskanen, T., Saarinen, J., Parkkonen, L., & Hari, R. (2008). From local to global: cortical dynamics of contour integration. *Journal of Vision, 8*(7).

Verleger, R. (2010). Markers of awareness? EEG potentials evoked by faint and masked events, with special reference to the "attentional blink". In I. Czigler & I. Winkler (Eds.), *Unconscious memory representations in perception: Processes and mechanisms in the brain* (pp. 37–70). Amsterdam: John Benjamins Publishing Company.

Wagemans, J., Elder, J. H., Kubovy, M., Palmer, S. E., Peterson, M. A., Singh, M., et al. (2012). A century of Gestalt psychology in visual perception: I. Perceptual grouping and figure-ground organization. *Psychological Bulletin, 138*(6), 1172–1217.

Attentional Control of Multisensory Integration is Preserved in Aging

Jyoti Mishra, Adam Gazzaley

Department of Neurology, Physiology and Psychiatry, Sandler Neurosciences Center,
University of California, San Francisco, San Francisco, CA, USA

INTRODUCTION

Integration of multisensory information concurrent in the auditory and visual modalities is a vital feature of sensory processing. While it has been consistently shown that unisensory processing degrades with age (Bayles & Kasniak, 1987; Chao and Knight, 1997; Clapp & Gazzaley, 2012; Corso, 1971; Craik & Salthouse, 2000, p. 755; Gazzaley, Cooney, Rissman, & D'Esposito, 2005; Gazzaley et al., 2008; Habak & Faubert, 2000; Keller, Morton, Thomas, & Potter, 1999; Lichtenstein, 1992; Nusbaum, 1999; Zanto, Hennigan, Ostberg, Clapp, & Gazzaley, 2010; Zanto, Toy, & Gazzaley, 2010; Zanto et al., 2011), there are very few studies and little consensus on the impact of aging on multisensory interactions (Cienkowski & Carney, 2002; Helfer, 1998; Stine, Wingfield, & Myers, 1990; Strupp, Arbusow, Borges Pereira, Dieterich, & Brandt, 1999). Laurienti, Burdette, Maldjian, and Wallace (2006) attributed the lack of consensus in the literature to ambiguities in research design that result in an inability to distinguish multisensory processing from higher-order cognitive operations, use of test conditions that do not resemble real-world stimulus environments, and variability in data analyses methods. While the fate of multisensory integration during aging remains somewhat undecided, to the best of our knowledge, it remains largely unknown as to how top-down attentional control interacts with multisensory information processing in older adults.

To date, multisensory research in aging has largely focused on performance in one task-relevant sensory modality while stimuli from another task-irrelevant modality are presented (Guerreiro & Van Gerven, 2011; Hugenschmidt, Mozolic, & Laurienti, 2009; Peiffer et al., 2009; Poliakoff, Ashworth, Lowe, & Spence, 2006; Townsend, Adamo, & Haist, 2006). Most of these studies have shown equivalent performance in older and younger adults (Hugenschmidt et al., 2009; Peiffer et al., 2009; Townsend et al., 2006), while others have observed that older adults suffer from greater interference to visual distractions relative to distractions in any other modality (auditory/tactile), and further that this differential modality impact is significantly larger in older than in younger adults (Guerreiro & Van Gerven, 2011; Poliakoff et al., 2006). While these studies used interspersed auditory/visual/tactile information streams, none of them employed concurrent multisensory (e.g., audiovisual) stimuli. Two behavioral investigations that did investigate concurrent audiovisual (av) processing in older and younger adults showed superior performance on av stimuli relative to unisensory auditory or visual stimuli in both younger and older adults (Laurienti et al., 2006; Strupp et al., 1999). In fact, the extent of the multisensory performance gain was found to be greater in the older age group. Importantly, this research suggested that in the face of age-related decline of unisensory processing capacities, older adults may benefit from multisensory environments such that their abilities are equivalent to or even surpass that of younger adults.

While research on multisensation and aging is still nascent, the intersection of attention and aging has been dissected to some extent in recent years (Gazzaley, 2013; Zanto and Gazzaley, in press). Specifically, selective attention paradigms have been used to assess attention to task-relevant information presented amidst other task-irrelevant stimuli that are to be ignored. Findings that older adults generally exhibit poor attention performance relative to younger adults are no surprise, given that the gamut of top-down cognitive abilities ranging from perception to attention to memory to action control is found to be deficient in older adults (Craik & Salthouse, 2000, p. 755; Greenwood, 2000). Recent neural evidence has further indicated that the observed age-related attention deficits in behavior specifically stem from an inability to effectively suppress the neural processing associated with the distracting information stream, while enhanced neural processing to attended stimuli is relatively well-preserved in older adults (Clapp & Gazzaley, 2012; Gazzaley et al., 2005, 2008; Zanto, Hennigan, et al., 2010; Zanto, Toy, et al., 2010; Zanto et al., 2011). Furthermore, this selective top-down suppression deficit during presentation of distracting information is correlated with the memory impairments subsequently probed in older adults (Clapp & Gazzaley, 2012; Wais, Rubens, Boccanfuso, & Gazzaley, 2010).

While unisensory selective attention has been studied in older adults, the mechanisms and outcomes of multisensory attention are not known for this age group. In a recent study in younger adults, we evaluated behavioral performance and neural processing of multisensory stimuli during two attention manipulations, (1) selective attention focused on one sensory modality (visual) vs (2) attention distributed across the visual and auditory modalities (Mishra & Gazzaley, 2012). The task design utilized spatio-temporally coincident audiovisual stimuli that were either semantically congruent (e.g., auditory: comb; visual: comb) or incongruent (e.g., auditory: rock; visual: comb) and were presented intermixed in a stream of isolated auditory and visual stimuli. Performance accuracies, response times, and event-related potentials (ERPs) were recorded as participants detected animal targets amongst nonanimal stimuli appearing in the visual and audiovisual stimuli streams, but not the auditory stream, during focused visual attention, and in either auditory/visual/audiovisual stimuli streams during distributed audiovisual attention. Importantly, the goals were never divided across different tasks (e.g., monitoring stimuli from multiple categories, such as animals and vehicles). Thus, we investigated selective attention toward a single task goal focused within vision or distributed across vision and audition. The two attentional variations (focused visual vs. distributed audiovisual) were, thus, compared under identical stimulus presentations to enable analysis of the impact of top-down goals on processing of identical bottom-up inputs; this is an important tenet of elegant attention experimental design as recommended for cognitive electrophysiology studies of attention by Steve Hillyard (Hillyard & Anllo-Vento, 1998).

Our study in younger adults generated novel findings that distributed audiovisual attention yield performance benefits over focused visual attention. These benefits during distributed relative to focused attention for congruent audiovisual stimuli were observed in the form of significantly faster reaction times with uncompromised accuracies. In the case of incongruent audiovisual stimuli, significantly improved target detection accuracies were observed under distributed relative to focused attention; in fact, performance deficits during focused visual attention due to stimulus incongruity were resolved under distributed audiovisual attention. Furthermore, consistent neural signatures emerged: early sensory processing of both auditory and visual constituents of the audiovisual stimuli had reduced amplitudes under distributed audiovisual relative to focused visual attention, for congruent as well as incongruent stimuli. Thus, the overall performance improvements under distributed attention were consistently associated with reduced neural processing.

Associations between improved performance and reduced neural processing have usually been observed in the perceptual learning literature. ERP recordings and functional magnetic resonance imaging (fMRI) studies of perceptual training have found that training-related behavioral improvements exhibit reduced post-training sensorineural signals (Alain & Snyder, 2008; Berry et al., 2010; Ding, Song, Fan, Qu, & Chen, 2003; Kelley & Yantis, 2010; Mukai et al., 2007). Further, individuals with trained attention expertise such as action video game players (Green & Bavelier, 2003) have been observed to have reduced neural responses to task-irrelevant stimuli relative to nonexperts (Mishra, Zinni, Bavelier, & Hillyard, 2011). The results of these plasticity studies have led to the interpretation that enhanced behavioral performance is associated with increased neural efficacy, as reflected in the reduced neural responses (Erickson et al., 2007). Hence, in our study with younger adults, we interpreted our findings of reduced neural processing associated with improved behavioral performance under distributed audiovisual relative to focused visual attention, to be suggestive of enhanced efficacy of multisensory processing underlying distributed audiovisual attention (Mishra & Gazzaley, 2012).

In the present study, we extend our novel paradigm investigating attentional control of multisensory integration in younger adults to healthy older individuals. Our paradigm is better suited for this research relative to previous designs in this domain (Degerman et al., 2007; Talsma, Doty, & Woldorff, 2007) as it explores multisensory integration in the context of spatio-temporal and semantic congruity, as well as incongruity of audiovisual stimuli that are often encountered in daily environments and thus has real-world relevance. Our goal was to assess if the interaction between attention and multisensory stimuli at the level of behavior, as well as underlying neural responses, is preserved with aging. Specifically, we investigated whether multisensory behavior is improved under distributed relative to focused attention and whether the concomitant underlying neural correlates suggest improved neural efficacy in older adults as previously found for younger adults.

MATERIALS AND METHODS

Participants

Twenty-two healthy older adults (mean age 68.5 years; range 60–82 years; nine females) gave informed consent to participate in the study approved by the Committee on Human Research at the University of California in San Francisco. All participants were screened to ensure they had no history of neurological, psychiatric, or vascular disease, were not depressed, were not taking any psychotropic medications, and had a minimum of 12 years of education. Participants were additionally screened using a 12 multiple-choice questionnaire to document no hearing problems in daily life situations. Prior to the experiment, all participants were examined for normal or corrected-to-normal vision using a Snellen chart, and for normal hearing tested in both ears in the 250–6 kHz frequency range as estimated by an audiometry software application UHear©. Individuals with poorer hearing sensitivities than in the "mild loss" range, as per UHear© results, were excluded from the study. Data from a cohort of 20 younger participants (mean age 23.4 years, range 19–29 years, 10 females) who previously engaged in the same experiment were utilized for age-group comparisons (Mishra & Gazzaley, 2012).

Neuropsychological Testing

Prior to the experiment, older adults were administered a battery of 13 neuropsychological tests. Participants were required to score within two standard deviations of published age-matched normative values on these tests to be included in the study. The neuropsychological evaluation consisted of tests designed to assess general intellectual function (Folstein, Folstein, & McHugh, 1975), verbal learning (CVLT-II), geriatric depression, visual-spatial function (modified Rey-Osterrieth figure), visual-episodic memory (memory for details of a modified Rey–Osterrieth Complex Figure (ROCF: Osterrieth, 1944; Rey, 1941), visual-motor sequencing (trail making tests A and B), phonemic fluency (words beginning with the letter "D"), semantic fluency (animals), calculation ability (arithmetic), executive functioning (Weschler, 2008), working memory and incidental recall, backward digit span and digit symbol, and WAIS-R.

Stimuli and Experimental Procedure

Stimuli were presented on presentation software (Neurobehavioral Systems, Inc.) run on a Dell Optiplex GX620 with a 22″ Mitsubishi Diamond Pro 2040U CRT monitor. Participants were seated with a chin rest in a dark room 80 cm from the monitor. Visual stimuli (v) were words presented as black text in Arial font in a gray square sized 4.8° at the fovea. Auditory words (a), were spoken in a male voice, normalized and equated in average power spectral density, and presented to participants at a comfortable sound level of 65 dB SPL using insert earphones (Cortech Solutions, LLC). Prior to the experiment, participants were presented with all auditory stimuli once, which they repeated to ensure 100% word recognition. All spoken and printed word nouns were simple, mostly monosyllabic everyday usage words, e.g., tree, rock, vase, bike, tile, book, plate, soda, ice, boat, etc. The experiment used 116 unique written and corresponding spoken words as visual and auditory stimuli, respectively; of these 46 words were animal names (cat, chimp, cow, deer, bear, hippo, dog, rat, toad, fish, etc.) and served as targets. Visual stimuli were presented for a duration of 100 ms, all auditory presentations had a 250 ms duration, and audiovisual stimuli (av) had simultaneous onset of the auditory and visual stimulus constituents. The spoken and written words were identical for congruent (av) stimuli and nonidentical for incongruent (av) stimuli. Each experimental run consisted of 360 randomized stimuli (shuffled from the set of 116 unique stimuli), with an equivalent 120 (v) alone, (a) alone, and (av) stimulus presentations. The interstimulus interval for all stimulus types was jittered at 800–1100 ms. Each experimental block run thus lasted 6 min, with a few seconds of a selfpaced break available to participants every quarter block. Stimuli were randomized at each block quarter to ensure equivalent distribution of (a), (v), and (av) stimuli in each quarter.

There were four unique block types randomly presented (Figure 15.1), with each block type repeated twice and the repeat presentation occurring after each block type had been presented at least once: Block type 1: Congruent—Focused Visual; Block type 2: Congruent—Distributed Audiovisual; Block type 3: Incongruent—Focused Visual; Block type 4: Incongruent—Distributed Audiovisual. Participants were briefed as per the upcoming block type, about the attention requirements (focused vs distributed) as well as stimulus congruency (congruent vs incongruent). Block type (1) had congruent (av) stimuli and participants were instructed to focus attention only on the visual stream and respond with a button press to visual animal targets, whether appearing as (v) alone or (av) stimuli (congruent focused visual attention block). In block type (2), (av) stimuli were again congruent and participants were instructed to distribute attention across both auditory and visual modalities and detect all animal names, appearing either in the (v), (a), or (av) stream (congruent distributed audiovisual attention block). In block type (3), (av) stimuli were

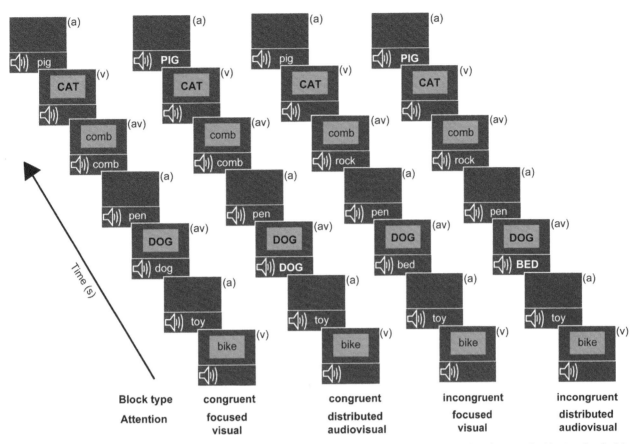

FIGURE 15.1 Overview of experimental block design. All blocks consisted of randomly interspersed auditory only (a), visual only (v), and simultaneous audiovisual (av) stimuli, labeled in each frame. The auditory and visual constituent stimuli of audiovisual trials matched during the two congruent blocks, and did not match on incongruent blocks. Target stimuli (animal words) in each block stream are depicted in uppercase (though they did not differ in actual salience during the experiment). During the focused visual attention blocks, participants detected visual animal word targets occurring in either the (v) or (av) stream. During the distributed audiovisual attention blocks, participants detected animal targets occurring in either of three stimulus streams.

incongruent and participants were instructed to focus attention on the visual stream only and respond to visual animal targets, either appearing alone or co-occurring with a conflicting nonanimal auditory stimulus (incongruent focused visual attention block). Lastly, in block type (4), (av) stimuli were incongruent and participants distributed attention to both (a) and (v) stimuli detecting animal names in either (v), (a), or incongruent (av) stream (incongruent distributed audiovisual attention block). Note that focused auditory block types were not included in the experiment in order to constrain the number of experimental manipulations and provide high quality neurobehavioral data minimally contaminated by fatigue effects.

Targets in the (a), (v), or (av) streams appeared at 20% probability. To further clarify, for the (av) stream in congruent blocks ((1) and (2)), visual animal targets were paired with identical auditory animal targets, while in incongruent blocks ((3) and (4)), visual animal targets were paired with auditory nonanimal stimuli, i.e., there were no visual nonanimal stimuli paired with auditory animal

targets in incongruent blocks ((3) and (4)). These particular aspects of the (av) stimuli pairing were unknown to participants (though, in general, participants knew whether an upcoming block was congruent or incongruent) and maintained the same number of visual constituent targets within the (av) streams across all blocks. Note that performance metrics were obtained for targets in the (v) and (av) streams in all blocks, while performance on targets in the (a) stream was only obtained in the distributed audiovisual attention blocks (2) and (4); targets in the (a) stream in the focused visual attention blocks (1) and (3) were not attended to and did not have associated responses.

Participants were instructed to fixate at the center of the screen at all times, and were provided feedback as per their average percent correct accuracy and RTs at the end of each block. Speed and accuracy were both emphasized in the behavior and correct responses were scored within a 200–1200 ms period after stimulus onset. Correct responses to targets were categorized as "hits" while responses to nontarget stimuli in either modality were classified as "false alarms". The hit and false alarm rates were used to derive the sensitivity estimate d' in each modality (MacMillan & Creelman, 1991).

EEG Data Acquisition

Data were recorded during eight blocks (two per block type) yielding 192 epochs of data for each standard (v)/(a)/(av) stimulus (and 48 epochs per target) per block type. Electrophysiological signals were recorded with a BioSemi ActiveTwo 64-channel electroencephalography (EEG) acquisition system in conjunction with BioSemi ActiView software (Cortech Solutions, LLC). Signals were amplified and digitized at 1024 Hz with a 24-bit resolution. All electrode offsets were maintained between ±20 mV.

The three-dimensional coordinates of each electrode and of three fiducial landmarks (the left and right pre-auricular points and the nasion) were determined by means of a BrainSight (Rogue Research, Inc.) spatial digitizer. The mean Cartesian coordinates for each site were averaged across all subjects and used for top-ographic mapping and source localization procedures.

Data Analysis

Raw EEG data were digitally rereferenced off-line to the average of the left and right mastoids. Eye arti-facts were removed through independent component analyses by excluding components consistent with topographies for blinks and eye movements and the elec-trooculogram time-series. Data were high-pass filtered at 0.1 Hz to exclude ultraslow DC drifts. This prepro-cessing was conducted in the Matlab (The Mathworks, Inc.) EEGLab toolbox (Swartz Center for Computational Neuroscience, UC San Diego). Further data analyses were performed using custom ERPSS software (Event-Related Potential Software System, UC San Diego). All ERP analyses were confined to the standard (nontarget) (v), (a), and (av) stimuli. Signals were averaged in 500 ms epochs with a 100 ms prestimulus interval. The averages were digitally low-pass filtered with a Gaussian finite impulse function (3 dB attenuation at 46 Hz) to remove high-frequency noise produced by muscle movements and external electrical sources. Epochs that exceeded a voltage threshold of ±75 μV were rejected.

Components of interest were quantified in the 0–300 ms ERPs over distinct electrode sets that corre-sponded to sites at which component peak amplitudes were maximal. Visual constituent processing of (av) stim-ulation was quantified in (av–a) difference waves over occipital sites corresponding to the peak topographies of the P1 and N1 latency components (P1: PO3/4, PO7/8, O1/2, N1: PO7/8, P7/P8). Auditory constituent pro-cessing was quantified in (av–v) difference waves over fronto-central electrodes corresponding to peak topog-raphies of the auditory P2 component (F1/2, FC1/2, Fz, FCz). Statistical analyses for ERP components as well as behavioral data utilized repeated-measures analyses of variance (ANOVAs) with a Greenhouse-Geisser cor-rection when appropriate. Post hoc analyses consisted of two-tailed t-tests. This ERP component analysis was additionally confirmed by conducting running point-wise two-tailed paired t-tests at all scalp electrode sites. In this analysis, a significant difference is considered if at least 10 consecutive data points meet the 0.05 alpha criterion and is a suitable alternative to Bonferroni cor-rection for multiple comparisons (Guthrie & Buchwald, 1991; Molholm et al., 2002; Murray, Foxe, Higgins, Javitt, & Schroeder, 2001). This analysis did not yield any new effects other than the components of interest described above.

Of note, here we refrained from analyses of later processes (>300 ms poststimulus onset) as it is not easy to distinguish whether such processes reflect a sen-sory/multisensory contribution or decision making/ response selection processes that are active at these latencies.

Modeling of ERP Sources

Inverse source modeling was performed to estimate the intracranial generators of the components within the grand-averaged difference waves that represented significant modulations in congruent and incongru-ent multisensory processing. Source locations were estimated by distributed linear inverse solutions based on a local auto-regressive average (LAURA: Grave de Peralta Menendez, Gonzalez Andino, Lantz, Michel, & Landis, 2001). LAURA estimates three-dimensional cur-rent density distributions using a realistic head model with a solution space of 4024 nodes equally distributed within the gray matter of the average template brain of the Montreal Neurological Institute. It makes no a priori assumptions regarding the number of sources or their locations and can deal with multiple simultaneously active sources (Michel et al., 2001). LAURA analyses were implemented using CARTOOL software by Denis Brunet (http://sites.google.com/site/fbmlab/cartool). To ascer-tain the anatomical brain regions giving rise to the differ-ence wave components, the current source distributions estimated by LAURA were transformed into the stan-dardized Montreal Neurological Institute (MNI) coordi-nate system using SPM5 software (Wellcome Department of Imaging Neuroscience, London, England).

RESULTS

Behavioral Performance

Detection performance is represented by sensitivity esti-mates (d') and by response times (RT (ms)) for (v), (a), and (av) target stimuli (Table 15.1). d' estimates were calculated

TABLE 15.1   Details of Behavioral Measures Observed for Target Stimuli During the Four Blocked Tasks

Block type/Attention	Target stimulus	d′ (sem)	Target hits % (sem)	Nontarget false alarms % (sem)	Reaction time ms (sem)
Congruent	(v)	4.8 (0.2)	96.9 (0.9)	0.5 (0.1)	599 (11)
Focused	(av)	5.4 (0.2)	97.8 (0.9)	0.5 (0.1)	587 (10)
Congruent	(v)	4.6 (0.2)	97.9 (0.5)	0.8 (0.1)	598 (13)
Distributed	(av)	5.1 (0.2)	98.3 (0.6)	0.9 (0.2)	568 (11)
	(a)	4.0 (0.3)	87.9 (2.4)	0.5 (0.1)	749 (17)
Incongruent	(v)	5.5 (0.2)	98.4 (0.7)	0.6 (0.1)	585 (11)
Focused	(av)	5.0 (0.2)	97.9 (0.7)	0.7 (0.1)	582 (10)
Incongruent	(v)	4.9 (0.3)	96.9 (0.8)	1.0 (0.3)	576 (10)
Distributed	(av)	5.5 (0.2)	98.5 (0.7)	0.9 (0.2)	578 (10)
	(a)	3.8 (0.3)	84.9 (3.9)	0.5 (0.1)	740 (18)

Values represented as means ± standard errors of mean. (v) = visual, (av) = audiovisual, and (a) = auditory.

in each modality from the hits and false alarm rates for target and nontarget stimuli in that modality, respectively (Table 15.1, MacMillan & Creelman, 1991). As previously analyzed in younger adults, the impact of focused vs. distributed attention on multisensory processing was compared using performance indices as the difference in performance between multisensory (av) and unisensory (v) stimuli, calculated for both attentional manipulations and separately for the congruent and incongruent blocks. Figure 15.2 shows differential (av–v) accuracy (d′) and RT metrics for distributed attention trials relative to focused attention trials (the line connecting data points in each graph portrays the relative performance trend between the two attention manipulations). The performance indices in the younger adults cohort are shown for comparison (with dashed trend lines). The zero horizontal baseline represents the relative performance on (v) trials in each attention manipulation. Of note, there is no parallel (av–a) performance comparison across the two attention manipulations as auditory targets were detected only in blocks with attention distributed to both auditory and visual inputs.

For either performance metric d′ or RT, 2 × 2 × 2 repeated measures ANOVAs with age as a between subjects factor and stimulus type ((av) vs (v)) and attention (focused vs. distributed) as within subject factors, were used to assess age-related changes in performance (Table 15.2). Importantly, a significant age × attention × stimulus type interaction would reveal differential attentional control of multisensation with aging.

Effects of Attention on Congruent Multisensory Performance

In congruent blocks, we recently showed that younger adults had significantly greater accuracy for (av) targets than for (v) targets independent of focused vs distributed attention goals (Mishra & Gazzaley, 2012, Figure 15.2(A): positive (av–v) indices). This result represented a stimulus congruency facilitation effect, and also extended to older adults, as no age interactions were found for the congruent d′ metric (Table 15.2). Post-hoc paired t-tests in the older age group confirmed that (av) accuracies were consistently superior to (v) accuracies in the focused ($t(21) = 3.47$, $p = 0.002$) as well as distributed attention condition ($t(21) = 3.05$, $p = 0.006$) (indicated by the square enclosed asterisks above the data in Figure 15.2(A), circle enclosed asterisks depict statistical significance in younger adults).

Congruent target RTs were generally slowed in older relative to younger adults and again results showed equivalent RT modulations in younger and older adults (Table 15.2, Figure 15.2(B): negative (av–v) indices). The overall stimulus type × attention interaction with relatively faster (av–v) RTs during distributed vs focused attention (Table 15.2) extended to older adults (attention × stimulus type interaction in older adults: $F(1, 21) = 17.33$, $p = 0.0004$). Post-hoc paired t-tests in older adults further confirmed that similar to younger adults, (av) RTs were significantly faster than (v) RTs during focused ($t(21) = 2.41$, $p = 0.025$) as well as distributed attention ($t(21) = 5.29$, $p < 0.0001$).

Thus, overall under congruent multisensory conditions, older adults matched performance in younger adults, with relatively faster (av–v) RTs under distributed audiovisual attention relative to focused visual attention. Of note, this RT speeding during distributed attention reflected improved performance relative to focused attention, as it was not accompanied by any decrements in accuracy (i.e., there was no speed-accuracy tradeoff).

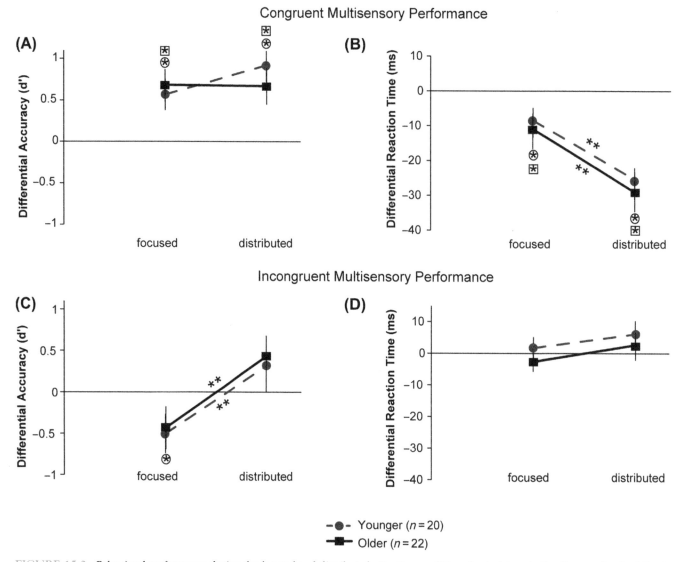

FIGURE 15.2   Behavioral performance during the focused and distributed attention conditions for (av) target stimuli normalized relative to performance on (v) targets. Measures are shown as differential d′ ((A), (C)) and differential RTs ((B), (D)) to depict (av–v) performance. Asterisks on plotted points (square and circle enclosed asterisks for older and younger adult data, respectively) represent significant (av) vs. (v) performance differences for that attention condition. Asterisks on trend lines indicate significant performance differences between the focused and distributed attention conditions.

TABLE 15.2   Outcomes of the $2 \times 2 \times 2$ Repeated Measures ANOVA Analyses Conducted on Multisensory Performance Data

Multisensory performance metric	Age effect (younger vs. older)	Attention effect (focused vs. distributed)	Stimulus effect (av) vs. (v)	Factor interactions
Congruent d′	$p = 0.28$	$p = 0.78$	$F(1,40) = 47.35, p < 0.0001$	None
Congruent RT	$F(1,40) = 11.04, p = 0.002$	$F(1,40) = 19.53, p < 0.0001$	$F(1,40) = 44.75, p < 0.0001$	Stimulus type × attention $F(1,40) = 32.08, p < 0.0001$
Incongruent d′	$p = 0.59$	$p = 0.26$	$p = 0.72$	Stimulus type × attention $F(1,40) = 9.92, p = 0.003$
Incongruent RT	$F(1,40) = 7.79, p = 0.008$	$p = 0.07$	$p = 0.49$	None

Effects of Attention on Incongruent Multisensory Performance

During incongruent blocks, we recently showed that younger adults had significantly diminished d' accuracy on incongruent (av) targets relative to (v) targets during focused visual attention. We further found that this incongruency related interference effect was resolved during distributed attention; equivalent (av) and (v) d' accuracies were observed in this case (Mishra & Gazzaley, 2012). This result also extended to older adults (Table 15.2, Fig. 15.2(C)) with a significant attention × stimulus type ANOVA interaction for the older participant data ($F(1,21) = 4.99$, $p = 0.037$). A post-hoc t-test within older adults showed that d' accuracy on incongruent (av) targets trended toward poorer performance relative to (v) targets during focused visual attention ($t(21) = 1.65$, $p = 0.11$). Of note, this interference effect was previously observed to be significant in younger adults (Figure 15.2(C) circle enclosed asterisks, Mishra & Gazzaley, 2012). Finally, as evidenced by the significant attention × stimulus type interaction above, this interference trend in older adults was significantly resolved under distributed audiovisual attention. The post-hoc t-test of (av) vs. (v) d' accuracy during distributed attention showed a trend for better performance on (av) targets ($t(21) = 1.70$, $p = 0.10$), similar to the result found in younger adults.

Incongruent target RTs were generally slowed in older relative to younger adults, but again no differential RT modulation were found with age (Table 15.2, Figure 15.2(D)). Overall, for both younger and older adults, distributed attention to incongruent audiovisual stimuli resulted in improved detection performance (d' measure) relative to focused visual attention, and notably without a speed-accuracy tradeoff.

Performance data on visual alone trials that served as a baseline measure (horizontal zero line: Figure 15.2) were also analyzed in 2 × 2 × 2 ANOVAs for d' and RT measures, respectively, with age as the between subjects factor, and attention (focused vs. distributed) and block type (congruent vs. incongruent) as the within subject factors. The ANOVA on d' measures neither showed a main effect of age nor any interactions of age with block type/attention. Post-hoc t-tests showed that d' accuracies for (v) targets were equivalent in the two attention manipulations during congruent blocks in either age group (older: $t(21) = 0.41$, $p = 0.68$, younger: $t(19) = 1.06$, $p = 0.30$). For incongruent blocks, the older participants showed somewhat reduced (v) target accuracies during distributed relative to focused attention (older: $t(21) = 3.41$, $p = 0.003$, younger: $t(19) = 0.94$, $p = 0.36$), but which did not result in significant age interactions in the larger ANOVA. A similar analysis of (v) target RTs showed a main effect of RT slowing with age ($F(1,40) = 10.11$, $p = 0.003$), but no between and/or within factor interactions.

Last, performance on isolated auditory (a) targets, which only occurred in the distributed attention conditions, was compared in 2 × 2 ANOVAs with age and block type (congruent vs. incongruent) as factors. For d' accuracies, there was no main effect age ($F(1,40) = 1.44$, $p = 0.24$) nor any age × block type interaction. For RTs, this ANOVA yielded slower RTs with age ($F(1,40) = 9.96$, $p = 0.003$), but no interaction between age and block type.

EVENT-RELATED POTENTIAL RESPONSES

Effects of Attention on Congruent Multisensory Processing

Behaviorally, we found that distributed audiovisual attention improved detection performance relative to focused visual attention for congruent audiovisual stimuli via more rapid RTs (Figure 15.2(B)). This was consistently found in both younger and older adults. Previously, we had investigated the underlying neural measures in younger adults by calculating the event-related processing of the visual and auditory constituents of the congruent (av) stimuli under distributed and focused attention. Visual constituent processing was obtained at occipital sites by subtracting the auditory alone ERP from the audiovisual ERP within each attention block (Calvert, Spence, & Stein, 2004; Molholm, Ritter, Javitt, & Foxe, 2004). In younger adults, this (av–a) difference wave revealed significantly reduced signal amplitudes at latencies of 130–140 ms and 160–190 ms in the distributed relative to focused attention condition (Figure 15.3(A) (positive µV plotted below horizontal axis)). Source estimates of the extracted visual processing signal at 130–140 ms and at 160–190 ms showed neural generators in extrastriate visual cortex in the region of BA 19, which respectively resembled the P1 and N1 components commonly elicited in the visual evoked potential (Gomez Gonzalez, Clark, Fan, Luck, & Hillyard, 1994; Di Russo, Martínez, Sereno, Pitzalis, & Hillyard, 2002, Di Russo, Martínez, & Hillyard, 2003).

A similar comparison as above in older adults showed exactly overlapping (av–a) difference waves under focused visual and distributed audiovisual attention (Figure 15.3(B)). To further unravel the neural data, we assessed the (av–a) difference waves for the higher and lower performing subgroups of older adults split by median RT gain from focused to distributed attention (Figure 15.3(C)). This performance split revealed an early P1-like effect at 100–110 ms with reduced amplitudes under distributed relative to focused attention observed in high performing older adults, similar to the early 130–140 ms latency results obtained in younger adults (age (younger vs high performing older) × attention

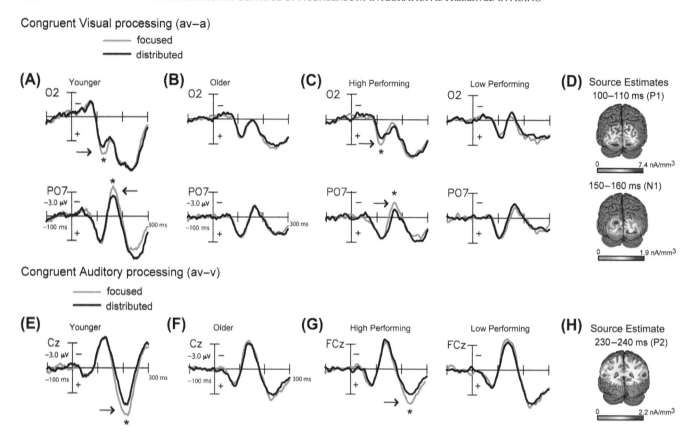

FIGURE 15.3 Grand-averaged difference waves ($n = 22$) depicting multisensory processing during the congruent trials compared for the focused and distributed attention conditions. (A) Extracted processing for the visual constituent of multisensory stimulation (av–a) at occipital sites (O2 and PO7) showing significant visual P1 and N1 latency amplitude differences in younger adults, (B) no differences in older adults, (C) differences similar to younger adults in high, but not low performing older adults, and (D) source estimates of the P1 and N1 latency modulations. (E–H) Parallel effects obtained for processing of the auditory constituent of multisensory stimulation (av–v) showing attention related differences at P2 latencies.

(focused vs. distributed): $F(1,29) = 0.02$, $p > 0.8$). Low performing adults did not show this signal modulation (age (younger vs. low performing older) × attention: $F(1,29) = 4.19$, $p = 0.05$). Similar to younger adults, high performing older adults also showed an N1-like modulation at 150–160 ms (age (younger vs. high performing older) × attention (focused vs. distributed): $F(1,29) = 1.05$, $p = 0.3$), while low performing older adults did not exhibit this effect (age (younger vs. low performing older) × attention: $F(1,29) = 12.29$, $p = 0.002$). These P1 and N1-like latency modulations in older adults localized to extrastriate visual cortex, BA18/19 (Figure 15.3(D)) in close proximity to their counterpart component sources found in the younger adult difference waves (MNI coordinates of the peaks of the source clusters in Table 15.3; Mishra & Gazzaley, 2012).

Previously in younger adults, we compared auditory constituent processing for the congruent (av) stimuli in (av–v) difference waves calculated during distributed audiovisual vs. focused visual attention. This analysis in younger adults showed a significant positive component difference at 175–225 ms or P200, which was larger when

the auditory information was task-irrelevant during focused visual attention relative to distributed audiovisual attention (Figure 15.3(E); Mishra & Gazzaley, 2012). Moreover, this (av–v) processing difference directly correlated with the (av–v) RT improvement observed for distributed vs. focused attention.

Grand-averaged (av–v) difference waves in older adults did not show any processing differences across distributed vs. focused attention (Figure 15.3(F)). Again, the RT-based performance split in older adults revealed a P2 positivity peaking at 230–240 ms latency that was larger in focused relative to distributed attention in high performing adults akin to the P200 findings in younger adults (age (younger vs. high performing older) × attention: $F(1,29) = 0.01$, $p > 0.9$), while low performing older adults did not show this P2 latency processing difference (age (younger vs. low performing older) × attention: $F(1,29) = 4.58$, $p = 0.04$) (Figure 15.3(G)). This 230–240 ms P2 positivity localized to superior temporal gyrus (STG, Figure 15.3(H)) in close proximity to the P200 source in younger adults (MNI coordinates of the peak of the source cluster in Table 15.3; Mishra & Gazzaley, 2012).

Overall, these results consistently show that, at least for high performing older adults, the neural modulations were similar to those observed in younger adults and underscore neural efficiency of responses with improved performance during distributed attention associated with reduced ERP component processing. Of note, the median RT performance splits further revealed that the congruent RT facilitation during distributed vs. focused attention was limited to the high performing older participants (high performing: $t(10) = 7.91$, $p < 0.0001$, low performing: $t(10) = 0.67$, $p = 0.52$).

TABLE 15.3   MNI Coordinates of the Peaks of the Source Clusters as Estimated in LAURA at Relevant Component Latencies Identified in the Extracted Visual (av–a) and Extracted Auditory (av–v) Difference Waveforms for Congruent and Incongruent Blocks. All Sources Were Modeled for Difference Waves in the Focused Visual attention Condition in High Performing Older Adults

Block type	Difference wave	Latency (ms)	x (mm)	y (mm)	z (mm)
Congruent	(av–a)	100–110	±24	−77	−2
	(av–a)	150–160	±26	−83	−7
	(av–v)	230–240	±53	−37	15
Incongruent	(av–a)	110–120	±12	−78	4
	(av–v)	235–245	±54	−33	7

Effects of Attention on Incongruent Multisensory Processing

In both younger and older adults we found that distributed attention improved (av–v) accuracies for incongruent audiovisual stimuli relative to focused visual attention (Figure 15.2(C)). Parallel to the ERP analysis for congruent stimuli, we first analyzed the visual constituent of incongruent (av) stimulus processing in (av–a) difference waves obtained for both focused and distributed attention conditions. In younger adults, the incongruent (av–a) difference waves had significantly reduced signal amplitudes at 110–130 ms during distributed relative to focused attention (Figure 15.4(A)). This P1-like component localized to extrastriate visual cortex (BA 19), in proximity to the P1 latency source in the congruent (av–a) difference waves. Again in older adults, the grand-averaged (av–a) difference waves yielded no difference across the two attention manipulations (Figure 15.4(B)). In this case, median performance splits based on d' accuracy improvements across distributed relative to focused attention revealed a 110–120 ms processing difference with reduced amplitudes during distributed relative to focused attention observed in high performing older adults akin to younger adults (age (younger vs. high performing older) × attention: $F(1,29) = 0.13$, $p = 0.72$), but not in low performing older adults (age (younger vs. low performing older) × attention: $F(1,29) = 4.2$, $p = 0.05$) (Figure 15.4(C)). This P1 latency

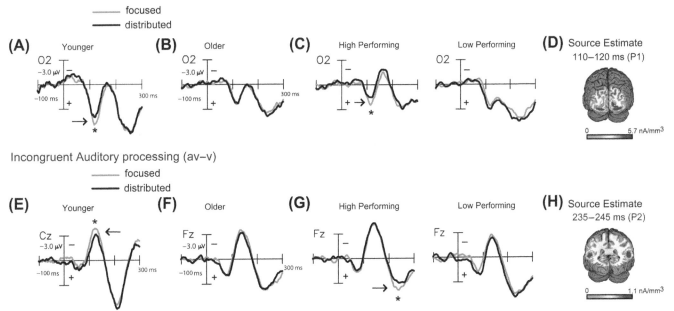

FIGURE 15.4   Grand-averaged difference waves ($n = 22$) depicting multisensory processing during the incongruent trials compared for the focused and distributed attention conditions. (A) Extracted processing for the visual constituent of multisensory stimulation (av–a) at occipital site (O2) showing significant visual P1 latency amplitude differences in younger adults, (B) no differences in older adults, (C) differences similar to younger adults in high, but not low performing older adults, and (D) source estimates of the P1 latency modulation. (E–H) Parallel effects obtained for processing of the auditory constituent of multisensory stimulation (av–v) showing attention related differences at P2 latencies.

difference wave component also localized to extrastriate visual cortex (BA18, Figure 15.4(D)) in proximity to the P1 latency source estimates in younger adults (MNI coordinates of the peak of the source cluster in Table 15.3; Mishra & Gazzaley, 2012).

In younger adults, auditory constituent processing calculated in (av–v) difference waves for incongruent audiovisual stimuli showed significantly reduced amplitudes during distributed relative to focused attention at early 110–120 ms latencies at fronto-central sites that localized to middle temporal gyrus (Figure 15.4(E); Mishra & Gazzaley, 2012). Again, the grand-averaged (av–v) waveforms in older adults were overlapping in the two attention conditions (Figure 15.4(F)). d′ accuracy dependent median performance splits revealed a 235–245 ms P2 latency processing difference for high performing, but not low performing older adults as analyzed in ANOVAs with attention as a factor (high performing: $F(1,10)=4.9$, $p=0.05$, low performing: $F(1,10)=0.97$, $p=0.3$) (Figure 15.4(G)). A comparison with younger adults was not possible in this case as the earlier N1 latency component was modulated in the younger age group; although mechanistically for both younger and high performing older adults distributed attention was associated with reduced signal amplitudes relative to focused attention. The P2 latency positivity in older adults localized to superior temporal gyrus (STG, BA22: Figure 15.4(H)) in close proximity to the P2 latency source found during congruent multisensory processing above (MNI coordinates of the peak of the source cluster in Table 15.3).

Thus for incongruent multisensory processing as well, high performing older adults continued to exhibit increased neural efficiency in the processing of the visual and auditory constituents. Again, the median d′ performance splits performed to reveal these neural results showed that the d′ facilitation during distributed vs. focused attention was highly significant for the high performers $(t(10)=6.78$, $p<0.0001)$ but only trended toward significance for the low performing older adults $(t(10)=2.05, p=0.07)$.

DISCUSSION

In a recent study, investigating two manipulations of attentional allocation: attention focused to a single sensory modality (visual) or attention distributed across modalities (auditory and visual) in the setting of semantically congruent and incongruent (av) stimuli, we found that younger adults consistently showed performance benefits during distributed attention (Mishra & Gazzaley, 2012). Here, we extended our findings to older adults and found on average parallel behavioral results: distributed relative to focused attention generated faster (av) reaction

times, without a compromise on accuracy in congruent stimulus settings; additionally distributed attention resulted in improved response accuracies for incongruent stimuli. Thus, at the behavioral level we generally found preserved attentional control of multisensation in aging. ERP recordings during the task revealed that early sensory processing of the auditory and visual constituents of (av) stimulation were consistently reduced during distributed relative to focused attention. Of note, these physiological findings, that resembled results in younger adults, were restricted to high but not low performing older adults, as divided by median performance gain from focused to distributed attention. Thus, the novel association recently found for younger adults between improved behavioral performance and increased neural efficiency, as reflected by reduced auditory and visual processing during distributed (av) attention, was replicated here, at least in high performing older adults. These findings lend support to the hypothesis that while age-related decline heavily impacts unisensory processing capacities, many older adults benefit from multisensory environments such that their abilities are equivalent to or even surpass that of younger adults (Guerreiro & Van Gerven, 2011; Hugenschmidt et al., 2009; Peiffer et al., 2009; Poliakoff et al., 2006; Townsend et al., 2006).

To the best of our knowledge, there is only one previous study that has reported that distributed audiovisual attention relative to focused attention to a single modality, either auditory or visual, differentially impacts multisensation in younger and older adults (Hugenschmidt et al., 2009). Multisensory stimuli in this study were always congruent, and similar to our results, the authors showed a greater multisensory to unisensory RT advantage during distributed attention conditions. Here, we further extend the findings of Hugenschmidt et al. to incongruent multisensory conditions, and show that distributed attention generates significantly better response accuracies than obtained under focused attention in older adults, similar to results in younger adults (Mishra & Gazzaley, 2012). Of note, our findings are consistent with those of Hugenschmidt et al. even though we use different stimuli types (spoken (a) and written (v) stimuli vs. spoken (a) and pictorial (v) stimuli in the prior study), different task designs (blocked attention vs. trial by trial cued attention in the prior study), and different response schemes (target detection vs. two-alternative forced choice in the prior study), speaking to the robustness of the findings.

The current study is the first to investigate the neural basis of the multisensory performance gains found in older adults. We compared early neural processing of both the visual and auditory constituents of (av) stimulation using difference wave calculations (Mishra & Gazzaley, 2012). Variance measures for the neural, but not behavioral, data were significantly greater in older relative to younger adults $(p=0.04)$, and neural data averaged across all older study participants were non-informative. A further separation of high performing older adults from low performers in median behavior splits, showed neural correlates similar to those previously observed in younger adults. The visual constituent of (av) stimulation showed reduced signal amplitudes during distributed relative to focused attention at visual P1 and N1 latencies for congruent stimuli, and only at P1 latencies for incongruent stimuli. This same pattern of results was previously found in younger adults. That distributed audiovisual attention was associated with reduced visual constituent processing compared to focused visual attention, is consistent with observations of sensory processing under unimodal divided attention (Beck & Kastner, 2009; Desimone, 1998; Desimone & Duncan, 1995; Kastner & Ungerleider, 2001; Reddy, Kanwisher, & VanRullen, 2009), and with the theory that limited attentional resources within a modality as available under distributed attention, are associated with reduced neural responses (Lavie, 2005).

The neural signal corresponding to the auditory constituent of (av) stimulation was also found to be reduced during distributed audiovisual relative to focused visual attention for high performing older adults. For both congruent and incongruent (av) stimuli, this amplitude modulation occurred at P2 component latencies and localized to the superior temporal region—a known site for multisensory integration (Beauchamp, 2005; Calvert, 2001; Calvert et al., 2004; Ghazanfar & Schroeder, 2006). Results for congruent stimuli matched those in younger adults, however, for incongruent stimuli an earlier N1 latency modulation was observed in younger adults. Of note, the direction of modulation, whether at N1 latencies in younger adults or P2 latencies in older adults, remained the same, i.e., reduced signal amplitudes during distributed attention. In this case, the P2 modulation during stimulus incongruency in older adults may be considered as "successful compensation" as per terminology suggested by Grady (2008, 2012), wherein distinct brain activity is recruited in older relative to younger adults that is associated with high task performance.

Of note, and also as previously noted in the younger adults' study, the reduced auditory constituent signal amplitudes during distributed audiovisual attention when auditory information is task-relevant vs. focused visual attention when auditory information is task-irrelevant, was unexpected. However, prior studies have shown that during a focused visual attention task, a concurrent stimulus in the auditory modality captures bottom-up attention such that auditory neural processing is enhanced relative to an inattentive baseline (Busse, Roberts, Crist, Weissman, & Woldorff, 2005; Fiebelkorn, Foxe, & Molholm, 2010; Zimmer, Itthipanyanan, et al., 2010; Zimmer, Roberts, et al., 2010). We interpret our findings as revealing that during distributed audiovisual attention, top-down control reduces the bottom-up capture by the interfering auditory stream and/or may even suppress the interfering stream, resulting in reduced early auditory processing and better performance accuracies as observed here and in our previous study (Mishra & Gazzaley, 2012).

Overall, our study extends prior age-related behavioral findings of generally preserved multisensory performance in older relative to younger adults. Additionally, we have generalized these results to incongruent, semantically conflicting audiovisual stimuli. We also provide a first report of early multisensory event-related processing in older adults, which importantly demonstrates preserved neural signal modulation mechanisms as observed in younger adults. Distributed audiovisual attention, which results in improved behavioral performance relative to focused visual attention, was found to be linked to reduced early sensory neural signals at least in high performing older adults. As noted in our previous study, improved behavior has been mostly linked to reduced sensorineural processing in training studies (Alain & Snyder, 2008; Berry et al., 2010; Ding et al., 2003; Kelley & Yantis, 2010; Mukai et al., 2007), which is interpreted as a reflection of increased neural efficiency impacting improved behavioral performance (Erickson et al., 2007). Here, we interpret reduced sensory signals in visual extrastriate and polysensory temporal cortices during distributed audiovisual attention as increased neural efficiency, which result in the multisensory performance gains.

AUTHOR CONTRIBUTIONS

J.M. and A.G. conceptualized the study. J.M. performed data collection and analysis. J.M. and A.G. wrote the paper.

Acknowledgments

This work was supported by the National Institute of Health Grant 5R01AG030395 (AG) and the Program for Breakthrough Biomedical Research grant (JM). We would like to thank Jacqueline Boccanfuso, Joe Darin, and Pin-wei Chen for their assistance with data collection.

References

Alain, C., & Snyder, J. S. (2008). Age-related differences in auditory evoked responses during rapid perceptual learning. *Clinical Neurophysiology*, 119(2), 356–366.

Bayles, A., & Kasniak, A. (1987). *Communication and cognition in normal aging and dementia*. Boston, MA: Little, Brown and Company.

Beauchamp, M. S. (2005). See me, hear me, touch me: multisensory integration in lateral occipital-temporal cortex. *Current Opinion in Neurobiology*, 15(2), 145–153.

Beck, D. M., & Kastner, S. (2009). Top-down and bottom-up mechanisms in biasing competition in the human brain. *Vision Research, 49*(10), 1154–1165.

Berry, A. S., Zanto, T. P., Clapp, W. C., Hardy, J. L., Delahunt, P. B., Mahncke, H. W., et al. (2010). The influence of perceptual training on working memory in older adults. N. Rogers, Ed., *PLoS ONE, 5*(7), e11537.

Busse, L., Roberts, K. C., Crist, R. E., Weissman, D. H., & Woldorff, M. G. (2005). The spread of attention across modalities and space in a multisensory object. *Proceedings of the National Academy of Sciences of the United States of America, 102*(51), 18751–18756.

Calvert, G. A. (2001). Crossmodal processing in the human brain: insights from functional neuroimaging studies. *Cerebral Cortex (New York, N.Y.: 1991), 11*(12), 1110–1123.

Calvert, G. A., Spence, C., & Stein, B. E. (2004). *The handbook of multisensory processing.* : University of Bath web-support@bath.ac.uk.

Chao, L. L., & Knight, R. T. (1997). Prefrontal deficits in attention and inhibitory control with aging. *Cerebral Cortex (New York, N.Y.: 1991), 7*(1), 63–69.

Cienkowski, K. M., & Carney, A. E. (2002). Auditory-visual speech perception and aging. *Ear and Hearing, 23*(5), 439–449.

Clapp, W. C., & Gazzaley, A. (2012). Distinct mechanisms for the impact of distraction and interruption on working memory in aging. *Neurobiology of Aging, 33*(1), 134–148.

Corso, J. F. (1971). Sensory processes and age effects in normal adults. *Journal of Gerontology, 26*(1), 90–105.

Craik, F. I. M., & Salthouse, T. A. (2000). *The handbook of aging and cognition.* Mahwah, NJ: Erlbaum.

Degerman, A., Rinne, T., Pekkola, J., Autti, T., Jääskeläinen, I. P., Sams, M., et al. (2007). Human brain activity associated with audiovisual perception and attention. *NeuroImage, 34*, 1683–1691.

Desimone, R. (1998). Visual attention mediated by biased competition in extrastriate visual cortex. *Philosophical transactions of the Royal Society of London. Series B, Biological Sciences, 353*(1373), 1245–1255.

Desimone, R., & Duncan, J. (1995). Neural mechanisms of selective visual attention. *Annual Review of Neuroscience, 18*, 193–222.

Di Russo, F., Martínez, A., & Hillyard, S. A. (2003). Source analysis of event-related cortical activity during visuo-spatial attention. *Cerebral Cortex (New York, N.Y.: 1991), 13*(5), 486–499.

Di Russo, F., Martínez, A., Sereno, M. I., Pitzalis, S., & Hillyard, S. A. (2002). Cortical sources of the early components of the visual evoked potential. *Human Brain Mapping, 15*(2), 95–111.

Ding, Y., Song, Y., Fan, S., Qu, Z., & Chen, L. (2003). Specificity and generalization of visual perceptual learning in humans: an event-related potential study. *Neuroreport, 14*(4), 587–590.

Erickson, K. I., Colcombe, S. J., Wadhwa, R., Bherer, L., Peterson, M. S., Scalf, P. E., et al. (2007). Training-induced plasticity in older adults: effects of training on hemispheric asymmetry. *Neurobiology of Aging, 28*(2), 272–283.

Fiebelkorn, I. C., Foxe, J. J., & Molholm, S. (2010). Dual mechanisms for the cross-sensory spread of attention: how much do learned associations matter? *Cerebral Cortex (New York, N.Y.: 1991), 20*(1), 109–120.

Folstein, M. F., Folstein, S. E., & McHugh, P. R. (1975). "Mini-mental state". A practical method for grading the cognitive state of patients for the clinician. *Journal of Psychiatric Research, 12*(3), 189–198.

Gazzaley, A. (2013). Top-down modulation deficit in the aging brain: an emerging theory of cognitive aging. In R. T. Knight & D. T. Stuss (Eds.), *Principles of frontal lobe function* (2nd ed.) (Vol. 35, pp. 593–608).

Gazzaley, A., Clapp, W., Kelley, J., McEvoy, K., Knight, R. T., & D' Esposito, M. (2008). Age-related top-down suppression deficit in the early stages of cortical visual memory processing. *Proceedings of the National Academy of Sciences of the United States of America, 105*(35), 13122–13126.

Gazzaley, A., Cooney, J. W., Rissman, J., & D'Esposito, M. (2005). Top-down suppression deficit underlies working memory impairment in normal aging. *Nature Neuroscience, 8*(10), 1298–1300.

Ghazanfar, A. A., & Schroeder, C. E. (2006). Is neocortex essentially multisensory? *Trends in Cognitive Sciences, 10*(6), 278–285.

Gomez Gonzalez, C. M., Clark, V. P., Fan, S., Luck, S. J., & Hillyard, S. A. (1994). Sources of attention-sensitive visual event-related potentials. *Brain Topography, 7*(1), 41–51.

Grady, C. L. (2008). Cognitive neuroscience of aging. *Annals of the New York Academy of Sciences, 1124*, 127–144.

Grady, C. (2012). The cognitive neuroscience of aging. Nature reviews. *Neuroscience, 13*(7), 491–505.

Grave de Peralta Menendez, R., Gonzalez Andino, S., Lantz, G., Michel, C. M., & Landis, T. (2001). Noninvasive localization of electromagnetic epileptic activity. I. Method descriptions and simulations. *Brain Topography, 14*(2), 131–137.

Green, C. S., & Bavelier, D. (2003). Action video game modifies visual selective attention. *Nature, 423*, 534–537.

Greenwood, P. M. (2000). The frontal aging hypothesis evaluated. *Journal of the International Neuropsychological Society: JINS, 6*, 705–726.

Guerreiro, M. J. S., & Van Gerven, P. W. M. (2011). Now you see it, now you don't: evidence for age-dependent and age-independent cross-modal distraction. *Psychology and Aging, 26*(2), 415–426.

Guthrie, D., & Buchwald, J. S. (1991). Significance testing of difference potentials. *Psychophysiology, 28*(2), 240–244.

Habak, C., & Faubert, J. (2000). Larger effect of aging on the perception of higher-order stimuli. *Vision Research, 40*(8), 943–950.

Helfer, K. S. (1998). Auditory and auditory-visual recognition of clear and conversational speech by older adults. *Journal of the American Academy of Audiology, 9*(3), 234–242.

Hillyard, S. A., & Anllo-Vento, L. (1998). Event-related brain potentials in the study of visual selective attention. *Proceedings of the National Academy of Sciences of the United States of America, 95*, 781–787.

Hugenschmidt, C. E., Mozolic, J. L., & Laurienti, P. J. (2009). Suppression of multisensory integration by modality-specific attention in aging. *Neuroreport, 20*(4), 349–353.

Hugenschmidt, C. E., Peiffer, A. M., McCoy, T. P., Hayasaka, S., & Laurienti, P. J. (2009). Preservation of crossmodal selective attention in healthy aging. Experimental brain research. Experimentelle Hirnforschung. *Expérimentation Cérébrale, 198*(2–3), 273–285.

Kastner, S., & Ungerleider, L. G. (2001). The neural basis of biased competition in human visual cortex. *Neuropsychologia, 39*(12), 1263–1276.

Keller, B. K., Morton, J. L., Thomas, V. S., & Potter, J. F. (1999). The effect of visual and hearing impairments on functional status. *Journal of the American Geriatrics Society, 47*(11), 1319–1325.

Kelley, T. A., & Yantis, S. (2010). Neural correlates of learning to Attend. *Frontiers in Human Neuroscience, 4*, 216.

Laurienti, P. J., Burdette, J. H., Maldjian, J. A., & Wallace, M. T. (2006). Enhanced multisensory integration in older adults. *Neurobiology of Aging, 27*(8), 1155–1163.

Lavie, N. (2005). Distracted and confused?: selective attention under load. *Trends in Cognitive Sciences, 9*(2), 75–82.

Lichtenstein, M. J. (1992). Hearing and visual impairments. *Clinics in Geriatric Medicine, 8*(1), 173–182.

Macmillan, N. A., & Creelman, C. D. (1991). *Detection theory: A user's guide.* New York: Cambridge University Press.

Michel, C. M., Thut, G., Morand, S., Khateb, A., Pegna, A. J., Grave de Peralta, R., et al. (2001). Electric source imaging of human brain functions. Brain research. *Brain Research Reviews, 36*(2–3), 108–118.

Mishra, J., Zinni, M., Bavelier, D., & Hillyard, S. A. (2011). Neural basis of superior performance of action videogame players in an attention-demanding task. *Journal of Neuroscience, 31*, 992–998.

Mishra, J., & Gazzaley, A. (2012). Attention distributed across sensory modalities enhances perceptual performance. *Journal of Neuroscience, 32*, 12294–12302.

Molholm, S., Ritter, W., Javitt, D. C., & Foxe, J. J. (2004). Multisensory visual-auditory object recognition in humans: a high-density electrical mapping study. *Cerebral Cortex (New York, N.Y.: 1991)*, *14*(4), 452–465.

Molholm, S., Ritter, W., Murray, M. M., Javitt, D. C., Schroeder, C. E., & Foxe, J. J. (2002). Multisensory auditory–visual interactions during early sensory processing in humans: a high-density electrical mapping study. *Brain Research. Cognitive Brain Research*, *14*(1), 115–128.

Mukai, I., Kim, D., Fukunaga, M., Japee, S., Marrett, S., & Ungerleider, L. G. (2007). Activations in visual and attention-related areas predict and correlate with the degree of perceptual learning. *The Journal of Neuroscience*, *27*(42), 11401–11411.

Murray, M. M., Foxe, J. J., Higgins, B. A., Javitt, D. C., & Schroeder, C. E. (2001). Visuo-spatial neural response interactions in early cortical processing during a simple reaction time task: a high-density electrical mapping study. *Neuropsychologia*, *39*(8), 828–844.

Nusbaum, N. J. (1999). Aging and sensory senescence. *Southern Medical Journal*, *92*(3), 267–275.

Osterrieth, P. (1944). Le test de copie d'une figure complexe. *Archiv Psychologie*, *30*, 206–356.

Peiffer, A. M., Hugenschmidt, C. E., Maldjian, J. A., Casanova, R., Srikanth, R., Hayasaka, S., et al. (2009). Aging and the interaction of sensory cortical function and structure. *Human Brain Mapping*, *30*(1), 228–240.

Poliakoff, E., Ashworth, S., Lowe, C., & Spence, C. (2006). Vision and touch in aging: crossmodal selective attention and visuotactile spatial interactions. *Neuropsychologia*, *44*(4), 507–517.

Reddy, L., Kanwisher, N. G., & VanRullen, R. (2009). Attention and biased competition in multi-voxel object representations. *Proceedings of the National Academy of Sciences of the United States of America*, *106*(50), 21447–21452.

Rey, A. (1941). L'examen psychologique dans les cas d'encephalopathie traumatique. *Archiv Psychologie*, *28*, 286–340.

Stine, E. A., Wingfield, A., & Myers, S. D. (1990). Age differences in processing information from television news: the effects of bisensory augmentation. *Journal of Gerontology*, *45*(1), P1–P8.

Strupp, M., Arbusow, V., Borges Pereira, C., Dieterich, M., & Brandt, T. (1999). Subjective straight-ahead during neck muscle vibration: effects of aging. *Neuroreport*, *10*(15), 3191–3194.

Talsma, D., Doty, T. J., & Woldorff, M. G. (2007). Selective attention and audiovisual integration: is attending to both modalities a prerequisite for early integration? *Cerebral Cortex*, *17*, 679–690.

Townsend, J., Adamo, M., & Haist, F. (2006). Changing channels: an fMRI study of aging and cross-modal attention shifts. *NeuroImage*, *31*(4), 1682–1692.

Wais, P. E., Rubens, M. T., Boccanfuso, J., & Gazzaley, A. (2010). Neural mechanisms underlying the impact of visual distraction on retrieval of long-term memory. *The Journal of Neuroscience: The Official Journal of the Society for Neuroscience*, *30*, 8541–8550.

Weschler, D. (2008). *Wechsler adult intelligence scale* (4th ed.). San Antonio, TX: The Psychological Corporation.

Zanto, T., Gazzaley, A. (in press). Attention and aging. In A. C. Nobre, S. Kastner (Ed.), Oxford Handbook of Attention. Oxford University Press.

Zanto, T. P., Hennigan, K., Ostberg, M., Clapp, W. C., & Gazzaley, A. (2010). Predictive knowledge of stimulus relevance does not influence top-down suppression of irrelevant information in older adults. *Cortex. A Journal Devoted to the Study of the Nervous System and Behavior*, *46*(4), 564–574.

Zanto, T. P., Pan, P., Liu, H., Bollinger, J., Nobre, A. C., & Gazzaley, A. (2011). Age-related changes in orienting attention in time. *The Journal of Neuroscience: The Official Journal of the Society for Neuroscience*, *31*(35), 12461–12470.

Zanto, T. P., Toy, B., & Gazzaley, A. (2010). Delays in neural processing during working memory encoding in normal aging. *Neuropsychologia*, *48*(1), 13–25.

Zimmer, U., Itthipanyanan, S., Grent-'t-Jong, T., & Woldorff, M. G. (2010). The electrophysiological time course of the interaction of stimulus conflict and the multisensory spread of attention. *European Journal of Neuroscience*, *31*(10), 1744–1754.

Zimmer, U., Roberts, K. C., Harshbarger, T. B., & Woldorff, M. G. (2010). Multisensory conflict modulates the spread of visual attention across a multisensory object. *NeuroImage*, *52*(2), 606–616.

ATTENTION AND COGNITIVE PROCESSES

Brain,
please help me find the connection -
the link to my mind to help explain
how it is my cells constrain
what I see
what I hear
what I think
what I fear
but dare not reveal in utterances aloud,
yet allow to be read
from sensors around my head:
Electrical and magnetic – empirically prophetic.

By Marta Kutas

An Evolutionary Perspective on Attentional Processes

Vincent P. Clark[1, 2, 3], Brian A. Coffman[1, 2, 3], Michael C.S. Trumbo[1, 2], Ashley R. Wegele[1, 4]

[1]Department of Psychology, University of New Mexico, Albuquerque, NM, USA, [2]Psychology Clinical Neuroscience Center, University of New Mexico, Albuquerque, NM, USA, [3]Mind Research Network and LBERI, Albuquerque, NM, USA, [4]Ronald E. McNair Post-Baccalaureate Achievement & Research Opportunity Program, University of New Mexico, Albuquerque, NM, USA

CRYPSIS AS AN ADAPTATION TO THE DEVELOPMENT OF SENSORY SYSTEMS

All sensory modalities we have today were likely developed in response to environmental pressures to find sources of food and other resources, and to avoid predation and other dangers that affected our ancestor's ability to survive and reproduce. Evolution is a process whereby genetically determined individual differences in physical and functional properties affect their reproductive success as they interact with their environment (Darwin, 1859). Successful changes or adaptations are passed on to future generations through genetic material, while unsuccessful changes leading to an early demise fail to be passed on and may die out. Therefore, an enhanced ability to identify and respond to predators and prey provides a survival advantage. Indeed, it has even been hypothesized that the immune system may have developed in order to identify other organisms chemically, and thus protect against predation at the cellular level (Semple, Cowlishaw, & Bennett, 2002).

Once sensory systems developed sufficiently, this likely resulted in evolutionary pressures for animals to conceal themselves from detection. This ability, called crypsis, is found to some degree in most animals (Endler & Greenwood, 1988). Figure 16.1 illustrates a number of examples. Crypsis was advantageous both for prey animals to avoid predators, and for predators to

avoid detection by prey before attacking. This can be achieved by adapting different physical properties, such as changes in shape to mimic other animals or objects, or changes in patterns of reflectance, transparency, and coloration to reduce the chance of detection by other animals. Prey animals have been observed to use a different form of locomotion or other behaviors in order to blend into their surroundings or to mimic an unpalatable object or animal, such as a poisonous type of prey, thereby concealing their true identity, whereas a predator may mimic a harmless animal or object (Endler & Greenwood, 1988).

There is evidence for crypsis in the fossil record going back over 160 million years. Cephalopod fossils similar to a cuttlefish have been found with what appears to be remnants of ink sacs filled with eumelanin, which modern squids and other cephalopods use as a screen when escaping predators (Glass et al., 2012). Chemical analyses suggest that this ancient form of eumelanin is identical to that used by cephalopods today, and may have been used for a similar purpose. There is evidence for crypsis used by many other animals that are alive today. As some examples, many animals that live either underwater or that fly have brighter coloration on their ventral surface than their dorsal surface, which may serve to mimic the general trend for greater light coming from above than below, so that they will blend in to their environment more effectively (Endler & Greenwood, 1988). One such

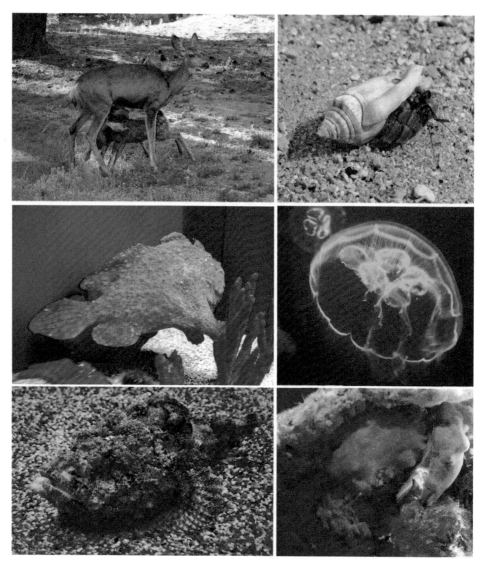

FIGURE 16.1   Different examples of crypsis found in nature. Top left: A deer with two fawns. The coloration of the deer is similar to the brown hues of dead foliage. The fawns have additional white spots, which serve to further disrupt their perception. Top right: A hermit crab, which lives inside a snail shell, in part to camouflage itself. Middle left: The frog fish, which mimics the color and texture of the brightly colored coral within which it lives. Middle right: A jellyfish that uses transparency to blend into the surrounding environment. Bottom left: A fish that mimics the color and texture of the ocean bottom. Bottom right: A crab that attaches sponges and other objects to its back, camouflaging itself from above.

species, the hatchet fish, lives in the deep ocean and has photophores on its ventral surface that are designed to mimic light from above, making them almost invisible from below (Fink, 1998). Also, animals living in climates with snow tend to be lighter in color than animals from warmer climates, and those that live in seasonal climates often change their coloration with the seasons (Figuerola & Senar, 2005). Many animals possess "disruptive" coloration that allows the animal to blend into their surroundings, such as stripes or mottled patterns. Certain animals, such as chameleons, octopi, and cuttlefish, have chromatophores in their skin that produce substantial changes to their visual appearance, allowing them to assume the appearance of their surroundings, or of other animals

at whim (Bagnara & Hadley, 1973). The *Octopus vulgaris* can match the visual pattern, color, brightness, and texture of its surroundings, and can control the movement of this coloration to mimic the speed and direction of waves, producing a degree of crypsis that is so complete it is nearly impossible to detect them visually (Froesch & Messenger, 1978).

Indeed, some degree of crypsis is the norm for almost all animals that do not actively advertise their presence. Exceptions include animals with other successful survival adaptations, such as those without natural enemies, birds that rely on flight to escape predation, and poisonous or venomous animals that advertise this ability using bright colors. Humans are also apparently without crypsis in our physical form; however, there are other forms of crypsis developed by our species. Human crypsis for survival is used mainly by subsistence hunters and by those in wartime environments, where threats such as explosive devises and snipers are hidden. Soldiers often wear camouflage whose design is adapted to the wartime environment (e.g., using patterns that match desert, forest or jungle). This is done both for protection and to maximize their ability to "sneak up" on enemy combatants.

In modern times, the need for humans to identify animals with crypsis in order to survive has been greatly diminished. We have removed many animals from our immediate environment that might do us harm. We have learned to breed animals for food, meaning that once captured and cared for, crypsis has little impact on their survival. Additionally, food now comes prepared, often in brightly colored and well-marked packaging, with little perceptual effort required on our part to identify the proper source of our next meal. Indeed, our attentional task has changed from identifying food sources hidden in the natural environment to seeking a desired product among the dizzying array of items competing for our attention in the modern grocery store. These modern methods for acquiring food for survival, and the nearly complete lack of predators that might use us for food, constitute a tremendous change in our environment. We must be aware that this change occurred very recently in evolutionary history, and our ancestors had to deal with a very different environment to survive for most of our evolutionary history. The perceptual and attentional systems we use today must have developed in a very different environment from that which we deal with now. To fully understand the characteristics of these systems, it is important to understand their history.

EVOLUTIONARY RESPONSES TO CRYPSIS

As the continuing evolution of prey and predator animals improved crypsis over time, the development of adequate perceptual capabilities to allow correct identification of cryptic animals improved as well. This might have occurred by developing improvements to sensory receptors, leading to increased spatial acuity and/or sensitivity to color or contrast among other properties. As one example, animals differ in the number of cell types in their retinas, which may be related to their ability to distinguish subtle differences in color (Roth, Lundström, Kelber, Kröger, & Unsbo, 2009). Most humans today have three types of cones, but it has been hypothesized that human ancestors lost their ability to recognize red hues at some point in history, and recovered this capability later. This has been hypothesized to be due to increased reliance on

fruits and other food items such as young leaves that tend to have a reddish tint (Dominy & Lucas, 2001). However, an alternative hypothesis is that this capability might have been lost and then recovered as other animals changed their methods of crypsis, making perception of reddish hues less useful for detecting crypsis for a time, and then more useful again later. While changes in receptor cell types are likely to have occurred during evolution, the genetic changes required to create such changes would likely be rare, and therefore unlikely to occur quickly.

By contrast, changes in the neural architecture specialized for processing of sensory stimuli could occur more easily than changes in sensory receptors themselves. This would not require genetic mutations to create new cell types, but would require alterations in synapses and modified strength of connections among existing cell types instead. Indeed, the type of perceptual learning used by endogenous attention to modify the perceptual interpretation of stimuli might occur very quickly after a prior exposure. Therefore, such changes in information processing performed at the neural level could lead to increased acuity and sensitivity, providing better detection accuracy, while requiring little or no evolutionary "work" to achieve these perceptual and behavioral changes required for survival once the ability to apply prior experiences to modify the interpretation of sensory stimuli was possible.

A number of hypotheses could be offered for how crypsis might take advantage of specific exogenous modes of sensory processing to produce its effects, and how the neural architecture of the brain could be modified in turn to perceive animals using crypsis with greater accuracy. First, many forms of crypsis, especially camouflage, seem designed to confuse perceptual systems that are exogenous, or purely bottom-up and sensory-based. Presenting features that match the background to obscure their outline serves to hide the presence of these animals. In addition, bottom-up or exogenous attentional systems designed to match lines, colors, and patterns in order to form the perception of objects might be fooled by well-executed camouflage, resulting in errors in the interpretation of the visual image. By contrast, top-down or endogenous attentional systems might offer an effective countermeasure to camouflage. This form of attention uses prior information to correct or supersede perceptually based sensory perceptions that could occur in error. In this scenario, one animal may use a form of crypsis, yet be revealed and accurately identified by another animal, and the perceiving animal survives to be better prepared for the next meeting. Alternatively, perceptual features that could be used to distinguish an animal using a specific form of crypsis might be encoded from birth.

This process of using past experience to interpret visual images is likely managed by brain regions outside of the lower-order visual areas that support bottom-up or exogenous visual processing. Areas specialized for encoding and recalling past experiences and specialized for imposing learned information for the interpretation rather than the perception of new experiences might include higher-order extrastriate regions, as well as attentional systems located in frontal, parietal, and cingulate cortices.

If it is true that there are specialized systems for identifying animals with crypsis, and that these systems developed in brain areas independent or semi-independent of purely perceptual areas, then it could be hypothesized that the ability to detect objects with crypsis could be modified, either enhanced or reduced, by altering activity in these regions. In order to test this hypothesis, we have performed a number of studies that have examined brain responses to camouflaged stimuli, and used brain stimulation designed to alter performance during camouflaged stimulus detection tasks (Clark et al., 2012; Coffman, Trumbo, Flores, et al., 2012; Falcone, Coffman, Clark, & Parasuraman, 2012) and on the relationship between different forms of attention and performance on camouflaged stimuli detection tasks (Coffman, Trumbo, & Clark, 2012).

EXAMINATION OF BRAIN REGIONS SUPPORTING THE DETECTION OF OBJECTS WITH CRYPSIS

The learning task used in these studies was designed in part to examine the brain basis of learning to perceive objects with crypsis. A naturalistic virtual environment was used. The task was designed to be similar to a video game in order to maintain the interest of the research subjects. Subjects did not actively engage in violence in this task, but rather were asked to detect evidence of possible threats, such as camouflaged bombs and snipers hidden in test images, in order to avoid them. This scenario was chosen in part as it represents one of the few realistic circumstances where crypsis is experienced in the modern day.

This task was presented as a discovery-learning paradigm (Bruner, 1961). Discovery learning is a naturalistic form of training, which involves subjects learning with minimal guidance, based on their ability to gain knowledge from interactions with the training environment. Before training, subjects were instructed that they would be placed in the role of a solider attempting to complete a mission in a middle-eastern country. In keeping with the discovery-learning paradigm, no specific information was given with regard to the nature of the camouflaged target objects that would be encountered throughout the mission—it was up to the participant to learn to recognize these objects and the perceptual cues predicting them via the training portion of the study.

Training consisted of a series of still images, presented for 2s each and followed by 1s of a blank screen with a fixation cross in the center, as illustrated in Figure 16.2. Following image presentation, subjects were given 3s during which they were required to press either a button indicating they detected a hidden object in the image, or a button indicating they did not believe an object was concealed within the image. After responding, a brief video clip was displayed showing the consequences of the decision made by the participant. As there were two possible responses that the participant could make (i.e., "hidden object present" or "no hidden object present") and two possibilities within the image (i.e., "hidden object present" or "no hidden object present") four potential feedback outcomes existed.

If a concealed object was present in the image and the subject failed to respond appropriately, the video displayed the outcome (e.g., a bomb blast occurring), which the subject could use to facilitate successful hidden object identification during future trials. During such a clip, the subject would be informed, via auditory feedback, that a hidden object had been missed and casualties had resulted, though no specific information regarding the identity of or precise nature of the threat presented by the hidden object was revealed by the voiceover. If the subject erroneously indicated the presence of a hidden object, they were chastised by the voiceover for delaying the mission. Correct identification of a hidden object resulted in words of praise and a video showed the mission progressing without incident. Correct indication of the absence of a hidden object likewise results in praise and an uneventful video clip. Each training trial lasted roughly 12s, including feedback, and there were four blocks of 60 trials each with brief breaks in between, resulting in approximately 15min per block and a total of 60min of training.

Testing occurred before training, and twice again after subjects reached intermediate and expert levels of expertise. Testing consisted of still images without feedback videos. Each image was presented for 2s followed by a jittered interstimulus interval of 4–8s during which a fixation cross appeared in the center of a gray background. Just as in training, subjects were given 3s following stimulus presentation to indicate via button press whether or not they believed a hidden object to be present in the image. Stimuli were grouped into blocks of 50 images each, for a total duration of 5min per block. For the functional magnetic resonance imaging (fMRI) obtained at novice, intermediate, and expert stages, six test blocks were used for each. During the transcranial direct current stimulation (tDCS) behavioral learning studies, two test blocks each were used for the pretest (prior to training), immediate posttest (just after completion of training), and delayed posttest.

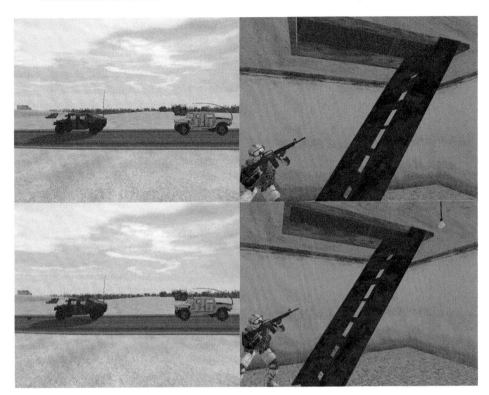

FIGURE 16.2   Examples of stimuli used in the camouflaged target object-learning task. The two top stimuli do not contain camouflaged target objects, while the two bottom stimuli using similar scenes contain camouflaged target objects, in this case a roadside improvised explosive device (IED) in the left image, and a sniper in the right image.

It was found that once learned, the greatest differences in blood oxygen level dependent (BOLD) fMRI responses between stimuli containing camouflaged objects with stimuli that did not was found in frontal, parietal, and cingulate regions, rather than brain regions supporting bottom-up processing such as posterior visual cortex (Clark et al., 2012). These regions showed a significantly greater response to stimuli containing camouflaged target objects when compared with stimuli without such targets. By contrast, occipital cortex showed the reverse effect, with a more negative response to stimuli containing camouflaged targets relative to standard stimuli. This supports the hypothesis that brain networks outside of posterior visual cortex may serve to increase our ability to perceive camouflaged objects, while those in posterior visual areas are actively suppressed, as if their contribution to sensory processing is reduced. Differences associated with training were found in overlapping regions frontal, parietal, and cerebellar regions, as illustrated in Figure 16.3.

This hypothesis was further tested in a series of studies by using anodal tDCS, which is thought to increase neural activity in regions below the stimulating electrode. The results of these studies are shown in Figure 16.4. Placing the anode over right inferior frontal or right parietal cortex led to increased performance on this task, with more than double the performance

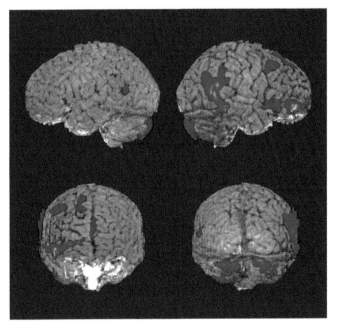

FIGURE 16.3   Brain regions that had a significant change during training from novice to intermediate stages of learning, in a re-analysis of data from Clark et al. (2012). Top row shows the left and right hemispheres on the left and right, respectively, and the bottom row shows the front and back of the brain on the left and right, respectively. Statistical threshold of $p < 0.01$ used and plotted onto a standard brain.

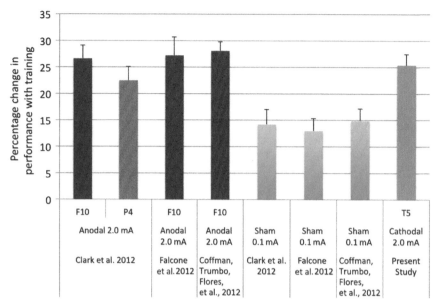

FIGURE 16.4 Results of two previously published studies from our laboratory (Clark et al., 2012; Coffman, Trumbo, & Clark, 2012) and another from a different laboratory (Falcone et al., 2012) using anodal current placed over right inferior frontal cortex, and an additional previously unpublished experiment with cathodal current placed over left occipital-temporal cortex, all using the same camouflaged target object-learning task illustrated in Figure 16.2. Bars indicate the increase in performance with 1 h of training to identify camouflaged target objects, using 2.0 mA of anodal current over F10 (red) or P4 (orange), 0.1 mA of sham current over F10 (blue), or 2.0 mA of cathodal current over T5 (green). For all experiments, the other electrode (cathode or anode) was placed on the right upper arm. Standard errors are indicated. Consistently greater increase in performance was found for 2.0 mA anodal stimulation over right frontal and parietal cortex and cathodal stimulation over left occipital–temporal cortex, when compared with 0.1 mA sham stimulation.

increase over the same amount of training when compared with a sham control (5% of the full current dose). Additionally, this effect increased over a 1 h rest period (Clark et al., 2012). A similar magnitude of effect of anodal tDCS on performance was found in two additional studies (Coffman, Trumbo, & Clark, 2012; Falcone et al., 2012). In Coffman, Trumbo, and Clark (2012), the differential effects of tDCS on performance accuracy were examined between test stimuli that varied by repetition vs. novelty between training and testing phases of the study. Accuracy for target detection discrimination sensitivity (d′) was greater for 2.0 mA current (1.77) compared with 0.1 mA (0.95), and no difference in response bias (β) was found. tDCS was associated with increased performance for all test stimuli, but was greatest for repeated test stimuli vs. novel test stimuli, and also for stimuli with hidden target objects present vs. those absent. This effect may be related to enhanced perception during training, leading to greater performance using learned perceptual strategies during later testing, particularly for previously detected cryptic target objects. Performance in single-blind task and double-blind task designs was not significantly different, suggesting that experimenter bias is not an important feature of this result. Individual differences in skin stimulation and mood also did not predict changes in accuracy. Falcone et al. (2012) used the same task, collecting data at a separate site, and also found a similarly large increase in d′ with active tDCS (1.86) vs sham control (0.73). In addition, a significant reduction in false alarm rate was found. Also, these differences were found to continue when tested again 24 h after stimulation was ended. The long duration of this effect suggested that once learned, the information needed to discriminate camouflaged stimuli was present in long-term memory.

These studies suggest that stimulation of frontal and parietal cortex leads to an increased ability to identify concealed objects in a virtual environment, as indicated by increased performance accuracy and (d′), and reduced false alarm rate. Our original hypothesis was confirmed by these studies; that stimulation of brain regions that mediate endogenous attention would lead to increased performance. An additional hypothesis was that reduction of activity in brain regions that mediate exogenous attentional-perceptual processing would also lead to increased performance. A recently completed study in our laboratory, as yet unpublished, was designed to test this hypothesis. In this study, cathodal current was administered to scalp site T5, above occipital–temporal cortex. Cathodal current is thought to reduce neural activity, and should thus reduce activity in left occipital–temporal cortex. While these regions should be involved in basic visual perception, their emphasis on bottom-up or exogenous processing, which may be confused by camouflage, suggests that reducing their activity should lead to improved performance.

For this study, 13 subjects received 2.0 mA of cathodal current for 30 min over location T5, with the anode placed on the left arm. Subjects were trained for 1 h to detect camouflaged target objects, and were tested before and after training for performance accuracy. This was compared with 23 subjects receiving sham tDCS (5% of the full current dose) published previously (Clark et al., 2012). The difference in performance accuracy found after training vs. before was computed as an indication of learning. For this analysis, subjects with learning scores greater than 1.5 SD from the mean of their condition were removed from further analysis. This included two subjects from the active condition, and three from the sham condition, leaving data from a total of 31 subjects for further analysis.

In this study, it was found that the amount of learning was greater for subjects receiving 2.0 mA of cathodal current over occipital–temporal cortex (25.4%, SD = 7.44%), relative to sham (13.35%, SD = 11.1%) with a significant difference between them (t (30) = 4.5, p = 0.00013). This suggests that suppression of activity in these brain regions may lead to enhanced performance. Taken together with our previous results, we conclude that both stimulation of frontal and parietal brain regions and inhibition of occipital and temporal brain regions leads to an increased ability to detect stimuli with crypsis hidden in complex images. These results are consistent with our hypothesis that endogenous attention and perception supports the accurate detection of camouflaged objects, while exogenous attention reduces this capability.

Other forms of attention may also be related to identifying camouflaged target objects. We performed an additional study to examine the relationship between different forms of attention, performance on this task, and the effects of brain stimulation on both. The Attention Network Task (ANT) was developed by Jin Fan, Michael Posner, and colleagues, and consists of a combination cued reaction time task (Posner, 1980) and flanker task (Eriksen & Eriksen, 1974) that examines the efficiency of three attentional networks—alerting, orienting, and executive attention. The alerting network has been defined as a network that is involved in achieving and maintaining an alert state; the orienting network is responsible for movement of attention through space; and the executive control network is thought to resolve conflict between expectation, stimulus, and response (Fan, McCandliss, Sommer, Raz, & Posner, 2002). Participants are required to indicate the direction (left or right) of a centrally located arrow; response times under various cue conditions (spatial cues, flankers, and alerting cues) are then used to determine network efficiency.

Using the ANT, the effect of tDCS on the aforementioned attentional networks was examined and then compared with performance on the hidden target object detection task. As in the previously described work, participants received either 0.1 mA (N = 10) or 2.0 mA (N = 9) tDCS during training, and test blocks were administered prior to training, immediately following training, and at a long delay. After the immediate test, participants completed the ANT. While orienting, executive network efficiency remained somewhat stable, alerting network efficiency was found to be significantly higher for those participants that received 2.0 mA of stimulation relative to the 0.1 mA group. Additionally, efficiency of the alerting network was found to correlate significantly with proportion of correct hidden target object identification (hits) in the 2.0 mA group (p < 0.01). These results demonstrate that alerting network efficiency may be related to the tDCS enhancement of performance on the hidden target object detection task. It is possible that increasing the efficiency of the alerting network leads to facilitation of initial identification, learning, and/or subsequent recognition of hidden target objects.

A third form of attention that might help to defeat crypsis is multimodal attention. By combining information from different sensory streams, such as auditory or olfactory information, specific combinations of sensory input might help to identify cryptic animals. Even a well-hidden animal might be given away by its scent, style of breathing, vibrations through the earth, or some other feature that could be perceived using a nonvisual sensory modality. Information encoded in the neural architecture could be used to increase identification accuracy by focusing on specific combinations of sensory characteristics that can be used to identify the animal, and/or to suppress the processing of features that tend to be confused by crypsis and reduce the chances of correct detection and identification of the animal.

LIMITATIONS

The proposed relationship between the evolution of crypsis and attention must remain hypothetical, as there are no methods that would allow us to determine the exact timing of the development of these qualities in separate cohabiting species through evolutionary history. However, there may be some options by which we could draw inferences regarding the development of these abilities. One would be to estimate the relative ages of genes associated with crypsis, and of other genes providing attentional and perceptual adaptations to crypsis. We would hypothesize that genes related to specific forms of crypsis that presented new perceptual challenges would occur first, followed by genes that alter brain function in a manner that would compensate for this change, such as an increase in the development of frontal and parietal cortically based visual perceptual and attentional processes. Another option would be to test the hypothesis directly, by developing an environment where a novel form of crypsis is presented, and then to watch as the subject animals improve their ability to detect this new form of crypsis through multiple generations. While this would not test human evolution directly, it would illustrate the progress of evolutionary change with regards to perceptual processing, and attest to the possibility that certain attentional processes were developed in response to new forms of crypsis.

The tDCS experiments described here used treatments designed to increase performance. It would also be interesting to examine treatments that reduce performance, such as applying cathodal tDCS to frontal or parietal cortex, or anodal tDCS to occipital or temporal cortex. We have collected some of the latter data in a limited sample, and find that these subjects do not perform any differently than sham. We are currently not approved by our Human Research Protections Office to perform studies that may lead to decreased capabilities relative to sham; therefore we must focus on studies that increase performance until we are approved to examine forms of stimulation that reduce performance.

Another limitation is the lack of certainty regarding the path of current through the brain. When tDCS is applied, the only certainty is the location of the electrodes and that current must flow from one electrode to another. However, the amount of current shunting through the skin vs that penetrating into the brain, the precise amplitude of current and associated fields within and across brain regions, and the exact properties of how brain tissue interacts with these is not known for certain. We are currently planning studies to quantify current amplitudes in vivo.

CONCLUSIONS

In this chapter, we propose that some aspects of our attentional and perceptual capabilities may have arisen in part as an evolutionary adaptation to the perceptual confusion created by crypsis used by other animals. While this hypothesis is difficult to test directly, we present indirect evidence here. First, we show that the identification of hidden target objects in complex scenes involves a number of brain networks independent of posterior visual cortex, including frontal, parietal, and cingulate brain regions. Their location outside of posterior visual cortex suggests that these networks may have arisen separately from the exogenous or bottom-up perceptual networks located in posterior visual cortex. These frontal–parietal networks may have developed to support endogenous or top-down attentional and perceptual processes. Second, behavioral performance during the hidden target object task, including target detection accuracy, false alarm rate and d′, was greatly improved by applying anodal stimulation to frontal and parietal cortex, and also cathodal stimulation to occipital–temporal cortex, relative to a sham control condition. While the precise effects of anodal and cathodal tDCS on neural activity are not completely understood, it is generally thought that anodal stimulation leads to greater neural excitation, while cathodal stimulation leads to less excitation. If true, we can conclude that excitation of frontal–parietal cortex and inhibition of occipital–temporal cortex both result in an increased ability to detect hidden target objects. Finally, we describe the results of a study whereby anodal stimulation of right frontal cortex leads to increased alerting attention, but without a significant change in orienting or executive attention, and enhanced alerting was also associated with better detection of camouflaged stimuli in this task. Taken together, these results agree with the hypothesis that both alerting and endogenous attentional processes are associated with detecting hidden target objects. These forms of attention supported by brain networks located in frontal and parietal cortex may have arisen through evolution at least in part as a response to crypsis, to augment perception or correct perceptual errors made by occipital–temporal networks that are more susceptible to the misperception created by crypsis. Endogenous attention may be more beneficial for detecting camouflaged target objects than exogenous or bottom-up forms of attentional and perceptual processes.

While primarily theoretical, the conclusion that a portion of our perceptual processes may have developed in response to the evolutionary pressures presented by crypsis, leads to a number of additional predictions. First, we would predict that the relative excitation and inhibition of frontal-parietal vs. occipital–temporal cortex would influence performance on other tasks designed to tap into endogenous vs. exogenous attention, in a crossed manner. If correct, then increased frontal–parietal relative to occipital–temporal activity would be associated with increased performance on endogenous attention tasks and reduced performance on exogenous attention tasks, while the reverse would be found for reversed polarity of stimulation (e.g., reduced frontal–parietal relative to occipital–temporal activity would be associated with increased performance on exogenous attention tasks and reduced performance on endogenous attention tasks). Another set of predictions relates to the possibility that, if our ancestors developed perceptual capabilities to increase the accuracy of identifying specific animals with crypsis (such as large predatory cats), our neural architecture might still retain some evidence of these adaptations. If true, then our ability to identify the specific perceptual characteristics by which ancient predators might be identified may still be greater, relative to other features that would not offer the same evolutionary advantages for our ancestors. Such vestigial aspects of our perceptual systems, designed to maximize our ancestors' survival in their ancient environment, may be stored in our genetic code. This might offer an explanation for a variety of findings from studies of attention and perception that have proven difficult to explain otherwise. Finally, another set of hypotheses relates to the relationship between environment and changes in our perceptual processes across generations. We have greatly modified our environment in a very short time, resulting in very different needs for survival than were experienced by our ancestors just a few generations ago. Our perceptual world has changed from purely natural, with crypsis prevalent in our day-to-day existence, to technological and digital. It is likely that with such changes, there may be a variety of new adaptations in our perceptual and attentional capabilities. Evidence of such changes is already being found. For instance, Daphne Bavelier and colleagues (Bavelier, Achtman, & Mani, 2012; Green & Bavelier, 2003, 2006, 2007) have found substantial differences in perceptual performance and neural activity between video game players and those who do not play, as well as changes within subjects associated with learning to play video games.

It is impossible to predict with certainty what ramifications will occur from the changes we have introduced to our environment for the perceptual and attentional systems of our descendants. However, it is likely that some other changes will occur over time as we adapt to new tools and circumstances we create. Regardless of what the outcome will be, it seems likely that remnants of our evolutionary history will be present for many generations to come, and it might be beneficial for us to consider the history of our species to date, as we develop a more complete understanding of the features of our brain organization that we study using cognitive electrophysiology and other methods available to us.

References

Bagnara, J. T., & Hadley, M. E. (1973). *Chromatophores and color change: The comparative physiology of animal pigmentation.* New Jersey: Prentice-Hall. Retrieved from http://www.getcited.org/pub/101320882.

Bavelier, D., Achtman, R. L., & Mani, M. (2012). Neural bases of selective attention in action video game players. *Vision Research, 61,* 132–143.

Bruner, J. S. (1961). The act of discovery. *Harvard Educational Review, 31,* 21–32.

Clark, V. P., Coffman, B. A., Mayer, A. R., Weisend, M. P., Lane, T. D. R., Calhoun, V. D., et al. (2012). TDCS guided using fMRI significantly accelerates learning to identify concealed objects. *NeuroImage, 59,* 117–128.

Coffman, B. A., Trumbo, M. C., & Clark, V. P. (2012). Enhancement of object detection with transcranial direct current stimulation is associated with increased attention. *BMC Neuroscience, 13,* 108.

Coffman, B. A., Trumbo, M. C., Flores, R. A., Garcia, C. M., van der Merwe, A. J., Wassermann, E. M., et al. (2012). Impact of tDCS on performance and learning of target detection: interaction with stimulus characteristics and experimental design. *Neuropsychologia, 50,* 1594–1602.

Darwin, C. (1859). *On the origin of species by means of natural selection, or the preservation of favoured races in the struggle for life.*

Dominy, N. J., & Lucas, P. W. (2001). Ecological importance of trichromatic vision to primates. *Nature, 410,* 363–366.

Endler, J. A., & Greenwood, J. J. D. (1988). Frequency-dependent predation, crypsis and aposematic coloration [and discussion]. *Philosophical Transactions of the Royal Society of London. B, Biological Sciences, 319,* 505–523.

Eriksen, B. A., & Eriksen, C. W. (1974). Effects of noise letters upon identification of a target letter in a nonsearch task. *Perception & Psychophysics, 16,* 143–149.

Falcone, B., Coffman, B. A., Clark, V. P., & Parasuraman, R. (2012). Transcranial direct current stimulation augments perceptual sensitivity and 24-hour retention in a complex threat detection task. *PLoS ONE, 7*(4), e34993.

Fan, J., McCandliss, B. D., Sommer, T., Raz, A., & Posner, M. I. (2002). Testing the efficiency and independence of attentional networks. *Journal of Cognitive Neuroscience, 14,* 340–347.

Figuerola, J., & Senar, J. C. (2005). Seasonal changes in carotenoid-and melanin-based plumage coloration in the Great Tit Parus major. *IBIS, 147,* 797–802.

Fink, W. L. (1998). Sternoptychidae. In J. R. Paxton & W. N. Eschmeyer (Eds.), *Encyclopedia of fishes.* (Vol. 121). San Diego: Academic Press.

Froesch, D., & Messenger, J. B. (1978). On leucophores and the chromatic unit of *Octopus vulgaris. Journal of Zoology, 186,* 163–173.

Glass, K., Ito, S., Wilby, P. R., Sota, T., Nakamura, A., Bowers, C. R., et al. (2012). Direct chemical evidence for eumelanin pigment from the Jurassic period. *National Academy of Science of the United States of America, 109,* 10218–10223.

Green, C. S., & Bavelier, D. (2003). Action video game modifies visual selective attention. *Nature, 423,* 534–537.

Green, C. S., & Bavelier, D. (2006). Effect of action video games on the spatial distribution of visuospatial attention. *Journal of Experimental Psychology of Human Perception and Performance, 32,* 1465–1478.

Green, C. S., & Bavelier, D. (2007). Action-video-game experience alters the spatial resolution of vision. *Psychological Science, 18,* 88–94.

Posner, M. I. (1980). Orienting of attention. *The Quarterly Journal of Experimental Psychology, 32,* 3–25.

Roth, L. S. V., Lundström, L., Kelber, A., Kröger, R. H. H., & Unsbo, P. (2009). The pupils and optical systems of gecko eyes. *Journal of Vision, 9,* 1–11.

Semple, S., Cowlishaw, G., & Bennett, P. M. (2002). Immune system evolution among anthropoid primates: parasites, injuries and predators. *Proceedings of the Royal Society of London. Series B: Biological Sciences, 269,* 1031–1037.

Stimulus-Preceding Negativity (SPN) and Attention to Rewards

Steven A. Hackley[1], Fernando Valle-Inclán[2], Hiroaki Masaki[3], Karen Hebert[1]

[1]University of Missouri, Columbia, MO, USA, [2]University of La Coruña, La Coruña, Spain, [3]Waseda University, Tokyo, Japan

ELECTROPHYSIOLOGY OF REWARD PROCESSING

Electrophysiology has played a central role in the investigation of the reward system since the discovery of this vital brain network by Olds and Milner (1954). The current prevalence of addiction and obesity gives impetus to this research. So far, the two most important contributions of surface electrophysiology have been the development of: (1) the error-related negativity (ERN) and closely related feedback negativity (FN) (ERN/Ne; Falkenstein, Hohnsbein, Hoorman, & Blanke, 1991; Gehring, Gross, Coles, Meyer, & Donchin, 1993; FN; Holroyd & Coles, 2002; Miltner, Braun, & Coles, 1997) as indices of the violation of reward expectation, and (2) probe-startle electromyography (EMG) as a measure of affective reactions to motivationally relevant stimuli (Vrana, Spence, & Lang, 1988). Research using these measures has enhanced our understanding of how the receipt of reward or punishment is processed in the brain.

Animal research using invasive electrophysiological methods has identified specific correlates of the anticipation as well as receipt of reinforcing stimuli. Schultz and colleagues (e.g., Schultz, Dayan, & Montague, 1997; Schultz, Tremblay, & Hollerman, 2000) report that midbrain dopaminergic cells fire in response to reward-predicting cues, especially when reward receipt is uncertain (Fiorillo, Tobbler, & Schultz, 2003). Neurons within dopamine-innervated cortical areas (e.g., orbitofrontal cortex) increase their firing rate as the action outcome draws near. The dopamine-secreting cells briefly discharge if the outcome is better than expected, but pause their firing if it is worse than expected. This phasic discharge is thought to serve as a diffusely broadcast teaching signal that enhances synaptic plasticity (Baldwin, Sadeghian, & Kelley, 2002; Tsai et al., 2009).

If this account is correct, and if the signal that mediates reinforcement-based learning reflects the difference between expected and received reward, then it is important to develop electrophysiological measures of this expectation in humans. To do so is critical, not just for addressing applied problems, but also because motivational processes are involved at least implicitly in nearly every attention-demanding task studied in the laboratory. In the case of animal research, Maunsell (2004) points out, attention and reward expectation are essentially indistinguishable. This is because the only tool available for controlling attention is the manipulation of immediate, primary rewards. In the case of human research, this possible isomorphism is less obvious because rewards and penalties are often indirect or social. A participant may reasonably expect that if he stops pressing the keys, the experimenter will enter the recording chamber and convey her concern and disappointment. By contrast, if he pays close attention and does his best, both he and the experimenter are likely to be pleased with his performance.

The event-related potential (ERP) that has been the focus of efforts to develop a measure of reward expectation is the stimulus-preceding negativity (SPN). This paper reviews the evidence for a specific association between the SPN and anticipatory activation within cortical portions of the reward system.

DECOMPOSITION OF THE CONTINGENT NEGATIVE VARIATION

The paradigms used for studying the SPN were developed during attempts to fractionate the contingent negative variation (CNV) (Walter, Cooper, Aldridge, McCallum, & Winter, 1964) into subcomponents reflecting motor preparation and perceptual attention. Discovery of the CNV marks the birth of cognitive neuroscience. The main experiment included a comparison across two conditions demonstrating that the component is purely endogenous: In a no-task control condition, subjects received a click followed 1 s later by a train of flashes. Both of these stimuli triggered modality-specific ERPs. In the task condition, the participants were told to make a speeded button press when the flashes began, in order to turn them off. Auditory and visual potentials were also evoked in this condition. In addition, though, a large, slow, negativity was observed that grew in amplitude during the interval between S1 and S2, terminating abruptly with the subject's key-press response.

What makes this the foundational study of cognitive neuroscience is the fact that the CNV is entirely endogenous. As one of the authors later put it: "It is important to note that CNV is not related to the characteristics of the stimuli themselves, but to the use that the subject makes of them—a link to cognitive psychology that has been very valuable" (Cooper, 1985). A specific link to the concept of attention was evident to two of the first neuroscientists to replicate Walter and colleagues, Hillyard and Galambos (1967). They stated that "The CNV could be an electrical component of the attention process, the function of which is to prepare the organism for reception and action".

Other researchers challenged this claim, arguing instead that the critical late portion of the CNV was solely due to preparation for action. Most notably, Rohrbaugh, Syndulko, and Lindsley (1976) attempted to decompose the CNV by separately estimating the early and late subcomponents. One condition measured the task-related response to S1 in isolation, the so-called "O-wave". The authors assumed that this component reflects an immediate response to the warning signal itself (e.g., perceptual interpretation) rather than expectation of the S2. This assumption is supported by recent evidence (Grent-'t-Jong & Woldorff, 2007). A second condition specifically assessed the motor readiness potential generated as the subject prepared an unwarned, key-press response identical to that used in the critical third condition. That third condition was a standard CNV paradigm in which S1 signaled the imminent arrival of S2, the imperative stimulus. Results showed that the algebraic sum of the O-wave and readiness potential obtained in the first two conditions closely matched the CNV obtained in the third condition. A subsequent review paper by Rohrbaugh and Gaillard (1983) summarized evidence that the CNV does not include a perceptual expectancy component. Rather, the early CNV comprises solely the immediate response to

S1, and the late CNV, preparation for the movement that will follow S2.

Even at the time of that review there was fragmentary evidence that the late CNV was not purely motoric. This evidence guided subsequent efforts to identify slow potentials that unambiguously reflect perceptual expectancy. By the early 1990s, two distinct programs of research emerged. One focuses on top-down, goal-directed control of selective perceptual processing. The other deals with motivationally relevant stimuli that draw attention automatically as their arrival is awaited.

GOAL-DIRECTED ATTENTION

Departing from conventional CNV trial structure, the top-down paradigm replaces the warning signal (S1) with a more specific, attention-directing cue. The cue does not just convey how attention should be oriented in time (e.g., the target will be presented in 900 ms), the cue also predicts the location or perceptual attributes of S2 (e.g., there is an 80% chance that the target will be displayed to the left of fixation). By contrast, the trial structure for studying motivational salience either incorporates a delayed feedback stimulus following the response, or else S2 is not a target but, rather, an intrinsically engaging event such as an electric shock or erotic photograph.

Beginning with a study by Harter, Miller, Price, LaLonde, and Keyes (1989), research on top-down control has emphasized lateralized difference potentials. The advantage of studying these brain waves is that they generally have well defined anatomical and cognitive correlates. Lateralized ERPs have been used to investigate such diverse processes as retention in working memory, retrieval from long-term memory, motor programming, response execution, and the automatic capture of attention (e.g., Gratton, 1998; Luck & Hillyard, 1994; Vogel, McCollough, & Machizawa, 2005).

The methods used by Harter et al. (1989) are representative. Each trial began with a left-pointing arrow or right-pointing arrow, which cued the side of the screen that the participant should shift their attention to, but without moving their eyes. One second after cue onset, a small square was flashed to the left or right of fixation. If it appeared on the cued side, the subjects (7-year-old boys) were to press a key with their right index finger.

To compute difference potentials, waveforms recorded at electrodes ipsilateral to the attended hemifield were subtracted from the corresponding waveforms at contralateral sites. Trials with left-pointing cues and right-pointing cues were then averaged. Among the lateralized components was a negativity at parietal and occipital sites opposite the attended hemifield, peaking about 180–220 ms following cue onset. Conforming to the (grammatically challenged) nomenclature that had been introduced by Deecke, Heise, Kornhuber, Lang, and Lang (1984), Harter et al. named this component the early directing attention negativity(EDAN).

Note that the S1–S2 trial structure was similar to that of the typical CNV experiment. The fact that EDAN was largest at sites overlying visual cortex and its laterality shifted in accordance with the focus of attention is compelling evidence against the hypothesis that the late CNV is purely motoric. Other research has further shown that attention-directing components can predict the size of target-evoked potentials, that they can be elicited by cues that direct attention cross-modally, and that they can reflect anticipation of nonspatial perceptual features (Dale, Simpson, Foxe, Luks, & Worden, 2008; Eimer, van Velzen, & Driver, 2002).

EARLY SPN RESEARCH

The second line of evidence against Rohrbaugh and Gaillard's hypothesis involves findings from research concerning anticipation of motivationally relevant stimuli. It seems likely that the attention-directing processes reflected in the components discussed above (e.g., EDAN, anterior directing attention negativity (ADAN)) contribute to the waveforms observed in this second group of studies, even though the visual stimuli they employ are almost always presented at fixation. Indeed, recent functional magnetic resonance imaging (fMRI) data indicate considerable overlap between the structures that underlie goal-directed attention and those that mediate anticipation of motivationally relevant stimuli (Krebs, Boehler, Roberts, Song, & Woldorff, 2012).

Some of the first papers that followed Walter et al.'s (1964) report emphasized the possibility that the CNV might reflect motivational processes. For example, the CNV was found to be larger prior to intense as compared to weak electro-cutaneous shocks (Irwin, Knott, McAdam, & Rebert, 1966). Sustained negativities were also observed prior to performance feedback (Weinberg, 1973) and slides of opposite-sex nudes (Simons, Öhman, & Lang, 1979). Because no overt response was required to the feedback or slides, these findings constituted evidence for the existence of nonmotoric slow waves. However, concerns remained: Might subjects prepare the oculomotor system to scan the erotic slides, thereby generating a Readiness Potential? Could negativity prior to feedback be caused by movement of the fingers to a resting posture in preparation for the intertrial interval (ITI)?

The first studies that convincingly isolated the SPN from movement-related components of the CNV were those of Damen and Brunia (1987). Their subjects performed a time estimation task, pressing a key when a certain number of seconds had elapsed after an imperative stimulus. Then, following a delay of 2 s, a feedback display indicated whether the interval was too short, too long, or just right. Movement-related potentials recorded in a control condition with repetitive, uncued, key presses were subtracted from ERPs in the main condition, to minimize the electrical potentials caused by repositioning the fingers to a resting posture prior to the ITI.

The subtraction procedure was successful in that the early portion of the interval extending from key press to feedback appeared flat. A large negative wave then developed, reaching a peak at the moment of arrival of the feedback display. Scalp topography also supported the assumption that the SPN was nonmotoric. Whereas ERPs associated with the key-press response were largest at sites overlying motor cortex contralateral to whichever hand responded—the SPN was consistently largest over the right hemisphere. Thus, by the late 1980s the existence of nonmotoric slow potentials reflecting stimulus anticipation was firmly established.

TWO ATTENTION NETWORKS

As the goal of early SPN research was to establish the existence of a *nonmotoric slow wave during stimulus anticipation*, this was essentially the definition of the SPN adopted in previous reviews (e.g., Brunia, 1988; Brunia, Hackley, van Boxtel, Kotani, & Ohgami, 2011; Van Boxtel & Böcker, 2004). Explicitly included within this category were slow potentials prior to probe stimuli in working memory and mental arithmetic tasks, prior to target stimuli requiring perceptual discrimination, and prior to trial-by-trial instructional displays. For most purposes, such a definition is nowadays too broad to be useful. Attention researchers who record ADAN and memory researchers who study the contralateral delay activity do not use the term *SPN* to refer to their measures. Consequently, we restrict the term SPN to negative slow waves preceding motivationally relevant stimuli, and focus our discussion specifically on the ERP that precedes feedback.

Following Brunia et al. (2011), we approach the problem of identifying SPN sources using Corbetta and Shulman's (2002) theory as a starting point. Under their account, attention is controlled by two partially segregated networks. The dorsal or goal-directed network is responsible for top-down control of perceptual resources—*active attention*, in James' (1890) terminology. Goal-directed control is implemented mainly by two bilateral regions of neocortex, roughly centered on the frontal eye fields and intraparietal sulci (IPS). The ventral or stimulus-driven network controls the automatic capture of attention by salient, novel, and other biologically relevant stimuli.

Although Corbetta and Shulman mainly review tasks involving arbitrary visual stimuli, they endorse James' broader perspective. He stated that *passive attention* is involuntarily captured when the stimulus is "intense, voluminous, or sudden; or it…appeals to some of our congenital impulses,… strange things, moving things, wild animals, bright things, pretty things, metallic things, blows, blood, etc." James' terminology has not been retained because in the late twentieth century it was shown that stimulus-driven (exogenous) attention is not passive or independent of task context (e.g., Folk, Remington, & Johnston, 1992; Yantis, 1993). A large, ferocious animal prowling only a few meters away might fail to capture the attention of a worker who has collected trash from that part of the zoo for several years.

A review of the relevant lesion and neuroimaging literature led Corbetta and Shulman to conclude that stimulus-driven attention is mediated mainly by two areas within the right hemisphere. One area comprises the inferior frontal gyrus, especially the operculum that overlies the right anterior insula, plus the portion of the middle frontal gyrus superior to the anterior insula. The other component of the ventral attention system is the temporo-parietal junction (TPJ). Subsequent research indicated that this region extends into the posterior insula (Fox, Corbetta, Snyder, Vincent, & Raichle, 2006).

Insular cortex is important because a source localization study of the pre-feedback SPN localized its main generators to the left and right insulae (Böcker, Brunia, & van den Berg-Lenssen, 1994). Topographic analyses are generally consistent with this. The SPN is broadly distributed over frontal, central and parietal sites. With regard to frontal and central electrodes, amplitudes are greater over the right hemisphere (e.g., Damen & Brunia, 1987). The right-hemisphere dominance is consistent with Corbetta and Shulman's (2002) account of the stimulus-driven attention network, as is the fact that the effect of monetary reward on the SPN is greatest at right prefrontal sites (Ohgami, Kotani, Hiraku, Aihara, & Ishii, 2004).

However, several SPN studies have reported a bilaterally symmetrical distribution. Ohgami et al. (2006) noted a methodological difference between monetary-incentive experiments that did and did not report right dominance. Studies that obtained the typical pattern included monetary penalties as well as rewards (e.g., Masaki, Takeuchi, Gehring, Takasawa, & Yamazaki, 2006; Masaki, Yamazaki, & Hackley, 2010), whereas those reporting bilaterally symmetrical negativity used only rewards (e.g., Kotani et al., 2003). Ohgami and coworkers interpreted this difference in terms of Davidson's theory (Davidson, Ekman, Saton, Senulis, & Friesen, 1990) that the left hemisphere is relatively specialized for approach and the right for withdrawal behavior. If this is the case, then a design favoring reward outcomes might lead to greater activation of the left hemisphere that could neutralize SPN's normal right dominance.

NEUROIMAGING DATA

Cognitive electrophysiologists are fortunate to be able to draw upon a rich neuroimaging literature in the attempt to identify likely generators of the SPN. The main challenge is that fMRI studies of reward anticipation generally use a trial structure that is more similar to that of a CNV than SPN experiment. The typical study follows the seminal methods of Knutson, Adams, Fong, and Hommer (2001). The precue (S1) signals the time of arrival of the imperative stimulus (S2), as well as the size and valence of the incentive (e.g., a chance to win $5.00). The display (S3) that conveys performance feedback and monetary outcome is presented soon after the key-press response. The pre-feedback interval is brief, unjittered, and not modeled by a unique regressor during data analysis. This poses an interpretive challenge because during the time period that is modeled, the pre-S2 interval, the subject is preparing to perceive and respond to the task stimulus. The incentive cue presumably alters these processes in addition to the ones that underlie reward anticipation. Obviously, the participant can be expected to try harder when more money is at stake.

An exception to this general approach is the study by Kotani et al. (2009), which was designed to analyze the pre-feedback interval. These investigators used the time-interval production task of Damen and Brunia (1987). Each trial began with an instructional cue that signaled the start of the time interval and indicated the duration of the interval to be produced, 4, 6, or 8s. The participants pressed a button with their right hand when they judged that this amount of time had elapsed. Three seconds later, feedback was presented that indicated whether the interval was too short, too long, or correct. The range of acceptable correct responses was adjusted across blocks to create easy, moderate, or difficult conditions. There was also a no feedback control condition.

Contrasts between difficult-vs.-easy conditions and difficult-vs.-moderate conditions were analyzed based on the assumption that attention to feedback would be enhanced in the more demanding tasks. A previous study by the Tokyo Tech group had shown that the SPN is larger when the feedback display conveys a greater degree of useful information (e.g., not just that the interval was incorrect, but that it specifically was too short by a certain amount; Kotani et al., 2003). This effect of informativeness was enhanced when positive feedback was supplemented by a monetary reward.

The fMRI contrasts revealed significant activation differences within the right anterior insula and the extra-striate visual cortex. This supports the assumption (Brunia et al., 2011) that the right-lateralized attention network of Corbetta and Shulman (2002) is a major source of the pre-feedback SPN. Corbetta and Shulman's ventral–dorsal dichotomy was more fully articulated in subsequent study (Fox et al., 2006) by the St. Louis group using a meta-analysis of their previous research, plus a new, resting-state, functional connectivity analysis. Comparing those findings (their Figure 5) to the pre-feedback data of Kotani et al. (2009), a number of tentative inferences can be drawn. Regarding the ventral attention network, Kotani and coworkers found pre-feedback activation within the left and right frontal opercula plus adjacent insular cortex, the middle frontal gyrus just above the right anterior insula, the anterior cingulate, and the right TPJ extending into the inferior parietal lobule. With respect to the dorsal attention system, there was a close match for the left and right IPS. No activation was identified in the other main constituent of the dorsal system, the frontal eye fields (see also Brunia, de Jong, van den Berg-Lenssen, & Paans, 2000).

It makes sense that both the dorsal and ventral attention networks would be activated as participants await arrival of a feedback display. Feedback includes both an affective, motivational component (positive feedback feels good; one strives to receive it), and also a cognitive component (feedback provides information that is needed to learn the task). A recent fMRI study (Krebs et al., 2012) directly compared the two attention networks. The cue indicated the hemifield in which the relevant target stimulus would be located, and it also signaled whether the perceptual task would be difficult or easy (dorsal system) and whether performance feedback would or would not be supplemented by a monetary incentive (ventral system). The findings were consistent with those of Kotani et al. (2009). A conjunction analysis for the S1–S2 interval showed that both types of cues activated the right IPS and the left and right anterior insulae, plus the overlying inferior frontal gyri. An interaction between the two cue types was observed in the antero-medial cingulate cortex.

Studies of the pre-feedback SPN have found inconsistent or negligible effects of perceptual difficulty (Bastiaansen, Böcker, & Brunia, 2002; Hillman, Apparies, & Hatfield, 2000; Kotani & Aihara, 1999). However, scalp topography does vary predictably as a function of the modality of the feedback stimulus (Brunia & van Boxtel, 2004; Ohgami et al., 2004) and left vs. right visual hemifield (Ohgami, Kotani, Yoshihiro, Tsukamoto, & Inoue, 2010). Consequently, it seems likely that the goal-directed attention network does contribute to the pre-feedback SPN.

By way of summary, the best evidence indicates that the generators of the SPN include the bilateral insulae, the inferior and middle frontal gyri directly above the right anterior insula; the middle or anterior cingulate gyrus; the bilateral IPS; the right TPJ; and the relevant modality-specific cortex. Current evidence supports the conclusion of previous reviews that, among neocortical structures, the anterior insulae are of paramount importance in the anticipation of feedback and monetary incentives (ERPs: Brunia et al., 2011; fMRI: Knutson & Greer, 2008).

PARKINSON'S DISEASE

These various cortical areas lie downstream from the heart of the reward system, the mesencephalic-striatal dopamine pathway. Although midbrain dopaminergic cells directly innervate cortical portions of the reward system (Lewis, Foote, Goldstein, & Morrison, 1988), their connections to the accumbens/caudate/putamen may be more important. It is via these connections that they modulate a set of parallel loops comprising partially overlapping regions of frontal cortex, striatum, pallidum, thalamus, and cortex (Alexander, DeLong, & Strick, 1986). The limbic loop is the most relevant to understanding reward expectation (Haber and Knutson, 2010), because it includes the nucleus accumbens, anterior cingulate, and orbitofrontal cortex.

It stands to reason, therefore, that attrition of dopamine-secreting neurons would compromise the function of the reward system, including the processes underlying reward anticipation. Parkinson's disease (PD) kills cells that have long, thin, poorly myelinated axons. Beginning about midway through the course of this disorder, large numbers of neurons that secrete dopamine die (Braak, Ghebremedhim, Rüb, Bratzke, & Del Tredici, 2004). Loss of dopaminergic cells that innervate the ventral striatum is delayed compared to attrition of the ones that supply the dorsal striatum. However, it is now recognized that the dorsal striatum also plays a vital role in reward processing (Haber & Knutson, 2010).

Two experiments at this laboratory assessed the SPN in patients with PD (Hebert, Valle-Inclán, Oh, Rolan, & Hackley, 2006; Mattox, Valle-Inclán, & Hackley, 2006). In the Mattox et al. study, 20 medication-withdrawn patients who had mild PD were compared to 32 age-matched control subjects using a reinforcement-learning paradigm. Performance of the *weather prediction task* is known to be slightly impaired by PD (Knowlton, Mangels, & Squire, 1996; Shohamy, Myers, Gluck, & Onlaor, 2004). As the task is learned, associations gradually develop based on repetition of triads comprising the stimulus, motor response, and reinforcement. The reinforcing feedback is probabilistic in nature. For example, pressing the key for "cloudy" rather than "sunny" in response to a card with purple circles would usually be followed by "Correct, + $0.75". Occasionally, though, the outcome would be "Incorrect, − $0.75".

Stimulus–response learning in the weather prediction task is associated with increased activation of the basal ganglia during both acquisition and performance phases, at least in people who are neurologically normal (Poldrack, Prabhakaran, Seger, & Gabrieli, 1999). Our behavioral results confirmed that people with PD do not perform as well as age-matched control subjects. More importantly, the results also showed that the SPN prior to the feedback was smaller in PD patients, but did not increase as a function of the size of rewards/penalties ($0.75 vs. $0.05), and was not larger on difficult as opposed to easy trials (3 cards vs. 1 card).

The follow-up study has only been published in abstract form (Hebert et al., 2006), so it will be described in more detail. The main purpose was to confirm the effect of PD on SPN amplitude, but in a group of patients in whom the disease was more advanced. A secondary goal was to test whether deep-brain stimulation (DBS) of the subthalamic nucleus (STN) would restore the SPN to normal levels. The apparatus delivers high frequency (~130 Hz) pulses 24 h a day. Whether the immediate effect within the STN should be considered as excitatory, inhibitory, frequency modulating, or patterned is still a matter of debate (Naskar, Sood, Goyal, & Dhara, 2010).

The downstream effects are more clearly established, as are the relevant anatomical connections. The STN is situated between the globus pallidus pars externa and the output nuclei of the basal ganglia, the substantia nigra pars reticulata (SNr) and globus pallidus pars interna (GPi), thereby comprising a portion of the "indirect pathway". Downstream effects include decreased activity within the supplementary motor area and sensorimotor cortex (Hershey et al., 2003; Thobois et al., 2002). Among putative SPN generators, effects of DBS are most reliably observed in the right inferior parietal lobule and anterior cingulate cortex.

The final sample comprised eight patients (two women) and 17 healthy controls (six women). The average illness duration was 13 years, and the time since their surgery was 1.5 years. A moderate degree of motor impairments persisted even when patients were on stimulation, as indicated by an average Hoehn and Yahr (1967) score of 3.97. On average, the patients were taking 50% of their presurgery dopaminergic medication dosage, but were not withdrawn from medication prior to participation (as subjects in the Mattox et al., 2006; study were).

Two versions of the reinforcement-learning task (Knowlton et al., 1994) that differed superficially were used, the "weather task" and the "stock market task". Cues consisted of four cards with different shapes. Each was associated with a given outcome at a fixed probability (0.2, 0.4, 0.6, and 0.8 for *sunny*, and the complementary probability for *cloudy*). There were four experimental blocks of 98 trials. Subjects completed testing over

2 days, with two experimental blocks per day (one block of the weather task, one of the stock market task). Task order was counterbalanced across subjects, with each task paired to a particular DBS state in the patient group (e.g., stock market task = DBS "on").

A trial began with the display of 1–3 cards on the screen. After the participant entered a response, the cards remained on the screen for 1000 ms. This was followed by a fixation-only screen for 2000 ms, the pre-feedback interval. If the subject's guess was a good one, the word "correct" was then displayed in green with the amount of money won (+ $1.00). For a wrong guess, the word "incorrect" was displayed in red along with the amount of money lost (− $1.00). The feedback screen remained on for 4000 ms, and was followed by an ITI of 4–6 s.

Electroencephalograms were recorded at F3, F4, C3, C4, FPz, Fz, Cz, and Pz, referred to the left mastoid (band pass, 0.01–30 Hz; digitization, 600 Hz). Eye movements were monitored by bipolar horizontal and vertical electro-oculograms. At least 70% of the experimental trials were retained for all subjects following rejection of those with artifacts. Epochs extended from 3000 ms preceding onset of the paired key press until 4000 ms later. Mean voltage of the first 500 ms within this 7000 ms epoch served as baseline. The measurement window for the SPN was 1000–3000 ms following the key press. There were no reliable differences in reaction time or accuracy between groups or, for patients, between on versus off DBS states.

Confirming the previous findings of Mattox et al. (2006), SPN amplitude was diminished or absent in participants whose dopaminergic system had been compromised by PD (Figure 17.1). The difference in amplitude was most reliable in the comparison of control subjects and patients when their DBS was turned on, $F(1, 23) = 6.55$, $p < 0.02$. Collapsing across DBS state, the effect of group was also significant, $F(1, 23) = 5.58$, $p < 0.04$.

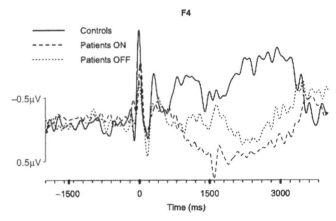

FIGURE 17.1 Grand average event-related potentials during the pre-feedback interval for healthy control subjects and PD patients who had deep brain stimulation (DBS) turned on or off.

There was no effect of DBS state. As expected, the SPN in control participants was larger over the right hemisphere ($F(1,15) = 5.35$, $p < 0.05$).

A likely explanation for SPN absence was loss of dopaminergic cells, but an alternative interpretation could be built upon some other pathological feature of PD, such as a loss of serotonergic or noradrenergic cells. However, a recent study of healthy young adults who differed with regard to dopamine genes (viz., catechol-O-methyltranferase) supports our original interpretation. Foti and Hajcak (2012) found that individuals of the Met/Met genotype generated larger SPN amplitudes prior to feedback in a gambling task than participants categorized either as Val/Met of Val/Val. Similarly, patients with schizophrenia—a dopaminergic disorder—exhibited reduced SPNs prior to emotion-inducing photographs that conveyed task feedback (Wynn, Horan, Kring, Simons, & Green, 2010).

RESPONSE-CONTINGENT INCENTIVES

In the language of everyday life as well that of science, the terms *reward*, *punishment*, and *penalty* refer to action outcomes. According to Skinner (1938) what becomes associated during instrumental learning is the triad of stimulus setting, action, and reinforcer. Therefore, a pleasant event that is not contingent on the subject's response (e.g., an erotic photo in an emotion study), is not a reward. It is not likely to fully engage the neural system that was created by evolution to reinforce adaptive behavior. This assertion is supported by a number of fMRI studies. Difference in activation patterns between response-contingent (instrumental) and noncontingent (Pavlovian) trial types reliably includes, for example, greater activation of the striatum in the former (e.g., Bjork & Hommer, 2007; Tricomi, Delgado, & Fiez, 2002, 2004).

Bjork and Hommer (2007) used a variant of the monetary incentive delay (MID; Knutson et al., 2001). As noted earlier, the MID can be characterized as a CNV paradigm in the sense that the measured interval involves brain activity associated with motor preparation and pretarget sensory attention as well as reward anticipation. This lack of specificity is less of a drawback if one's goal is to understand how triads of cue, response, and reinforcer become bound together during instrumental learning. For the present purpose, we can simply ignore visual, motor, and subcortical findings as being of marginal relevance to understanding neocortical activity that is specific to the pre-feedback SPN.

On each trial of their study, the cue indicated both the probability of a reward ($1.00; $p = 0$, 0.5, or 1.0) and whether the participant should or should not make a speeded key-press response when the target (a white square) was presented. Onset asynchrony of the cue and target was 2500 ms, and of the target and feedback, 2000 ms, with no jitter. Among putative SPN generators, greater activation for $p = 1.0$ vs 0 was found for the left and right insulae, the left superior and inferior parietal lobules, and the left cingulate motor area (mid-cingulate cortex). These activations were only observed during active trials, those for which the subject was required to make a response. During the passive condition, little effect of the probability manipulation was observed.

Critics might argue that the requirement of making a motor response simply increases the salience of the target and feedback stimuli. The observed increase in activation might have nothing to do with response contingency or, for that matter, reward expectation. However, Tricomi et al. (2002, 2004) obtained similar results using a paradigm that equated perceptual and motor factors across conditions. On both active and passive trials, participants performed a perceptual discrimination task in which the key press was followed by a monetary gain or loss. On half of the trials, a cue correctly indicated that the monetary outcome was randomly determined by the computer. Gain or loss was also random on the other trials, but it was implied otherwise. The cue on these trials signaled that the subject should try to guess the correct response. A postexperimental questionnaire indicated that the participants believed that they had more control in the active condition. The striatum was the region of interest in Tricomi et al.'s (2004) article, but a preliminary report including whole-brain analyses (Tricomi et al., 2002) showed that the anterior insulae were more strongly activated when participants believed that the monetary gains and losses were contingent upon their key-press responses.

This method of equating perceptual and motor factors across conditions was adopted in a study of the SPN by Masaki et al. (2010). Subjects performed a gambling task in which each trial began with a cue indicating whether they had a choice or whether the computer would make the guess for them. On choice trials the participant pressed one of two buttons with fingers of their right hand to indicate whether their guess was the box to the left of fixation or the one to the right. An arrow immediately appeared at the fixation that pointed toward the selected box. Two and a half seconds later, the boxes were replaced by a picture of an intact or a broken 50-yen coin (about U.S. $0.50) to indicate whether they won or lost. No-choice trials were similar, but the cue indicated that the participant should press a single, designated button with their thumb.

Using a translated version of Tricomi's questionnaire, subjects indicated that they believed (incorrectly) that there was a pattern to the correct answers in the choice condition and that they had a degree of control over the outcome. Congruent with fMRI data described above, Masaki and colleagues found that the SPN was more than twice as large in the choice than in the no-choice condition. The fact that a motor response was required in both conditions argues that the SPN enhancement was not due to greater salience or nonspecific arousal associated with making a movement. Rather, the SPN appears to reflect anticipation of action-dependent outcomes, in other words, reinforcers.

VALENCE SPECIFICITY

In Masaki and colleagues' experiment, as in most SPN studies, the subjects did not know whether they would receive positive or negative feedback. Ohgami et al. (2006), by contrast, used a blocked manipulation of feedback type that allowed them to assess valence specificity of the SPN. The task was to press a key when 3s had elapsed following onset of a cue. Two seconds later, a feedback display informed the participant as to whether the interval was correct, too short, or too long. The feedback display also indicated the monetary reward or penalty, which varied across four types of trial blocks. In the reward condition, the subject received 50 yen for a correct response, but there was no penalty for mistakes. In the punishment condition, there were no rewards, but penalties resulted in a 50-yen loss. In the combined condition, each response resulted in either a 50-yen penalty or reward. Finally, in the control condition, the feedback was not supplemented with a monetary incentive.

The results were straightforward in showing that SPN topography exhibits at least a modest degree of valence specificity (Figure 17.2). Amplitude of the SPN was largest at fronto-central sites just above the temples. It was also larger over the right hemisphere than the left hemisphere in all conditions except the reward-only trial blocks. As noted earlier, Ohgami and colleagues interpreted their results in terms of Davidson et al. (1990) frontal asymmetry theory: Trial blocks with rewards but no punishment are associated with relatively greater left hemisphere activation, thereby canceling out the normal right dominance.

Neuroimaging studies have made extensive use of such reward-only designs and punishment-only designs. In a 2008 review of the literature, Knutson and Greer performed a meta-analysis that included 12 previous experiments, all of which separately assessed expectation of possible monetary gain and loss. The only cortical regions to reliably index reward anticipation were the right anterior insula and a mesial prefrontal site ($x, y, z = 2, 26, 36$). Greater activation during loss anticipation than gain anticipation was found for bilateral insulae and the left superior temporal gyrus (focused at -50, $-32, 8$). Further research will be needed to reconcile SPN and fMRI lateralization findings.

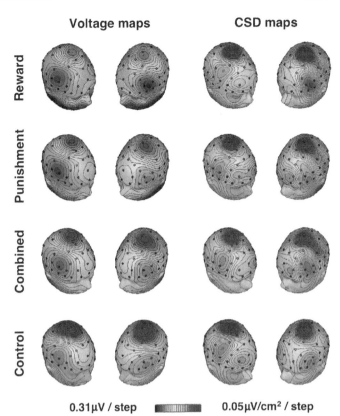

Voltage maps   **CSD maps**

Reward

Punishment

Combined

Control

0.31µV / step ▬▬▬ 0.05µV/cm² / step

FIGURE 17.2 Statistical parameter maps portraying topographical variation in voltage and current source density (CSD) at conclusion of the pre-feedback interval in the four conditions of Ohgami et al. (2006). *Source: Reprinted with permission from Ohgami et al. (2006).*

In the half century since Grey Walter founded cognitive electrophysiology, the field has generated a wealth of knowledge with regard to anticipatory attention. With wealth and maturity, it is natural that the discipline should strive for a more balanced portfolio, one with greater investments in applied topics. An investment of resources in the study of attention to rewards could pay off handsomely in terms of a much needed understanding of cue-elicited cravings, instrumental learning, and other processes that bring about addiction and obesity.

References

Alexander, G. E., DeLong, M. R., & Strick, P. L. (1986). Parallel organization of functionally segregated circuits linking basal ganglia and cortex. *Annual Review of Neuroscience, 9*, 357–381.

Baldwin, A. E., Sadeghian, K., & Kelley, A. E. (2002). Appetitive instrumental learning requires coincident activation of NMDA and dopamine D1 receptors within the medial prefrontal cortex. *Journal of Neuroscience, 22*, 1063–1071.

Bastiaansen, M. C., Böcker, K. B., & Brunia, C. H. (2002). ERD as an index of anticipatory attention? Effects of stimulus degradation. *Psychophysiology, 39*, 16–28.

Bjork, J. M., & Hommer, D. W. (2007). Anticipating instrumentally obtained and passively-received rewards: a factorial fMRI investigation. *Behavioral Brain Research, 177*, 165–170.

Böcker, K. B., Brunia, C. H., & van den Berg-Lenssen, M. M. (1994). A spatiotemporal dipole model of the stimulus preceding negativity (SPN) prior to feedback stimuli. *Brain Topography, 7,* 71–88.

Braak, H., Ghebremedhin, E., Rüb, U., Bratzke, H., & Del Tredici, K. (2004). Stages in the development of Parkinson's disease-related pathology. *Cell and Tissue Research, 318,* 121–134.

Brunia, C. H. M. (1988). Movement and stimulus preceding negativity. *Biological Psychology, 26,* 165–178.

Brunia, C. H. M., de Jong, B. M., van den Berg-Lenssen, M. M., & Paans, A. M. (2000). Visual feedback about time estimation is related to a right hemisphere activation measured by PET. *Experimental Brain Research, 130,* 328–337.

Brunia, C. H. M., Hackley, S. A., van Boxtel, G. J. M., Kotani, Y., & Ohgami, Y. (2011). Waiting to perceive: reward or punishment? *Clinical Neurophysiology, 122,* 858–868.

Brunia, C. H. M., & van Boxtel, G. J. (2004). Anticipatory attention to verbal and non-verbal stimuli is reflected in a modality-specific SPN. *Experimental Brain Research, 156,* 231–239.

Cooper, R. (1985). This week's citation classic. *Citation Classics, 21,* 25.

Corbetta, M., & Shulman, G. L. (2002). Control of goal-directed and stimulus-driven attention in the brain. *Nature Reviews: Neuroscience, 3,* 201–215.

Dale, C. L., Simpson, G. V., Foxe, J. J., Luks, T. L., & Worden, M. S. (2008). ERP correlates of anticipatory attention: spatial and nonspatial specificity and relation to subsequent selective attention. *Experimental Brain Research, 188,* 45–62.

Damen, E. J., & Brunia, C. H. (1987). Changes in heart rate and slow brain potentials related to motor preparation and stimulus anticipation in a time estimation task. *Psychophysiology, 24,* 700–713.

Davidson, R. J., Ekman, P., Saton, C. D., Senulis, J. A., & Friesen, W. V. (1990). Approach-withdrawal and cerebral asymmetry: emotional expression and brain physiology. *Journal of Personality and Social Psychology, 58,* 330–341.

Deecke, L., Heise, B., Kornhuber, H. H., Lang, M., & Lang, W. (1984). Brain potentials associated with voluntary manual tracking. *Annals of the New York Academy of Sciences, 425,* 450–464.

Eimer, M., van Velzen, J., & Driver, J. (2002). Cross-modal interactions between audition, touch and vision in endogenous spatial attention: ERP evidence on preparatory states and sensory modulation. *Journal of Cognitive Neuroscience, 14,* 1–18.

Falkenstein, M., Hohnsbein, J., Hoormann, J., & Blanke, L. (1991). Effects of cross-modal divided attention on late ERP components. II. Error processing in choice reaction tasks. *Electroencephalography and Clinical Neurophysiology, 78,* 447–455.

Fiorillo, C. D., Tobbler, P. N., & Schultz, W. (2003). Discrete coding of reward probability and uncertainty by dopamine neurons. *Science, 299,* 1898–1902.

Folk, C. L., Remington, R. W., & Johnston, J. C. (1992). Involuntary covert orienting is contingent on attentional control settings. *Journal of Experimental Psychology: Human Performance and Perception, 18,* 1030–1044.

Foti, D., & Hajcak, G. (2012). Genetic variation in dopamine moderates neural response during reward anticipation and delivery: evidence from event-related potentials. *Psychophysiology, 49,* 617–626.

Fox, M. D., Corbetta, M., Snyder, A. Z., Vincent, J. L., & Raichle, M. E. (2006). Spontaneous neuronal activity distinguishes human dorsal and ventral attention systems. *Proceedings of the National Academy of Science, 103,* 10046–10051.

Gehring, W. J., Gross, B., Coles, M. G. H., Meyer, D. E., & Donchin, E. (1993). A neural system for error detection and correction. *Psychological Science, 4,* 385–390.

Gratton, G. (1998). The contralateral organization of visual memory: a theoretical concept and a research tool. *Psychophysiology, 35,* 638–647.

Grent-'t-Jong, T., & Woldorff, M. (2007). Timing and sequence of brain activity in top-down contral of visual-spatial attention. *PLoS Biology, 5,* 114–126.

Haber, S. N., & Knutson, B. (2010). The reward circuit: linking primate anatomy and human imaging. *Neuropsychopharmacology Reviews, 35,* 4–26.

Harter, M. R., Miller, S. L., Price, N. J., LaLonde, M. E., & Keyes, A. L. (1989). Neural processes in directing attention. *Journal of Cognitive Neuroscience, 1,* 223–237.

Hebert, K. R., Oh, M., Valle-Inclán, F., Rolan, T., & Hackley, S. A. (2006). Deep brain stimulation impairs reward-based learning in Parkinson's disease. *Psychophysiology, 43*(Suppl.), S44.

Hershey, T., Revilla, F. J., Wernle, A. R., McGee-Minnich, L., Antenor, J. V., Videen, T. O., et al. (2003). Cortical and subcortical blood flow effects of subthalamic nucleus stimulation in PD. *Neurology, 61,* 816–821.

Hillman, C. H., Apparies, R. J., & Hatfield, B. D. (2000). Motor and non-motor event-related potentials during a complex processing task. *Psychophysiology, 37,* 731–736.

Hillyard, S. A., & Galambos, R. G. (1967). Effects of stimulus and response contingencies on a surface negative slow potential in man. *Electroencephalography and Clinical Neurophysiology, 22,* 297–304.

Hoehn, M. M., & Yahr, M. D. (1967). Parkinsonism: onset, progression and mortality. *Neurology, 17,* 427–442.

Holroyd, C. B., & Coles, M. G. H. (2002). The neural basis of human error processing: reinforcement learning, dopamine and error-related negativity. *Psychological Review, 109,* 679–709.

Irwin, D. A., Knott, J. R., McAdam, D. W., & Rebert, C. S. (1966). Motivational determinants of the "contingent negative variation". *Electroencephalography and Clinical Neurophysiology, 21,* 538–543.

James, W. (1890). *The principles of psychology.* New York: Holt & Co.

Knowlton, B. J., Mangels, J. A., & Squire, L. R. (1996). A neostriatal habit learning system in humans. *Science, 273,* 1399–1402.

Knowlton, B. J., Squire, L. R., & Gluck, M. A. (1994). Probabilistic classification learning in amnesia. Learning & Memory, 1, 106–120.

Knutson, B., Adams, C., Fong, G., & Hommer, D. (2001). Anticipation of increasing monetary reward selectively recruits nucleus accumbens. *Journal of Neuroscience, 21,* 1–5.

Knutson, B., & Greer, S. M. (2008). Anticipatory affect: neural correlates and consequences for choice. *Philosophical Transactions of the Royal Society, London: B. Biological Science, 363,* 3771–3786.

Kotani, Y., & Aihara, Y. (1999). The effect of stimulus discriminability on stimulus-preceding negativities prior to instructive and feedback stimuli. *Biological Psychology, 50,* 1–18.

Kotani, Y., Kishida, S., Hiraku, S., Suda, K., Ishii, M., & Aihara, Y. (2003). Effects of information and reward on stimulus-preceding negativity prior to feedback stimuli. *Psychophysiology, 40,* 818–826.

Kotani, Y., Ohgami, Y., Kuramoto, Y., Tsukamoto, T., Inoue, Y., & Aihara, Y. (2009). The role of the right anterior insular cortex in the right hemisphere preponderance of stimulus-preceding negativity (SPN): an fMRI study. *Neuroscience Letters, 450,* 75–79.

Krebs, R. M., Boehler, C. N., Roberts, K. C., Song, A. W., & Woldorff, M. (2012). The involvement of the dopaminergic midbrain and cortico-striatal-thalamic circuits in the integration of reward prospect and attentional task demands. *Cerebral Cortex, 22,* 607–615.

Lewis, D. A., Foote, S. L., Goldstein, M., & Morrison, J. H. (1988). The dopaminergic innervations of monkey prefrontal cortex: a tyrosine hydroxylase immunohistochemical study. *Brain Research, 449,* 225–243.

Luck, S. J., & Hillyard, S. A. (1994). Electrophysiological correlates of feature analysis during visual search. *Psychophysiology, 31,* 291–308.

Masaki, H., Takeuchi, S., Gehring, W., Takasawa, N., & Yamazaki, K. (2006). Affective-motivational influences on feedback-related ERPs in a gambling task. *Brain Research, 1105,* 110–121.

Masaki, H., Yamazaki, K., & Hackley, S. H. (2010). Stimulus-preceding negativity is modulated by action-outcome contingency. *NeuroReport, 21,* 277–281.

Mattox, S. T., Valle-Inclán, F., & Hackley, S. A. (2006). Psychophysiological evidence for impaired reward anticipation in Parkinson's disease. *Clinical Neurophysiology, 117,* 2144–2153.

Maunsell, J. H. R. (2004). Neuronal representations of cognitive states: reward or attention? *Trends in Cognitive Sciences, 8,* 261–265.

Miltner, W. H. R., Braun, C. H., & Coles, M. G. H. (1997). Event-related brain potentials following incorrect feedback in a time-estimation task: evidence for a "generic" neural system for error detection. *Journal of Cognitive Neuroscience, 9,* 788–798.

Naskar, S., Sood, S. K., Goyal, V., & Dhara, M. (2010). Mechanism(s) of deep brain stimulation and insights into cognitive outcomes in Parkinson's disease. *Brain Research Reviews, 65,* 1–13.

Ohgami, Y., Kotani, Y., Hiraku, S., Aihara, Y., & Ishii, M. (2004). Effects of reward and stimulus modality on stimulus-preceding negativity. *Psychophysiology, 41,* 729–738.

Ohgami, Y., Kotani, Y., Tsukamoto, T., Omura, K., Inoue, Y., Aihara, Y., et al. (2006). Effects of monetary reward and punishment on stimulus-preceding negativity. *Psychophysiology, 43,* 227–236.

Ohgami, Y., Kotani, Y., Yoshihiro, T., Tsukamoto, T., & Inoue, Y. (2010). Stimulus-preceding negativity (SPN) prior to unilateral visual feedback stimulus: a combined EEG/fMRI study. *Psychophysiology, 47(Suppl. 1),* S60.

Olds, J., & Milner, P. (1954). Positive reinforcement produced by electrical stimulation of the septal area and other regions of the rat brain. *Journal of Comparative and Physiological Psychology, 47,* 419–427.

Poldrack, R. A., Prabhakaran, V., Seger, C. A., & Gabrieli, J. D. E. (1999). Striatal activation during acquisition of a cognitive skill. *Neuropsychology, 13,* 564–574.

Rohrbaugh, J. W., & Gaillard, A. W. K. (1983). Sensory and motor aspects of the contingent negative variation. In A. W. K. Gaillard & W. Ritter (Eds.), *Tutorials in ERP research: Endogenous components.* Netherlands: North-Holland Publishing Co.

Rohrbaugh, J. W., Syndulko, K., & Lindsley, D. B. (1976). Brain wave components of the contingent negative variation in humans. *Science, 191,* 1055–1057.

Schultz, W., Dayan, P., & Montague, P. R. (1997). A neural substrate of prediction and reward. *Science, 275,* 1593–1599.

Schultz, W., Tremblay, L., & Hollerman, J. R. (2000). Reward processing in primate orbitofrontal cortex and basal ganglia. *Cerebral Cortex, 10,* 272–283.

Shohamy, D., Myers, C., Gluck, M., & Onlaor, S. (2004). Role of the basal ganglia in category learning: how to patients with Parkinson's disease learn. *Behavioral Neuroscience, 118,* 676–686.

Simons, R. F., Öhman, A., & Lang, P. L. (1979). Anticipation and response set: cortical, cardiac and electrodermal correlates. *Psychophysiology, 16,* 222–233.

Skinner, B. F. (1938). *The behavior of organisms: An experimental analysis.* Oxford: Appleton-Century.

Thobois, S., Dominey, P., Fraix, V., Mertens, P., Guenot, M., Zimmer, L., et al. (2002). Effects of sub thalamic nucleus stimulation on actual and imagined movement in Parkinson's disease: a PET study. *Journal of Neurology, 249,* 1689–1698.

Tricomi, E. M., Delgado, M. R., & Fiez, J. A. (2002). Modulation of caudate activity by action contingency [abstract]. *Proceedings of the Society for Neuroscience.*

Tricomi, E. M., Delgado, M. R., & Fiez, J. A. (2004). Modulation of caudate activity by action contingency. *Neuron, 41,* 281–292.

Tsai, H. C., Zhang, F., Adamantidis, A., Stuber, G. D., Bonci, A., de Lecea, L., et al. (2009). Phasic firing in dopaminergic neurons is sufficient for behavioral conditioning. *Science, 32,* 1080–1084.

Van Boxtel, G. J. M., & Böcker, K. B. E. (2004). Cortical measures of anticipation. *Journal of Psychophysiology, 18,* 61–76.

Vogel, E. K., McCollough, A. W., & Machizawa, M. G. (2005). Neural measures reveal individual differences in controlling access to working memory. *Nature, 438,* 500–503.

Vrana, S. R., Spence, E. L., & Lang, P. J. (1988). The startle probe response: a new measure of emotion? *Journal of Abnormal Psychology, 97,* 487–491.

Walter, W. G., Cooper, R., Aldridge, V. J., McCallum, W. C., & Winter, A. L. (1964). Contingent negative variation: an electric sign of sensori-motor association and expectation in the human brain. *Nature, 203,* 380–384.

Weinberg, H. (1973). The contingent negative variation: its relation to feedback and expectant attention. In W. C. McCallum & J. R. Knott (Eds.), *Event-related slow potentials of the brain: Their relation to behavior* (pp. 219–228). Amsterdam: Elsevier. EEG Supplement 33.

Wynn, J. K., Horan, W. P., Kring, A. M., Simons, R. F., & Green, M. F. (2010). Impaired anticipatory event-related potentials in schizophrenia. *International Journal of Psychophysiology, 77,* 141–149.

Yantis, S. (1993). Stimulus-driven attentional capture and attention control settings. *Journal of Experimental Psychology: Human Perception and Performance, 19,* 676–681.

A Neural Measure of Item Individuation

David E. Anderson, Edward K. Vogel, Edward Awh

Department of Psychology, University of Oregon, Eugene, OR, USA

A typical visual scene contains more information than the visual system can process at any given time, requiring observers to selectively encode only a limited amount of information. Multiple studies have asserted processing capacity limits in: (1) *perception* (Duncan, 1980; Fisher, 1982; Hoffman, 1978; Prinzmetal & Banks, 1983); (2) *attention* (Bundesen, 1990; Desimone & Duncan, 1995; Duncan & Humphreys, 1989; Fisher, 1982; Pashler, 1987; Treisman & Gelade, 1980; Wolfe, 1994); and (3) *working memory* (WM) (Cowan, 2001; Luck & Vogel, 1997; Palmer, 1990; Pashler, 1988; Phillips, 1974). Thus, sharp capacity limits permeate all levels of visual cognition. As will be discussed in this review, various stages of visual processing share quantitatively similar limits in the number of items that can be simultaneously apprehended and maintained, as well as a common electrophysiological signature that covaries with behavioral success. These findings underlie our thesis that multiple stages of visual processing may depend on the success of a common processing resource.

Our working hypothesis is that this resource is required when observers needed to *individuate*—or form distinct representations of – multiple items at the same time. For example, imagine finding a friend in a crowded stadium without the ability to individually inspect each person to determine their status as friend or stranger. Failures to individuate would result in "blended" representations, yielding the kind of confusion errors often associated with visual crowding (Levi, 2008), a form of interference that is observed when targets are surrounded by nearby distractors. Moreover, we suggest that this individuation process is important not just during the initial apprehension of stimuli, but also during the subsequent maintenance of those representations in WM (Ester, Vogel, & Awh, 2012). This "individuation thread" may explain why similar item limits have been inferred across a wide range of tasks that require internal

and external selection, such as visual search (Anderson, Vogel, & Awh, 2013), multiple object tracking (MOT) (Drew & Vogel, 2008; Pylyshyn & Storm, 1988), rapid enumeration (Ester, Drew, Klee, Vogel, & Awh, 2012; Ester, Vogel, et al., 2012; Halberda, Sires, & Feigenson, 2006; Pagano & Mazza, 2012), and storage in visual WM (Cowan, 2001; Luck & Vogel, 1997).

OVERVIEW OF SELECTION-DEPENDENT ELECTROPHYSIOLOGICAL ACTIVITY

While similar capacity limits provide one link between the diverse set of paradigms described above, we will focus this review on another common signature of individuation that has been identified for these tasks. Specifically, each of these forms of visual selection has been shown to evoke an event-related potential waveform known as the N2pc. The N2pc is a phasic negativity over posterior electrode sites contralateral to the attended location approximately 200–300 ms after stimulus onset (Luck & Hillyard, 1994), with contributions from lateral extrastriate, inferotemporal, and posterior parietal cortices (Hopf et al., 2000). N2pc amplitudes are estimated by subtracting ipsilateral activity from contralateral activity evoked in lateral occipital electrodes. The N2pc has been associated with the visual selection of items amongst competing distractors (Eimer, 1996; Luck & Hillyard, 1994; Luck, Girelli, McDermott, & Ford, 1997) and rapid shifts of spatial attention across visual hemifields (Woodman & Luck, 1999). In this discussion, the key point is that the amplitude of the N2pc provides a sensitive measure of the number of items each observer can successfully process in a wide array of paradigms. Specifically, the amplitude of the N2pc component increases monotonically with the number of targets during MOT (Drew & Vogel, 2008), rapid enumeration

(Ester, Drew, et al., 2012; Pagano & Mazza, 2012), visual search, (Anderson et al., 2013) and encoding into WM (Anderson & Awh, 2012; Anderson, Vogel, & Awh, 2011); moreover, the shape of this N2pc amplitude by set size function is a robust predictor of behavioral success in each of these tasks. These findings suggest that this diverse set of tasks is constrained by a common neural process, and that this neural process may be critical for item individuation. The central goal of this review, therefore, is to outline how this common neural signature may reveal a common cognitive resource for item individuation that constrains performance across multiple stages of processing.

INDIVIDUATION LIMITS IN RAPID ENUMERATION

Rapid enumeration, or subitization, requires observers to quickly and accurately count the number of stimuli present in a visual display (Kaufman, Lord, Reese, & Volkmann, 1949). Although this simple task seems to require only the most elementary visual analysis—to register the existence of the counted items—multiple studies have demonstrated a limit in the number of items than can be simultaneously enumerated (Mandler & Shebo,

1982; Piazza, Fumarola, Chinello, & Melcher, 2011; Trick & Pylyshyn, 1993, 1994; Revkin, Piazza, Izzard, Cohen, & Dehaene, 2008; Trick & Pylyshyn, 1994). Evidence for item limits in enumeration has primarily come from behavioral studies. Performance in these tasks is typically characterized by very low error rates for reporting the number of relevant items at smaller set sizes, followed by a monotonic increase in error rates for set sizes exceeding three to four items. This piecewise linear pattern of errors with rising set size has been interpreted to reflect a relatively low item limit for the number of items that can be simultaneously apprehended.

To further test the hypothesis that apparent limits in enumeration capacity are constrained by fixed item limits in individuation, Ester, Drew, et al. (2012) recorded electroencephalogram (EEG) during a subitizing task (Figure 18.1(A)). After a spatial cue was presented to indicate which visual hemifield should be attended, an array of squares was presented in random spatial positions. While the number of square items (12 or 14) was kept constant across trials, the number of relevant (green or blue) items to be enumerated varied, where set size ranged from one to twelve, inclusive. In line with previous research, error rates remained stable at earlier set sizes, then increased sharply after the putative item limit

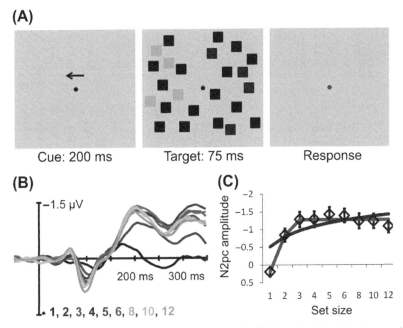

(A)

Cue: 200 ms   Target: 75 ms   Response

(B)

-1.5 μV

200 ms   300 ms

• 1, 2, 3, 4, 5, 6, 8, 10, 12

(C)

N2pc amplitude

Set size

FIGURE 18.1   Electrophysiological response patterns during a subitization task. (A) On each trial, subjects were given a spatial cue (for 200 ms) to attend either the left or right visual hemifield of a bilateral display. Following this cue, a bilateral array of items was presented for 75 ms, and subjects were instructed to count the number of target items (e.g., green items) present within the display while ignoring nontargets in black. Total display size was kept constant, while the number of target items varied between 1 and 12 items across trials. Subjects were then to indicate how many targets were present in the display. (B) Grand averaged difference waves (contralateral minus ipsilateral activity) for each set size (negative voltages plotted up by convention). The N2pc was apparent in lateral occipital (OL/OR) electrodes 200–300 ms after stimulus onset. (C) N2pc amplitude increased monotonically with set size, then reached a stable plateau after exceeding set size three. N2pc by set size functions were better fit with the predicted piecewise linear function indicative of a fixed item limit (red) than a logarithmic function with no apparent item limits (blue).

was exceeded; estimated enumeration spans, which were determined by calculating the set size at which error rates began to increase, ranged between two to four items. Thus, behavioral performance reported by Ester, Drew, et al. (2012) was similar to previous studies (Mandler & Shebo, 1982; Piazza et al., 2011; Pylyshyn & Storm, 1993, 1994; Revkin et al., 2008; Trick & Pylyshyn, 1994).

During the N2pc epoch (~200–300 ms), a monotonic rise in amplitude was observed with increasing set size (Figure 18.1(B)), suggesting that the N2pc component indexed the number of items that were being simultaneously apprehended. Supporting the hypothesis that observed behavioral limits in enumeration were constrained by individuation limits, N2pc amplitude showed a stable plateau after only about three items (Figure 18.1(C)). Critically, individual differences in the set size at which the N2pc by set size function reached asymptote predicted the set size at which behavioral enumeration performance began to decline, such that individuals with higher enumeration spans reached asymptote in the N2pc by set size function at a larger set size. Thus, individuation limits, as indexed by the N2pc by set size function, determine the number of items that can be simultaneously enumerated (see also Mazza & Caramazza, 2011).

INDIVIDUATION LIMITS IN VISUAL SEARCH

In addition to enumeration, individuation is critical for visual search behavior. The process of visual search requires the apprehension and discrimination of target items embedded among multiple distractors. Thus, although this task requires a much more in-depth encoding of the items than does rapid enumeration, the same core individuation process is a key component of visual search. Multiple models have suggested that the initial apprehension of search items is followed by the inspection of each item within an online workspace to evaluate target status (Bundesen, 1990; Desimone & Duncan, 1995; Duncan & Humphreys, 1989; Fisher, 1982; Pashler, 1987; Treisman & Gelade, 1980; Wolfe, 1994). More specifically, multiple authors have suggested that search items are selected and inspected in small clusters, with serial shifts of visual selection from one cluster to the next (e.g., Fisher, 1982; Pashler, 1987; Wolfe, 2005). Our proposal is that the number of items in each cluster may be determined by the number of items that each observer can individuate in parallel. In a recent study, we tested this hypothesis by measuring N2pc amplitude during a visual search task (Anderson et al., 2013; Figure 18.2(A)). After a spatial

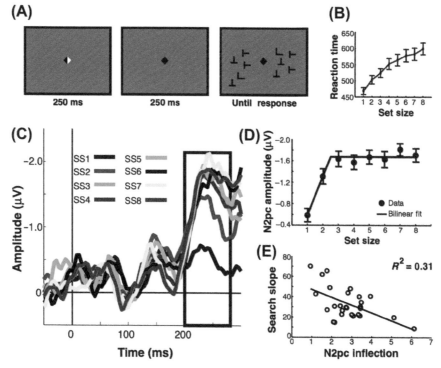

FIGURE 18.2 Electrophysiological response patterns during a visual search task. (A) On each trial, subjects were given a spatial cue (e.g., white arrow) to attend either the left or right visual hemifield of a bilateral display. Subjects were instructed to identify the direction of the target L as quickly as possible. (B) Mean reaction time by set size function. (C) Grand averaged difference waves for each set size. The N2pc was apparent in lateral occipital (OL/OR) electrodes 200–300 ms after stimulus onset. (D) N2pc amplitude increased monotonically with set size, then reached a stable plateau after exceeding set size three. N2pc by set size functions were well described by a piecewise linear function (black line). (E) A strong correlation was observed between search slope (estimated as the slope of individual reaction time by set size functions in B) and the set size at which the N2pc by set size function reached asymptote.

cue was presented to indicate which visual hemifield should be attended, a search array (set sizes ranged from one to eight) was presented in random spatial positions. The distractors were randomly oriented (i.e., 0°, 90°, 180°, or 270°) Ts, and the target item was an L that was either leftward or rightward facing; these heterogeneous displays ensured that the search task was sufficiently difficult and would require the individual inspect of each item (Duncan & Humphreys, 1989). In line with previous research, these displays led to relatively "inefficient search" as demonstrated by an average search slope of 20.8 ms/item (Figure 18.2(B)).

During the N2pc epoch (~200–300 ms), a monotonic rise in amplitude was observed with concurrent increases in set size (Figure 18.2(C)), suggesting that the N2pc component indexed the number of items that can be simultaneously apprehended during search. Supporting the hypothesis that the distribution of attention is constrained to a handful of items during search, a stable plateau was observed after the putative item limit was exceeded (Figure 18.1(D)). Models of visual search positing that search is performed online among a handful of individuated representations (e.g., Bundesen, 1990; Duncan & Humphreys, 1989; Fisher, 1982; Wolfe, 1994) make a clear prediction: individuals who can individuate a greater number of representations should be more efficient when performing a visual search task because each shift of attention encompasses a greater number of items. Confirming this prediction, individual differences in the set size at which the N2pc by set size function reached asymptote predicted search slopes measured from reaction time by set size functions (Figure 18.2(E)) such that observers who demonstrated a smaller search slope reached asymptote in their N2pc by set size functions at a larger set size. This observation confirms the hypothesis that observers who can individuate more items within a given shift of attention can more efficiently search among multiple items. Thus, the Anderson et al. (2013) findings demonstrate that visual search is constrained by relatively sharp limits in the number of items that can be simultaneously individuated.

INDIVIDUATION LIMITS IN SPATIOTEMPORAL UPDATING

The purpose of individuating an external representation typically extends beyond its initial apprehension. Generally speaking, the objective of individuation is to impose some goal-directed behavior on the representations to which we have invested limited resources in selecting. One such behavior involves updating the spatial position of an individuated representation as it moves through space. Watching a basketball game, for example, requires the updating of player position as they move across the court; in order to successfully attend to the player with possession of the ball, observers must first individuate this player from among others, then update, or track the position of this player as he moves across the court. Thus, if you fail to individuate an object, it follows that you will also fail to track or update its spatial position.

MOT is a process that recruits both individuation and updating processes (Alvarez & Cavanagh, 2005; Pylyshyn & Annan, 2006; Yantis, 1992). MOT tasks typically involve cueing a subset of static items in a display, after which observers are instructed to track the spatial position of each cued item as they move randomly among identical distractors (Pylyshyn & Storm, 1988). The ability to track multiple items is extremely limited, with tracking limits constrained to approximately four items (Cavanagh & Alvarez, 2005; Pylyshyn & Storm, 1988; Scholl, Pylyshyn, & Feldman, 2001). At first glance, performance during both enumeration (i.e., selection) and tracking (i.e., updating) appears to be constrained by a similar fixed item limit.

To understand the neural mechanisms of spatiotemporal updating, Drew and Vogel (2008) recorded EEG waveforms during an MOT task. In their experiment (Figure 18.3(A)), a subset of framed squares was cued (red or green) in one visual hemifield, indicating which items were to be attended during the tracking period. While the number of total items was held constant, the number of targets varied across trials. Following the tracking period, a single item was probed, and observers indicated whether the probed item was one of the cued items. Performance in this task varied as a function of how successful the observer was at tracking each cued item.

In order to successfully track a moving object, an observer must first individuate the item from among distractors, and then update its spatial position during online tracking. In line with this two-component process view of spatiotemporal updating (Alvarez & Cavanagh, 2005; Pylyshyn & Annan, 2006; Yantis, 1992), Drew and Vogel (2008) observed two distinct electrophysiological components during online tracking. Following the onset of the cue array, a clear N2pc component was observed between 200 and 300 ms (Figure 18.3(B)). N2pc amplitude increased monotonically with increasing set size and, as was demonstrated in a later experiment, this rise in N2pc amplitude reached a stable plateau after approximately three items; thus, N2pc amplitude during MOT reflects individuation demands, where larger amplitudes are observed when more items are individuated. Consistent with the hypothesis that the individuation of object representations determines the successful updating of their spatial positions, the change in N2pc amplitude across set sizes predicted individual tracking limits, where individuals with high tracking spans elicited a larger increase in N2pc amplitude from set sizes

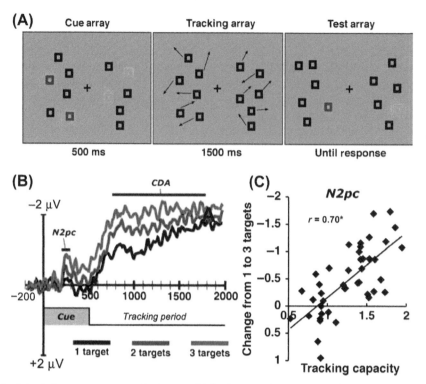

FIGURE 18.3 Electrophysiological response patterns during a multiple object tracking (MOT) task. (A) On each trial, subjects were cued to attend to the target items (e.g., red items) presented in either the left or right visual hemifield. Total display size was kept constant, while the number of target items varied from one to three items across trials. After the 500 ms cue array, target information (i.e., color) was removed, and each item in the display began to move randomly for 1500 ms. Following the tracking array, a single item was probed, and subjects were to indicate if the probed item was one of the target items. (B) Grand averaged difference waves for each set size. Both the N2pc and CDA components were apparent, and each increased monotonically with set size. (C) An individual differences analysis revealed that observers with larger tracking capacities evoked a larger increase in N2pc amplitude when going from one to three items.

one to three (Figure 18.3(C)). This pattern of results confirms the view that individuation is a necessary step for spatiotemporal updating, and provides further evidence favoring the N2pc as a neural measure of individuation.

In addition to the N2pc, Drew and Vogel (2008) measured the contralateral delay activity (CDA) (McCollough, Machizawa, & Vogel, 2007; Vogel & Machizawa, 2004). In contrast to the N2pc, which is an early phasic negativity, the CDA is a later sustained negativity in posterior electrode sites, contralateral to the tracked items, beginning approximately 300 ms after the motion onset. In addition to being temporally distinct components, the topography of these components is also dissimilar. Relative to the N2pc, which has a more ventral focus, the scalp distribution of the CDA is significantly more dorsal (McCollough et al., 2007). Finally, the N2pc and CDA components are functionally distinct. On the one hand, the N2pc component tracks moment-to-moment fluctuations in the allocation of external attention (Woodman & Luck, 1999). On the other hand, the CDA component is sensitive to online storage load during periods of sustained internal attention (Vogel & Machizawa, 2004).

In Drew and Vogel (2008), the profile of CDA amplitude was similar to that observed in the N2pc. Specifically, CDA amplitudes were strongly modulated by set size, with increases in CDA amplitude occurring with concurrent increases in set size. Also similar to the pattern of results observed in the N2pc, Drew and Vogel (2008) observed a strong link between the shape of the CDA by set size function and tracking capacity, indicating that online storage capacity predicts how many items can be simultaneously tracked.

These findings provide further converging evidence for interpreting the N2pc as a neural measure of individuation by demonstrating a link between the N2pc, an early component sensitive to the allocation of attention, and sustained tracking performance. Furthermore, the demonstrated correspondence between the pattern of N2pc and CDA amplitudes, as well as their relationship to behavior, provides support for the hypothesis that external and internal attention are constrained by a common discrete item limit.

INDIVIDUATION LIMITS IN WM STORAGE

So far, we have reviewed evidence that visually selecting stimuli during rapid enumeration, visual search, or online tracking requires the active individuation of the

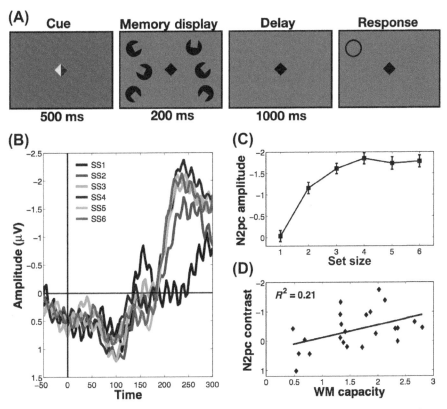

FIGURE 18.4 Electrophysiological response patterns during a working memory (WM) task. (A) On each trial, subjects were given a spatial cue (e.g., yellow arrow) to attend either the left or right visual hemifield of a bilateral display. Subjects were instructed to remember the orientation of each randomly oriented item within the cued display. After a 1000 ms delay period, a single location was probed, and subjects were to respond with the remembered orientation of the probed item by clicking on the perimeter of the ring. (B) Grand averaged difference waves for each set size measured lateral occipital (OL/OR) electrodes 200–300 ms after stimulus onset (C) N2pc amplitude increased monotonically with set size, then reached a stable plateau after exceeding set size three. (D) An individual differences analysis revealed that observers with larger working memory capacities evoked a larger increase in N2pc amplitude when going from two to four items.

selected items, and that this process evokes a common electrophysiological response. Moreover, we postulate that the same individuation process may be required to maintain distinct internal representations in WM. In the following section, we will review evidence supporting this link between internal and external item individuation. Importantly, individual difference analyses show strong links between the number of items that can be individuated during the initial apprehension of visual items and the internal storage of visual items in WM.

WM is a limited capacity system that stores information in an online state. In typical visual WM tasks, observers are asked to remember the specific feature values of items distributed across visual space. During test, observers must either determine whether the feature of a single item changed (Luck & Vogel, 1997) or recall the specific feature value of a probed item (Wilken & Ma, 2004; Zhang & Luck, 2008). Across both change detection and recall paradigms, a similar capacity limit of approximately three to four items is observed. Two broad classes of models have emerged to characterize the nature of this capacity limit. Discrete resource models

propose that WM capacity is constrained by a fixed item limit, such that no information can be gleaned from additional items once this item limit has been exceeded. Alternatively, flexible resource models propose that WM constraints are determined by a single resource that is distributed among a larger number of items, with each item receiving fewer resources as storage load increases; here, capacity limits are a consequence of increased interference between noisy, low-quality representations at larger storage loads. While both models agree that each item must be individuated to maintain a clear representation, each model offers a qualitatively different explanation for the emergence of capacity limits in WM.

Recently, we reported evidence in favor of discrete resource limits in WM storage during the recording of selection—and storage-related neural activity (Anderson et al., 2011). Our WM task required observers to remember from one to six orientations presented within a cued hemifield (Figure 18.4(A)). Similar to Drew and Vogel (2008), we observed a prominent N2pc approximately 200 ms following the onset of the memory display (Figure 18.4(B)). N2pc amplitude increased monotonically with set size and reached a stable plateau when set size exceeded approximately three items (Figure 18.4(C)). This piecewise linear N2pc by set size function suggests that observers could no longer select additional items once this putative item limit was exceeded. Critically, the shape of this N2pc by set size function predicted WM capacity, such that N2pc amplitude reach asymptote at larger set sizes for higher capacity individuals (Figure 18.4(D)).

While the N2pc indexed the number of items that could be apprehended during external attention, the CDA reflected the number of items that could be maintained online during periods of internal attention. Approximately 400 ms after memory onset, the CDA emerged. A pattern similar to the N2pc results was observed in the CDA: the amplitude of this sustained negativity rose monotonically with set size, reaching a stable plateau once putative item limits were exceeded. Furthermore, the shape of the CDA by set size function provided a strong link with individual WM capacity estimates. Thus, the sustained neural activity observed during the delay period of the WM task strongly predicted individual differences in this fixed item limit in WM.

These data provide an important demonstration of apparent links between external and internal attention (Awh & Jonides, 2001; Chun, 2012). The N2pc component, which we argue to provide a neural index of individuation, suggested a selection limit of about three items, and this selection limit was a robust predictor of WM capacity. Importantly, this link between initial selection capacity and storage capacity was not simply an artifact of an encoding limited task. We showed this by measuring memory performance in both a simultaneous condition (eight items at a time) and a sequential condition (four items at a time) that halved the encoding load; the probability of storage and the precision of the stored representations was equivalent in the simultaneous and sequential conditions, showing that encoding was not a limiting factor in this procedure (see also, Anderson & Awh, 2012, experiment 2, for a comprehensive follow-up experiment that corroborates this conclusion). Thus, the reviewed evidence so far suggests that individuation is a central capacity limit that determines the number of items that can be simultaneously selected and stored.

SENSITIVITY TO PERCEIVED NUMBER OF ITEMS

This review, thus far, has provided strong evidence favoring the N2pc component as a neural measure of individuation. The piecewise linear shape of the N2pc by set size function, which serves as an index of the number of items that can be simultaneously

individuated, predicted performance across enumeration, visual search, MOT, and WM tasks. In these tasks the target items are either presented alone, (Anderson et al., 2011) or are distinct from the distractor items (Drew & Vogel, 2008; Ester, Drew, et al., 2012) during selection. We have argued that selection-related processes modulate N2pc amplitude, which scales with set size because observers would select more items as set size increased. This argument is further supported by the strong link between the shape of N2pc by set size functions and performance.

An alternative explanation is that N2pc amplitudes are modulated simply by the number of relevant items without imposing an individuation account on the observed increase in N2pc amplitude as a function of set size. This account might explain observed N2pc amplitude modulations as an interaction between relevant stimulus intensities within attended hemifields and attention-related processes. For example, attending to a hemifield in which three items are presented might elicit a greater activation of neural responses in attention-related cortical regions because neural responses in these regions are sensitive to the overall stimulus intensity of the attended set.

In recent work, we have developed a task that addresses this alternative explanation. Using the same orientation stimuli as in Anderson et al. (2011), we held constant the number of stimulus elements presented while manipulating the number of *perceived* items. Memory items were presented in pairs, and the orientation of each item was either random with respect to each other or collinear with respect to each other; in the random condition, the number of perceived items was identical to the number of presented items, whereas in the collinear condition, the number of perceived items was half that of the number of presented items (see Figure 18.5(A)). For example, when the two items in the pair were presented randomly with respect to each other, the perceived set size was two; when the two items were collinear and facing each other, the resulting illusory contour led to a perceived set size of one. The key result was that N2pc amplitude was determined by the number of perceived items rather than by the number of elements in the memory display (Figure 18.5(B)). N2pc amplitudes were identical between set size four grouped and set size two random conditions, in which perceived set sizes were identical (Figure 18.5(C)). A similar pattern was observed in the CDA (Figure 18.5(E)), and both electrophysiological measures predicted WM performance (Figure 18.5(D) and (F)). This pattern of results suggests that the number of perceived items, rather than the number of image elements or stimulus intensity, modulates N2pc amplitude. Thus, we conclude that the N2pc provides a sensitive neural index of the number of perceived items.

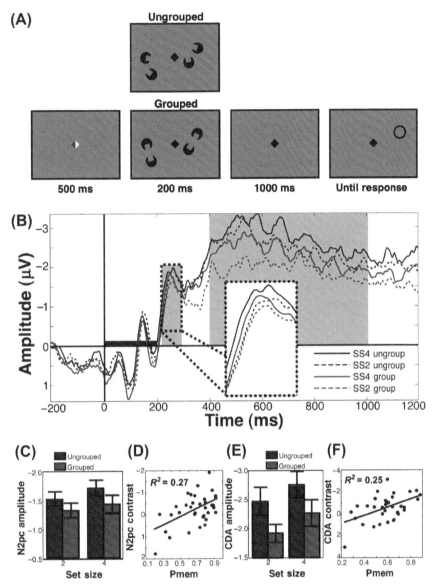

FIGURE 18.5 Electrophysiological response patterns during a working memory (WM) task in which pairs of elements formed two distinct items (ungrouped condition) or a single perceptual group (grouped condition). (A) The structure of each trial was similar to that in Figure 18.4, with the only exception being that pairs of items were arranged in either a grouped or ungrouped fashion such that each item within a pair was collinear or randomly oriented, respectively. (B) Grand averaged difference waves for each set size and condition measured from lateral occipital (OL/OR) electrodes. (C) N2pc amplitude was sensitive to both set size and grouping. Selection of two ungrouped items elicited N2pc amplitudes statistically indistinguishable from two grouped pairs, suggesting the N2pc is sensitive to the number of perceived items. (D) A significant relationship was observed between WM capacity and the slope of N2pc amplitudes as a function of set size. (E) CDA amplitude was sensitive to both set size and grouping; storage of two ungrouped items elicited CDA amplitudes statistically indistinguishable from two grouped pairs. (F) A significant relationship was observed between WM capacity and the slope of CDA amplitudes as a function of set size.

GENERAL DISCUSSION

In this chapter, we reviewed evidence from a wide array of studies that converges on the conclusion that the N2pc component provides a neural measure of item individuation. Across a wide variety of tasks that varied dramatically in the types of stimuli and the kinds of discriminations required, we observed a common empirical pattern. N2pc amplitude rose with the number of selected or stored items, and reached a plateau at a set size that predicted individual performance. We argue that this common neural response, taken together with its link to behavioral success, argues for a common processing stage that determines performance across multiple stages of processing; we propose that this neural response reflects the cognitive process of item individuation.

In the reviewed studies, we also demonstrated that the N2pc is sensitive to the number of individuated items, rather than the total number of elements or distractors.

For example, both Drew and Vogel (2008) and Ester, Drew, et al. (2012) kept display sizes constant while manipulating the number of relevant target items. If the N2pc was sensitive to the number of total items within an attended hemifield, these authors should have observed a flat N2pc by set size component. Instead, they found that N2pc amplitude was sensitive to the number of target items, which varied independent of the number of total items. More conclusively, Anderson, Vogel, and Awh (2012) employed perceptual grouping to manipulate the number of perceived items while holding constant the number of stimulus elements in the display. N2pc amplitude was determined by the number of distinct items that were perceived, despite large variations in the physical properties (e.g., total number of elements, physical area occupied, total luminance change) of the grouped and ungrouped displays. Thus, N2pc amplitude is determined by the number of individuated representations formed by the observer.

CONCLUSIONS

We have reviewed recent electrophysiological work that has provided substantial evidence favoring the N2pc component as a neural measure of item individuation. The response profile of this component is sensitive to apparent item limits across multiple task contexts, and supports discrete resource models of visual cognition. Our broad conclusion is that a common individuation thread determines capacity across multiple stages of processing, determining the maximum number of items that can be simultaneous apprehended or stored, and evoking a common neural signature. Our hope is that this may provide a productive perspective for exploring the core capacity limits in visual cognition.

References

Alvarez, G. A., & Cavanagh, P. (2005). Independent resources for attentional tracking in the left and right visual hemifields. *Psychological Science*, 16, 637–643.

Anderson, D. E., & Awh, E. (2012). The plateau in mnemonic resolution across large set sizes indicates discrete resource limits in visual working memory. *Attention, Perception, and Psychophysics*, 74, 891–910.

Anderson, D. E., Vogel, E. K., & Awh, E. (2011). Precision in visual working memory reaches a stable plateau when individual item limits are exceeded. *Journal of Neuroscience*, 31, 1128–1138.

Anderson, D. E., Vogel, E. K., & Awh, E. (2012). The selection and storage of perceptual groups is constrained a discrete resource in working memory. *Journal of Experimental Psychology: Human Perception and Performance*. http://dx.doi.org/10.1037/a0030094. Advance online publication.

Anderson, D. E., Vogel, E. K., & Awh, E. (2013). A common discrete resource for visual working memory and visual search. *Psychological Science*. DOI:10.1177/0956797612464380. Published online 9 April 2013.

Awh, E., & Jonides, J. (2001). Overlapping mechanisms of attention and spatial working memory. *Trends in Cognitive Science*, 5, 119–126.

Bundesen, C. (1990). A theory of visual attention. *Psychological Review*, 97, 523–547.

Cavanagh, P., & Alvarez, G. A. (2005). Tracking multiple targets with multifocal attention. *Trends in Cognitive Science*, 9, 349–354.

Chun, M. M. (2012). Visual working memory as visual attention sustained over time. *Neuropsychologia*, 49, 1407–1409.

Cowan, N. (2001). The magical number 4 in short-term memory: a reconsideration of mental storage capacity. *Behavioral and Brain Sciences*, 24, 87–185.

Desimone, R., & Duncan, J. (1995). Neural mechanisms of selective visual attention. *Annual Review of Neuroscience*, 18, 193–222.

Drew, T., & Vogel, E. K. (2008). Neural measures of individual differences in selecting and tracking multiple moving objects. *Journal of Neuroscience*, 28, 4183–4191.

Duncan, J. (1980). The locus of interference in the perception of simultaneous stimuli. *Psychological Review, 87*, 272–300.

Duncan, J., & Humphreys, G. W. (1989). Visual search and stimulus similarity. *Psychological Review, 96*, 433–458.

Eimer, M. (1996). The N2pc component as an indicator of attentional selectivity. *Electroencephalography and Clinical Neurophysiology, 99*, 225–234.

Ester, E. E., Drew, T. W., Klee, D., Vogel, E. K., & Awh, E. (2012). Neural measures reveal a fixed item limit in subitizing. *Journal of Neuroscience, 32*, 7169–7177.

Ester, E., Vogel, E. K., & Awh, E. (2012). Discrete resource limits in working memory and attention. In M. I. Posner (Ed.), *Cognitive neuroscience of attention*. New York: Guilford Press.

Fisher, D. L. (1982). Limited-channel models of automatic detection: capacity and scanning in visual search. *Psychological Review, 89*, 662–692.

Halberda, J., Sires, S. F., & Feigenson, L. (2006). Multiple spatially overlapped sets can be enumerated in parallel. *Psychological Science, 17*, 572–576.

Hoffman, J. E. (1978). Search through a sequentially presented visual display. *Perception and Psychophysics, 23*, 1–11.

Hopf, J. M., Luck, S. J., Girelli, M., Hagner, T., Mangun, G. R., Scheich, H., Heinze, H. J. (2000). Neural sources of focused attention in visual search. *Cerebral Cortex, 10*, 1233–1241.

Kaufman, E. L., Lord, M. W., Reese, T. W., & Volkmann, J. (1949). The discrimination of visual number. *American Journal of Psychology, 62*, 498–525.

Levi, D. M. (2008). Crowding—an essential bottleneck for object recognition: a mini review. *Vision Research, 48*, 635–654.

Luck, S. J., Girelli, M., McDermott, M. T., & Ford, M. A. (1997). Bridging the gap between monkey neurophysiology and human perception: an ambiguity resolution theory of visual selective attention. *Cognitive Psychology, 33*, 64–87.

Luck, S. J., & Hillyard, S. A. (1994). Spatial filtering during visual search: evidence from human electrophysiology. *Journal of Experimental Psychology: Human Perception and Performance, 20*, 1000–1014.

Luck, S. J., & Vogel, E. K. (1997). The capacity of visual working memory for features and conjunctions. *Nature, 390*, 279–281.

Mandler, G., & Shebo, B. J. (1982). Subitizing: an analysis of its component processes. *Journal of Experimental Psychology: General, 111*, 1–22.

Mazza, V., & Caramazza, A. (2011). Temporal brain dynamics of multiple object processing: the flexibility of individuation. *PLoS One, 6*, e17453.

McCollough, A. W., Machizawa, M. G., & Vogel, E. (2007). Electrophysiological measures of maintaining representations in visual working memory. *Cortex, 43*, 77–94.

Pagano, S., & Mazza, V. (2012). Individuation of multiple targets during visual enumeration: new insights from electrophysiology. *Neuropsychologia, 50*(5), 754–761.

Palmer, J. (1990). Attentional limits on the perception and memory of visual information. *Journal of Experimental Psychology: Human Perception and Performance*, 16, 332–350.

Pashler, H. (1987). Detecting conjunctions of color and form: reassessing the serial search hypothesis. *Perception and Psychophysics*, 41, 191–201.

Pashler, H. (1988). Familiarity and visual change detection. *Perception and Psychophysics*, 44, 369–378.

Phillips, W. A. (1974). On the distinction between sensory storage and short-term visual memory. *Perception and Psychophysics*, 16, 283–290.

Piazza, M., Fumarola, A., Chinello, A., & Melcher, D. (2011). Subitizing reflects visuo spatial object individuation capacity. *Cognition*, 121, 147–153.

Prinzmetal, W., & Banks, W. P. (1983). Perceptual capacity limits in visual detection and search. *Bulletin of the Psychonomic Society*, 21, 263–266.

Pylyshyn, Z. W., & Annan, V. (2006). Dynamics of target selection in multiple object tracking (MOT). *Spatial Vision*, 19, 485–504.

Pylyshyn, Z. W., & Storm, R. W. (1988). Tracking multiple independent targets: evidence for a parallel tracking mechanism. *Spatial Vision*, 3, 179–197.

Revkin, S. K., Piazza, M., Izzard, V., Cohen, L., & Dehaene, S. (2008). Does subitizing reflect numeral estimation? *Psychological Science*, 19, 607–614.

Scholl, B. J., Pylyshyn, Z. W., & Feldman, J. (2001). What is a visual object? Evidence from target merging in multiple object tracking. *Cognition*, 80, 159–177.

Treisman, A. M., & Gelade, G. (1980). A feature-integration theory of attention. *Cognitive Psychology*, 12, 97–136.

Trick, L. M. & Pylyshyn, Z. W. (1993). What enumeration studies can show us about spatial attention: evidence for limited capacity preattentive processing. *Journal of Experimental Psychology: Human Perception and Performance*, 19, 331–351.

Trick, L. M., & Pylyshyn, Z. W. (1994). Why are small and large numbers enumerated differently? A limited capacity preattentive stage in vision. *Psychological Review*, 101, 80–102.

Vogel, E. K., & Machizawa, M. G. (2004). Neural activity predicts individual differences in visual working memory capacity. *Nature*, 428, 748–751.

Wilken, P., & Ma, W. J. (2004). A detection theory account of change detection. *Journal of Vision*, 4, 1120–1135.

Wolfe, J. M. (1994). Guided search 2.0: a revised model of visual search. *Psychonomic Bulletin and Review*, 1, 202–238.

Wolfe, J. M. (2005). Guidance of visual search by preattentive information. In L. Itti, G. Rees & J. Tsotsos (Eds.), *Neurobiology of attention* (pp. 101–104). San Diego, CA: Academic Press.

Woodman, G. F., & Luck, S. J. (1999). Electrophysiological measures of rapid shifts of attention during visual search. *Nature*, 400, 867–869.

Yantis, S. (1992). Multi-element visual tracking: attention and perceptual organization. *Cognitive Psychology*, 24, 295–340.

Zhang, W., & Luck, S. J. (2008). Discrete fixed-resolution representations in visual working memory. *Nature*, 453, 233–235.

Selective Attention, Processing Load, and Semantics: Insights from Human Electrophysiology

Cyma Van Petten

Department of Psychology, Binghamton University, State University of New York, Binghamton, NY, USA

In a paper published in *Science* in 1973, Hillyard and colleagues used a simple but elegant paradigm to isolate selective attention in the human brain (Hillyard, Hink, Schwent, & Picton, 1973). Tone pips were played to the right and left ears in a rapid unpredictable sequence, as subjects attempted to detect slightly higher-pitched tones in one ear while ignoring stimuli on the opposite side. A sensory component of the auditory event-related potential (ERP) – the N100 – was enhanced for all tones presented to the attended side. Only later in time did the ERP differentiate the rare, higher-pitched targets from the frequent standard tones—eliciting a larger P300, a typical response to rare and task-relevant events. The target P300 response occurred only for tones on the attended side, showing a hierarchical process in which an easy-to-differentiate feature (left or right side) was used to select some stimuli for the additional processing necessary to make the more difficult frequency discrimination. In the 40 years since this groundbreaking work, many sophisticated variants of this basic selective attention paradigm have been developed in the laboratories of Hillyard and his trainees, leading to an ever more detailed picture of how the sensory systems represent fundamental stimulus properties and how those properties can be amplified or suppressed by top-down attentional processes.

In the current chapter, I summarize progress on how attention influences language processing and the parallels between attentional modulation of perceptual and linguistic processes. The studies reviewed here were inspired by the success of the Hillyardian approach to examining interactions between perception and attention, yet they tackle somewhat different and often less

well-defined questions. Although words have perceptual properties like any other stimuli (spatial locations, colors, auditory frequencies, etc.), the more important features of words are symbolic. The defining property of a symbol is the association between a physical stimulus and stored knowledge—information that is accessible only via a learned mapping between the physical form and some internal representation. It might be argued that many stimuli are associated with stored knowledge (e.g., a familiar face is associated with information about that person), but symbolic information is distinct from such idiosyncratic associations in two fundamental ways. First, individual symbols are not independent entities but elements of a structured system. The number system provides a particularly clear example. In addition to serving as a sign for a specific quantity, the numeral "8" occupies a specific position in an ordered sequence, is the cube of 2, the square root of 64 (etc.), and can be subject to the same mathematical operations as any other positive whole integer. In an analogous way, animate nouns can occupy some semantic roles but not others—"panther" or "Steven" or "the fisherman" can all serve as the agent of an action, but cannot specify the time of an action in the way that "yesterday", "later", or "5 min ago" can. Second, many symbol systems can be represented in alternate surface forms without altering the internal structure of the system. To return to our numerical example, the symbolic properties of "VIII" are identical to "8" despite the difference in surface representation. The semantic and syntactic properties of language can similarly be divorced from surface representation, so that an utterance has the same denotation in auditory, visual, and haptic (Braille) formats.

Numerous ERP experiments have been designed to uncover how attention operates on the symbolic or abstract features of words. In contrast to the studies of perceptual attention reviewed elsewhere in this volume, this enterprise is complicated by the fact that the inventory of such features is neither brief nor universally agreed upon. A group of vision researchers might, for instance, agree that location, brightness, size, edge orientation, binocular disparity, color, spatial frequency, direction and speed of motion are basic features and argue about how this small set of features are combined to yield object recognition. A group of linguists or psycholinguists are likely to converge on only a handful of basic semantic and syntactic features (such as animacy and number), while agreeing that a proper listing should be much longer.

Fortunately, some fundamental questions about attention and language can still be addressed in the absence of a canonical feature list. For instance, we can wonder about the separability of a word's perceptual and abstract features—does attending to a given spatial location or color necessitate processing the meaning of a word presented in that location or color? Or, conversely, can the meaning of a word be accessed even if some of its physical features have been designated as to-be-ignored? We can also ask whether a semantic feature can define an attentional channel, i.e., can someone attend to words denoting animate objects in the same way that he can attend to words printed in blue? It has been possible to experimentally address these questions (and others) because the ERP includes a signature of semantic processing, namely, the N400 component. The N400 was discovered and developed as a tool in Hillyard's laboratory during his partnership with Marta Kutas in the 1980s. Here, I summarize progress on four issues: (1) how selective attention to physical features influences semantic processing, (2) whether preparatory attention can be tuned to words and/or the semantic features of words, (3) whether word meanings must be relevant to a subject's assigned task for semantic processing to occur, and (4) the impact of general processing load on semantic processing. I begin with a synopsis of the N400's sensitivity to the abstract properties of words to provide background for the attention studies (see Duncan et al., 2009; Kutas, Van Petten, & Kluender, 2006; Kutas & Federmeier, 2011; Van Petten & Luka, 2012 for more thorough reviews).

THE N400 AS AN INDEX OF CONCEPTUAL AND LEXICAL PROCESSING

Conceptual Manipulations

Kutas and Hillyard (1980a, 1980b, 1980c) discovered the N400 when comparing responses to sentence-final words that formed predictable completions to those that were semantically incongruent. While predictable endings elicited a broad positive waveform from 200 to 600 ms, the incongruent words elicited a large negative wave in this time range, peaking at about 400 ms after stimulus onset. Shortly thereafter, it became clear that neither incongruent endings nor even sentences were required to observe contextual modulation of N400 amplitude. Kutas and Hillyard (1984) found that congruent sentence completions also elicited N400s if the words were not completely predictable, and that N400 amplitude was closely and inversely correlated with an off-line measure of predictability, *cloze* probability (see Thornhill & Van Petten, 2012; Van Petten & Luka, 2012 for review and update). Examination of the ERPs elicited by congruent intermediate words showed large N400s for early words, which became progressively smaller as the sentence proceeded and provided semantic constraints for subsequent words (Van Petten & Kutas, 1990; Van Petten, 1993). Furthermore, the second words of semantically related pairs also elicit smaller N400s than the second words of unrelated pairs (Bentin, McCarthy, & Wood, 1985), as illustrated in Figure 19.1. The N400 is also sensitive to discourse-level context from preceding sentences and real-world knowledge in the form of arbitrary facts (Hagoort, Hald, Bastiaansen, & Peterson, 2004; van Berkum, Hagoort, & Brown, 1999; Van Petten, 1995). For our present purpose of using the N400 to examine the vulnerability of semantic processing to attentional biases and processing load, it is relevant that most of these early experiments did not require any behavioral responses from the subjects.

The N400 semantic context effect is evident in printed, spoken, and signed language (Kutas, Neville, & Holcomb, 1987). N400-like potentials are also evident in response to other meaningful stimuli—line drawings, photos, and environmental sounds like footsteps or glass shattering—and also reduced in amplitude when these nonverbal stimuli are preceded by conceptually related stimuli. I refer to these potentials as "N400-like" because they closely resemble the verbal N400 in waveshape and timing, but have slightly different spatial distributions across the scalp (Ganis, Kutas, & Sereno, 1996; Holcomb & McPherson, 1994; Plante, Van Petten, & Senkfor, 2000; Van Petten & Rheinfelder, 1995). These data suggest that verbal and nonverbal N400s reflect similar cortical computations occurring in different, although perhaps overlapping, populations of neurons (see Van Petten & Luka, 2006 for review of the neural bases of the N400). Figure 19.2 shows that verbal and nonverbal N400 semantic context effects can be, however, dissociated within the same subjects.

In addition to the pervasive effect of conceptual context on N400 amplitude, the content of what is retrieved also influences the amplitude and topographic distribution of ERP activity in the N400 latency range. Holcomb and colleagues first noted that concrete words (e.g., DAISY)

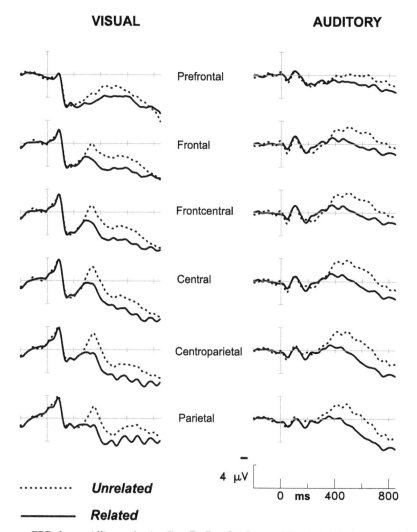

VISUAL   **AUDITORY**

.... **Unrelated**

———— **Related**

FIGURE 19.1   Grand average ERPs from midline scalp sites Fpz, Fz, Fcz, Cz, Cpz, and Pz, elicited by the second words of visual and auditory English word pairs. Subjects performed a lexical decision task on the eliciting words. Visual data from Luka and Van Petten (unpublished, $N=24$); auditory data from Macizo, Van Petten, and O'Rourke (2012, $N=34$). Negative voltage is plotted in the upward direction.

elicited more negative potentials than abstract words (e.g., FUN), but also that the "concreteness effect" had a more anterior scalp distribution than the typical centro-parietal N400 effect (Holcomb, Kounios, Anderson, & West, 1999; West & Holcomb, 2000). Huang et al. have recently suggested that the concreteness effect can be decomposed into a standard posterior N400 plus a somewhat later frontal negativity (Huang, Lee, & Federmeier, 2010). Most authors attribute the larger N400 to the retrieval of more visual or sensory detail for concrete than for abstract words. For visual words, a reliable difference in the lateral asymmetry of N400 context effects may also be tied to the content of what is retrieved. The standard semantic context effect is typically slightly larger at right than left scalp sites (Kutas, Van Petten, & Besson, 1988). When visual word pairs are presented for a rhyming/nonrhyming decision, rhyming words elicit smaller N400s (Barrett & Rugg, 1989; Kramer & Donchin, 1987; Rugg, 1984a, 1984b). This effect shows a more dramatic right-greater-than-left asymmetry than the semantic effect, which may reflect a

shift in the nature of the information accessed from long-term store—greater phonological than conceptual detail (see Van Petten & Luka, 2006; Van Petten & Rheinfelder, 1995 for discussion of the paradoxical asymmetry of the N400).

In addition to more obviously conceptual factors, N400 amplitude is reliably influenced by word frequency in that low-frequency (less commonly used) words elicit larger N400s than high-frequency words. It is possible that the N400 word frequency effect has a semantic basis; compatible with this idea is the finding that the N400 word frequency effect is attenuated or eliminated when words are placed in a supportive semantic context (Van Petten, 1993, 1995; Van Petten, Kutas, Kluender, Mitchener, & McIsaac, 1991). Alternatively, the word frequency effect may be more lexical in origin, reflecting the difficulty of mapping a rare letter string onto a concept. However, below, I will suggest that this semantic vs. lexical dichotomy may not be a particularly fruitful one for thinking about the N400.

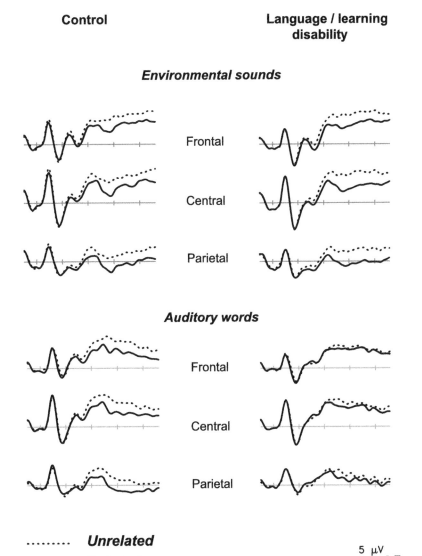

Control

Language / learning disability

Environmental sounds

Frontal

Central

Parietal

Auditory words

Frontal

Central

Parietal

········· **Unrelated**

——— **Related**

5 μV

0   400   800 ms

FIGURE 19.2   Top: Grand average ERPs from midline scalp sites Fz, Cz, and Pz, elicited by nonlinguistic but meaningful sounds (dripping faucet, horse hooves striking pavement, animal vocalizations, etc.) that were preceded by conceptually related or unrelated pictures. Bottom: ERPs elicited by spoken words that were preceded by semantically related or unrelated printed words. The left column shows ERPs from healthy college students; the right column shows ERPs from other college students who had received a diagnosis of developmental language/learning disability (LD). In an off-line test, the LD participants were able to discriminate related from unrelated word pairs with 98% accuracy. The two groups showed equivalent nonlinguistic N400 context effects, but the word-elicited N400 effect was significant only in the control group. Negative voltage is plotted in the upward direction. *Source: Adapted from Plante et al. (2000).*

Lexical Manipulations

Studies of visual word recognition show several ERP components that differentiate orthographic from nonorthographic stimuli and occur within 200 ms of stimulus onset, prior to the onset of the N400. These include a left-lateralized negativity peaking between 140 and 180 ms that is larger for letter strings than for many types of visual stimuli (variably called the visual N1, N170, N180); intracranially recorded ERPs suggest that this scalp potential is likely to receive some contribution from a posterior

fusiform region considered to be the "visual form area" (Appelbaum, Liotti, Perez, Fox, & Woldorff, 2009; Nobre, Allison, & McCarthy, 1994; Schendan, Ganis, & Kutas, 1998; see Barber & Kutas, 2007 for review). A negative peak at about 250 ms has proven sensitive to some varieties of orthographic priming and is also dissociable from the N400 (Grainger & Holcomb, 2009). Finally, a somewhat later negative peak varies in latency (from roughly 280–340 ms) with word length and the frequency of a word's occurrence in natural language use

(King & Kutas, 1998; Osterhout, Bersick, & McKinnon, 1997). These earlier components reflect the perceptual processes that transform visual input into more abstract orthographic representations, and which are sensitive to the familiarity of orthographic patterns.

In contrast to the components described above, the N400 has been argued to index a more purely conceptual stage of analysis in which the retrieved meaning of an item is integrated with prior context (Hagoort, Baggio, & Willems, 2009). However, closer consideration of the data indicates that the N400 continues to be influenced by processes that precede the analysis of the conceptual/semantic content retrieved from long-term memory. Recall that although N400s elicited by visual, auditory, verbal, and nonverbal stimuli are similarly responsive to prior conceptual context, these potentials have subtly different scalp distributions in healthy adults, and can be differentially affected by developmental language disorders (Duncan et al., 2009; Plante et al., 2000; see Figure 19.2). Although this component of the ERP can be called multimodal, it is not amodal, but instead reflects the physical nature of the input (see Van Petten & Luka, 2006 for review). Moreover, numerous studies have shown orderly variation in the amplitude of the N400 elicited by various types of meaningless stimuli. Larger N400s are elicited by unpronounceable letter strings than by false-font stimuli that are similar in visual complexity to alphabetic stimuli (Appelbaum et al., 2009; Bentin, Mouchetant-Rostaing, Giard, Echallier, & Pernier, 1999). In turn, pronounceable pseudowords elicit larger N400s than strings of consonants or alphanumeric symbols (Bentin et al., 1999; Rugg & Nagy, 1987). Finally, both real words and pseudowords with more orthographic neighbors (real words that can be formed by changing one letter) elicit larger N400s than words and pseudowords with fewer neighbors (Holcomb, Grainger, & O'Rourke, 2002; Laszlo & Federmeier, 2011; Müller, Duñabeitia, & Carreiras, 2010). All three groups of authors attribute this latter effect to greater global activation in a lexico-semantic network when a letter string from a dense neighborhood is encountered, because of partial activation of numerous words that are near matches to the actual input. The orthographic neighborhood effect is consistent with the letter-string-vs.-false-font and pseudoword-vs.-consonant-string results in suggesting a general principle: as a visual stimulus becomes more wordlike—more similar to more items in one's vocabulary and thus more likely to be potentially meaningful—it elicits a larger N400. One report shows that the influence of orthographic neighborhood size on N400 amplitude is like the word frequency effect—attenuated or eliminated when words are placed in supportive semantic context (Molinaro, Conrad, Barber, & Carreiras, 2010, but see also Laszlo & Federmeier, 2009).

Some investigators (see for instance, Lau, Phillips, & Poeppel, 2008) have argued that the neural processes reflected in the scalp-recorded N400 should be categorized according to a dichotomy proposed by psycholinguists some decades ago: either *prelexical*, referring to processes that yield identification of a word in order to access information stored with that letter-string (meaning, pronunciation, possible syntactic roles) or *postlexical*, referring to processes that act on the retrieved information (semantic and/or syntactic integration with prior context, inferences, predictions about upcoming words, etc.). The results briefly reviewed above do not comfortably fit within this dichotomy given that N400 amplitude is influenced by both the effort expended in assessing stimuli that ultimately prove to have no stored meaning (e.g., consonant strings) and by the nature of what is retrieved when a stimulus does prove to be meaningful (e.g., the concreteness effect). Interactions between factors typically assigned to one or the other side of this division, such as those between semantic context and orthographic neighborhood density or between semantic context and word frequency, are particularly problematic for the proposed dichotomy.

The long temporal duration of most N400 effects (several hundred milliseconds) and apparent generation within a large region of cerebral cortex (a substantial portion of the left temporal lobe with some contribution from the right temporal lobe; Halgren et al., 2002; Van Petten & Luka, 2006) allows for the possibility that "the N400" is divisible into subcomponents and subfunctions occurring in different latency ranges and different cortical areas. The attention and processing-load studies reviewed below have largely considered the N400 as a single entity, but further work may aid in identifying subcomponents.

IS ATTENTION TO PERCEPTUAL FEATURES NECESSARY FOR SEMANTIC PROCESSING?

As described at the outset of this chapter, the selective attention paradigm pioneered by Hillyard and colleagues incorporates the principle of hierarchical selection of stimuli for further processing: when processing capacity is taxed, items meeting a simple criterion will be further processed to determine if they meet some second criterion, but items that fail the initial criterion will receive only minimal processing. The paradigm itself is, of course, agnostic as to the origin of the hierarchy. Imagine stimuli with two dimensions (A and B), each with two feature values (e.g., location left vs. right, and color red vs. reddish-orange). Initial attentional selection might be based on dimension A rather than dimension B because: (1) the instructions or reward structure for the task give priority to dimension A; (2) the two feature values for A are easier to discriminate than the two values of dimension B; or (3) the two dimensions are processed sequentially by the nervous system, such that information about dimension A always becomes available sooner than information about dimension B. The first two possibilities will be peculiar to individual experiments, whereas results that bear on possibility (3) will be more informative about human neurophysiology. ERP studies of visual selective have suggested that although people can bias the processing of stimuli based on spatial location, color, edge orientation and direction of motion, selection on the basis of location has temporal priority (Anllo-Vento & Hillyard, 1996; Bengson, Lopez-Calderon, & Mangun, 2012; Hillyard & Münte, 1984). Initial attention effects based on location appear to be enhancements of obligatory ERP components elicited by all stimuli, beginning with the occipito-temporal P1 at roughly 70 ms after stimulus onset. In contrast, responses to stimuli with other attended features typically differ from their unattended counterparts only after 150 ms, and the attention effects do not always appear to be enhancements of obligatory ERP components.

Selective attention paradigms that include word meaning as a "dimension" can, in principle, tell us something about where meaning extraction falls in the temporal stream of neural processing. The onset latency of the visual N400 at roughly 200 ms suggests that meaning extraction lags behind analysis of most basic visual properties, but it is logically possible that some earlier semantic analysis is not reflected in the N400. The experiments reviewed below do not depend on any interpretation of N400 latency, but only on the presence or absence of N400 amplitude differences between conditions.

Spatial Attention is Necessary for Semantic Processing

McCarthy and Nobre (1993) evaluated the relationship between visuospatial attention and semantic processing by presenting words to the right and left of fixation, with instructions to attend to one side on a given block of trials. As in previous experiments with nonlinguistic stimuli, words on the attended side elicited a larger P1 component than words on the unattended side. The target dimension was semantic: participants were instructed to press a button for body-part words (EYE, ARM, etc.) appearing on the designated side. As expected, these low-probability targets elicited P300s, whereas body-part words on the unattended side did not. However, McCarthy and Nobre included a second manipulation to evaluate the possibility of semantic processing in the absence of spatial attention. On both attended and unattended sides, sequential words were sometimes semantically related (e.g., CAT followed by DOG, both on the attended side, or TABLE followed by CHAIR, both on the unattended side). When falling on the attended side, semantically related words elicited a smaller N400 component than unrelated words. On the unattended side, there was no difference between related and unrelated trials (no N400 effect), indicating that semantic relationships were not noticed. A second result suggested that semantic processing was simply not engaged for words outside of the "spatial spotlight"—words on the unattended side elicited little sign of a negative peak in the N400 latency range (i.e., no N400). These results indicate that attentional selection on the basis of visual location precedes semantic processing, so that application of an early spatial filter can block subsequent semantic processing.

Vogel and colleagues confirmed the importance of spatial attention for semantic processing with a trial-by-trial cueing procedure (Vogel, Woodman, & Luck, 2005). Participants first viewed a context word, then a central arrow cue signaling the likely location of an upcoming word, and finally a briefly presented array of four letter strings in four spatial quadrants (one word and three nonwords). Participants indicated whether the word target was related to the context word. Note that, in contrast to the experiments above, the attentional cue was probabilistic (75% valid) rather than absolute, and the instructions mandated some attempt at semantic processing even for uncued locations. We might thus expect attenuation rather than elimination of semantic processing for uncued locations, and this is what was observed. When target words appeared in validly cued locations, accuracy was high, and the N400 context effect was large. When words appeared in uncued locations, accuracy dropped to ~65%, and the N400 context effect was severely reduced as well. However, this experiment also made the important point that similar patterns of behavior can mask distinct attentional processes. In a separate block of trials, the spatial cue was simultaneously presented with the target array, so that participants were not able to shift their attentional focus in advance. The simultaneous cue still yielded a substantial accuracy benefit for validly cued locations, but validly and invalidly cued locations yielded equivalent N400 context effects. The contrasting ERP results of the two cueing conditions indicate that attentional selection can take place at different times (or levels) of the processing stream, which can either precede or follow semantic processing. In the case of a simultaneous cue, spatial attention was not engaged early enough to block semantic processing in unattended locations, but did influence some later stage of processing useful for the behavioral task. I return to this point about the timing of attentional processes just below, and in the section entitled Preparing to Process Words.

Auditory spatial attention

Bentin, Kutas, and Hillyard (1995) examined spatial attention and semantic processing in the auditory modality. Different words were simultaneously presented to the right and left ears; consecutive words within each channel of input were either related or unrelated. The participants in this study were instructed to memorize the words on one side for a subsequent test, but were given no ongoing target detection task. A robust difference in N400 amplitude was observed between related and unrelated words presented to an attended ear, whether left or right, despite a larger pathway from the right ear to the language-dominant left hemisphere. Related and unrelated items elicited essentially identical ERPs when presented to an ignored left ear. In contrast, participants reported greater difficulty in ignoring words presented to their right ear, and a weak but significant N400 context effect was observed in the unattended right ear. The small N400 effect for nominally unattended words may indicate that spatial attention is less effective in the auditory than visual modality, or may have reflected slippage of attention to the wrong ear on a small proportion of trials. An argument in favor of the "slippage" account is that a different dichotic listening experiment found no differences between first and repeated presentations of words unless both were in the attended ear (Okita & Jibu, 1998).

Attentional Selection by Color Attenuates, but Does Not Eliminate Semantic Processing

Attention to color also modulates ERPs, but with a latency delay relative to visuospatial attention. Early studies with nonlinguistic stimuli reported no impact of color-based attention prior to 150 ms or even 200 ms after stimulus onset,[1] a latency that is very close to our best estimates of when access to word meaning might begin (based on both the onset latencies of N400 context effects and gaze-duration measures during reading). The Stroop color-word interference effect also suggests close temporal competition between the processing of color and meaning. These estimates suggest that semantic processing might occur regardless of attentional biases toward or away from a word's color.

[1]Color-based attention effects that begin earlier (~100 ms after stimulus onset) have been observed in two studies with unusual stimuli that consisted of discontinuous colored elements—clouds of colored dots (Zhang & Luck, 2009) or checkerboards with gray and colored checks (Anllo-Vento, Luck, & Hillyard, 1998). Although printed words also consist of discontinuous elements (letters) these have consistently yielded substantially later differences between attended and unattended colors (Kellenbach & Michie, 1996; Nobre, Allison, & McCarthy, 1998; Otten et al., 1993).

Kellenbach and Michie (1996) thus intermixed red and green words with red and green nonword letter strings and asked their participants to make lexical decisions only for items in a single color. Robust ERP differences between attended and unattended colors were observed beginning ~200 ms. The design allowed four contrasts between semantically related and unrelated words: both words of a sequentially presented pair in the attended color (AA), both in the unattended color (UU), first word in the attended color and the second word in the unattended color (AU), and the reverse (UA). Two experiments yielded the same pattern of ERP results: robust N400 semantic context effects in the AA condition (as expected), null effects in the UU and UA conditions, but a detectable effect for unattended targets following attended context words (AU). Semantically related words are typically remembered better than unrelated items (Besson, Kutas, & Van Petten, 1992; Olichney et al., 2000), but semantic processing in the AU condition was apparently too weak to lead to effective memory encoding as these words could not be discriminated from new items in a subsequent recognition test. Overall, the results showed that attentional selection based on color occurred early enough to attenuate (but not completely block) semantic processing. This conclusion has been confirmed by three additional studies from different laboratories (Heil & Rolke, 2004; Otten, Rugg, & Doyle, 1993; Phillips & Lesperance, 2003). Echoing the findings of Kellenbach and Michie (1996), Phillips and Lesperance also observed a dissociation between the immediate measure of semantic processing offered by the N400 and slightly delayed memory tests. This finding indicates that semantic processing can occur without leaving a durable memory trace, a point I return to later under the section entitled Semantic Access and Processing Load.

PREPARING TO PROCESS WORDS: HOW ABSTRACT IS PREPARATORY ATTENTION?

The experiments reviewed above document the downstream consequences of having oriented attention to a fundamental visual feature—enhanced semantic processing of words possessing those features (or alternatively, suppressed semantic processing of those that do not). In most of these experiments, the initial process of orienting attention occurred well in advance of the actual stimuli, at the outset of a block of trials. The orienting process itself is thought to be governed by a frontal-parietal network that is relatively independent of sensory modality, and which acts to up- or down-regulate activity in other cortical areas depending on what aspects of the environment are relevant to current goals, expectations about what is likely to occur in the immediate future, etc. Several functional magnetic resonance imaging (fMRI) experiments have shown that predictive cues about the nature of an upcoming stimulus activate this frontal–parietal network, but also lead to anticipatory activity in cortical areas that will process the predicted stimulus. For instance, Hopfinger, Buonocore, and Mangun (2000) observed enhanced activity in visual cortex contralateral to the expected location of an upcoming stimulus, although the predictive cue was centrally presented. Langner et al. (2011) observed increased activity in unimodal visual, auditory, and somatosensory cortices after cues that suggested that the next stimulus would occur in the respective modality. These neural preparatory attentional processes are likely to make some contribution to the superior perception and semantic processing of items whose physical features have been designated as to-be-attended. However, we can wonder about what kinds of features are amenable to preparatory attention, in particular, whether it is possible to predispose brain activity toward words as a class of stimuli, or, in a more extreme case, toward specific semantic features. A handful of ERP studies have begun to approach these questions.

On each trial, the subjects of Miniussi, Marzi, and Nobre (2005) saw one of two novel geometric shapes that predicted whether the next stimulus would be a letter string or an angle within a circle. If the imperative stimulus was a letter string, it called for a lexical decision (word/nonword); if the imperative stimulus was an angle, it called for an acute/obtuse judgment. The cues were informative about both the perceptual nature of the upcoming stimulus and the task to be performed, so that this design combines preparatory attention with task-set configuration. The two cues elicited different ERPs, showing differential preparation for the letter-strings vs angles (or their associated tasks); letter-string cues elicited a larger posterior N1 whereas angle cues elicited a prolonged parietal positivity beginning ~280 ms. The cues validly predicted the type of upcoming stimulus on 80% of the trials but were invalid for the other 20%, so that comparisons between validly and invalidly cued items reveal the impact of differential preparation. As expected, behavioral responses were faster for validly cued items, but early visual components (P1, N1) were unaffected. For the letter strings, validly cued items elicited more negative ERPs in the N400 latency range, suggestive of enhanced lexical processing due to preparation to process letter strings. This validity effect had a more frontal scalp distribution than the typical N400, but two other aspects of the results support the conclusion that it indexed lexical processing. First, the validity effect appeared to be qualitatively identical to the ERP difference between words and nonwords (as shown in Figure 19.3), strongly suggesting an origin in the processes that attempt to derive meaning from letter strings. Second, the validity effect for angle stimuli was qualitatively distinct from the letter-string validity effect, primarily consisting of a larger P300 for the surprising occurrence of an unpredicted stimulus type.

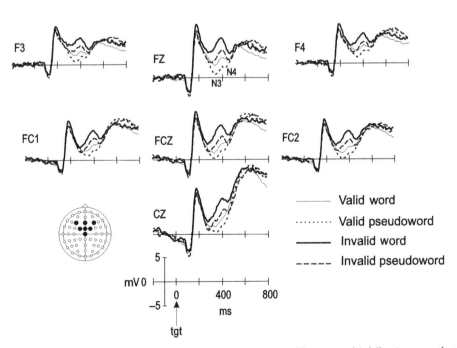

FIGURE 19.3 Grand average ERPs elicited by letter-strings (word or pronounceable nonwords) following cues that validly predicted the occurrence of a letter-string or were invalid cues because they predicted the occurrence of an angle stimulus. Positive voltage is plotted in the upward direction. *Source: Reprinted from Miniussi, Marzi and Nobre (2005).*

The inclusion of both cue- and target-elicited ERPs in this experiment was particularly persuasive in showing that people can selectively prepare for linguistic stimuli or linguistic tasks.

Cristescu and Nobre (2008) used a similar trial-by-trial cueing procedure, but all of the target stimuli were letter strings and all required the same task of lexical decision, so that the design focused on preparatory attention. For one group of subjects, cues predicted whether the target words (or nonwords) were more likely to appear on the right or left side of the screen; these spatial cueing results replicated McCarthy and Nobre's (1993) results in showing larger early visual potentials (P1) and larger N400-like potentials for items appearing in validly cued locations.[2] For other subjects, the cue predicted the likely semantic category of upcoming words but was always uninformative about its location. One cue specified that an animal word was likely; the other specified that a tool word was likely. This particular contrast is interesting given (contentious) suggestions that these two categories differ in visual and action/motoric semantic features associated with different brain regions (Martin, Wiggs, Ungerleider, & Haxby, 1996; Tyler & Moss, 2001). Unfortunately, Cristescu and Nobre did not compare the ERPs elicited by animal and tool cues. In an fMRI version of this experiment, semantic cues (collapsed across category) produced greater brain activity than spatial cues in cortical areas generally considered critical for language processing: the posterior part of the left middle temporal gyrus, left inferior frontal gyrus, as well as the left angular gyrus (Cristescu, Devlin, & Nobre, 2006). The fMRI results thus show that preparatory attention is not restricted to preactivation of sensory cortices, but extends to language cortex. In the ERP experiment, words preceded by invalid semantic cues (collapsed across categories) elicited more negative potentials in the N400 latency range than validly cued words, suggesting that an unpredicted category was more difficult to process. The contrast between larger late negative potentials for cued vs. uncued spatial locations, but smaller negativities for cued vs. uncued semantic categories (as well as different scalp distributions for the two effects) indicates that there were at least two distinct preparatory processes at work. The former resembled the validity effect in Minuissi et al. (2005) and may have reflected the benefit of preparing for lexical processing per se, while the latter may have reflected the benefit of expecting a class of semantic features.

Kanske, Plitschka, and Kotz (2011) have pursued the benefits and costs of expectations for semantic content by cueing subjects to expect animal vs tool words in one

block, or words with negative vs neutral emotional content (e.g., TUMOR vs. PEA) in another block. Words were frequently repeated across the course of the experiment, so that the "×" and "+" cues may also have led to expectations for specific words as well as their semantic features. Both varieties of valid cueing led to faster response times (RTs) in the nonsemantic task of judging grammatical gender of the German words. As in Christecu and Nobre's (2008) experiment, semantic cues did not influence early visual potentials, but did lead to larger late negative potentials for words from invalidly cued categories, as shown in Figure 19.4. The validity effects had more frontal scalp distributions than the typical N400 semantic context effect, reminiscent of Miniussi et al.'s frontal validity effect.

The broad results of two studies with categorical cues (Cristescu & Nobre, 2008; Kanske et al., 2011) are in accord with a larger body of work using single words, phrases, and sentence contexts to manipulate expectations about upcoming words. Multiple experiments show that presentation of a category description ("type of furniture") yields smaller N400s for subsequent exemplars of that category than for out-of-category words (Federmeier, Kutas, & Schul, 2010; Heinze, Münte, & Kutas, 1998; Kutas & Iragui, 1998; Olichney et al., 2000). However, a closer comparison of the two literatures also shows differences that are not yet understood. The category-label experiments lead to N400 effects that are invariably largest over centro-parietal scalp, whereas the cue-validity effects often seem to have frontal scalp distributions. These topographic differences hint at the possibility that semantic or lexical expectations derived during routine language processing differ from more purely top-down expectations driven by arbitrary cues. It remains for future work to more closely integrate these two literature.

TASK RELEVANCE OF SEMANTIC INFORMATION

In visual attention research, there has been some debate about whether attention purely operates at the level of features (color, orientation, etc.) or also at the level of whole objects. Theories of object-based attention suggest that it is difficult to selectively process only some attributes of a coherent visual object and that processing one feature of an object entails processing of its other features as well (Duncan, 1996; Kahneman, Treisman, & Gibbs, 1992). The results of some fMRI experiments suggest that when attention is directed to one feature of an object, brain regions that process other, task-irrelevant aspects of the same object also show increased activity (O'Craven, Downing, & Kanwisher, 1999; Schoenfeld et al., 2003). ERP experiments from Hillyard's group

---

[2]Only stimuli presented in the right visual field were analyzed in this ERP experiment, although the fMRI version (Cristescu et al., 2006) analyzed items from both visual fields.

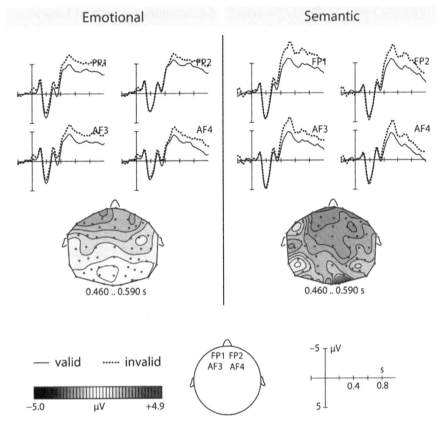

FIGURE 19.4 Left: Grand average ERPs elicited by emotionally negative and neutral words, after "×" and "+" cues that validly or invalidly predicted emotional valence. Right: ERPs elicited by words denoting tools and animals, after cues that validly or invalidly predicted semantic category. Topographic maps at bottom display the amplitudes of difference waves formed by subtracting validly cued ERPs from invalidly cued ERPs. Negative voltage is plotted in the upward direction. *Source: Adapted from Kanske et al. (2011).*

have demonstrated that spatial attention spreads to all parts of an object even when the assigned task demands attention to only a small part of the object, but these have not examined whether other dimensions of the object (color, motion, etc.) are also facilitated (Martínez, Teder-Salejarvi, & Hillyard, 2007; Martínez et al., 2006). One recent experiment has made this claim for stimuli that are object-like (dot clouds with coherent motion; Snyder, Fiebelkorni, & Foxe, 2012).

In the psycholinguistic literature, an analogous question has received considerable attention: what properties of words are accessed when they are irrelevant to the assigned task? It is possible that words behave like atomic units such that even the most abstract of properties are accessed whenever any of its dimensions is attended. The alternative is that word-processing is at least partially hierarchical and that the extent of processing is under voluntary control. Note that intermediate positions are also possible, that some lexical attributes form inseparable bundles whereas others are dissociable. For instance, it is possible that orthographic processing necessarily entails phonological processing, but not access to semantic or syntactic properties. In this section, I take up only one question: whether attending to

a physical feature of a word necessitates access to its meaning.

The purely behavioral literature emphasizes a single task combination: subjects are asked to process the letters (only) of some context word, followed by a lexical decision on a subsequent target word. Lexical decisions are generally faster for semantically related than unrelated targets, but the logic here is that if subjects truly restrict their processing to the physical letters of the context word, such context–target relationships will go unnoticed. Smith and colleagues first reported exactly this result: if subjects had to decide whether a context word contained a simultaneously presented letter, the standard RT advantage for related targets was eliminated (Smith, Theodore, & Franklin, 1983). Stolz and Besner (1998, 1999) have suggested that semantic processing of the context word does not occur if the letter-search task diverts resources at a critical moment.

A wider variety of tasks and stimuli have been used across the ERP literature. Brain activity measures provide a different window into the manner in which semantic processing is governed by attention, because the link between instruction and task performance can be broken. A subject's overt behavior may indicate perfect adherence to task instructions, but his or her brain activity may indicate engagement in other processes (like semantic analysis) that were neither requested nor useful for task performance. As summarized below, the bulk of the evidence indicates that N400 semantic context effects are observed during the performance of nonsemantic tasks.

Kutas and Hillyard (1989) first reported that a letter-search task yielded reliable semantic context effects on N400 amplitude; in this experiment a probe letter followed a pair of words and subjects judged whether the letter had been present in at least one of the preceding words. My laboratory has similarly observed robust semantic context effects during physical probe-matching tasks after pairs of stimuli consisting of printed and spoken words, environmental sounds and spoken words, and environmental sounds and pictures (Plante et al., 2000; Van Petten & Rheinfelder, 1995). For pairs consisting of printed words and environmental sounds, Orgs and colleagues directly compared a semantic and physical task; the color of a printed word signaled whether the following sound should be judged for its semantic match to the word or merely whether it was presented to the right or left ear. N400-like context effects were observed for both tasks and were indistinguishable in amplitude (Orgs, Lange, Dombrowski, & Heil, 2007). However, in a follow-up experiment in which the same tasks were blocked rather than randomly interleaved, these investigators observed a smaller (but significant) context effect in the physical task as compared to the semantic task (Orgs, Lange, Dombrowski, & Heil, 2008).

In a design more like that of the purely behavioral studies, Heil and colleagues asked subjects to perform a letter-detection task on a context word (decide if a simultaneously presented letter is present in the word), followed by a lexical decision on a target word that was either unrelated, semantically related, or a repetition of the context word. Lexical decisions were fastest for repetitions, but identical for related and unrelated words. An N400 semantic context effect was observed despite the absence of an RT effect, leading Heil et al. to conclude that N400 amplitude is a more sensitive metric of semantic processing than lexical decision time (Heil, Rolke, & Pecchinenda, 2004; Küper & Heil, 2009). An alternative interpretation is that the behavioral and brain measures in this paradigm reflect different processes. Although semantic information typically contributes to lexical decisions, judgments of lexicality can (a priori) be made on the basis of memory for word forms alone. Engaging in letter search for the first word of a pair may shift the basis for a subsequent lexical decision toward word forms and away from semantics. Under this account, lexical decisions based on this strategy would be speeded by orthographic overlap between context and target, and thus yield faster RTs for repeated targets, but not

for semantically related targets, as observed. However, breaking the link between semantics and the lexical decision task need not imply that semantic information is not accessed merely that semantic information now makes no contribution to task performance. This account is very similar to that proposed by Stolz and Besner (1998), except that it emphasizes the role of transfer-appropriate processing between tasks, and does not assume that lexical decision times need reflect all of the cognitive processes engendered by presentation of a word. Under this account, the modulation of N400 amplitude observed by Heil et al. (2004) reflected task-irrelevant semantic processing.

Other studies have explicitly compared the magnitude of semantic context effects across tasks. Besson and colleagues compared orthographic to semantic judgments on visual words. In the orthographic task, subjects indicated if the two preceding words shared a common pattern of initial and final letters (vowel initial and consonant final, consonant initial and consonant final, etc.). Semantic relationship did not influence RT during the orthographic task, but a reliable N400 context effect was observed that was nonsignificantly smaller than in the semantic task of judging whether the two words matched on animacy (Besson, Fischler, Boaz, & Raney, 1992). Besson et al.'s results are consistent with our proposal that semantics can be disconnected from task performance but continue to show an influence on brain activity. Chwilla and colleagues contrasted related and unrelated word pairs (sequentially presented) in lexical decision and font judgment (upper- vs. lower-case) tasks and observed ERP differences between the related and unrelated items even during the font judgment. This experiment also manipulated the probability of related and unrelated pairs, such that the observed semantic effect clearly included a modulation of P300 amplitude; it is difficult to determine if N400 amplitude also varied, but the results clearly demonstrated task-irrelevant processing of word meaning (Chwilla, Brown, & Hagoort, 1995). West and Holcomb (2000) compared abstract to concrete words during true/false judgments. Some of the stimuli required an orthographic judgment (e.g., "There is a letter E in the word ELEPHANT"); some required an imagery judgment (e.g., "It is easy to form a mental image of an APTITUDE"); and some required a semantic judgment (e.g., "It is unusual for people to have an ELEPHANT"). As in previous reports, concrete words elicited a larger N400 than abstract words, and this was true even in the orthographic task (albeit with reduced amplitude relative to the semantic task), indicating that word meanings were accessed. Echoing some other reports, reaction times did not differentiate concrete and abstract words in the orthographic task despite the continued presence of an N400 difference (West & Holcomb, 2000). In an experiment using word pairs, Perrin and García-Larrea (2003) found that semantically related words elicited smaller N400s than unrelated although participants were asked to decide if the pairs rhymed, although this effect was smaller than during a semantic relationship judgment. Hohlfeld and Sommer (2005) presented auditory context words followed by target words that had been digitally edited to be higher or lower in pitch than the talker's natural voice. Semantically related words elicited smaller N400s and faster RTs during a pitch judgment task, although the ERP effect was smaller than a prior experiment with semantic judgments (Hohlfeld, Sangals, & Sommer, 2004). A later experiment from the same lab examined the N400 word frequency effect (smaller N400s for commonly used than rarely used words), with very similar results suggesting intact (although slower) lexical access during a nonlexical task (Rabovsky, Álvarez, Hohlfeld, & Sommer, 2008).

Overall, ERP studies that have directed participants' attention toward words but away from their semantic properties, appear to lie on a continuum with the selective attention experiments reviewed above. The usual reduction in N400 amplitude produced by a related semantic context is attenuated when a task encourages processing of nonsemantic properties of the stimuli, much like perceptual attention attenuates semantic processing of words in an unattended color. Both effects are weaker than directing attention away from the spatial location of a word.

A general conclusion from the task-relevance experiments reviewed here is that semantic processing is spontaneously engaged by meaningful material, whether or not such processing is required by explicit task instructions. However, it is important to note that spontaneous is by no means equivalent to an older term used in the cognitive psychology literature—*automatic*—a term suggesting a resource-free process that never competes with other cognitive activities. The nonsemantic tasks above were performed with high accuracy, implying that they were not especially demanding and were likely to leave plenty of "spare capacity" for subjects to pursue their natural interest of comprehending the stimuli. Below, I examine experiments in which participants were deliberately overloaded with multiple tasks during rapid stimulus presentation.

SEMANTIC ACCESS AND PROCESSING LOAD

A rapidly accumulating literature uses the N400 to examine interactions between semantic processing and nonlinguistic processing load. As summarized below, these experiments have yielded a variety of results, from very good preservation of semantic processing in the face of other demands, to complete elimination of N400 effects under a high processing load, so that many details remain to be clarified. The methodologies are of some interest for understanding cognitive limitations and the level(s) at which language comprehension interacts with other brain processes.

When a rapid stream of simple stimuli (letters or numbers, at a rate of ~10/s) contains two targets, observers are usually impaired at reporting the second target (T2), as compared to conditions with only one target. This *attentional blink* effect has attracted considerable interest because of its peculiar time course. Accuracy in detecting T2 typically suffers little impairment when it immediately follows the first target (T1), drops to a low point at a T1–T2 lag of three items, and then recovers by a lag of six to eight items (Chun & Potter, 1995). This time course suggests that the attentional blink does not arise from purely perceptual factors (masking, for instance, should be the greatest at the shortest lag), but from interference between T1 and T2 at some other stage of processing. Several lines of evidence suggest that this stage is one of storage in working memory (Vogel, Luck, & Shapiro, 1998).

Luck, Vogel, and Shapiro (1996) examined the fate of semantic processing during the attentional blink by presenting a context word at the beginning of each trial, followed by a stream of stimuli mostly consisting of consonant strings, at a rate of 12/s. Within this rapid stream were two critical stimuli: a numeric target (T1, e.g., 3333333) and a word (T2) that could be semantically related or unrelated to the context word for that trial. After another 10 consonant strings, participants were asked to make two binary judgments, indicating whether the number was even or odd, and if the word was related or unrelated to the context word. Performance showed the typical attentional blink pattern: T2 accuracy of ~90% when the number and word occurred in immediate succession or with a lag of six intervening items, but only 66% with a lag of two intervening items. N400 amplitude was smaller when T2 was related to the initial context word, and neither the amplitude nor latency of this semantic context effect was affected by T1–T2 lag, as shown in Figure 19.5. The ERP data thus showed that the meanings of words could be extracted and compared with other semantic information without reaching a stage at which the results of this comparison could be retained in working memory for even one to 2s. These results are consistent with other reports that semantic processing can be evident in the immediate reflection of brain activity offered by ERPs without leaving a memory record (Kellenbach & Michie, 1996; Olichney et al., 2000; Phillips & Lesperance, 2003), but extend the previous dissociations between semantic processing and long-term memory to working memory as well. A subsequent experiment showed that although

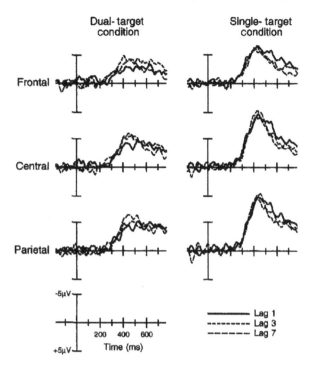

FIGURE 19.5 Grand average N400 difference waves (unrelated minus related) from the attentional blink experiment reported in Luck et al., 1996 and as Exp. 2 in Vogel et al. (1998), see text for description. In the "dual target condition", words served as second targets (T2, see text) and occurred 83 ms (Lag 1), 249 ms (Lag 3), or 581 ms (Lag 7) after a number target (T1). The "single target" condition included the same sequence of stimuli, but subjects were not instructed to make any decision or response to T1. Negative voltage is plotted in the upward direction. *Source: Reprinted from Vogel et al. (1998).*

neither the N400 nor earlier components were sensitive to the attentional blink, a different component of the ERP tracked behavioral performance. The P3, typically elicited by target stimuli in a string of nontargets and traditionally associated with the updating of working memory (Donchin, 1981; Donchin & Coles, 1988), was suppressed for targets presented during the attentional blink as compared to targets at shorter or longer lags outside the critical time frame (Vogel et al., 1998).

Rolke and colleagues reported the other half of the attentional blink story: that N400 context effects are observed when targets are preceded by contexts that occurred during the attentional blink (Rolke, Heil, Streb, & Henninghausen, 2001). This latter finding poses more of a challenge to conventional psycholinguistic thought, which would suppose that contexts must be stored in working memory to be effective. Indeed, the psycholinguistic literature shows that low working memory capacity and external memory loads impair comprehension (Blackwell & Bates, 1995; King & Just, 1991). The attentional blink results might then indicate the existence of distinct short-term buffers that serve conceptual processing vs explicit decisions about stimuli (as proposed by Vogel et al., 1998). The psycholinguistic literature

has, however, primarily addressed sentential processing rather than the simpler word-pair relationships used in attentional blink experiments. Using N400 measures, we have shown that semantic context effects between associated words are much less sensitive to working memory limitations than sentential semantics (Federmeier, Van Petten, Schwartz, & Kutas, 2003; Van Petten, 1993; Van Petten, Weckerly, McIsaac, & Kutas, 1997). One can imagine that processing word-pair relationships need not involve explicit storage of the first word as a discrete item, but a mechanism more like that proposed in some network models. In attractor (Hopfield) networks, processing of one word causes the system to "settle" in a particular state; if a second item shares semantic features, less change in the state of the network is required than for dissimilar words, analogous to faster responses and less neural activity (McRae, de Sa, & Seidenberg, 1997). Because it does not include a working memory store separate from the processing system, such a system might be able to accommodate the observation of semantic context effects for words that cannot be reported. However, such a system would still need to be paired with a working memory system that allows for explicit readout of recent stimuli under some conditions and for the extra demands of combining words during sentence processing.

Other studies have found more deleterious consequences for semantic processing when multiple tasks must be performed on rapidly presented stimuli. Hohlfeld and colleagues presented an auditory context word, followed by a visual letter at the offset of this word, followed by a second auditory word that could be related or unrelated to the first (Hohlfeld et al., 2004). Participants first indicated the left/right location of the visual letter with a foot-pedal response and then made a relationship judgment about the word pair. Two processing load manipulations were included: the stimulus-onset asynchrony (SOA) between the visual letter and the second word (100, 400, or 700 ms), and the spatial compatibility of the location response (compatible, right-sided letter called for right-foot response, or incompatible, right-sided letter called for left-foot response). As expected from previous studies of the psychological refractory period (PRP), RTs for the second response—the relationship judgment—were slowed by shorter SOAs between the two target stimuli, especially when the first response was spatially incompatible with the first target. Such PRP effects on reaction time are often attributed to overlap between two tasks at a "central bottleneck", such that some stage in processing of the second target must wait for the first target to clear the bottleneck (Pashler, 1994). Response selection is typically offered as a strong candidate for a central bottleneck that will be required by any overt task. By this logic, we might have expected no impact of Hohlfeld's difficulty manipulations on N400 latency, because N400 semantic context effects can be observed with no overt response at all, such that response selection would seem to have little relevance. However, both the SOA and response-compatibility manipulations did influence the latency of the N400 semantic context effect. It is unclear whether onset latency was affected, but the duration of the context effect was prolonged in the more difficult conditions, resulting in a delayed peak. Total amplitude of the context effect was equivalent across conditions, but spread out over a longer time frame, indicating that at least the completion (if not the initiation) of semantic processing was delayed by the requirement to complete the other task. A second study used the same sequence of stimuli but made the semantic relationship between the two auditory words task irrelevant; participants instead judged the relative pitch of the two words after the spatial location response (Hohlfeld & Sommer, 2005). These latter task requirements had a much more severe impact on the N400 context effect, eliminating the effect altogether when the location task included an incompatible stimulus–response mapping.

More recent experiments have returned to the attentional blink paradigm pioneered by Luck et al. (1996). These have used the same metric of meaning access, namely N400 responses to visual words (second targets, T2s) that differ depending on their semantic relationship to a pretrial context word. In contrast to the initial study, the recent reports include delays and/or reductions of the N400 context effect on T2 when T2 was presented shortly after a first target (T1) (Batterink, Karns, Yamada, & Neville, 2010; Giesbrecht, Sy, & Elliott, 2007; Lien, Ruthruff, Cornett, Goodin, & Allen, 2008; Vachon & Jolicoeur, 2011, 2012). Such delays and reductions are apparent even when T1 and T2 tasks appear to have very little in common. Lien et al. (2008), for instance, asked subjects to discriminate pure tones from white noise with a foot-pedal response, yet observed slow and small N400 effects for subsequent visual words requiring a manual response. In other words, meaning access seemed to be impaired after processing another stimulus that was nonsymbolic, in a different sensory modality, and required a nonoverlapping motor response. However, one can wonder if handling the first target really impairs semantic processing of T2, or instead causes the pretrial context word to become (at least temporarily) inaccessible. Under this scenario, there is no deficit in accessing the meaning of T2, only an inability to compare that meaning with the context word. One of the experiments in Lien et al. (2008) partly addressed this possibility by dropping the pretrial context word and instead examining whether the ERP elicited by T2 words varied according to their frequency of usage. The impact of word frequency[3] was substantially reduced when T2 words

occurred shortly after an initial target, suggesting that the processing deficit was localized to T2 itself, rather than the comparison between T2 and some prior context. As suggested earlier in this chapter, the origin of word frequency effects may be semantic or may include other factors. Lien et al.'s "no-context" variant of the attentional blink paradigm could be altered to more definitively isolate access to meaning. Recall that under standard conditions (slow presentation, single task), words with concrete meanings elicit larger N400s than words with abstract meanings. If processing an initial target led to a reduction in the concreteness effect for T2 words, there would be little question that the deficit arose from a failure of meaning access.

In recent studies, the exact time lags between T1 and T2 that have yielded the most severe semantic deficits do not always appear to be identical to the classic attentional blink phenomenon. The most severe reductions in the N400 context effect have often occurred with a 100 ms lag—earlier than the standard "blink" observed in behavioral data. This has led to the proposal that multiple processing bottlenecks arise at different times with more or less severe impacts on semantic processing. For instance, Vachon and Jolicoeur (2011, 2012) have argued that semantic processing cannot be initiated during time periods of task set reconfiguration when participants are preparing to switch over from the task assigned for T1 to the task assigned for T2. Such task-switching effects will be most severe when targets occur in close temporal proximity. With short lags between T1 and T2, these authors observed much smaller and later N400 context effects on T2 if subjects performed different tasks on the two targets, as compared to a condition with the same task for T1 and T2, as shown in Figure 19.6. Surprisingly, task-switching reduced the N400 context effect even when both tasks were semantic in nature—judging T1 as natural/artifact and T2 as related/unrelated to the context word presented at the beginning of the trial. Vachon and Jolicoeur's emphasis on task-set configuration appears consistent with the impact of incompatible stimulus–response mappings observed by Hohlfeld et al. (2004), given that establishing the correct relationship between a decision and a response is one aspect of a task set. Task-set reconfiguration cannot be the whole story however, as Luck et al. (1996) observed no attenuation of N400 context effects despite different tasks for T1 and T2, and Giesbrecht, Sy, and Elliot (2007) observed variable amounts of N400 suppression in conditions that always included two different tasks, with the degree of suppression dependent on the perceptual demands of the T1 task.

The experiments reviewed earlier under the section entitled Task Relevance of Semantic Information led to the conclusion that healthy literate adults access the meanings of words as a default procedure, without the explicit prodding needed for laboratory tasks that are neither as well-practiced nor as generally useful in

---

[3]These authors discussed the observed word frequency effect as a modulation of P300 amplitude. The direction of the effect—more negative ERPs for low-frequency than high-frequency words—is equally consistent with a modulation of N400 amplitude.

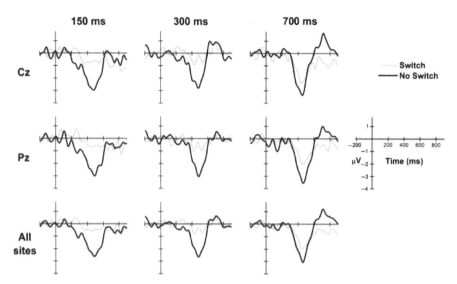

FIGURE 19.6 Grand average N400 difference waves (unrelated minus related) for second target words, depending on whether they were semantically related to a pretrial context word. On each trial, the eliciting word (T2) followed another target word (T1) in a rapid stream of items; the three columns show results from three different stimulus-onset-asynchronies between the two targets. In the No Switch condition (black line), T1 and T2 were both judged for their relationship to the context word. In the Switch condition, the T1 word was instead judged as natural or artifactual. Positive voltage is plotted in the upward direction. *Source: Reprinted from Vachon and Jolicoeur (2012).*

daily life. The more recent multitasking experiments reviewed in this section indicate that, although meaning access is a relatively quick process, semantic processing can be delayed or prevented if other demands crop up at the wrong time. The exact number and nature of the demands that interfere with meaning access are still under investigation. However, at least some of these demands must be very generic, given that interfering tasks need not share a sensory modality or a motor effector, and perhaps not even require symbolic processing. A more elaborate characterization of the relevant central bottlenecks will be very pertinent to a long-standing controversy in psycholinguistics and neurolinguistics. This controversy is whether the functional resources or brain areas critical for language are used solely for language, or instead implement domain-general functions that are necessary for language and at least some other cognitive activities (see e.g., Just & Carpenter, 1992 vs Waters & Caplan, 1996 for the psycholinguistic debate, and Fedorenko, Behr, & Kanwisher, 2011 vs Makuuchi, Bahlmann, & Friederici, 2012 for the neurolinguistic debate).

Acknowledgments

I am grateful to Barbara Luka for comments on a draft of this chapter.

References

Anllo-Vento, L., & Hillyard, S. A. (1996). Selective attention to the color and direction of moving stimuli: electrophysiological correlates of hierarchical feature selection. *Perception and Psychophysics, 58,* 191–206.

Anllo-Vento, L., Luck, S. J., & Hillyard, S. A. (1998). Spatio-temporal dynamics of attention to color: evidence from human electrophysiology. *Human Brain Mapping, 6,* 216–238.

Appelbaum, L. G., Liotti, M., Perez, R., III, Fox, S. P., & Woldorff, M. G. (2009). The temporal dynamics of implicit processing of non-letter, letter, and word-forms in the human visual cortex. *Frontiers in Human Neuroscience, 3,* 56.

Barber, H., & Kutas, M. (2007). Interplay between computational models and cognitive electrophysiology in visual word recognition. *Brain Research Reviews, 53,* 98–123.

Barrett, S. E., & Rugg, M. D. (1989). Asymmetries in event-related potentials during rhyme matching: confirmation of the null effects of handedness. *Neuropsychologia, 27,* 539–548.

Batterink, L., Karns, C., Yamada, Y., & Neville, H. (2010). The role of awareness in semantic and syntactic processing: an ERP attentional blink study. *Journal of Cognitive Neuroscience, 22,* 2514–2529.

Bengson, J. J., Lopez-Calderon, J., & Mangun, G. R. (2012). The spotlight of attention illuminates failed feature-based expectancies. *Psychophysiology, 49,* 1101–1108.

Bentin, S., Kutas, M., & Hillyard, S. A. (1995). Semantic processing and memory for attended and unattended words in dichotic listening: behavioral and electrophysiological evidence. *Journal of Experimental Psychology: Human Perception and Performance, 21,* 54–67.

Bentin, S., McCarthy, G., & Wood, C. C. (1985). Event-related potentials associated with semantic priming. *Electroencephalography and Clinical Neurophysiology, 60,* 343–355.

Bentin, S., Mouchetant-Rostaing, Y., Giard, M. H., Echallier, J. F., & Pernier, J. (1999). ERP manifestations of processing printed words at different psycholinguistic levels: time course and scalp distribution. *Journal of Cognitive Neuroscience, 11,* 235–260.

Besson, M., Fischler, I., Boaz, T., & Raney, G. (1992). Effects of automatic associative activation on explicit and implicit memory tests. *Journal of Experimental Psychology: Learning, Memory, and Cognition, 18,* 89–105.

Besson, M., Kutas, M., & Van Petten, C. (1992). An event-related potential analysis of semantic congruity and repetition effects in sentences. *Journal of Cognitive Neuroscience, 4,* 132–149.

Blackwell, A., & Bates, E. (1995). Inducing agrammatic profiles in normals: evidence for the selective vulnerability of morphology under cognitive resource limitation. *Journal of Cognitive Neuroscience, 7,* 228–257.

Christecu, T. C., & Nobre, A. C. (2008). Differential modulation of word recognition by semantic and spatial orienting of attention. *Journal of Cognitive Neuroscience, 20,* 787–801.

Chun, M. M., & Potter, M. C. (1995). A two-stage model for multiple target detection in rapid serial visual presentation. *Journal of Experimental Psychology: Human Perception and Performance, 21,* 109–127.

Chwilla, D. J., Brown, C. M., & Hagoort, P. (1995). The N400 as a function of the level of processing. *Psychophysiology, 32,* 274–285.

Cristescu, T. C., Devlin, J. T., & Nobre, A. C. (2006). Orienting attention to semantic categories. *Neuroimage, 33,* 1178–1187.

Donchin, E. (1981). Surprise!… Surprise? *Psychophysiology, 18,* 493–513.

Donchin, E., & Coles, M. G. H. (1988). Is the P300 component a manifestation of context updating? *Behavioral and Brain Sciences, 11,* 357–374.

Duncan, J. (1996). Cooperating brain systems in selective perception and action. In T. Inui & J. L. McClelland (Eds.), *Attention and performance XVI: Information integration in perception and communication* (pp. 549–578). Cambridge, MA: MIT Press.

Duncan, C. C., Barry, R. J., Connolly, J. F., Fischer, C., Michie, P. T., Näätänen, R., et al. (2009). Event-related potentials in clinical research: guidelines for eliciting, recording, and quantifying Mismatch Negativity, P300, and N400. *Clinical Neurophysiology, 120,* 1883–1908.

Federmeier, K. D., Kutas, M., & Schul, R. (2010). Age-related and individual differences in the use of prediction during language comprehension. *Brain and Language, 114,* 149–161.

Federmeier, K. D., Van Petten, C., Schwartz, T. J., & Kutas, M. (2003). Sounds, words, sentences: age-related changes across levels of language processing. *Psychology and Aging, 18,* 858–872.

Fedorenko, E., Behr, M. K., & Kanwisher, N. (2011). Functional specificity for high-level linguistic processing in the human brain. *Proceedings of the National Academy of Sciences of the United States of America, 108,* 16428–16433.

Ganis, G., Kutas, M., & Sereno, M. I. (1996). The search for common sense: an electrophysiological study of the comprehension of words and pictures in reading. *Journal of Cognitive Neuroscience, 8,* 89–106.

Giesbrecht, B., Sy, J. L., & Elliot, J. E. (2007). Electrophysiological evidence for both perceptual and post-perceptual selection during the attentional blink. *Journal of Cognitive Neuroscience, 19,* 2005–2018.

Grainger, J., & Holcomb, P. J. (2009). An ERP investigation of orthographic priming with relative-position and absolute-position primes. *Brain Research, 270,* 45–53.

Hagoort, P., Baggio, G., & Willems, R. M. (2009). Semantic unification. In M. Gazzaniga (Ed.), *The cognitive neurosciences* (4th ed., pp. 819–836). Boston: MIT Press.

Hagoort, P., Hald, L., Bastiaansen, M., & Peterson, K. M. (2004). Integration of word meaning and world knowledge in language comprehension. *Science, 304,* 438–441.

Halgren, E., Dhond, R., Christensen, N., Van Petten, C., Marinkovic, K., Lewine, J. D., et al. (2002). N400-like MEG responses modulated by semantic context, word frequency, and lexical class in sentences. *Neuroimage, 17,* 1101–1116.

Heil, M., & Rolke, B. (2004). Unattended distractor-induced priming in a visual selective attention task. *Journal of Psychophysiology, 18,* 164–169.

Heil, M., Rolke, B., & Pecchinenda, A. (2004). Automatic semantic activation is no myth: semantic context effects on the N400 in a letter-search task in the absence of response time effects. *Psychological Science, 15,* 852–857.

Heinze, H. J., Münte, T. F., & Kutas, M. (1998). Context effects in a category verification task as assessed by event-related brain potential (ERP) measures. *Biological Psychology, 47,* 121–135.

Hillyard, S. A., Hink, R. F., Schwent, V. L., & Picton, T. W. (1973). Electrical signs of selective attention in the human brain. *Science, 182,* 177–179.

Hillyard, S. A., & Münte, T. F. (1984). Selective attention to color and locational cues: an analysis with event-related brain potentials. *Perception and Psychophysics, 36,* 185–198.

Hohlfeld, A., Sangals, J., & Sommer, W. (2004). Effects of additional tasks on language perception: an event-related brain potential investigation. *Journal of Experimental Psychology: Learning, Memory, and Cognition, 30,* 1012–1025.

Hohlfeld, A., & Sommer, W. (2005). Semantic processing of unattended meaning is modulated by additional task load: evidence from electrophysiology. *Cognitive Brain Research, 24,* 500–512.

Holcomb, P. J., Grainger, J., & O'Rourke, T. (2002). An electrophysiological study of the effects of orthographic neighborhood size on printed word perception. *Journal of Cognitive Neuroscience, 14,* 938–950.

Holcomb, P. J., Kounios, J., Anderson, J. E., & West, W. C. (1999). Dual-coding, context-availability, and concreteness effects in sentence comprehension: an electrophysiological investigation. *Journal of Experimental Psychology: Learning, Memory, and Cognition, 25,* 721–742.

Holcomb, P. J., & McPherson, W. B. (1994). Event-related brain potentials reflect semantic priming in an object decision task. *Brain and Cognition, 24,* 259–276.

Hopfinger, J. B., Buonocore, M. H., & Mangun, G. R. (2000). The neural mechanisms of top-down attentional control. *Nature Neuroscience, 3,* 284–291.

Huang, H. W., Lee, C. L., & Federmeier, K. D. (2010). Imagine that! ERPs provide evidence for distinct hemispheric contributions to the processing of concrete and abstract concepts. *Neuroimage, 49,* 1116–1123.

Just, M. A., & Carpenter, P. A. (1992). A capacity theory of comprehension: individual differences in working memory. *Psychological Review, 99,* 122–149.

Kahneman, D., Treisman, A., & Gibbs, B. J. (1992). The reviewing of object files: object-specific integration of attention. *Cognitive Psychology, 24,* 175–219.

Kanske, P., Plitschka, J., & Kotz, S. A. (2011). Attentional orienting towards emotion: P2 and N400 ERP effects. *Neuropsychologia, 49,* 3121–3129.

Kellenbach, M. I., & Michie, P. T. (1996). Modulation of event-related potentials by semantic priming: effects of color-cued selective attention. *Journal of Cognitive Neuroscience, 8,* 155–173.

King, J., & Just, M. A. (1991). Individual differences in syntactic processing: the role of working memory. *Journal of Memory and Language, 30,* 580–602.

King, J. W., & Kutas, M. (1998). Neural plasticity in the dynamics of human visual word recognition. *Neuroscience Letters, 244,* 61–64.

Kramer, A. F., & Donchin, E. (1987). Brain potentials as indexes of orthographic and phonological interaction during word matching. *Journal of Experimental Psychology: Learning, Memory and Cognition, 13,* 86–86.

Küper, K., & Heil, M. (2009). Electrophysiology reveals semantic priming at a short SOA irrespective of depth of prime processing. *Neuroscience Letters, 453,* 107–111.

Kutas, M., & Federmeier, K. (2011). Thirty years and counting: finding meaning in the N400 component of the event-related potential (ERP). *Annual Review of Psychology, 62,* 621–647.

Kutas, M., & Hillyard, S. A. (1980a). Reading senseless sentences: brain potentials reflect semantic incongruity. *Science, 207,* 203–205.

Kutas, M., & Hillyard, S. A. (1980b). Reading between the lines: event-related brain potentials during natural speech processing. *Brain and Language, 11,* 354–373.

Kutas, M., & Hillyard, S. A. (1980c). Event-related brain potentials to semantically inappropriate and surprisingly large words. *Biological Psychology, 11,* 99–116.

Kutas, M., & Hillyard, S. A. (1984). Brain potentials during reading reflect word expectancy and semantic association. *Nature, 307,* 161–163.

Kutas, M., & Hillyard, S. A. (1989). An electrophysiological probe of incidental semantic association. *Journal of Cognitive Neuroscience, 1,* 38–49.

Kutas, M., & Iragui, V. (1998). The N400 in a semantic categorization task across 6 decades. *Electroencephalography and Clinical Neurophysiology: Evoked Potentials, 108,* 456–471.

Kutas, M., Neville, H. J., & Holcomb, P. J. (1987). A preliminary comparison of the N400 response to semantic anomalies during reading, listening, and signing. *Electroencephalography and Clinical Neurophysiology, Supplement, 39*, 325–330.

Kutas, M., Van Petten, C., & Besson, M. (1988). Event-related potential asymmetries during the reading of sentences. *Electroencephalography and Clinical Neurophysiology, 69*, 218–233.

Kutas, M., Van Petten, C., & Kluender, R. (2006). Psycholinguistics electrified II: 1995–2005. In M. Traxler & M. A. Gernsbacher (Eds.), *Handbook of psycholinguistics* (2nd ed., pp. 659–724). New York: Elsevier.

Langner, R., Kellermann, T., Boers, F., Sturm, W., Wilmes, K., & Eickhoff, S. B. (2011). Modality-specific perceptual expectations selectively modulate baseline activity in auditory, somatosensory, and visual cortices. *Cerebral Cortex, 21*, 2850–2862.

Laszlo, S., & Federmeier, K. D. (2009). A beautiful day in the neighborhood: an event-related potential study of lexical relationships and prediction in context. *Journal of Memory and Language, 61*, 326–338.

Laszlo, S., & Federmeier, K. D. (2011). The N400 as a snapshot of interactive processing: evidence from regression analyses of orthographic neighbor and lexical associate effects. *Psychophysiology, 48*, 176–186.

Lau, E., Phillips, C., & Poeppel, D. (2008). A cortical network for semantics: (de)constructing the N400. *Nature Reviews Neuroscience, 9*, 920–933.

Lien, M. C., Ruthruff, E., Cornett, L., Goodin, Z., & Allen, P. A. (2008). On the nonautomaticity of visual word processing: electrophysiological evidence that word processing requires central attention. *Journal of Experiment Psychology: Human Perception and Performance, 34*, 751–773.

Luck, S. J., Vogel, E. K., & Shapiro, K. L. (1996). Word meanings can be accessed but not reported during the attentional blink. *Nature, 383*, 616–618.

Macizo, P., Van Petten, C., & O'Rourke, P. L. (2012). Semantic access to embedded words? Electrophysiological and behavioral evidence from Spanish and English. *Brain and Language, 113*, 123–134.

Makuuchi, M., Bahlmann, J., & Friederici, A. D. (2012). An approach to separating the levels of hierarchical structure building in language and mathematics. *Philosophical Transactions of the Royal Society B, 367*, 2033–2045.

Martínez, A., Teder-Salejarvi, W., & Hillyard, S. A. (2007). Spatial attention facilitates selection of illusory objects: evidence from event-related brain potentials. *Brain Research, 1139*, 142–153.

Martínez, A., Teder-Salejarvi, W., Vazquez, M., Molholm, S., Foxe, J. J., Javitt, D. C., et al. (2006). Objects are highlighted by spatial attention. *Journal of Cognitive Neuroscience, 18*, 298–310.

Martin, A., Wiggs, C. L., Ungerleider, L. G., & Haxby, J. V. (1996). Neural correlates of category-specific knowledge. *Nature, 379*, 649–652.

McCarthy, G., & Nobre, A. C. (1993). Modulation of semantic processing by spatial selective attention. *Electroencephalography and Clinical Neurophysiology, 88*, 210–219.

McRae, K., de Sa, V., & Seidenberg, M. S. (1997). On the nature and scope of featural representations of word meaning. *Journal of Experimental Psychology: General, 126*, 99–130.

Miniussi, C., Marzi, C. A., & Nobre, A. C. (2005). Modulation of brain activity by selective task sets observed using event-related potentials. *Neuropsychologia, 43*, 1514–1528.

Molinaro, N., Conrad, N., Barber, H. A., & Carreiras, M. (2010). On the functional nature of the N400: contrasting effects related to visual word recognition and contextual semantic integration. *Cognitive Neuroscience, 1*, 1–7.

Müller, O., Duñabeitia, J. A., & Carreiras, M. (2010). Orthographic and associative neighborhood density effects: what is shared, what is different? *Psychophysiology, 47*, 455–466.

Nobre, A. C., Allison, T., & McCarthy, G. (1994). Word recognition in the human inferior temporal lobe. *Nature, 372*, 260–263.

Nobre, A. C., Allison, T., & McCarthy, G. (1998). Modulation of human extrastriate visual processing by selective attention to colours and words. *Brain, 121*, 1357–1368.

Okita, T., & Jibu, T. (1998). Selective attention and N400 attenuation with spoken word repetition. *Psychophysiology, 35*, 260–271.

Olichney, J., Van Petten, C., Paller, K., Salmon, D., Iragui, V., & Kutas, M. (2000). Word repetition in amnesia: electrophysiological evidence of spared and impaired memory. *Brain, 23*, 1948–1963.

Orgs, G., Lange, K., Dombrowski, J. H., & Heil, M. (2007). Is conceptual priming for environmental sounds obligatory? *International Journal of Psychophysiology, 65*, 162–166.

Orgs, G., Lange, K., Dombrowski, J. H., & Heil, M. (2008). N400-effects to task-irrelevant environmental sounds: further evidence for obligatory conceptual processing. *Neuroscience Letters, 436*, 133–137.

Osterhout, L., Bersick, M., & McKinnon, R. (1997). Brain potentials elicited by words: word length and frequency predict the latency of an early negativity. *Biological Psychology, 46*, 143–168.

Otten, L. J., Rugg, M. D., & Doyle, M. C. (1993). Modulation of event-related potentials by word repetition: the role of visual selective attention. *Psychophysiology, 30*, 559–571.

O'Craven, K. M., Downing, P. E., & Kanwisher, N. (1999). FMRI evidence for objects as the units of attentional selection. *Nature, 401*, 584–587.

Pashler, H. (1994). Dual-task interference in simple tasks: data and theory. *Psychological Bulletin, 116*, 220–244.

Perrin, F., & García-Larrea, L. (2003). Modulation of the N400 potential during auditory phonological/semantic interaction. *Cognitive Brain Research, 17*, 36–47.

Phillips, N. A., & Lesperance, D. (2003). Breaking the waves: age differences in electrical brain activity when reading text with distractors. *Psychology and Aging, 18*, 126–139.

Plante, E., Van Petten, C., & Senkfor, A. J. (2000). Electrophysiological dissociation between verbal and nonverbal processing in learning disabled adults. *Neuropsychologia, 38*, 1669–1684.

Rabovsky, M., Álvarez, C. J., Hohlfeld, A., & Sommer, W. (2008). Is lexical access autonomous? Evidence from combining overlapping tasks with recording event-related brain potentials. *Brain Research, 1222*, 156–165.

Rolke, B., Heil, M., Streb, J., & Hennighausen, E. (2001). Missed prime words within the attentional blink evoke an N400 semantic priming effect. *Psychophysiology, 38*, 165–174.

Rugg, M. D. (1984a). Event-related potentials in phonological matching tasks. *Brain and Language, 23*, 225–240.

Rugg, M. D. (1984b). Event-related potentials and the phonological processing of words and nonwords. *Neuropsychologia, 22*, 435–443.

Rugg, M. D., & Nagy, M. E. (1987). Lexical contribution to nonword-repetition effects: evidence from event-related potentials. *Memory and Cognition, 15*, 473–481.

Schendan, H., Ganis, G., & Kutas, M. (1998). Neurophysiological evidence for visual perceptual organization of words and faces within 150 ms. *Psychophysiology, 35*, 240–251.

Schoenfeld, M. A., Templemann, C., Martinez, A., Hopf, J. M., Sattler, C., Heinze, H. J., et al. (2003). Dynamics of feature binding during object-selective attention. *Proceedings of the National Academy of Sciences of the United States of America, 100*, 11806–11811.

Smith, M. C., Theodor, L., & Franklin, P. E. (1983). The relationship between contextual facilitation and depth of processing. *Journal of Experimental Psychology: Learning, Memory, and Cognition, 9*, 697–712.

Snyder, A. C., Fiebelkorni, I. C., & Foxe, J. J. (2012). Pitting binding against selection – electrophysiological measures of feature-based attention are attenuated by Gestalt object grouping. *European Journal of Neuroscience, 35*, 960–967.

Stolz, J. A., & Besner, D. (1998). Levels of representation in visual word recognition: a dissociation between morphological and semantic processing. *Journal of Experimental Psychology: Human Perception and Performance, 24*, 1642–1655.

Stolz, J. A., & Besner, D. (1999). On the myth of automatic semantic activation in reading. *Current Directions in Psychological Science, 8,* 61–65.

Thornhill, D. E., & Van Petten, C. (2012). Lexical versus conceptual anticipation during sentence processing: frontal positivity and N400 ERP components. *International Journal of Psychophysiology, 83,* 382–392.

Tyler, L. K., & Moss, H. E. (2001). Towards a distributed account of conceptual knowledge. *Trends in Cognitive Science, 5,* 244–252.

Vachon, F., & Jolicoeur, P. (2011). Impaired semantic processing during task-set switching: evidence from the N400 in rapid serial visual presentation. *Psychophysiology, 48,* 102–111.

Vachon, F., & Jolicoeur, P. (2012). On the automaticity of semantic processing during task switching. *Journal of Cognitive Neuroscience, 24,* 611–626.

van Berkum, J. J. A., Hagoort, P., & Brown, C. M. (1999). Semantic integration in sentences and discourse: evidence from the N400. *Journal of Cognitive Neuroscience, 11,* 657–671.

Van Petten, C. (1993). A comparison of lexical and sentence-level context effects and their temporal parameters. *Language and Cognitive Processes, 8,* 485–532.

Van Petten, C. (1995). Words and sentences: event-related brain potential measures. *Psychophysiology, 32,* 511–525.

Van Petten, C., & Kutas, M. (1990). Interactions between sentence context and word frequency in event-related brain potentials. *Memory and Cognition, 18,* 380–393.

Van Petten, C., Kutas, M., Kluender, R., Mitchiner, M., & McIsaac, H. (1991). Fractionating the word repetition effect with event-related potentials. *Journal of Cognitive Neuroscience, 3,* 131–150.

Van Petten, C., & Luka, B. J. (2006). Neural localization of semantic context effects in electromagnetic and hemodynamic studies. *Brain and Language, 97,* 279–293.

Van Petten, C., & Luka, B. J. (2012). Prediction during language comprehension: benefits, costs, and ERP components. *International Journal of Psychophysiology, 83,* 176–190.

Van Petten, C., & Rheinfelder, H. (1995). Conceptual relationships between spoken words and environmental sounds: event-related brain potential measures. *Neuropsychologia, 33,* 485–508.

Van Petten, C., Weckerly, J., McIsaac, H. K., & Kutas, M. (1997). Working memory capacity dissociates lexical and sentential context effects. *Psychological Science, 8,* 238–242.

Vogel, E. K., Luck, S. J., & Shapiro, K. L. (1998). Electrophysiological evidence for a postperceptual locus of suppression during the attentional blink. *Journal of Experimental Psychology: Human Perception and Performance, 24,* 1656–1674.

Vogel, E. K., Woodman, G. F., & Luck, S. J. (2005). Pushing around the locus of selection: evidence for the flexible selection hypothesis. *Journal of Cognitive Neuroscience, 17,* 1907–1922.

Waters, G. S., & Caplan, D. (1996). The capacity theory of sentence comprehension: critique of Just and Carpenter (1992). *Psychological Review, 103,* 761–772.

West, W. C., & Holcomb, P. J. (2000). Imaginal, semantic, and surface-level processing of concrete and abstract words: an electrophysiological investigation. *Journal of Cognitive Neuroscience, 12,* 1024–1037.

Zhang, W., & Luck, S. J. (2009). Feature-based attention modulates feedforward visual processing. *Nature Neuroscience, 12,* 24–25.

Altered N400 Congruity Effects in Parkinson's Disease without Dementia

Marta Kutas[1, 2], Vicente J. Iragui[1], Yu-Qiong Niu[3, 4], Tanya J. D'Avanzo[5], Jin-Chen Yang[3, 4], David P. Salmon[1], Lin Zhang[3], John M. Olichney[3, 4]

[1]Department of Neurosciences, University of California, San Diego, La Jolla, CA, USA, [2]Department of Cognitive Science, University of California, San Diego, La Jolla, CA, USA, [3]Department of Neurology, University of California, Davis, Sacramento, CA, USA, [4]Center for Mind and Brain, University of California, Davis, Davis, CA, USA, [5]Department of Psychology, Rehabilitation Hospital of the Pacific, Honolulu, HI, USA

INTRODUCTION

Cognitive impairments are common in Parkinson's disease (PD) even in the absence of the global cognitive deficits characteristic of dementia. For example, in the Sydney Multicenter Study of PD, 84% of patients exhibited some cognitive decline (Hely, Morris, Reid, & Trafficante, 2005). Other studies likewise have found that 20–50% of PD patients are present with mild cognitive impairment (PD-MCI) (Barone et al., 2011). The specific domains of cognition affected in nondemented PD patients are varied including abnormalities and/or deficits in executive functions, attention, semantic fluency and more generally semantic processing, visual-spatial processing, and memory (Kudlicka, Clare, & Hindle, 2011; Williams-Gray et al., 2009). Semantic memory deficits in nondemented individuals with PD seem to cover the entire spectrum of processes from encoding to retrieval (e.g., Mahurin, Feher, Nance, Levy, & Pirozzolo, 1993) to executive functions (Bronnick, Alves, Aarsland, Tysnes, & Larsen, 2011).

In the past two decades, a number of investigators have employed priming tasks of various sorts to examine semantic activation and semantic processing in patients with PD (with and without dementia). In a priming task, a prior experience (prime) biases subsequent performance (with respect to a target item) indicating that at least some fragment of the priming experience has been retained—though not necessarily via conscious or intentional recollection of the priming episode (encoding). PD patients (demented or not) have been found to exhibit normal lexical priming in word stem completion tasks (Bondi & Kaszniak, 1991; Heindel, Salmon, Shults, Walicke, & Butters, 1989). The results for direct and indirect semantic priming especially using lexical decision tasks (LDTs) (i.e., is the stimulus a real word or not) are mixed, likely implicating multiple contributors to the semantic priming patterns observed (e.g., Arnott, Chenery, Murdoch, & Silburn, 2001; Copland, 2003; Copland, Sefe, Ashley, Hudson, & Chenery, 2009; Heindel et al., 1989; McDonald, Brown, & Gorell, 1996). Perhaps most surprisingly, in several studies using LDTs in which the nature of the relationship between primes and targets (e.g., identity, associate, semantically related, categorical) was manipulated, individuals with PD (but without dementia) have been reported to show hyperpriming (specifically, significantly greater facilitation by related primes) compared to normal controls (e.g., Filoteo et al., 2003; Marí-Beffa, Hayes, Machado, & Hindle, 2005; Spicer, Brown, & Gorell, 1994). One hypothesis attributes the hyperpriming to insufficient inhibition of the activation of irrelevant semantic information. Another, not mutually exclusive suggestion attributes the hyperpriming to overactivation of the prime (although this is more a restatement of the result rather than an account of any specific mechanism). Yet another qualitatively different account of the hyperpriming in PD positions responsibility in some postlexical decision making stage (e.g., Brown et al., 2002; Spicer et al., 1994). As we will explain shortly, it may be possible to help adjudicate

METHODS 255

among some of these alternatives using event-related brain potentials (ERPs).

Of particular use in this context is the N400 component of the ERP (Kutas & Hillyard, 1980). The N400 refers to a relative negativity between 200 and 600 ms poststimulus onset, often peaking around 400 ms, that is present in the ERP to any potentially meaningful item (e.g., written or spoken words, pseudowords, acronyms, pictures, faces, smells, among other stimuli, see Kutas & Federmeier, 2000 for a review). The N400 has been linked to semantic access based on its functional properties and neural generators in the anterior temporal cortex (reviewed in Kutas & Federmeier, 2011). N400 amplitude is highly sensitive to a variety of semantic manipulations and insensitive to a whole host of nonsemantic (e.g., physical or syntactic) manipulations (see Kutas & Hillyard, 1980, for absence of an N400 to font size violations in semantically congruous sentences). More specifically, N400 amplitude systematically varies with semantic congruity in isolated sentences (Kutas & Hillyard, 1984) as well as in discourse (Van Berkum, Hagoort, & Brown, 1999), being significantly smaller in the ERP for congruous than incongruous words. N400 amplitude is also reliably smaller for semantic associates than nonassociates (e.g., to the target word "cat" following "dog" than "table") as for primed category exemplars relative to nonmembers (e.g., "table" following "furniture" than "fruit"). Importantly, N400 amplitude to written words is sensitive to semantic expectancy (operationalized in terms of off-line cloze probabilities, i.e., the relative probability of an individual continuing and/or completing the context with that word), even when all experimental sentences are unarguably congruent (Kutas & Hillyard, 1984). N400 amplitude is also sensitive to an item's concreteness, being smaller for abstract than concrete words (Kounios & Holcomb, 1994; West & Holcomb, 2000). Indeed, at least in the reading of isolated words, the N400 amplitude provides a viable index of the number of semantic features activated in response to a particular input (e.g., Laszlo & Federmeier, 2007, 2010). Especially strong evidence for this claim comes from the findings that the strongest predictors of the N400 amplitude to any given item is its orthographic neighborhood size (number of words that can be created by changing one letter at a time) and neighbor frequency; regression analyses of single item ERPs revealed that N400 amplitudes were greater for items with more neighbors, and increase for items with more lexical associates and with higher frequency neighbors or associates (see also Holcomb, Grainger, & O'Rourke, 2002). In short, the N400 reflects stimulus-induced semantic activity in long term memory, which is sometimes correlated, but also dissociable from reaction time measures (Kutas & Federmeier, 2011; Laszlo & Federmeier, 2010).

We thus chose to use the N400 potential as a means of investigating the effect of Parkinson's disease on semantic representations and processing. Specifically, we compared the N400s of nondemented individuals with PD and age-matched, elderly controls in a paradigm known to yield a reliable N400 effect. In this paradigm, each trial consists of a spoken context followed by a briefly flashed written word that was either congruent or incongruent with the context. We chose this particular paradigm because we know what ERP patterns to expect, how they behave with the manipulations, and have published normative data on the N400 effects (incongruous minus congruous ERPs) as a function of healthy aging in adults (Kutas & Iragui, 1998). Moreover, we have found that this task can be performed even by patients with compromised mental capabilities (e.g., Iragui, Kutas, & Salmon, 1996).

Since the N400 amplitude is reduced with increasing strength of semantic association and degree of contextual constraint, we manipulated these variables by using two different types of context—one that was highly constraining (e.g., antonyms or opposites, for which there is only one correct answer) and one that was of more moderate constraint (e.g., category membership). Antonymic and categorical relations also map onto the distinction that has been made between associative and semantic priming as well as the distinction between prediction-based vs. expectancy-based strategies for utilizing contextual information, respectively. Thus, while we expect to obtain N400 effects for both context types (although smaller than typically observed for younger adults), the proposed differences in the lexical and contextual mechanisms underlying priming with opposites and categories would predict smaller N400 effects for categories. The question at issue is whether the size (and/or perhaps the latency) of the N400 effect would be reliably different from those in the normal elderly controls. We expect different outcomes depending on what accounts for the observed hyperpriming effects. Under the assumption that the N400 reflects activation in semantic memory, if the behavioral hyperpriming reflects postlexical decision making, we would not expect to see any differences in the size of the N400 effects (incongruous minus congruous ERPs between 300 and 600 ms poststimulus onset) for PD vs. normal elderly. However, if the behavioral priming reflects greater normal activation of semantic features in semantic memory, then we would expect larger N400 congruity effects in PD (compared to elderly controls).

METHODS

Participants

Eleven individuals with PD (nine men and two women) and 11 healthy elderly controls participated in the experiment. The groups were matched on age, gender, handedness, and numbers of years of education. The mean age of the PD group was 66.4 years (range 53–80), mean education 16.6 years (range 12–20), and the mean duration of illness was 10.75 years (range 5–18 years); the mean age of the elderly control group was 65.7 years, with mean education 15.7 years. All PD patients were receiving L-dopa (mean daily dosage = 631 mg), and only one patient was also receiving anticholinergic drugs. The diagnosis of idiopathic PD was made by a senior staff neurologist prior to ERP recordings. Patients with a history of alcoholism, psychiatric illness, stroke, or other neurological illnesses were excluded from the study. The overall cognitive abilities of PD patients were assessed via the Mini-Mental State Examination (MMSE) (Folstein, Folstein, & McHugh, 1975) and the Dementia Rating Scale (DRS) (Mattis, 1988). Their average MMSE score was 29.0 (range 25–30) and their average DRS score was 141.3 (range 137–144). PD patients with evidence of global cognitive impairment (MMSE scores less than 25, or DRS scores less than 137) were excluded from the present study. None of the patients were taking psychiatric medications nor enrolled in experimental drug protocols.

Normal elderly controls were paid participants free of a history of alcoholism, drug abuse, learning disabilities, neurological, psychiatric, and significant medical diseases. The study was approved by the Human Subjects Committee of the University of California, San Diego. Monocular corrected visual acuity was better than 20/30 in all participants.

Event-Related Brain Potential Recordings

Procedure

Participants sat in a comfortable reclining chair in an electrically shielded room, facing a CRT monitor. The screen was occluded except for a rectangular slit in the center through which the words were viewed. Each word consisted of white letters against a dark background. The monitor was 100 cm from the participant. Words subtended 0.3° visual angle vertically and 0.3–2.9° visual angle horizontally.

Participants participated in four blocks of 80 context–target pairs each for a total of 320 trials. Half of the phrases defined antonymic relationships, that is, opposites (e.g., "the opposite of tall") and half indicated category membership relations (e.g., "a type of flower"). Half of the target words were semantically congruent with the sense of the preceding phrase (see Table 20.1 for sample stimuli) while the remaining half was not.

On each trial, a context phrase was read aloud by the investigator. Approximately 1 s later, the target word was flashed in the center of a CRT for a 265 ms duration. About 1.5 s after target word presentation, the

TABLE 20.1 Examples of Context–Target Pair Stimuli

Condition	Context–target pair
Congruent antonym	"The opposite of black"—"**white**"
Incongruent antonym	"The opposite of hot"—"**peach**"
Congruent category	"A member of royalty"—"**king**"
Incongruent category	"A type of animal"—"**table**"

participant was asked to indicate whether or not the target was appropriate given the sense of the preceding phrase by saying yes or no. Regardless of the correctness of their answer, the participant was then asked to report the word that she/he actually read.

Electrophysiological data collection

The electroencephalogram (EEG) was recorded using Ag/AgCl electrodes placed at 13 scalp sites and the right mastoid, each referred to an electrode over the left mastoid. Each scalp site was re-referenced off-line to an average of the left and the right mastoid recordings. Vertical eye movements were monitored via an electrode placed on the right inferior orbital ridge, referred to the left mastoid; horizontal eye movements were monitored via a right to left bipolar montage at the external canthi. Participants were asked to keep eye movements, blinks, and body movements to a minimum.

Seven of the 13 scalp electrodes were placed according to the International 10–20 system at Cz, F7, F8, T5, T6, O1 and O2 sites. In addition, symmetrical left and right anterior temporal electrodes (BL, BR) were placed halfway between F7-T3 and F8-T4, respectively (the left hemisphere site corresponded approximately to Broca's area). Symmetrical right and left posterior temporal (WL, WR) electrodes were placed laterally to the vertex by 30% of the interaural distance and posteriorly to the vertex by 12.5% of the nasion–inion distance (over the left hemisphere, this electrode sat approximately over Wernicke's area). Symmetrical left and right midtemporal electrodes were placed 33% of the interaural distance laterally to the vertex (L41, R41).

The EEG and electrooculogram (EOG) were amplified using Grass P511 amplifiers with 8 s time constant. The high frequency half amplitude cut off was 300 Hz (−6 dB). The amplified signals were digitized online at a sampling rate of 167 Hz and for subsequent averaging.

Data Analysis

Separate ERP averages were obtained for congruous and incongruous target words for the opposite and category stimuli. Each waveform consisted of a 1500 ms epoch including 100 ms prior to stimulus onset (pre-stimulus baseline). Trials contaminated by eye blinks or movements, excessive muscle activity or amplifier blocking were automatically rejected by computer algorithm prior to averaging (about 8% of trials were rejected). Peak amplitude, peak latency, and mean amplitude of N100 (70–170 ms) and P200 (120–220 ms) were measured from the ERPs to the target words (all four conditions). N400 peak latency and mean amplitude measurements were calculated from the ERPs to the congruous and incongruous words per se as well as from the difference ERPs derived from a point-by-point subtraction of the congruous from the incongruous word ERPs. Latencies were measured relative to stimulus onset, and amplitudes were measured relative to 100 ms prestimulus baseline voltage. The peak of N400 was identified as the maximum negativity between 300 and 500 ms poststimulus. Mean amplitudes were measured between 300 and 400 ms (surrounding the N400 peak).

Amplitude and latency values were subjected to repeated measures analysis of variance (ANOVA) with the two experimental groups (normal controls, PD patients) as a between subject variable and three within subject variables: target type (congruous or incongruous), stimulus type (opposite or categories), and electrode site (13 locations). Greenhouse-Geisser correction was applied whenever appropriate.

RESULTS

Grand-average ERPs ($N = 11$) elicited by congruous and incongruous words for the PD and control groups are shown in Figures 20.1 and 20.2 (for the opposite and category conditions, respectively). As is evident in these figures, ERPs to all words were characterized by early sensory components—a posterior N1 component and an anteriorly distributed P2 followed by a broad negativity between 200 and 600 ms peaking around 350–400 ms (N400) that was larger for incongruous than congruous words, in both stimulus conditions. The N400 congruity effect is best seen in the difference ERPs derived from point-by-point subtraction of congruous word ERPs from the incongruous word ERPs as shown in Figure 20.3, in which the opposite and category difference ERPs are overlapped. Visual inspection of these ERP data seems to indicate that both groups elicit similar N400 congruity effects in the category decision task. However, the PD group had larger amplitude N400 effects in the opposite condition. Indeed, as can be seen in the individual participant difference ERPs from the right Wernicke's site for the opposite condition (Figure 20.4), this group amplitude difference is not driven by only a few individuals.

N1 and P2

Analyses of N1 measures (at O1/O2) and P2 measures (at Cz and F7/8) revealed no significant group differences, but marginal trends suggested slower N1 latencies (means = 148 vs 137 ms, $F_{(1,20)} = 4.09$, $p = 0.057$), and smaller P2 peak amplitudes ($F_{(1,20)} = 4.10$, $p = 0.057$) in the PD group. The trend for reduced P2 amplitude in PD was not confirmed by the mean amplitude analysis (group effect: $F_{(1,20)} = 1.40$, $p = 0.25$), a measurement less vulnerable to noise and temporal variability (e.g., intertrial "jitter") (Luck, 2005).

N400 Latency

The peak latency of the N400 congruity effect was measured in the difference ERPs. An analysis revealed that the two groups did not reliably differ in the peak latencies of the N400 congruity effects ($p = 0.96$; PD patients = 344 ± 49 ms vs normal controls = 344 ± 54 ms, collapsed across the opposite and category conditions).

N400 Peak Amplitude

The peak amplitude of the N400 congruity effect was also measured in the difference ERPs. Across all electrode sites, there was a significant 3-way interaction of group × condition × electrode ($F_{(12, 240)} = 1.82$, Greenhouse-Geisser epsilon (ε) = 0.41, $p = 0.047$). Since the N400 is typically larger (and most sensitive to various lexical manipulations) over posterior sites, we conducted an additional analysis including only the posterior (central, temporal, and occipital) sites. As expected, this analysis reveals a significant group × condition interaction ($F_{(1, 20)} = 5.18$, $p = 0.03$). Follow-up tests support our observation based on visual inspection, namely that the PD patients have significantly larger N400 peak congruity effects than the normal control participants for both the categories ($F_{(1, 10)} = 5.47$, $p = 0.04$) and opposites ($F_{(1, 10)} = 21.84$, $p = 0.0009$). Figure 20.5 illustrates the relative enlargement of the N400 effects amplitude at the vertex for each condition.

N400 Mean Amplitude and Scalp Distribution

We also analyzed the mean amplitude of the N400 congruity effect (300–400 ms) in the difference ERPs. There was a main effect of condition ($F_{(1, 20)} = 18.44$, $p = 0.0004$), with the opposite N400 congruity effect being significantly larger than that for categories. There was also a significant stimulus condition × electrode interaction: ($F_{(12, 240)} = 5.87$, $\varepsilon = 0.32$, $p = 0.0004$),

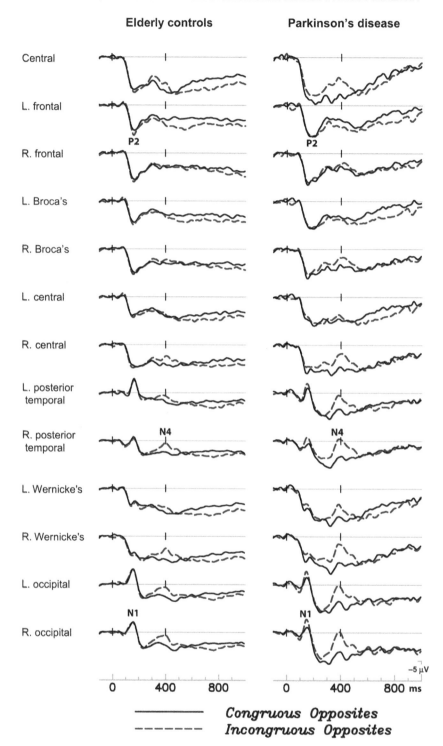

FIGURE 20.1   Grand-average ($N = 11$) ERP waveforms elicited by congruous and incongruous antonyms. Negative is plotted up in this and all subsequent figures.

reflecting that the posterior N400 congruity effect is bilaterally symmetric for the opposites and has a slight right hemisphere bias for categories ($F_{(1,\ 65)} = 24.49$, $p < 0.0001$). Neither of these effects interacted with group.

Consistent with the peak amplitude analyses, there was a nonsignificant trend of group × electrode interaction with all sites included ($F_{(12,\ 240)} = 2.65$, $\varepsilon = 0.25$, $p = 0.057$). Follow-up tests including only measures taken at posterior electrode sites demonstrated a

ELDERLY CONTROLS   **PARKINSON'S DISEASE**

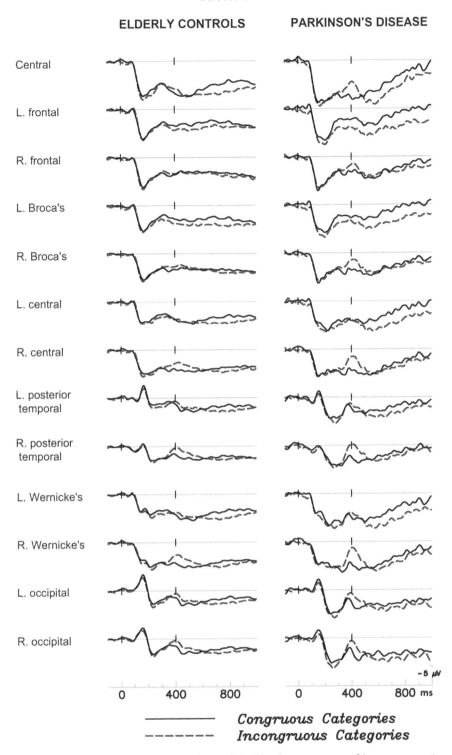

Central

L. frontal

R. frontal

L. Broca's

R. Broca's

L. central

R. central

L. posterior temporal

R. posterior temporal

L. Wernicke's

R. Wernicke's

L. occipital

R. occipital

0   400   800   0   400   800 ms

−5 μV

———— *Congruous Categories*
- - - - - *Incongruous Categories*

FIGURE 20.2   Grand-average ($N=11$) ERP waveforms elicited by the congruous and incongruous category stimuli.

significant group × condition interaction ($F_{(12, 20)}=7.80$, $p=0.01$). Post-hoc analyses revealed that the Parkinson's patients demonstrate greater N400 mean amplitude than controls for the opposite condition ($F_{(1, 20)}=9.31$, $p=0.01$), but not for the category condition ($F_{(1, 20)}=0.32$, $p=0.58$).

DISCUSSION

Previously we have reported that, on average, adults of all ages show a larger N400 to written words that do not fit with the meaning of the immediately preceding spoken phrase than to those that do. More precisely, we

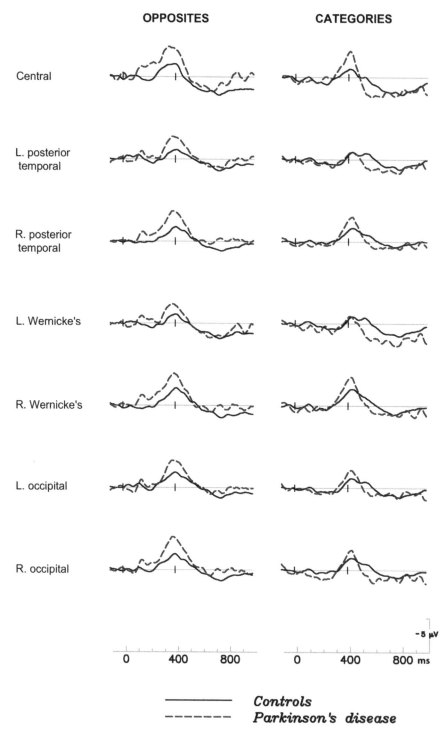

FIGURE 20.3   Difference ERPs (point-by-point subtraction of incongruous ERPs minus congruous ERPs) of seven channels.

have found that the N400 congruity effect (difference between ERPs in N400 time window to contextually incongruent minus congruent words) shows a reliable linear decrease in amplitude between 0.05 and 0.09 μV per year with advancing age (Kutas & Iragui, 1998). In short, the N400 semantic congruity effect at the scalp gets smaller with normal aging. Moreover, we also found that N400 amplitudes take an especially large hit when the aging is accompanied by Alzheimer's disease (AD), as we had previously discussed (Iragui et al., 1996). In the current study we find that, at least when it comes to the N400 congruity effect, elderly individuals with Parkinson's disease (and without dementia), resemble younger adults more than their age-matched

ELDERLY CONTROLS   PARKINSON'S DISEASE

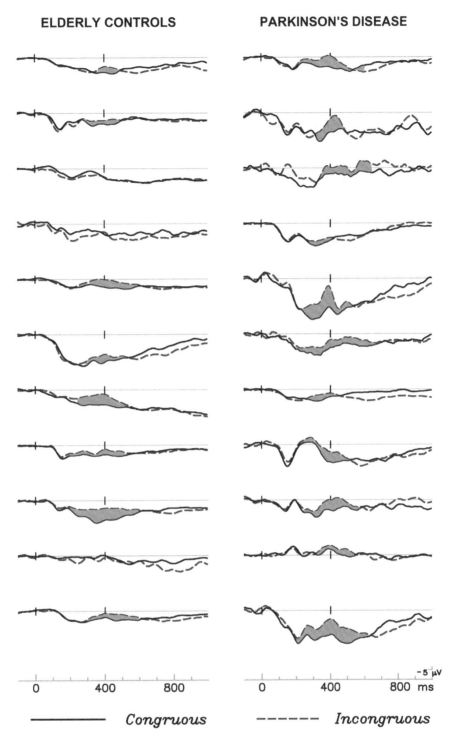

——————— *Congruous*   – – – – – *Incongruous*

FIGURE 20.4   ERP waveforms from the right Wernicke's channel for each individual participant in the two subject groups elicited by congruous and incongruous antonyms.

controls. That is, the size of the N400 congruity effect is about 2 μV larger in the Parkinson patient group than in the normal elderly (age-matched) control group. This is a remarkable finding, and although we do not (yet) have a ready explanation we will explore some of our thoughts and points worthy of further consideration. As

Hillyard, Iragui, and Kutas learned early on in their clinical collaborations, working with brain-compromised patients is more eye opening and exhilarating than clean and easy!

The larger N400 congruity effect in individuals with PD is a novel finding. To the minimal extent that others

ELDERLY CONTROLS   PARKINSON'S DISEASE

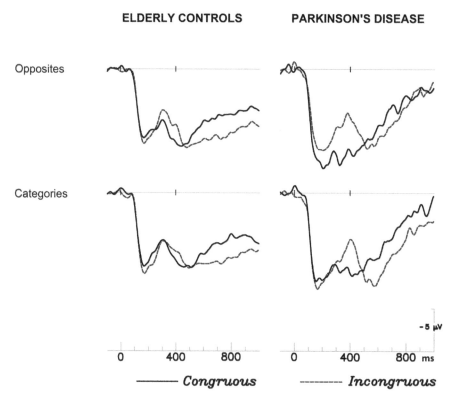

FIGURE 20.5   Grand-average (*N* = 11) ERP waveforms at the central site.

have studied PD with N400-eliciting phrase/sentence-context priming paradigms, they have reported no reliable N400 amplitudes differences between individuals with PD and age-matched elderly controls. Friederici, Kotz, Werheid, Hein, and von Cramon (2003), for example, investigated the lexico-semantic and syntactic processing in PD patients using ERP measures. Their participants listened to sentences that were both syntactically correct and semantically congruent or either semantically anomalous or syntactically incorrect. Friederici's focus was on whether the degeneration of the dopaminergic neurons in the basal ganglia (BG; characteristic of PD) and its impact on the frontal cortex would influence early automatic and later integrative syntactic processes similarly, their theory predicting a difference. To that end, Friederici and her colleagues elicited and then measured three specific ERP components: the early left-anterior negativity (Neville et al., 1991) hypothetically linked to automatic first-pass parsing processes (e.g., Friederici, Pfeifer, & Hahne, 1993), the P600 elicited by syntactic violations and/or difficult syntactic operations (Hagoort et al., 1993; Kaan, Harris, Gibson, & Holcomb, 2000; Osterhout & Holcomb, 1992), and the N400 primarily as a lexico-semantic control (e.g., Kutas & Hillyard, 1980, 1984). Their results were clear: PD patients exhibited N400 semantic congruity effects (as well as early LANs) that were statistically indistinguishable from those of the elderly controls, but did show

reliably smaller than normal P600s. These results were taken to mean that semantic processing (and for that matter automatic syntactic processes), at least as tested with passive sentences, were intact in PD whereas late integrative syntactic processes were somehow compromised. Experimental differences between that study and ours might account for the fact that they observed comparable N400s in their PD and age-matched controls whereas we observed a group difference: they could include, but are not limited to, the nature of the stimuli (passive sentences vs category verification), the different modalities (auditory), and/or the different medication protocols. Still, even in Friederici et al., unlike the auditory P6, the auditory N400 though not enhanced, was not diminished.

The larger than normal visual N400 semantic congruity effect in individuals with PD in our study is consistent with the observations of behavioral hyperpriming described in the introduction. Because interpreting direct raw ERP comparisons across subject groups can be problematic, we restricted our analyses to effects (i.e., to ERP congruity difference ERPs). Taken at face value, however, it may be noteworthy that the PD and control ERPs do differ for both the congruent and the incongruent conditions—e.g., as evident in the potentials at the vertex recording site (Figure 20.5) which are more positive in the N400 region of the congruent ERPs and more negative in the N400 region of the incongruent ERPs in the PD group relative to their counterparts in the elderly controls. On the view that N400 amplitude reflects overall amount of semantic activation (Kutas & Federmeier, 2011), our results do not provide support for an account of hyperpriming in PD due to a postlexical decision making stage, which would have modulated potentials post N400. Instead, our N400 patterns are more in line with the suggestion that hyperpriming arises from insufficient inhibition of irrelevant semantic information and perhaps greater activation of the target. Both the greater positivity to congruent responses and greater negativity to incongruent ones in principle could be explained in terms of insufficient inhibition in the computational model of the N400 built by Laszlo and Plaut (2012). This model is in a development phase, but already nicely accounts for neighborhood effects on N400 amplitude, and importantly for present purposes has been found to reproduce the key dynamics of the N400 in visual word recognition only when it includes neurally plausible excitatory and inhibitory connections (i.e., separate excitatory and inhibitory connections with any given unit having one or the other and only excitatory connections going across levels and inhibitory connections remaining within level).

N400 amplitudes to words in a sentence are correlated with the word's cloze probability; the higher a word's cloze probability, the smaller the N400 it elicits (Kutas & Hillyard, 1984). In fact, very high cloze items in the context of highly constraining contexts where only one response is expected (e.g., facts) show no N400 activity, being instead quite positive in the N400 region. The opposites in the present study behave much the same way; they are highly predictable and elicit positivities in the N400 time window.

The sensitivity of the N400 to semantic/associative relationships in the context of prime-target word pairs was first demonstrated using lexical decision tasks (Bentin, McCarthy, & Wood, 1985; Holcomb, 1988) and category membership verification tasks (Boddy, 1981; Neville, Kutas, Chesney, & Schmidt, 1986). When directly compared, the N400 effect appears larger for (incongruent vs. congruent) words in sentences than unassociated vs. associated words in lists or word pairs (Kutas & Van Petten, 1988), presumably because sentences provide more contextual constraint. In addition, although the relationship between the N400 and attention has proven to be quite nuanced (Kutas & Federmeier, 2011), in word pair tasks, as more attention is deliberately paid to semantic relationships, the larger the associated N400 relatedness effect (Deacon & Shelley-Tremblay, 2000; Holcomb, 1988). Our finding of larger N400 congruity effects in the PD group than in the control group then could conceivably reflect abnormally heavy reliance upon external cues and/or attention to integrate words into context. On the clinical level, patients with PD may

appear to be "stimulus bound", and deficits in forward planning and attentional set-shifting have been well described (Kehagia, Barker, & Robbins, 2010).

Larger than normal anomalous word N400s and/or N400 congruity effects also have been reported for groups who find language processing difficult. Neville et al. (1993), for example, investigated sentence processing in language impaired (LI) and reading-disabled (RD) children. Their participants were asked to read a series of sentences ending with either an appropriate (congruent) or a semantically anomalous (incongruent) word. All of the LI and RD children demonstrated unusually large N400s to sentence-final words that were semantically anomalous. These increased N400 amplitudes were hypothesized to reflect children's greater reliance on context for word recognition, presumably compensating for sensory and/or syntactic processing deficits. More generally, Holcomb et al. (1992) found a marked decline in N400 amplitude across normal childhood and into adulthood; they also interpreted this as evidence for decreasing reliance on context for word recognition with age and experience. If this interpretation is correct, then the increased N400s (and N400 effect) in PD patients likewise may be due to difficulties they encounter integrating words with a mental representation of the preceding context.

What could be the pathophysiological basis of this finding? Evidence supports a multifactorial origin of the cognitive deficits in PD that implicate dysfunctional subcortical neurochemical systems in addition to dysfunctions in regions of the cerebral cortex (Cooper et al., 1992; Picconi, Piccoli, & Calabresi, 2012). The major neurochemical abnormality in PD, namely, dopamine deficiency, may be responsible for some of these cognitive impairments (Lange, Paul, Naumann, & Gsell, 1995; Picconi et al., 2012; Williams-Gray et al., 2009). Since PD is characterized by major loss of nigro-striatal dopamine on the one hand, and deficits in executive functioning on the other, it has been proposed that the disturbance in executive functioning results from disruption due to striatal damage of the reciprocal connections between the striatum and frontal cortex, known essential for proper executive functioning (Alexander, DeLong, & Strick, 1986; Kudlicka et al., 2011; Taylor, Saint-Cyr, & Lang, 1990; Zgaljardic, Borod, Foldi, & Mattis, 2003). In a lexical decision study on 18 PD patients undergoing surgery for deep brain stimulation, Castner et al. (2007) demonstrated that stimulation of the subthalamic nucleus restored the otherwise compromised controlled semantic priming at long stimulus onset asynchrony (SOA). These results suggest that the basal ganglia-thalamocortical circuit is involved in at least some aspects of semantic processing. In patients with unilateral basal ganglia (BG) lesions, Kotz, Frisch, Von Cramon, and Friederici (2003) observed an extended duration (up to 700 ms) N400-like negativity in response to grammatical violations (with absent P600s). The results were interpreted as showing a role of the basal ganglia in supporting controlled semantic processes, supplementing their critical role in syntactic processes.

One of the major functions of prefrontal cortex is considered to be coordinating higher-level processes to execute the appropriate behavior given task demands and/or goals (Banich, 2009; Gilbert & Burgess, 2008; Miyake et al., 2000). Indeed, PD patients do seem to make less use of spontaneous organizational strategies than their age-matched peers (e.g., Bondi, Kaszniak, Bayles, & Vance, 1993; Brown & Marsden, 1988; Taylor et al., 1990); this executive dysfunction is commonly recognized as the most pronounced cognitive impairment in PD (Kudlicka et al., 2011). Both clinical and experimental data suggest that PD patients, by contrast, place a heavier reliance upon external guidelines to circumvent the cognitive difficulties they experience, presumably as the result of their neuropathology. In his book *Awakenings*, Oliver Sacks (1990) describes the Parkinson patient as suffering "abulia", or the absence of will: "Parkinsonian patients….would sit for hours not only motionless, but apparently without any impulse to move: they were, seemingly, content to do nothing, and they lacked the 'will' to enter upon or continue any course of activity, although they might move quite well if the stimulus or command or request to move came from another person-from the outside (p. 11)" (also see Ingvar, 1994). Sack's narrative of his Parkinsonian patients is striking: "Thus one may see such patients, rigid, motionless, seemingly lifeless, as statues, abruptly called into normal life and action by some sudden exigency which catches their attention (p. 12)". As mentioned above, the larger N400 in PD observed in the present study may conceivably reflect compensatory activation of external cue information, (and if so) likely modulated by prefrontal cortex, in which stronger activation was associated with a larger N4-like component in an integrated ERP-fMRI study of healthy adults (Opitz, Mecklinger, Friederici, & von Cramon, 1999).

It has been proposed that the localization of dopamine D1 receptors in cerebral cortex on dendritic spines and distal dendrites rather than at proximal synapses implicates them in the modulation of excitatory (glutaminergic) input to cortical pyramidal cells (Smiley, Williams, Szigeti, & Goldman-Rakic, 1992; Smiley, Levey, Ciliax, & Goldman-Rakic, 1994). Individuals with PD, by virtue of their dopamine depletion, may be faced with lower "signal-to-noise ratios" as information within their frontostriatal circuits is being processed (Cools, Stefanova, Barker, Robbins, & Owen, 2002; Rolls, Thorpe, Boytim, Szabo, & Perrett, 1984). In a lexical decision task with masked prime, in healthy volunteers, the semantic priming effect at 500 ms SOA of the levodopa group

was significantly reduced by L-DOPA compared to the placebo control group, suggesting a mediating role for dopamine in lexico-semantic priming (Angwin et al., 2004). Kischka et al. (1996) examined the mediating role of dopamine in healthy adults using LDT and found only marginal effects of L-DOPA ingestion (vs. placebo) on direct semantic priming, but a significantly reduced indirect priming effect. They concluded that their results support the hypothesis that dopamine increases the signal-to-noise ratio in semantic networks by reducing the spread of semantic processing, thereby leading to a focusing of activation and reduced indirect priming. Others also have found evidence for dopamine mediation of semantic priming (Angwin et al., 2004; Pederzolli et al., 2008).

Another factor which may prove crucial for the understanding of the cognitive profile of our PD group is their medication status. All of the PD participants were on L-DOPA medication. It has been hypothesized that dopamine replacement therapy in individuals with PD may counteract the increased noise in their cortical networks (Cools et al., 2002; Kischka et al., 1996). In nonhuman primates, for example, dopamine depletion in the frontal lobes leads to deficits in delayed alternation tasks, which are reversed with L-DOPA treatment (Brozoski, Brown, Rosvold, & Goldman, 1979). Moreover, individuals with PD on L-DOPA have been reported to not only make fewer errors (Cooper et al., 1992), but also to exhibit an increase in the number of categories achieved in the Wisconsin Card Sorting Test (Bowen et al., 1975). These findings are consistent with the possibility that L-DOPA promotes effective attentional shifting (Lange et al., 1995). On this account, the robust and peaked N400 congruity effects we observed could be related to L-DOPA's effect on attention to incoming stimuli.

Perhaps L-DOPA not only counteracts some of the deleterious effects of Parkinson's disease on the availability of dopamine, but also some of the known loss of dopamine as a consequence of normal aging, as well. There is evidence for the degeneration of the dopamine system in aged monkeys (Arnsten, Cai, Murphy, & Goldman-Rakic, 1994), and in normally aging humans, as well (De Keyser, Ebinger, & Vauquelin, 1990). Moreover, treatment with D1 dopamine agonist has been found to improve working memory performance in aged, but not in young monkeys (Castner & Goldman-Rakic, 2004). In humans, dopaminergic neurotransmission is impaired with age due to degeneration of the substantia nigra pars compacta neurons, as well as decreases in the density of postsynaptic D1 and D2 dopamine receptors in the striatum (Levey et al., 1993).

While we cannot be certain that the L-DOPA medication of the participants in our PD group was sufficient to wholly counteract their dopamine deficiency, there are some indications that dopamine circuits may be involved in N400 generation. Studies of individuals with schizophrenia—characterized by hyperactive dopaminergic transmission—have reported abnormal N400 activity, with increased amplitudes in some cases (e.g., Nestor et al., 1997; Salisbury, Shenton, Nestor, & McCarley, 2002) and decreased in others (Grillon, Ameli, & Glazer, 1991; Hokama, Hiramatsu, Wang, O'Donnell, & Ogura, 2003; Olichney, Iragui, Kutas, Nowacki, & Jeste, 1997). Most of these studies, however, are confounded as these patients were on various antipsychotic medications which block dopamine receptors. The scalp-recorded N400 potential is assumed to represent overlapping activity from multiple neural generators (Van Petten & Luka, 2006). Intracranial recordings have implicated the neocortex of the anterior medial temporal lobe in the region of the anterior fusiform gyri (McCarthy, Nobre, Bentin, & Spencer, 1995; Smith, Stapleton, & Halgren, 1986). These areas are known to have a high density of dopaminergic receptors (Smiley et al., 1992) and are targets of mesolimbic and mesocortical pathways, both of which are routinely affected in PD.

Not all of the cognitive changes in PD are due to a loss of central dopaminergic function. Cholinergic deficits, for instance, also seem to play a role (Perry et al., 1985). Reductions in cortical choline acetyl-transferase correlate with the degree of neuronal loss in the nucleus basalis, the main source of widespread cholinergic innervation of the neocortex and hippocampus (Jellinger, 1991). The severity of this neuronal loss, however, is much greater in demented than in nondemented Parkinsonian patients. It is relatively unlikely that the cholinergic deficit plays a role in the enhanced N400 effect amplitudes observed in our nondemented Parkinsonian patients, since individuals with AD, who also have severe cholinergic deficits, have markedly reduced or absent N400 in this same paradigm (Iragui et al., 1996). Preliminary unpublished observations in our laboratory indicate that demented PD patients, where the severity of neuronal loss in the nucleus basalis is similar to that of AD, do not exhibit these larger than normal N400 congruity effects, showing instead reduced N400 amplitudes similar to those observed in AD.

Overall, the results of this study are intriguing, though at present without a fully satisfactory explanation. If dopamine—crucial for optimizing the signal-to-noise ratio of local cortical circuits via the D1- and D2-receptors on pyramidal neurons—is somehow involved, then it is important to know whether it is dopamine deficiency or the dopamine replacement (L-DOPA) that is key. If practical, this could be tested by examining elderly Parkinson patients prior to (and then after) L-DOPA treatment, and/or examining healthy young and elderly adults who have ingested L-DOPA or a placebo. Even if dopamine is a major contributor to the enhanced congruity effect, additional research is needed to determine whether the responsible mechanisms indeed have their impact

through the mediation of neuronal excitability and/or recurrent inhibition that contributes to the stability of cortical representations of stimuli (in cortical microcircuits). Whatever the pathophysiological changes in the brain, we need to consider the possibility that these may result not only in dysfunction, but in adaptation as well. In the case of PD, one adaptive response to the changes that take place in cognitive functioning may be an undue reliance upon external command to help guide information processing. Disruption of normal frontal functioning may make internal control of semantic integration difficult, even for nondemented patients—and this difficulty may be what we see in the enhancement of the N400 congruity effect. There are too many unknowns to fully understand the nature of the increased N400 effects observed herein, but these results offer a reliable effect that any viable model of Parkinson's disease will need to accommodate, just as PD patients learn to accommodate to the internal and external environment they face with less endogenous dopamine and/or its pharmacological replacement.

References

Alexander, G. E., DeLong, M. R., & Strick, P. L. (1986). Parallel organization of functionally segregated circuits linking basal ganglia and cortex. *Annual Review Neuroscience*, 9, 357–381.

Angwin, A. J., Chenery, H. J., Copland, D. A., Arnott, W. L., Murdoch, B. E., & Silburn, P. A. (2004). Dopamine and semantic activation: an investigation of masked direct and indirect priming. *Journal of the International Neuropsychological Society*, 10, 15–25.

Arnott, W. L., Chenery, H. J., Murdoch, B. E., & Silburn, P. A. (2001). Semantic priming in Parkinson's disease: evidence for delayed spreading activation. *Journal of Clinical and Experimental Neuropsychology*, 23, 502–519.

Arnsten, A. F. T., Cai, J. X., Murphy, B. L., & Goldman-Rakic, P. S. (1994). Dopamine D1 receptor mechanisms in the cognitive performance of young adult and aged monkeys. *Psychopharmacology (Berlin)*, 116, 143–151.

Banich, M. T. (2009). Executive function: the search for an integrated account. *Current Directions in Psychological Science*, 18, 89–94.

Barone, P., Aarsland, D., Burn, D., Emre, M., Kulisevsky, J., & Weintraub, D. (2011). Cognitive impairment in nondemented Parkinson's disease. *Movement Disorders*, 26, 2483–2495.

Bentin, S., McCarthy, G., & Wood, C. C. (1985). Event-related potentials, lexical decision and semantic priming. *Electroencephalography and Clinical Neurophysiology*, 60, 343–355.

Boddy, J. (1981). Evoked potentials and the dynamics of language processing. *Biological Psychology*, 13, 125–140.

Bondi, M. W., & Kaszniak, A. W. (1991). Implicit and explicit memory in Alzheimer's disease and Parkinson's disease. *Journal of Clinical and Experimental Neuropsychology*, 13, 339–358.

Bondi, M. W., Kaszniak, A. W., Bayles, K. A., & Vance, K. T. (1993). Contribution of frontal system dysfunction to memory and perceptual abilities in Parkinson's disease. *Neuropsychology*, 7, 89–102.

Bowen, F. P., Kamienny, R. S., Burns, M. M., & Yahr, M. D. (1975). Parkinsonism: effects of levodopa treatment on concept formation. *Neurology*, 25, 701–704.

Bronnick, K., Alves, G., Aarsland, D., Tysnes, O. B., & Larsen, J. P. (2011). Verbal memory in drug-naive, newly diagnosed Parkinson's disease. The retrieval deficit hypothesis revisited. *Neuropsychology*, 25, 114–124.

Brown, G. G., Brown, S. J., Christenson, G., Williams, R. E., Kindermann, S. S., Loftis, C., et al. (2002). Effects of task structure on category priming in patients with Parkinson's disease and in healthy individuals. *Journal of Clinical and Experimental Neuropsychology*, 24, 356–369.

Brown, R. G., & Marsden, C. D. (1988). Internal versus external cues and the control of attention in Parkinson's disease. *Brain*, 111, 323–345.

Brozoski, T. J., Brown, R. M., Rosvold, H. E., & Goldman, P. S. (1979). Cognitive deficit caused by regional depletion of dopamine in prefrontal cortex of rhesus monkey. *Science*, 205, 929–932.

Castner, J. E., Chenery, H. J., Copland, D. A., Coyne, T. J., Sinclair, F., & Silburn, P. A. (2007). Semantic and affective priming as a function of stimulation of the subthalamic nucleus in Parkinson's disease. *Brain*, 130, 1395–1407.

Castner, S. A., & Goldman-Rakic, P. S. (2004). Enhancement of working memory in aged monkeys by a sensitizing regimen of dopamine D1 receptor stimulation. *Journal of Neuroscience*, 24, 1446–1450.

Cools, R., Stefanova, E., Barker, R. A., Robbins, T. W., & Owen, A. M. (2002). Dopaminergic modulation of high-level cognition in Parkinson's disease: the role of the prefrontal cortex revealed by PET. *Brain*, 125, 584–594.

Cooper, J. A., Sagar, H. J., Doherty, S. M., Jordan, N., Tidswell, P., & Sullivan, E. V. (1992). Different effects of dopaminergic and anticholinergic therapies on cognitive and motor function in Parkinson's disease. A follow-up study of untreated patients. *Brain*, 115, 1701–1725.

Copland, D. A. (2003). The basal ganglia and semantic engagement: potential insights from semantic priming in individuals with subcortical vascular lesions, Parkinson's disease, and cortical lesions. *Journal of the International Neuropsychological Society*, 9, 1041–1052.

Copland, D. A., Sefe, G., Ashley, J., Hudson, C., & Chenery, H. J. (2009). Impaired semantic inhibition during lexical ambiguity repetition in Parkinson's disease. *Cortex*, 45, 943–949.

De Keyser, J., Ebinger, G., & Vauquelin, G. (1990). Age-related changes in the human nigrostriatal dopaminergic system. *Annals of Neurology*, 27, 157–161.

Deacon, D., & Shelley-Tremblay, J. (2000). How automatically is meaning accessed: a review of the effects of attention on semantic processing. *Frontiers in Bioscience*, 5, E82–E94.

Filoteo, J. V., Friedrich, F. J., Rilling, L. M., Davis, J. D., Stricker, J. L., & Prenovitz, M. (2003). Semantic and cross-case identity priming in patients with Parkinson's disease. *Journal of Clinical and Experimental Neuropsychology*, 25, 441–456.

Folstein, M. F., Folstein, S. E., & McHugh, P. R. (1975). "Mini-mental state". A practical method for grading the cognitive state of patients for the clinician. *Journal of Psychiatric Research*, 12, 189–198.

Friederici, A. D., Kotz, S. A., Werheid, K., Hein, G., & von Cramon, D. Y. (2003). Syntactic comprehension in Parkinson's disease: investigating early automatic and late integrational processes using event-related brain potentials. *Neuropsychology*, 17, 133–142.

Friederici, A. D., Pfeifer, E., & Hahne, A. (1993). Event-related brain potentials during natural speech processing: effects of semantic, morphological and syntactic violations. *Brain Research. Cognitive Brain Research*, 1, 183–192.

Gilbert, S. J., & Burgess, P. W. (2008). Executive function. *Current Biology*, 18, R110–R114.

Grillon, C., Ameli, R., & Glazer, W. M. (1991). N400 and semantic categorization in schizophrenia. *Biological Psychiatry*, 29, 467–480.

Hagoort, P., Colin., B., & Groothusen, J. (1993). The syntactic positive shift (SPS) as an ERP measure of syntactic processing. *Language and Cognitive Processes*, 8, 439–483.

Heindel, W. C., Salmon, D. P., Shults, C. W., Walicke, P. A., & Butters, N. (1989). Neuropsychological evidence for multiple implicit memory systems: a comparison of Alzheimer's, Huntington's, and Parkinson's disease patients. *Journal of Neuroscience*, 9, 582–587.

Hely, M. A., Morris, J. G. L., Reid, W. G. J., & Trafficante, R. (2005). Sydney Multicenter Study of Parkinson's disease: non-L-dopa-responsive problems dominate at 15 years. *Movement Disorders*, 20, 190–199.

Hokama, H., Hiramatsu, K. I., Wang, J., O'Donnell, B. F., & Ogura, C. (2003). N400 abnormalities in unmedicated patients with schizophrenia during a lexical decision task. *International Journal of Psychophysiology*, 48, 1–10.

Holcomb, P. J. (1988). Automatic and attentional processing: an event-related brain potential analysis of semantic priming. *Brain and Language*, 35, 66–85.

Holcomb, P. J., Coffey, S. A., & Neville, H. J. (1992). Visual and auditory sentence processing: a developmental analysis using event-related potentials. *Developmental Neuropsychology*, 8, 203–241.

Holcomb, P. J., Grainger, J., & O'Rourke, T. (2002). An electrophysiological study of the effects of orthographic neighborhood size on printed word perception. *Journal of Cognitive Neuroscience*, 14, 938–950.

Ingvar, D. H. (1994). The will of the brain: cerebral correlates of willful acts. *Journal of Theoretical Biology*, 171, 7–12.

Iragui, V., Kutas, M., & Salmon, D. P. (1996). Event-related brain potentials during semantic categorization in normal aging and senile dementia of the Alzheimer's type. *Electroencephalography and Clinical Neurophysiology/Evoked Potentials Section*, 100, 392–406.

Jellinger, K. A. (1991). Pathology of Parkinson's disease. Changes other than the nigrostriatal pathway. *Molecular and Chemical Neuropathology*, 14, 153–197.

Kaan, E., Harris, A., Gibson, E., & Holcomb, P. (2000). The P600 as an index of syntactic integration difficulty. *Language and Cognitive Processes*, 15, 159–201.

Kehagia, A. A., Barker, R. A., & Robbins, T. W. (2010). Neuropsychological and clinical heterogeneity of cognitive impairment and dementia in patients with Parkinson's disease. *The Lancet Neurology*, 9, 1200–1213.

Kischka, U., Kammer, T. H., Maier, S., Weisbrod, M., Thimm, M., & Spitzer, M. (1996). Dopaminergic modulation of semantic network activation. *Neuropsychologia*, 34, 1107–1113.

Kotz, S. A., Frisch, S., Von Cramon, D. Y., & Friederici, A. D. (2003). Syntactic language processing: ERP lesion data on the role of the basal ganglia. *Journal of the International Neuropsychological Society*, 9, 1053–1060.

Kounios, J., & Holcomb, P. J. (1994). Concreteness effects in semantic processing: ERP evidence supporting dual-coding theory. *Journal of Experimental Psychology. Learning, Memory, and Cognition*, 20, 804–823.

Kudlicka, A., Clare, L., & Hindle, J. V. (2011). Executive functions in Parkinson's disease: systematic review and meta-analysis. *Movement Disorders*, 26, 2305–2315.

Kutas, M., & Federmeier, K. D. (2000). Electrophysiology reveals semantic memory use in language comprehension. *Trends in Cognitive Sciences*, 4, 463–470.

Kutas, M., & Federmeier, K. D. (2011). Thirty years and counting: finding meaning in the N400 component of the event-related brain potential (ERP). *Annual Review of Psychology*, 62, 621–647.

Kutas, M., & Hillyard, S. A. (1980). Reading senseless sentences: brain potentials reflect semantic incongruity. *Science*, 207, 203–205.

Kutas, M., & Hillyard, S. A. (1984). Brain potentials during reading reflect word expectancy and semantic association. *Nature*, 307, 161–163.

Kutas, M., & Iragui, V. (1998). The N400 in a semantic categorization task across 6 decades. *Electroencephalography and Clinical Neurophysiology/Evoked Potentials Section*, 108, 456–471.

Kutas, M., & Van Petten, C. (1988). Event-related brain potential studies of language. In P. K. Ackles, J. R. Jennings & M. G. H. Coles (Eds.), *Advances in psychophysiology* (Vol. 3, pp. 139–187). Greenwich, Connecticut: JAI Press Inc.

Lange, K. W., Paul, G. M., Naumann, M., & Gsell, W. (1995). Dopaminergic effects on cognitive performance in patients with Parkinson's disease. *Journal of Neural Transmission [Supplementum]*, 46, 423–432.

Laszlo, S., & Federmeier, K. D. (2007). Better the DVL you know: acronyms reveal the contribution of familiarity to single-word reading. *Psychological Science, 18*, 122–126.

Laszlo, S., & Federmeier, K. D. (2010). The N400 as a snapshot of interactive processing: evidence from regression analyses of orthographic neighbor and lexical associate effects. *Psychophysiology, 48*, 176–186.

Laszlo, S., & Plaut, D. C. (2012). A neurally plausible parallel distributed processing model of event-related potential word reading data. *Brain and Language, 120*, 271–281.

Levey, A. I., Hersch, S. M., Rye, D. B., Sunahara, R. K., Niznik, H. B., Kitt, C. A., et al. (1993). Localization of D1 and D2 dopamine receptors in brain with subtype-specific antibodies. *Proceedings of the National Academy of Sciences of the United States of America, 90*, 8861–8865.

Luck, S. J. (2005). *An Introduction to the Event-Related Potential Technique.* Cambridge (MA): MIT Press.

Mahurin, R. K., Feher, E. P., Nance, M. L., Levy, J. K., & Pirozzolo, F. J. (1993). Cognition in Parkinson's disease and related disorders. In R. W. Parkes, R. F. Zec & R. S. Wilson (Eds.), *Neuropsychology of Alzheimer's disease and related disorders* (pp. 308–349). New York: Oxford University Press.

Marí-Beffa, P., Hayes, A. E., Machado, L., & Hindle, J. V. (2005). Lack of inhibition in Parkinson's disease: evidence from a lexical decision task. *Neuropsychologia, 43*, 638–646.

Mattis, S. (1988). *Dementia Rating Scale professional manual.* Odessa (FL): Psychological Assessment Resources.

McCarthy, G., Nobre, A. C., Bentin, S., & Spencer, D. D. (1995). Language-related field potentials in the anterior-medial temporal lobe: I. Intracranial distribution and neural generators. *Journal of Neuroscience, 15*, 1080–1089.

McDonald, C., Brown, G. G., & Gorell, J. M. (1996). Impaired setshifting in Parkinson's disease: new evidence from a lexical decision task. *Journal of Clinical and Experimental Neuropsychology, 18*, 793–809.

Miyake, A., Friedman, N. P., Emerson, M. J., Witzki, A. H., Howerter, A., & Wager, T. D. (2000). The unity and diversity of executive functions and their contributions to complex "frontal lobe" tasks: a latent variable analysis. *Cognitive Psychology, 41*, 49–100.

Nestor, P. G., Kimble, M. O., O'Donnell, B. F., Smith, L., Niznikiewicz, M., Shenton, M. E., et al. (1997). Aberrant semantic activation in schizophrenia: a neurophysiological study. *The American Journal of Psychiatry, 154*, 640–646.

Neville, H. J., Coffey, S. A., Holcomb, P. J., & Tallal, P. (1993). The neurobiology of sensory and language processing in language-impaired children. *Journal of Cognitive Neuroscience, 5*, 235–253.

Neville, H. J., Kutas, M., Chesney, G., & Schmidt, A. L. (1986). Event-related brain potentials during initial encoding and recognition memory of congruous and incongruous words. *Journal of Memory and Language, 25*, 75–92.

Neville, H. J., Nicol, J. L., Barss, A., Forster, K. I., & Garrett, M. F. (1991). Syntactically based sentence processing classes: evidence from event-related brain potentials. *Journal of Cognitive Neuroscience, 3*, 151–165.

Olichney, J. M., Iragui, V. J., Kutas, M., Nowacki, R., & Jeste, D. V. (1997). N400 abnormalities in late life schizophrenia and related psychoses. *Biological Psychiatry, 42*, 13–23.

Opitz, B., Mecklinger, A., Friederici, A. D., & von Cramon, D. Y. (1999). The functional neuroanatomy of novelty processing: integrating ERP and fMRI results. *Cerebral Cortex, 9*, 379–391.

Osterhout, L., & Holcomb, P. J. (1992). Event-related brain potentials elicited by syntactic anomaly. *Journal of memory and language, 31*, 785–806.

Pederzolli, A. S., Tivarus, M. E., Agrawal, P., Kostyk, S. K., Thomas, K. M., & Beversdorf, D. Q. (2008). Dopaminergic modulation of semantic priming in Parkinson disease. *Cognitive and Behavioral Neurology, 21*, 134–137.

Perry, E. K., Curtis, M., Dick, D. J., Candy, J. M., Atack, J. R., Bloxham, C. A., et al. (1985). Cholinergic correlates of cognitive impairment in Parkinson's disease: comparisons with Alzheimer's disease. *Journal of Neurology, Neurosurgery and Psychiatry, 48*, 413–421.

Picconi, B., Piccoli, G., & Calabresi, P. (2012). Synaptic dysfunction in Parkinson's disease. *Advances in Experimental Medicine and Biology, 970*, 553–572.

Rolls, E. T., Thorpe, S. J., Boytim, M., Szabo, I., & Perrett, D. I. (1984). Responses of striatal neurons in the behaving monkey. 3. Effects of iontophoretically applied dopamine on normal responsiveness. *Neuroscience, 12*, 1201–1212.

Sacks, O. (1990). *Awakenings.* New York: HarperPerennial.

Salisbury, D. F., Shenton, M. E., Nestor, P. G., & McCarley, R. W. (2002). Semantic bias, homograph comprehension, and event-related potentials in schizophrenia. *Clinical Neurophysiology, 113*, 383–395.

Smiley, J. F., Levey, A. I., Ciliax, B. J., & Goldman-Rakic, P. S. (1994). D1 dopamine receptor immunoreactivity in human and monkey cerebral cortex: predominant and extrasynaptic localization in dendritic spines. *Proceedings of the National Academy of Sciences of the United States of America, 91*, 5720–5724.

Smiley, J. F., Williams, S. M., Szigeti, K., & Goldman-Rakic, P. S. (1992). Light and electron microscopic characterization of dopamine-immunoreactive axons in human cerebral cortex. *The Journal of Comparative Neurology, 321*, 325–335.

Smith, M. E., Stapleton, J. M., & Halgren, E. (1986). Human medial temporal lobe potentials evoked in memory and language tasks. *Electroencephalography and Clinical Neurophysiology, 63*, 145–159.

Spicer, K. B., Brown, G. G., & Gorell, J. M. (1994). Lexical decision in Parkinson disease: lack of evidence of generalized bradyphrenia. *Journal of Clinical and Experimental Neuropsychology, 16*, 457–471.

Taylor, A. E., Saint-Cyr, J. A., & Lang, A. E. (1990). Memory and learning in early Parkinson's disease: evidence for a "frontal lobe syndrome". *Brain and Cognition, 13*, 211–232.

Van Berkum, J. J., Hagoort, P., & Brown, C. M. (1999). Semantic integration in sentences and discourse: evidence from the N400. *Journal of Cognitive Neuroscience, 11*, 657–671.

Van Petten, C., & Luka, B. J. (2006). Neural localization of semantic context effects in electromagnetic and hemodynamic studies. *Brain and Language, 97*, 279–293.

West, W. C., & Holcomb, P. J. (2000). Imaginal, semantic, and surface-level processing of concrete and abstract words: an electrophysiological investigation. *Journal of Cognitive Neuroscience, 12*, 1024–1037.

Williams-Gray, C. H., Evans, J. R., Goris, A., Foltynie, T., Ban, M., Robbins, T. W., et al. (2009). The distinct cognitive syndromes of Parkinson's disease: 5 year follow-up of the CamPaIGN cohort. *Brain, 132*, 2958–2969.

Zgaljardic, D. J., Borod, J. C., Foldi, N. S., & Mattis, P. (2003). A review of the cognitive and behavioral sequelae of Parkinson's disease: relationship to frontostriatal circuitry. *Cognitive and Behavioral Neurology, 16*, 193–210.

Oscillations and Behavior: The Role of Phase–Amplitude Coupling in Cognition

Boaz Sadeh[1, 2, *], Sara M. Szczepanski[1, 2, *], Robert T. Knight[1, 2]

[1]Helen Wills Neuroscience Institute, University of California, Berkeley, Berkeley, CA, USA, [2]Department of
Psychology, University of California, Berkeley, Berkeley, CA, USA

*These two authors contributed equally to this work.

INTRODUCTION

Phase–amplitude cross-frequency coupling (PAC) refers to a neural mechanism in which the phase of an oscillation at a lower frequency modulates the occurrence of activity at a higher frequency. For example, spiking activity or broadband high-gamma (HG; 80–200 Hz) power can be periodically enhanced during certain phases of an underlying local field potential (LFP) oscillation and reduced during the remainder of the oscillation cycle (Figure 21.1(A) and (B)). In other words, the higher-frequency component activity is nested within the cyclic changes of the lower-frequency rhythm. Such dynamics of neural activity has been observed in the hippocampus, basal ganglia, and neocortex of the mammalian brain (e.g., Bragin et al., 1995; Buzsaki et al., 2003; Canolty et al., 2006; Lakatos et al., 2005; Tort, Komorowski, Manns, Kopell, & Eichenbaum, 2009; Tort et al., 2008), and has been proposed to constitute a mechanism of neuronal integration, computation, and communication (Canolty & Knight, 2010). In this chapter, we attempt to shed light on the neural mechanisms underlying PAC. We review evidence for the participation of PAC in different cognitive functions as well as how PAC may serve as a marker for certain neurological disorders.

Mechanisms Underlying Cortical Communication through Oscillations and PAC

Electrical or magnetic stimulation applied to neurons does not result in identical single-unit responses across all repetitions (Arieli, Sterkin, Grinvald, & Aertsen, 1996; Bishop, 1933; Romei et al., 2008). This single-unit response variability was long suggested to reflect a mechanism for controlling neural excitability rather than a random noise process. Bishop (1933) first reported that the excitability of the optic pathway of a rabbit follows rhythmic changes between depolarizing and hyperpolarizing states, at the speed of the theta frequency (~4–8 Hz). Cyclical transitions between up and down states of the membrane resting potential were also found during slow-wave sleep (Sanchez-Vives & McCormick, 2000). It is increasingly accepted that intrinsic cortical oscillations, which are a property of neural networks, reflect these cyclic changes in synaptic excitability (Burchell, Faulkner, & Whittington, 1998; Buzsaki & Draguhn, 2004; Fries, 2005; Gregoriou, Gotts, Zhou, & Desimone, 2009; Holcman & Tsodyks, 2006; Schroeder & Lakatos, 2009; Siegel, Donner, & Engel, 2012; Volgushev, Chistiakova, & Singer, 1998). The cyclic changes create time windows during which synaptic input is favored, since spiking activity sent from one neuron to another will have a higher likelihood of eliciting a synaptic response if the membrane of the receiving neuron is in an excitable state. In this way, neural activity can be chunked or parsed into discrete units according to time windows of favored synaptic processing. The activity units have a temporal frequency dictated by the oscillation that creates them, and this frequency can differ across cortical areas and cognitive tasks.

One possible use of this mechanism is for scaling the oscillation and aligning it with the temporal modulations of the incoming information, so that the information is tracked and encoded properly across time

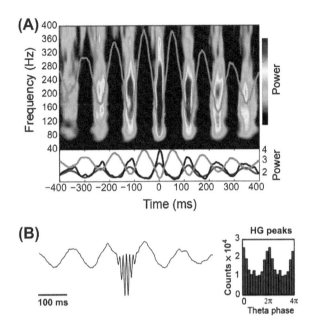

FIGURE 21.1 **Phase–amplitude cross-frequency coupling (PAC).** (A) PAC in the deep layers of the rat's hippocampus (CA1). The spectrogram shows mean normalized power of the local field potential (LFP; color coded) time-locked to the trough of a 7–12 Hz theta oscillation (gray trace; note that 7–12 Hz includes theta and alpha). The amplitude of the LFP oscillations in the high gamma (HG) range is maximal around the troughs of the theta rhythm. Lower panel: mean normalized power at 80 Hz (red) and 160 Hz (blue). (B) Left: averaged LFP trace from the rat's CA1, time-locked to the HG peaks, centered around 80 Hz. Right: histogram of theta phases during which these peaks occurred. *Source: Adapted with permission from Tort et al. (2008).*

(Ahissar & Arieli, 2001; Giraud & Poeppel, 2012). For instance, it has been proposed that in the auditory cortex, theta and low gamma (30–50 Hz) rhythms are predominant in speech processing, since they match the temporal characteristics of human vocalization (Giraud & Poeppel, 2012; Lehongre, Ramus, Villiermet, Schwartz, & Giraud, 2011; for more details, see the section below on entrainment of neuronal oscillations and PAC). Neuronal oscillations in sensory cortices can thus be entrained by sensory input, so that the stimulus structure and time of arrival reset the occurrence of these rhythmic processing time windows (Giraud & Poeppel, 2012; Lakatos, Karmos, Mehta, Ulbert, & Schroeder, 2008; Schroeder & Lakatos, 2009).

Neuronal groups oscillating in synchrony (the difference in their phases is constant across time) are able to send and receive information more effectively than neuronal groups whose membrane oscillatory activities are not coordinated (Fries, 2005; Miltner, Braun, Arnold, Witte, & Taub, 1999; Siegel et al., 2012). This enables areas to effectively transfer action potentials by coordinating oscillatory changes in membrane potential across a network. Although each neuron has multiple anatomical connections with other neurons, instantaneous modulations of oscillatory synchronization can be used to achieve a finer, more flexible, control on the effective

functional connectivity, based upon attention, volition, memory, or psychological state (Buzsaki & Draguhn, 2004; Fries, 2005; Fries, Reynolds, Rorie, & Desimone, 2001; Gregoriou et al., 2009). Phase synchronization is a plausible mechanism for enhancing network communication since neural responses are facilitated or inhibited as a function of cycle phase. The phase can thus be employed as a coordination system for activity pairing across two or more distant neuronal ensembles that process the same information.

Brain rhythms are not only temporally scaled, but also spatially scaled. Neuronal oscillations vary from slow oscillations created by distributed neuronal groups to faster oscillations confined to a more local region, up to the resonance and oscillations of single neurons. In general, low-frequency rhythms are created by large neuronal populations and serve to coordinate activity across distant brain regions, whereas higher frequencies, such as gamma-band oscillations, reflect information integration in a more localized area (Buzsaki & Draguhn, 2004; Canolty et al., 2007; Llinas, 1988; von Stein & Sarnthein, 2000). Slower oscillations, which can shift and reset their phase according to external or internal events, organize faster local computational processes and coordinate communication and integration across cortical locations (Canolty & Knight, 2010).

PAC as a Possible Mechanism for Information Coding and Integration

Coupling between high-frequency power and the phase of lower-frequency rhythms can serve as an information integration mechanism across the temporal and spatial scales discussed above. HG power has been proposed to represent local cortical activation. Evidence supporting this link is provided by optogenetic studies, which demonstrate that broadband HG is generated by recurrent inhibitory neural activity that is linked to increased single-unit spiking activity (Cardin et al., 2009; Yizhar, Fenno, Davidson, Mogri, & Deisseroth, 2011). Further, Ray and Maunsell (Ray & Maunsell, 2011) nicely showed that unlike sustained oscillations in the lower gamma range, HG activity in the monkey brain has a transient character and is related to local spiking activity. An interdependence between such local activity (spike probability or HG power) and the phase of LFP oscillations has been established in several animal studies (e.g., Bragin et al., 1995; Tort et al., 2008; Volgushev et al., 1998). For example, Volgushev et al. (1998) showed that synaptically evoked spiking activity is precisely locked to the phase of injected sinusoidal currents. Further, the probability of spike generation following subthreshold synaptic activation changes as a function of the phase of the induced oscillations. In the rat hippocampus, gamma power was found to increase close to the positive phase of local theta rhythms, and the spiking activity of inter-neurons was found to be greater on the ascending phase of local gamma oscillations (Bragin et al., 1995). More-over, these changes in PAC strength are tied to behavior. Tort et al. (2008) demonstrated that PAC strength could quickly change from no coupling to strong coupling in a matter of milliseconds. The increase in PAC occurred at different timing intervals, depending on the brain region, as rodents navigated through a T-maze. These data indicate that the coupling between the phase of slow oscillations and the power of higher oscillations or spiking activity is behaviorally relevant, rather than just epiphenomenal.

It was recently suggested that cortical rhythms are nested in a hierarchical manner across pairs of increas-ingly high-frequency bands, e.g., gamma power nests within alpha or theta phase and theta power nests within delta phase (Lakatos et al., 2005). Oscillations can thus facilitate information integration over multiple temporal and spatial scales in order to coordinate network interac-tions. Additionally, as mentioned previously, the instan-taneous phase of an oscillation can be modulated by the input characteristics. PAC can thus reflect a supplemen-tary level of coupling, in which the output function of neuronal assemblies is systematically chunked accord-ing to the temporal frame that is dictated by the oscilla-tory phase of the input function. This may be used as a method for PAC to reorganize high frequency or spiking activity according to the characteristics of the informa-tion that needs to be processed (for example, see the sec-tion below about entrainment of oscillations).

Taken together, interactions between neuronal oscil-lations in different frequency bands are increasingly viewed as an essential characteristic of neural process-ing, playing fundamental roles in information integra-tion, computation, and communication across short and long distances (Buzsaki & Draguhn, 2004; Canolty & Knight, 2010; Engel, Fries, & Singer, 2001; Fries, 2005; Gray & Singer, 1989; Jensen, Kaiser, & Lachaux, 2007; Klimesch, 1996; Miltner et al., 1999; Siegel et al., 2012; Ward, 2003). In the current chapter, we focus on the role of PAC in cognition, discussing evidence for PAC in both the human and the animal brain.

PAC AND VISUAL PERCEPTION

Low-frequency neuronal oscillations at the alpha and theta range are ubiquitous in human scalp and intracra-nial recordings and are generated in numerous cognitive tasks. These two rhythms are characterized by the distinct distributions and tasks that elicit them, suggesting a func-tional dissociation between their roles in neural process-ing (Klimesch, 1999; Voytek et al., 2010). Although widely distributed over cortical regions, the theta rhythm is often

reported at frontal recording sites and in the hippocam-pus, and it has been related to attention, cognitive control, and memory (Gevins, Smith, McEvoy, & Yu, 1997; Kahana, Seelig, & Madsen, 2001; Onton, Delorme, & Makeig, 2005). The alpha rhythm has a more posterior distribu-tion and is observed extensively in visual perception and visual attention tasks (Hari, Salmelin, Makela, Salenius, & Helle, 1997; Palva & Palva, 2007; Romei, Gross, & Thut, 2010; Sauseng et al., 2005). Given the predominance of the alpha rhythm over the visual cortex and the role of oscillations in modulating membrane excitability, we can hypothesize that the phase of the alpha rhythm may play an important role in the visual modality for modu-lating higher frequencies in PAC measures. Indeed, new evidence from human intracranial recordings and mag-netoencephalography (Osipova, Hermes, & Jensen, 2008; Voytek et al., 2010) show coupling between alpha phase and gamma amplitude during visual tasks. Voytek et al. (2010) demonstrated that the preferred coupling phase shifts to alpha in posterior electrode sites as the task changes from nonvisual to visual, independently of alpha power changes. This strengthens the idea that synchro-nous rhythms change according to the type of cognitive task being executed (Ward, 2003).

Neuronal oscillations occurring at the time of sensory input arrival can modulate the cortical response to that input, and, as a consequence, affect our perception. It has been suggested that the overall recorded cortical evoked response is an interaction between the stimulus-driven potential and the changing dynamics of cortical excit-ability reflected in background oscillations (Arieli et al., 1996; Lakatos et al., 2005). In line with this idea, numerous studies have shown that the power of the alpha rhythm measured over a short period of time just before stimulus presentation can predict the probability of visual detec-tion, with reduced power favoring enhanced perception (Ergenoglu et al., 2004; Hanslmayr et al., 2007; Romei et al., 2008; van Dijk, Schoffelen, Oostenveld, & Jensen, 2008). This is in agreement with the notion that posterior alpha power suppression reflects an increase in attention and alertness (e.g., Pfurtscheller, 2001; Sauseng et al., 2005; Worden, Foxe, Wang, & Simpson, 2000; see also the section below about PAC and attention). The power of the oscillation, however, is not the only parameter found to modulate visual perception. In fact, the instantaneous phase of the alpha fluctuation at the time when visual input arrives has a critical influence on the brain's evoked response and on the formation of a conscious percept. Studies report that the probability of perceiving a near-threshold stimulus (Busch, Dubois, & VanRullen, 2009) or a masked image (Mathewson, Gratton, Fabiani, Beck, & Ro, 2009) changes as a function of the alpha phase at stimulus onset (see Lakatos et al., 2005 for similar find-ings in audition). In other words, if we compare trials in which a low intensity visual stimulus is detected with trials in which such a stimulus is not detected, we will find that one major difference between the two is the phase of background occipital alpha that coincides with stimulus appearance. One step toward demonstrating a causal relationship between the phase of occipital alpha and conscious perception was made using transcranial magnetic stimulation (TMS). Dugue and colleagues showed that the probability of phosphene perception in near-threshold TMS to the occipital cortex depends on the phase of the alpha rhythm at the time when stimulation is applied (Dugue, Marque, & VanRullen, 2011). The alpha rhythm therefore modulates visual awareness on different time scales: changes in power can control visual awareness fluctuations on the level of seconds and distinguish between more vigilant and less vigilant observers, whereas phase changes underlie more rapid and rhythmic fluctuations in visual perception threshold (Hanslmayr et al., 2007; Mathewson et al., 2009).

This relationship between the phase of a background oscillation and local neural processing is reflected in PAC. In a scalp electroencephalography (EEG) study by Demiralp and colleagues (Demiralp et al., 2007), gamma power was modulated by a slow oscillation (although by theta, not alpha, phase) over occipital electrodes in a visual decision task. This correlation was found only during the first 300 ms following stimulus onset, and it was absent at later latencies, although the stimulus was presented for a second. It may be argued that this transient PAC, reflecting the co-occurrence of an evoked potential and a transient induced gamma-band response, does not have a function beyond reflecting time-locking of both activity components to the stimulus appearance. The induced gamma response has, in addition to the transient burst, a sustained rhythmic component. One possible way to demonstrate a functional relationship between the phase of a background oscillation and gamma power modulations would be by detecting PAC over longer periods of information processing, reflecting a recurrence of the higher-frequency activity at successive cycles of the lower-frequency activity. Preliminary data from our laboratory show this type of sustained PAC over occipital scalp electrodes, between the phase of the visual alpha rhythm and gamma oscillations (40–70 Hz) throughout prolonged visual input. During a 4 s visual stimulus presentation, PAC was sustained, reappearing at the same phase across oscillation cycles throughout the entire stimulus presentation time (Figure 21.2(A) and (B)). This coupling was restricted to occipital electrode sites and to the alpha oscillation, as predicted for visual information processing. Correspondingly, Osipova and colleagues found gamma power modulation by alpha phase while subjects were at rest (Osipova et al., 2008). Although no task was performed, alpha–gamma PAC showed a posterior distribution similar to the visual alpha. The authors proposed that occipital alpha, which mediates the functional

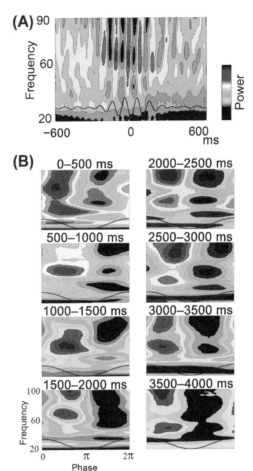

FIGURE 21.2 **Alpha (8–12 Hz) modulation of gamma power during visual perception**. PAC at occipital scalp electrode Oz of a representative subject, during prolonged presentation (4 s) of faces. Gamma power is higher around the descending, relative to the ascending, phase of the alpha cycle. (A) Spectrogram representing power modulation time-locked to the trough of the alpha oscillation. The trough-locked average of the alpha trace is superposed on the spectrogram (black trace). The first 500 ms after stimulus onset was rejected to avoid transients, leaving only sustained gamma and alpha comodulation. (B) The 4 s stimulus presentation divided into eight windows of 500 ms each. Presented are spectrograms of the averaged alpha cycle for each time-window. It can be seen that PAC is refreshed across alpha cycles throughout the entire stimulus presentation period.

excitation-inhibition balance of the visual cortex and favors conscious visual perception at lower power time windows (see above), allows sustained gamma rhythms to occur during the alpha resting state only at particular values of its phase (such as the troughs), thus leading to functional alpha–gamma PAC during rest.

PAC AND ATTENTION

Attention is a critical component of perception and goal-directed behavior that allows the brain to allocate its limited resources depending on current task demands.

Attention can operate on any modality, with attentional enhancement effects observed in sensory areas throughout the brain. Evidence from functional neuroimaging and lesion studies in humans and physiology studies in monkeys suggests that these attention-related modulatory signals are derived from higher-order areas in the frontal cortex and the posterior parietal cortex (PPC) and are transmitted via feedback projections to the sensory cortex (Barcelo, Suwazono, & Knight, 2000; Corbetta & Shulman, 2002; Kastner & Ungerleider, 2000; Mesulam, 1981; Moore & Armstrong, 2003; Saalmann, Pigarev, & Vidyasagar, 2007). Thus, attentional enhancement is also observed in the lateral prefrontal cortex, the frontal eye field, and the supplementary eye field in the frontal cortex, and the superior parietal lobule and portions of the intraparietal sulcus in the PPC. In the current chapter, we chose to focus on visual experiments that provide evidence for the use of PAC as a means of communication during attentional allocation, since vision is the most extensively studied sensory modality.

Two frequency bands in particular, gamma and alpha, have been linked to visuospatial attention processing in humans based upon the human EEG literature (see Jensen et al., 2007; Palva & Palva, 2007 for reviews). Increases in broadband gamma power and coherence over sensory, parietal, and prefrontal cortex (PFC) regions are associated with active, attentive aspects of visual processing (Bauer, Oostenveld, Peeters, & Fries, 2006; Doesburg, Roggeveen, Kitajo, & Ward, 2008; Gruber, Muller, Keil, & Elbert, 1999; Landau, Esterman, Robertson, Bentin, & Prinzmetal, 2007; Ray, Niebur, Hsiao, Sinai, & Crone, 2008). Changes in alpha power and coherence are thought to reflect an active attentional suppression mechanism over the parietal–occipital cortex, with increases and synchronization contralateral to distracting, ignored stimuli, and decreases and desynchronization with anticipation of contralateral visual targets (Capotosto, Babiloni, Romani, & Corbetta, 2009; Kelly, Lalor, Reilly, & Foxe, 2006; Worden et al., 2000).

Although some oscillatory dynamics, such as power and coherence changes, have been examined with attentional paradigms, considerably less is known about how attentional networks may utilize PAC as a means of communication. Lakatos et al. (2008) investigated PAC in the primary visual cortex while monkeys were trained to attend to either visual or auditory stimuli that were presented in a rhythmic stream in an intermixed fashion. They found that the neural activity entrained to the stimulus rhythm (in this case, a frequency in the delta band) and that the delta oscillatory synchrony was enhanced by attention. In addition, the amplitude of the multiunit responses and LFPs was systemically related to the phase of the delta oscillation during attention to both modalities. This result suggests coupling between the delta phase and a high-frequency amplitude in the

visual cortex during attention, although multiple cycles of the coupling were not demonstrated.

Evidence for PAC within two other visual areas, V4 and TEO, was also demonstrated by Saalmann, Pinsk, Wang, Li, and Kastner (2012). They trained monkeys to perform a modified version of a flanker task, which required attention to a cued target that was surrounded by an array of distracting stimuli. Attention to a stimulus enhanced alpha synchronization as well as coupling between the phase of the alpha oscillation and gamma power, compared to when attention was directed away from a stimulus. This increase in alpha synchronization during attentional allocation is in contrast to reports from the human EEG literature, which find alpha synchronization and power increases contralateral to distracting, unattended stimuli (Kelly et al., 2006; Worden et al., 2000).

Recently, we examined the temporal dynamics and interactions within and between regions of the human fronto-parietal attention network and the visual cortex using electrocorticography (ECoG; Szczepanski, Parvizi, Auguste, Kuperman, & Knight, 2012). ECoG signals were measured directly from subdural electrode arrays that were implanted in patients undergoing intracranial monitoring for localization of epileptic foci. Subjects performed a dynamic reaction time task, in which they allocated visuospatial attention to either the right or left visual field and responded when a target eventually appeared somewhere in the visual field. In each individual subject, we found increases in PAC between HG power (70–180 Hz) and the delta/theta phase (2–5 Hz) within electrodes over the lateral frontal, posterior parietal, and occipital cortex during allocation of spatial attention, which was attenuated in the unattended condition (Figure 21.3). The increases in coupling across frontal–parietal areas tracked attentional behavioral performance (reaction time) on a trial-by-trial basis. These results are compatible with those reported by Lakatos et al. (2008, 2005) in the nonhuman primate.

These results highlight the potential role for PAC as a selective mechanism for communication within and between fronto-parietal and visual areas, which adjusts parameters on a subsecond basis depending on momentary attentional demands. However, based upon the reviewed studies, it is evident that no single frequency band is solely related to attentional processes, perhaps because attention is not a unitary function (Fan et al., 2007).

PAC AND MEMORY

Oscillatory activity in the theta and gamma bands has been proposed to mediate the processing of newly acquired memories (Axmacher et al., 2010, 2007;

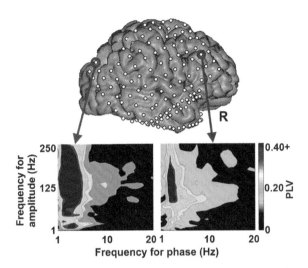

FIGURE 21.3 **Phase–amplitude coupling in the human frontal and posterior parietal cortex (PPC) during allocation of visuospatial attention.** An example is given from one subject who had an implanted subdural grid for the localization of epileptic foci, which covered portions of the frontal and PPC in the right hemisphere. Subjects performed a spatial attention task in which they were cued to attend to either the right or left visual field and to respond when a target appeared in the periphery. Allocation of attention to the contralateral visual field produced significant coupling between the phase of the delta/theta (~2–5 Hz) oscillation and broadband high gamma amplitude (~70–180 Hz). Examples of significant coupling are shown for two electrodes, one near the intraparietal sulcus in PPC (left) and one in the dorsolateral prefrontal cortex (right). Each comodulogram plots the phase locking value (PLV) across a wide range of frequencies (x axis = frequency for phase signal, y axis = frequency for amplitude signal). Contour lines represent p-values (outer to inner: p = 0.50, 0.10, 0.05, 0.01, 0.001).

Axmacher, Mormann, Fernandez, Elger, & Fell, 2006; Fell & Axmacher, 2011; Kahana et al., 2001). Animal studies report prominent theta and gamma activity in the hippocampus of rodents, a structure implicated in memory and learning (Bragin et al., 1995; Csicsvari, Jamieson, Wise, & Buzsaki, 2003), and human scalp EEG studies established a correlation between memory and activity in the theta band (Klimesch, 1999; Klimesch, Doppelmayr, Russegger, & Pachinger, 1996). Researchers have proposed that the phase synchrony and PAC of two frequency ranges, namely gamma and theta, are important for information encoding in memory. Evidence for such theta gamma PAC during learning was recently provided by human (Rutishauser, Ross, Mamelak, & Schuman, 2010; Sauseng et al., 2009) and animal (Tort et al., 2009) studies. Tort et al. (2009) further demonstrated that the strength of the theta–gamma PAC in the rat hippocampus positively correlated with successful learning. The modulation of spike timing by the gamma cycle may be particularly well suited for long-term potentiation (LTP). Given that an action potential will occur when the cycle of the membrane oscillation becomes excitable enough, phase synchronization will ensure that both synchronized cells fire in temporal proximity. Memory models suggest that synchronization in a high rhythm (e.g., gamma) between pre- and postsynaptic activity increases spike-time precision, allowing for a Hebbian learning process (Axmacher et al., 2006; Fell & Axmacher, 2011; Miltner et al., 1999). Hebbian learning results from the pairing of pre- and postsynaptic cellular activity, which leads to synaptic enhancement. The theta phase and its modulation of synaptic activity also play a role in LTP. It was shown that the synchronization of high-frequency gamma activity with the phase of theta oscillations in the hippocampus promotes LTP (Pavlides, Greenstein, Grudman, & Winson, 1988). This idea was directly tested through electrical stimulation studies, which successfully induced LTP and LTD (long-term depression) through stimulation at distinct phases of a hippocampal theta oscillation. Trains of high-frequency pulses applied during theta peaks induced synaptic potentiation, while stimulation trains given during theta troughs reversed this potentiation or had no effect (Holscher, Anwyl, & Rowan, 1997; Pavlides et al., 1988).

How do high-frequency oscillations nested in the phase of the theta frequency oscillations underlie short-term memory (STM)? In an attempt to explain the neural mechanism behind multiple item maintenance in STM, Lisman and Idirat proposed an influential model that incorporates theta–gamma nested oscillations (Lisman & Buzsaki, 2008; Lisman & Idiart, 1995). In their model, each unique item held in STM is represented by neurons firing at different subcycles of an ongoing background theta oscillation (5–10 Hz) in the hippocampus and possibly in the prefrontal cortex. Multiple memories can be serially represented if gamma bursts, coding for the items to memorize, appear at successive phases (subcycles) of the theta oscillation. This precise subcycle representation could renew itself from cycle to cycle throughout a prolonged retention period (Lisman & Idiart, 1995). The temporal order of represented objects can thus be encoded by distinct subgroups of neurons, each responding to a different object identity, which lock to a particular phase of an ongoing oscillation (Figure 21.4(A)). The theta cycle serially chunks gamma-represented items. This phase-dependent coding of information goes beyond spiking rate information alone, since both the identity and the temporal order of mnemonic items can be coded efficiently (Kahana et al., 2001).

Compelling evidence for this type of serial encoding of items in different subcycles was found in the monkey prefrontal cortex (Siegel, Warden, & Miller, 2009). Siegel and colleagues trained monkeys to hold two visual objects presented one after the other in memory while performing a delayed match-to-sample task. Siegel found that nested oscillations carry precise information about the items that were being held in STM and their presentation order, although the most informative

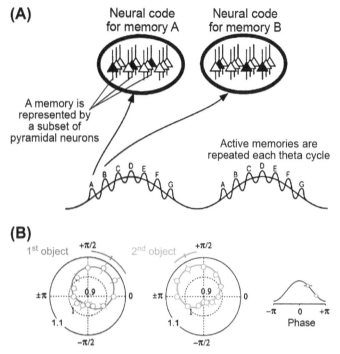

FIGURE 21.4 **Coupling between gamma activity and the phase of a lower-frequency oscillation may index item order in short-term memory (STM).** (A) A theta–gamma discrete code model of STM by Lisman and Idirat (1995). Each item is represented by a different pattern of neurons, which then couples with a specific subcycle of the slow oscillation. The order of representation is held throughout multiple cycles of the oscillation. *Source: Adapted with permission from Lisman and Buzsaki (2008).* (B) Optimal information about each one of two memorized objects is encoded using a different phase of a ~30 Hz oscillation in the monkey prefrontal cortex. *Source: Adapted with permission from Siegel et al. (2009).*

nesting frequency was gamma (at 30 Hz), rather than theta. First, each of the two object identities was specifically encoded by a difference in average spiking level in the prefrontal cortex. Further, this object-selective spiking activity, which was conserved during the delay period, was phase-dependent. That is, activity carrying information about an object's identity was distributed across the phase of the ~30 Hz oscillation as a function of the presentation order of the two objects. Activity related to the identity of the initially presented object was centered at an earlier phase than the activity related to the object presented second (Figure 21.4(B)). Thus, the phase of the 30 Hz oscillations encoded the memorized objects throughout the delay period according to their presentation order. This neural mechanism can account for behavioral results suggesting that STM is a serial scanning process (Sternberg, 1966). Indeed, the order dependence of the phase was lost for trials in which the monkey did not remember the object order (Siegel et al., 2009).

The average capacity of human STM was traditionally thought to be 7 ± 2 items (Miller, 1956). It is tempting to assume that the cycle length of the theta oscillation

determines this capacity, since we can think of it as a window into which gamma cycles should fit (Demiralp et al., 2007; Lisman & Buzsaki, 2008). The model by Lisman can account for STM capacity by applying this logic, and there are some data to support this notion. For example, Axmacher and colleagues found that the theta cycle peak that modulates gamma power in the human hippocampus decreases with an increase of memory load. That is, an increase in the number of items to memorize is associated with longer theta cycles (Axmacher et al., 2010). Additionally, the scanning time for items held in STM was previously proposed to be around 30 ms per item, a time that fits the separation interval of gamma cycles that are nested within subcycles of a theta oscillation (see, for review, Lisman & Buzsaki, 2008; Sternberg, 1966). Note, however, that these are not direct demonstrations of the theta cycle defining STM capacity. Further research is needed to elucidate the precise role of oscillations and PAC in the various stages of learning and memory retrieval (see Axmacher et al., 2010 for discussion).

ENTRAINMENT OF NEURONAL OSCILLATIONS AND PAC AS A CODING MECHANISM

It has been suggested that the phase of neuronal oscillations can be entrained by, as well as track, the modulation of rhythmic external, or internal events (Lakatos et al., 2008; Schroeder & Lakatos, 2009). Here we review two examples of models that emphasize the importance of locking high-frequency activity to a slower oscillation phase as a means for efficient information integration.

Speech Processing by Neuronal Oscillations (Giraud & Poeppel, 2012)

Speech has a rhythmic, although complex and irregular, structure. Information at the phonemic level of the speech has a high-frequency modulation time scale of about 30–50 Hz. Slower acoustic modulations may characterize the syllable unit rate, and intonation or prosody rhythms of whole words embedded in the sentence level are even slower (Ghitza, 2011; Giraud & Poeppel, 2012). It is hypothesized that the neural activity in the human cortical speech network is well suited to process the rhythmic information in the specific temporal scales that compose speech using neuronal oscillations at the frequencies that correspond to them. The gamma, theta, and delta rhythms observed in the auditory cortex have cycle-lengths corresponding to these hierarchical acoustic modulations, and therefore may be associated with the corresponding units within an utterance (Ghitza, 2011; Giraud & Poeppel, 2012; Poeppel, 2003). A recent model by Giraud and Poeppel proposed a precise sequence of operations, including phase-coding and theta–gamma PAC, by which the parsing, or discretization, of continuous speech into effective temporal units is accomplished (Giraud & Poeppel, 2012). According to the model, the input information first phase-resets theta oscillations in the auditory cortex, leading to its tracking of, or entrainment to, the speech envelope. In other words, the theta oscillation phase-tracks the speech envelope (see also Luo & Poeppel, 2007). The phase resetting of the theta oscillation, in turn, reshapes gamma activity (related to the fast-modulating information components) through theta–gamma PAC. According to Giraud, the excitable period for the gamma interneuron network set by each theta oscillation allows for about four gamma cycles, which fits a syllable duration. These gamma oscillations would modulate spiking activity in the superficial (output) cortical layers, generating appropriately time-scaled "packages" of spikes for subsequent processing. In summary, this model suggests that phase information in oscillations helps to shape neural activity in language processing.

Dynamic Theory of Vision (Ahissar & Arieli, 2001)

Another theory that makes use of phase-coding of rhythmic modulations in input provides an approach to visual information coding in the early visual cortex (Ahissar & Arieli, 2001). Contrary to speech, visual information is not naturally rhythmic except under circumscribed conditions such as a flashing light. However, the retinal image fades rapidly, and information coding in the eye seems to be especially suited for temporal changes (Nirenberg & Meister, 1997). It was suggested that constant eye movements play a role in a temporal coding mechanism, with some features that are reminiscent of the speech processing model discussed above.

Our eyes constantly move, using fixational eye movements (FEMs) of different frequency ranges, going from small drifts to rapid saccades. Interestingly, the distribution of FEM frequencies matches to a surprising degree the cortical rhythms observed in the visual cortex, namely the alpha and gamma ranges. Ahissar and Arieli (2001) proposed that the constantly moving retina uses temporal coding of spatial information, while the visual cortex uses a phase-based decoding system to read the information coded by the retina. Consider the shape depicted in Figure 21.5, featuring a spatial offset (misalignment of the gray rectangles). To encode this offset, receptive fields (RFs) move across the image as the eye saccades, and when encountering a contrast change, their respective ganglion cells fire a spike burst. The offset will be encoded as a time lag between the outputs of two RFs (Figure 21.5). This time-based spatial coding can,

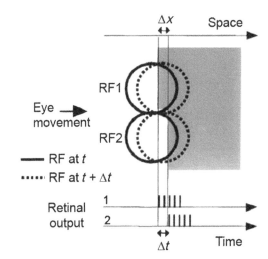

FIGURE 21.5 **Encoding of an offset by the retina during fixational eye movements (FEMs).** Each circle represents a receptive field (RF), moving rightward during a horizontal FEM. When each of the ganglion cells crosses the contrast change border, represented here by the gray square, it fires. The time lag (delta t) between the bursts of the two ganglion cells is encoded as a relative spatial offset (delta x) of the contour. In order for the cortex to read this code, the eye velocity needs to be known. This is done using a phase reset by the FEM and the entrainment of oscillations in V1. *Source: Adapted with permission from Ahissar and Arieli (2001).*

according to the model by Ahissar and Arieli, explain the higher spatial precision (acuity) observed, as compared to what may be expected from the retinal receptor distribution and size. How does the visual cortex read these spikes? The model proposes phase-locking between the incoming spikes and intrinsic cortical oscillations. Phase-locking of the cortical oscillations to the FEM will be used to parse the input and provide the necessary information about the time lag between FEM-induced retinal bursts (needed in order to extract spatial relations between contrast edges).

Although PAC is not specifically discussed in the model, spiking activity locked to slow oscillatory phase is a form of PAC. Furthermore, there is evidence for HG phase-locking to slow oscillations in V1 (Mazzoni, Brunel, Cavallari, Logothetis, & Panzeri, 2011; Montemurro, Rasch, Murayama, Logothetis, & Panzeri, 2008). One may speculate that these PAC measures reflect spiking activity indexed by HG oscillations reorganized in time via alpha oscillations that are reset by FEMs. Such a hypothesis, however, is yet to be empirically tested.

NEURAL DYNAMICS IN THE ABNORMAL BRAIN

Compared to the vast number of studies that have investigated oscillatory dynamics in an intact, healthy brain, relatively fewer studies have focused on how these dynamics might be compromised or lead to dysfunction in pathological brain states, such as schizophrenia, epilepsy, dyslexia, and Alzheimer's disease (AD). Studies have begun to investigate how abnormal neuronal synchrony may be used as a marker for disease. This is important, since certain brain diseases, such as schizophrenia and AD, have long been characterized to result from the disconnection of neuronal regions, leading to malfunctions in the coordination of neural activity between and within areas. Given that the brain has been hypothesized to use synchronization of oscillatory activity across neural systems as a means of network coordination, a breakdown in this synchronization may contribute a key neurophysiological deficit in multiple disorders.

Schizophrenia is a severe mental disorder that is characterized by psychotic symptoms (delusions, hallucinations), negative symptoms (flattened affect), and disorganized thoughts and behaviors. This disorder has been associated with abnormal synchronization in the higher-frequency range. Numerous studies have found abnormal beta and gamma synchronization while patients perform visual (Green et al., 2003; Haig et al., 2000; Spencer et al., 2003; Uhlhaas et al., 2006; Wynn, Light, Breitmeyer, Nuechterlein, & Green, 2005) and auditory (Gallinat, Winterer, Herrmann, & Senkowski, 2004) tasks. Abnormalities in rhythm-generating networks of GABAergic inhibitory neurons (Lewis, Hashimoto, & Volk, 2005) and glutamatergic neurons that mediate long-distance synchronization (Moghaddam, 2003) may contribute to this irregular synchronization observed in the schizophrenic brain, although no study thus far has directly connected neurotransmitter system malfunction to changes in neuronal synchrony.

Epilepsy arises from a diverse set of disorders leading to abnormal (too high and too extended) neuronal synchronization that is the hallmark of a seizure. Because of the heterogeneity of subtypes, there is not just one abnormal mechanism characterizing epilepsy. High-frequency oscillations, especially in the gamma band, have been frequently associated with epileptic events (Bragin, Engel, Wilson, Fried, & Mathern, 1999; Jirsch et al., 2006; Rampp & Stefan, 2006). However, these increases in synchrony occur in highly localized areas presaging a focal onset of a seizure (Garcia Dominguez et al., 2005; van Putten, 2003). Le Van Quyen, Navarro, Martinerie, Baulac, and Varela (2003) also report beta band desynchronization preceded ictal periods in sites that were close to the epileptic focus. These observations indicate that epilepsy is characterized by complicated patterns of both synchronization and desynchronization across multiple frequency bands, depending on the type of seizure and the brain regions involved.

Dyslexia is a developmental disorder that affects how patients properly recognize and process certain symbols, leading to reading impairments. It has been hypothesized that a phonological deficit may be the underlying cause of the impairment. For example, dyslexic children are proposed to have a deficit in the representation of the processing of speech sounds (Vellutino, Fletcher, Snowling, & Scanlon, 2004). In the normal brain, the most prevalent oscillations in the auditory cortex are in the delta/theta and low gamma bands (Giraud et al., 2007; Morillon et al., 2010). As discussed above, these oscillations are at frequencies that match the rates of the strongest modulations in speech (the syllabic, 4 Hz, and phonemic, 30 Hz rates) and are well suited to process rhythmic information at these temporal scales. Additionally, these rhythms are stronger in the left than the right hemisphere (Poeppel, 2003), matching the left hemisphere dominance for language (Knecht et al., 2000). Recently, Lehongre et al. (2011) found that entrainment of acoustic modulations in the 25–35 Hz (low gamma) range was significantly reduced in the left hemisphere of dyslexics compared to controls. These decreases in the entrainment of frequencies predictive of phonemic processing were accompanied by increases of entrainment at higher frequencies relative to controls, which suggests that phonemes are sampled in a higher rate than optimally needed in dyslexics. This inability of the auditory cortex to phase-lock to acoustic features similar to speech provides a potential mechanism to explain deficient phonological processing in dyslexia. Furthermore, this study provides evidence that one of the key features of dyslexia is abnormal neuronal synchronization.

AD is the most common type of dementia and is characterized by a progressive decline in certain cognitive abilities, including memory, visuospatial, and executive functions. Multiple studies conducted by Stam, Jones, Nolte, Breakspear, and Scheltens (2007), Stam et al. (2005) and Stam, van der Made, Pijnenburg, and Scheltens (2003) have demonstrated decreased alpha and beta synchronization in patients with AD, which is most pronounced for synchronization between distant areas (Stam et al., 2007). Pijnenburg et al. (2004) confirmed these results by demonstrating that AD patients showed a reduction in alpha and beta synchronization as compared to controls during working memory maintenance. Perhaps one of the most convincing studies to link AD to abnormal neural processing was conducted by Stern et al. (2004), who demonstrated that the timing of evoked action potentials in the neocortex of transgenic mice with increased expression of amyloid precursor protein was jittered compared to that of wild-type mice. Amyloid beta plaques are one of the hallmarks of AD, making this an appropriate animal model for AD. This study suggests that proteins specifically associated with AD may have specific effects on spike timing and synchronization within and between brain areas.

A few studies have begun to examine the relationship between abnormal PAC and brain dysfunction.

One might hypothesize that a brain disorder linked to abnormal changes in synchrony might also manifest abnormal changes in PAC, since oscillatory phase changes contribute to measures of both synchronization and PAC. A recent EEG study compared PAC while schizophrenic patients and healthy controls performed an auditory oddball task (Allen et al., 2011). An independent component analysis was used to isolate specific PAC profiles that were each associated with a unique spatial profile. Two components were found to differ between schizophrenics and healthy controls. First, the total global amount of PAC (across all frequencies and across the entire brain) was significantly greater in controls than in schizophrenic patients. Second, beta phase–HG amplitude (60–160 Hz) coupling was higher over fronto-temporal regions in schizophrenic patients than controls. While none of these PAC components significantly correlated with behavior, there was a significant correlation between negative symptoms of schizophrenia and PAC, where more severe negative symptoms were related to decreases in low-frequency (1–8 Hz) phase–HG amplitude (150–200 Hz) coupling centered over frontal electrodes. This is particularly interesting since coupling between the theta phase and the HG amplitude is robust over frontal electrode sites in control patients, who do not manifest schizophrenic symptoms (Canolty et al., 2006; Voytek et al., 2010). Perhaps the loss of this theta–HG PAC over the frontal cortex could serve as a liability marker for schizophrenia. More studies are needed to replicate this finding, especially since the reliability of measuring broadband HG with scalp EEG is contentious (see below).

Recently, changes in PAC patterns were also found to predict seizure onset. A recent study by Alvarado-Rojas, Valderrama, Witon, Navarro, and Le Van Quyen (2011) examined fluctuations in coupling between the phase of low-frequency rhythms (delta and theta) and the amplitudes of high-frequency activity (broadband gamma) throughout a 3400 h recording period in 20 patients who were undergoing intracranial monitoring for the localization of epileptic foci. They found that in 50% of the patients, increases in PAC between the delta or theta phase and broadband gamma amplitude reliably predicted pre-ictal changes up to 10 min before seizure onset. However, the phase and amplitude frequencies that served as indicators varied substantially from patient to patient (e.g. delta phase–low gamma amplitude, delta phase–HG amplitude, theta phase–low gamma amplitude, and theta phase–HG amplitude all served as indicators in different patients). No one phase–amplitude frequency pair dominated. In addition, multiple electrodes, sometimes within and sometimes outside the seizure focus, were used to predict seizure onset based upon PAC increases.

The few studies reviewed here suggest that changes in PAC may serve as a possible marker for disease in the clinical domain. However, little work to date has investigated the relationship between PAC and brain dysfunction. In addition, is not yet known how abnormal mechanisms of PAC and synchronization may interact or reinforce one another in each of these brain diseases. These are areas ripe for future research and have the potential to improve detection, diagnosis, and treatment of numerous brain diseases.

CAN PAC BE RELIABLY MEASURED USING SCALP EEG?

Phase–amplitude coupling is increasingly being investigated in human subjects. Since the first reports of PAC in human ECoG (Canolty et al., 2006; Mormann et al., 2005), numerous studies have begun to explore the role of PAC in cognitive, sensory, and motor functions. However, only a few studies have investigated PAC using scalp-recorded EEG (e.g., Allen et al., 2011; Burgess & Ali, 2002; Demiralp et al., 2007; Sauseng et al., 2009; Schack, Vath, Petsche, Geissler, & Moller, 2002). One reason for this may lie in the limited spectral content in signals recorded from the scalp. Many ECoG reports of PAC focus on HG rhythms (e.g., >70 Hz), while scalp EEG is traditionally considered unsuitable for reliable collection of high-frequency data. Electrophysiological signals crossing the skull undergo a reduction in power for all frequencies, with stronger dampening as frequencies rise, making it difficult for surface contacts to detect these high-frequency oscillations (e.g., Davidson, Jackson, & Larson, 2000). Additionally, artifacts of muscular origin, as well as microsaccadic eye movements, contaminate the scalp data in the gamma range, further impairing the already low signal-to-noise ratio (SNR) at these frequencies (Yuval-Greenberg, Tomer, Keren, Nelken, & Deouell, 2008).

Despite these limitations, an increasing number of studies report HG activity recorded over the scalp, sometimes up to 250 Hz (Ball et al., 2008; Hipp, Engel, & Siegel, 2011; Lenz et al., 2008; Onton & Makeig, 2009), suggesting that reliable measurements of PAC, including high-frequency oscillations, may be obtained using scalp EEG. Furthermore, even though human ECoG and animal studies reporting PAC often concentrate on the coupling of HG with slower oscillations, PAC may be hierarchically observed across numerous frequency bands (Lakatos et al., 2005) including lower ranges of gamma (e.g., Axmacher et al., 2010; Burgess & Ali, 2002; Demiralp et al., 2007; Mormann et al., 2005; Sauseng et al., 2009), and can be observed across two low frequencies (e.g., alpha or theta power nesting in the delta phase, Cohen, Elger, & Fell, 2009; Lakatos et al., 2005). Moreover, one large advantage for scalp EEG when studying PAC as a possible mechanism for hierarchical long-range information integration across brain regions is its distribution of electrodes across the whole scalp. In comparison, ECoG electrodes usually have restricted coverage.

Scalp EEG measures of PAC can also have substantial contributions in clinical research and may possibly serve as a future diagnostic aid. Abnormal PAC is increasingly reported in the context of neurological and psychiatric disorders, as reviewed earlier in this chapter. Measuring PAC over the scalp can be readily used in a clinical setting, since EEG is noninvasive and widely available. Thus, it is possible for scalp-recorded PAC to become a tool for neurological evaluation of certain diseases. However, the reliability of measuring PAC over the scalp is not yet well established. The few scalp EEG studies of PAC cited above used different coupling estimates, and most did not eliminate the possibility of confounds from saccadic eye movements, muscular activity, or sharp-edge noise, particularly relevant in scalp EEG data (Kramer, Tort, & Kopell, 2008). We have recently conducted a study to assess the use of scalp EEG to measure PAC (Sadeh & Knight, 2012; see Figure 21.2). We found reliable coupling between gamma amplitude and alpha phase in the visual system during a visual target detection task. The coupling was not the result of microsaccade-induced gamma artifacts coupled with alpha phase-resetting at occipital sites, since gamma power taken from frontal electrodes was not coupled with the alpha phase at occipital electrodes, indicating that the gamma component of the PAC is a local cortical phenomenon in occipital regions. We then introduced sharp-edge noise into real data to examine whether coupling-like patterns produced by this noise may be confounded with authentic cortical PAC. When filtered and then averaged across overlapping trough-locked windows, high-frequency noise can appear in the spectrogram mimicking phase-locked gamma bursts (Kramer et al., 2008). However, these coupling-like patterns differ from our data in important ways. For example, coupling-like noise appeared with any of the tested slow oscillations, whereas our data showed specificity for the alpha rhythm. Additionally, there was no reliable coupling on a single-cycle level and no consistency across channels of the subcycles within the slow oscillation with which the gamma power was coupled, whereas the data showed phase consistency across occipital electrodes and across subjects. This indicated that combined with the use of proper artifact reduction procedures and controls, PAC may be reliably recorded in scalp EEG settings.

CONCLUSIONS

There is an increasing interest in PAC as a common mechanism for information phase-coding and integration for various cognitive functions. This interest is fed by recent findings elucidating the functional role that PAC plays in memory, visual processing, attention, language, and other cognitive functions. A few recent models have incorporated PAC as a computational principle in a progression of complex brain operations underlying information encoding or decoding (e.g., Giraud & Poeppel, 2012; Lisman & Idiart, 1995). These models, in turn, may lead to further interest and analyses using PAC as a metric for neural processing. In the clinical domain, PAC has been suggested as a metric to assess neurological and psychiatric diseases, and evidence for the feasibility and reliability of this measure for diagnostic purposes has begun to emerge.

A challenge still remains in demonstrating that the comodulation of phase and amplitude within a complex signal has a functional role in information processing by the brain, or a causal directionality (i.e., whether the amplitude of a higher frequency is modulated by the phase of the lower frequency, or whether the higher-frequency activity resets the phase of an oscillation, creating a feedback process). A functional role for PAC can be studied, for example, by looking for correlations between PAC measures and behavior in even more domains than previously demonstrated, by assessing PAC modulation as a function of task demands and psychological or neurological states, or by functionally intervening with normal brain activity (e.g., by using TMS or transcranial direct current stimulation in humans) and measuring the impact on PAC and behavior. Another question is to what extent and under what circumstances long-range phase coherence is related to PAC. We would benefit from a better characterization of the relationship between these two neural mechanisms. Lastly, whether and how PAC occurs during consciousness or the sleep–wake cycle, or how it changes throughout the course of development, will be important directions for future research.

Acknowledgments

This research was supported by NINDS Grant NS21135 and the Nielsen Corporation.

References

Ahissar, E., & Arieli, A. (2001). Figuring space by time. *Neuron, 32*(2), 185–201.

Allen, E. A., Liu, J., Kiehl, K. A., Gelernter, J., Pearlson, G. D., Perrone-Bizzozero, N. I., et al. (2011). Components of cross-frequency modulation in health and disease. *Frontiers in Systems Neuroscience, 5*, 59.

Alvarado-Rojas, C., Valderrama, M., Witon, A., Navarro, V., & Le Van Quyen, M. (2011). Probing cortical excitability using cross-frequency coupling in intracranial EEG recordings: a new method for seizure prediction. *Conference Proceedings: Annual International Conference of the IEEE Engineering in Medicine and Biology Society, 2011*, 1632–1635.

Arieli, A., Sterkin, A., Grinvald, A., & Aertsen, A. (1996). Dynamics of ongoing activity: explanation of the large variability in evoked cortical responses. *Science, 273*(5283), 1868–1871.

Axmacher, N., Henseler, M. M., Jensen, O., Weinreich, I., Elger, C. E., & Fell, J. (2010). Cross-frequency coupling supports multi-item working memory in the human hippocampus. *Proceedings of the National Academy of Sciences of the United States of America, 107*(7), 3228–3233.

Axmacher, N., Mormann, F., Fernandez, G., Cohen, M. X., Elger, C. E., & Fell, J. (2007). Sustained neural activity patterns during working memory in the human medial temporal lobe. *Journal of Neuroscience*, 27(29), 7807–7816.

Axmacher, N., Mormann, F., Fernandez, G., Elger, C. E., & Fell, J. (2006). Memory formation by neuronal synchronization. *Brain Research Reviews*, 52(1), 170–182.

Ball, T., Demandt, E., Mutschler, I., Neitzel, E., Mehring, C., Vogt, K., et al. (2008). Movement related activity in the high gamma range of the human EEG. *Neuroimage*, 41(2), 302–310.

Barcelo, F., Suwazono, S., & Knight, R. T. (2000). Prefrontal modulation of visual processing in humans. *Nature Neuroscience*, 3(4), 399–403.

Bauer, M., Oostenveld, R., Peeters, M., & Fries, P. (2006). Tactile spatial attention enhances gamma-band activity in somatosensory cortex and reduces low-frequency activity in parieto-occipital areas. *Journal of Neuroscience*, 26(2), 490–501.

Bishop, G. H. (1933). Cyclic changes in excitability of the optic pathway of the rabbit. *American Journal of Physiology*, 103(1), 213–224.

Bragin, A., Engel, J., Jr., Wilson, C. L., Fried, I., & Mathern, G. W. (1999). Hippocampal and entorhinal cortex high-frequency oscillations (100–500 Hz) in human epileptic brain and in kainic acid-treated rats with chronic seizures. *Epilepsia*, 40(2), 127–137.

Bragin, A., Jando, G., Nadasdy, Z., Hetke, J., Wise, K., & Buzsaki, G. (1995). Gamma (40–100 Hz) oscillation in the hippocampus of the behaving rat. *Journal of Neuroscience*, 15(1 Pt 1), 47–60.

Burchell, T. R., Faulkner, H. J., & Whittington, M. A. (1998). Gamma frequency oscillations gate temporally coded afferent inputs in the rat hippocampal slice. *Neuroscience Letters*, 255(3), 151–154.

Burgess, A. P., & Ali, L. (2002). Functional connectivity of gamma EEG activity is modulated at low frequency during conscious recollection. *International Journal of Psychophysiology*, 46(2), 91–100.

Busch, N. A., Dubois, J., & VanRullen, R. (2009). The phase of ongoing EEG oscillations predicts visual perception. *Journal of Neuroscience*, 29(24), 7869–7876.

Buzsaki, G., Buhl, D. L., Harris, K. D., Csicsvari, J., Czeh, B., & Morozov, A. (2003). Hippocampal network patterns of activity in the mouse. *Neuroscience*, 116(1), 201–211.

Buzsaki, G., & Draguhn, A. (2004). Neuronal oscillations in cortical networks. *Science*, 304(5679), 1926–1929.

Canolty, R. T., Edwards, E., Dalal, S. S., Soltani, M., Nagarajan, S. S., Kirsch, H. E., et al. (2006). High gamma power is phase-locked to theta oscillations in human neocortex. *Science*, 313(5793), 1626–1628.

Canolty, R. T., & Knight, R. T. (2010). The functional role of cross-frequency coupling. *Trends in Cognitive Sciences*, 14(11), 506–515.

Canolty, R. T., Soltani, M., Dalal, S. S., Edwards, E., Dronkers, N. F., Nagarajan, S. S., et al. (2007). Spatiotemporal dynamics of word processing in the human brain. *Frontiers in Neuroscience*, 1(1), 185–196.

Capotosto, P., Babiloni, C., Romani, G. L., & Corbetta, M. (2009). Frontoparietal cortex controls spatial attention through modulation of anticipatory alpha rhythms. *Journal of Neuroscience*, 29(18), 5863–5872.

Cardin, J. A., Carlen, M., Meletis, K., Knoblich, U., Zhang, F., Deisseroth, K., et al. (2009). Driving fast-spiking cells induces gamma rhythm and controls sensory responses. *Nature*, 459(7247), 663–667.

Cohen, M. X., Elger, C. E., & Fell, J. (2009). Oscillatory activity and phase–amplitude coupling in the human medial frontal cortex during decision making. *Journal of Cognitive Neuroscience*, 21(2), 390–402.

Corbetta, M., & Shulman, G. L. (2002). Control of goal-directed and stimulus-driven attention in the brain. *Nature Reviews Neuroscience*, 3(3), 201–215.

Csicsvari, J., Jamieson, B., Wise, K. D., & Buzsaki, G. (2003). Mechanisms of gamma oscillations in the hippocampus of the behaving rat. *Neuron*, 37(2), 311–322.

Davidson, R. J., Jackson, D. C., & Larson, C. L. (2000). Human electroencephalography. In J. T. Cacioppo, L. G. Tassinary & G. Berntson (Eds.), *Handbook of psychophysiology* (2nd ed., pp. 27–52). Cambridge: Cambridge University Press.

Demiralp, T., Bayraktaroglu, Z., Lenz, D., Junge, S., Busch, N. A., Maess, B., et al. (2007). Gamma amplitudes are coupled to theta phase in human EEG during visual perception. *International Journal of Psychophysiology*, 64(1), 24–30.

Doesburg, S. M., Roggeveen, A. B., Kitajo, K., & Ward, L. M. (2008). Large-scale gamma-band phase synchronization and selective attention. *Cerebral Cortex*, 18(2), 386–396.

Dugue, L., Marque, P., & VanRullen, R. (2011). The phase of ongoing oscillations mediates the causal relation between brain excitation and visual perception. *Journal of Neuroscience*, 31(33), 11889–11893.

Engel, A. K., Fries, P., & Singer, W. (2001). Dynamic predictions: oscillations and synchrony in top-down processing. *Nature Reviews Neuroscience*, 2(10), 704–716.

Ergenoglu, T., Demiralp, T., Bayraktaroglu, Z., Ergen, M., Beydagi, H., & Uresin, Y. (2004). Alpha rhythm of the EEG modulates visual detection performance in humans. *Brain Research Cognitive Brain Research*, 20(3), 376–383.

Fan, J., Byrne, J., Worden, M. S., Guise, K. G., McCandliss, B. D., Fossella, J., et al. (2007). The relation of brain oscillations to attentional networks. *Journal of Neuroscience*, 27(23), 6197–6206.

Fell, J., & Axmacher, N. (2011). The role of phase synchronization in memory processes. *Nature Reviews Neuroscience*, 12(2), 105–118.

Fries, P. (2005). A mechanism for cognitive dynamics: neuronal communication through neuronal coherence. *Trends in Cognitive Sciences*, 9(10), 474–480.

Fries, P., Reynolds, J. H., Rorie, A. E., & Desimone, R. (2001). Modulation of oscillatory neuronal synchronization by selective visual attention. *Science*, 291(5508), 1560–1563.

Gallinat, J., Winterer, G., Herrmann, C. S., & Senkowski, D. (2004). Reduced oscillatory gamma-band responses in unmedicated schizophrenic patients indicate impaired frontal network processing. *Clinical Neurophysiology*, 115(8), 1863–1874.

Garcia Dominguez, L., Wennberg, R. A., Gaetz, W., Cheyne, D., Snead, O. C., 3rd, & Perez Velazquez, J. L. (2005). Enhanced synchrony in epileptiform activity? Local versus distant phase synchronization in generalized seizures. *Journal of Neuroscience*, 25(35), 8077–8084.

Gevins, A., Smith, M. E., McEvoy, L., & Yu, D. (1997). High-resolution EEG mapping of cortical activation related to working memory: effects of task difficulty, type of processing, and practice. *Cerebral Cortex*, 7(4), 374–385.

Ghitza, O. (2011). Linking speech perception and neurophysiology: speech decoding guided by cascaded oscillators locked to the input rhythm. *Frontiers in Psychology*, 2, 130.

Giraud, A. L., Kleinschmidt, A., Poeppel, D., Lund, T. E., Frackowiak, R. S., & Laufs, H. (2007). Endogenous cortical rhythms determine cerebral specialization for speech perception and production. *Neuron*, 56(6), 1127–1134.

Giraud, A. L., & Poeppel, D. (2012). Cortical oscillations and speech processing: emerging computational principles and operations. *Nature Neuroscience*, 15(4), 511–517.

Gray, C. M., & Singer, W. (1989). Stimulus-specific neuronal oscillations in orientation columns of cat visual cortex. *Proceedings of the National Academy of Sciences of the United States of America*, 86(5), 1698–1702.

Green, M. F., Mintz, J., Salveson, D., Nuechterlein, K. H., Breitmeyer, B., Light, G. A., et al. (2003). Visual masking as a probe for abnormal gamma range activity in schizophrenia. *Biological Psychiatry*, 53(12), 1113–1119.

Gregoriou, G. G., Gotts, S. J., Zhou, H., & Desimone, R. (2009). High-frequency, long-range coupling between prefrontal and visual cortex during attention. *Science*, 324(5931), 1207–1210.

Gruber, T., Muller, M. M., Keil, A., & Elbert, T. (1999). Selective visual-spatial attention alters induced gamma band responses in the human EEG. *Clinical Neurophysiology*, 110(12), 2074–2085.

Haig, A. R., Gordon, E., De Pascalis, V., Meares, R. A., Bahramali, H., & Harris, A. (2000). Gamma activity in schizophrenia: evidence of impaired network binding? *Clinical Neurophysiology*, 111(8), 1461–1468.

Hanslmayr, S., Aslan, A., Staudigl, T., Klimesch, W., Herrmann, C. S., & Bauml, K. H. (2007). Prestimulus oscillations predict visual perception performance between and within subjects. *Neuroimage, 37*(4), 1465–1473.

Hari, R., Salmelin, R., Makela, J. P., Salenius, S., & Helle, M. (1997). Magnetoencephalographic cortical rhythms. *International Journal of Psychophysiology, 26*(1–3), 51–62.

Hipp, J. F., Engel, A. K., & Siegel, M. (2011). Oscillatory synchronization in large-scale cortical networks predicts perception. *Neuron, 69*(2), 387–396.

Holcman, D., & Tsodyks, M. (2006). The emergence of up and down states in cortical networks. *PLoS Computational Biology, 2*(3), e23.

Holscher, C., Anwyl, R., & Rowan, M. J. (1997). Stimulation on the positive phase of hippocampal theta rhythm induces long-term potentiation that can be depotentiated by stimulation on the negative phase in area CA1 in vivo. *Journal of Neuroscience, 17*(16), 6470–6477.

Jensen, O., Kaiser, J., & Lachaux, J. P. (2007). Human gamma-frequency oscillations associated with attention and memory. *Trends in Neurosciences, 30*(7), 317–324.

Jirsch, J. D., Urrestarazu, E., LeVan, P., Olivier, A., Dubeau, F., & Gotman, J. (2006). High-frequency oscillations during human focal seizures. *Brain, 129*(Pt 6), 1593–1608.

Kahana, M. J., Seelig, D., & Madsen, J. R. (2001). Theta returns. *Current Opinion in Neurobiology, 11*(6), 739–744.

Kastner, S., & Ungerleider, L. G. (2000). Mechanisms of visual attention in the human cortex. *Annual Review of Neuroscience, 23*, 315–341.

Kelly, S. P., Lalor, E. C., Reilly, R. B., & Foxe, J. J. (2006). Increases in alpha oscillatory power reflect an active retinotopic mechanism for distracter suppression during sustained visuospatial attention. *Journal of Neurophysiology, 95*(6), 3844–3851.

Klimesch, W. (1996). Memory processes, brain oscillations and EEG synchronization. *International Journal of Psychophysiology, 24*(1–2), 61–100.

Klimesch, W. (1999). EEG alpha and theta oscillations reflect cognitive and memory performance: a review and analysis. *Brain Research Brain Research Reviews, 29*(2–3), 169–195.

Klimesch, W., Doppelmayr, M., Russegger, H., & Pachinger, T. (1996). Theta band power in the human scalp EEG and the encoding of new information. *Neuroreport, 7*(7), 1235–1240.

Knecht, S., Deppe, M., Drager, B., Bobe, L., Lohmann, H., Ringelstein, E., et al. (2000). Language lateralization in healthy right-handers. *Brain, 123*(Pt 1), 74–81.

Kramer, M. A., Tort, A. B. L., & Kopell, N. J. (2008). Sharp edge artifacts and spurious coupling in EEG frequency comodulation measures. *Journal of Neuroscience Methods, 170*(2), 352–357.

Lakatos, P., Karmos, G., Mehta, A. D., Ulbert, I., & Schroeder, C. E. (2008). Entrainment of neuronal oscillations as a mechanism of attentional selection. *Science, 320*(5872), 110–113.

Lakatos, P., Shah, A. S., Knuth, K. H., Ulbert, I., Karmos, G., & Schroeder, C. E. (2005). An oscillatory hierarchy controlling neuronal excitability and stimulus processing in the auditory cortex. *Journal of Neurophysiology, 94*(3), 1904–1911.

Landau, A. N., Esterman, M., Robertson, L. C., Bentin, S., & Prinzmetal, W. (2007). Different effects of voluntary and involuntary attention on EEG activity in the gamma band. *Journal of Neuroscience, 27*(44), 11986–11990.

Le Van Quyen, M., Navarro, V., Martinerie, J., Baulac, M., & Varela, F. J. (2003). Toward a neurodynamical understanding of ictogenesis. *Epilepsia, 44*(Suppl. 12), 30–43.

Lehongre, K., Ramus, F., Villiermet, N., Schwartz, D., & Giraud, A. L. (2011). Altered low-gamma sampling in auditory cortex accounts for the three main facets of dyslexia. *Neuron, 72*(6), 1080–1090.

Lenz, D., Jeschke, M., Schadow, J., Naue, N., Ohl, F. W., & Herrmann, C. S. (2008). Human EEG very high frequency oscillations reflect the number of matches with a template in auditory short-term memory. *Brain Research, 1220*, 81–92.

Lewis, D. A., Hashimoto, T., & Volk, D. W. (2005). Cortical inhibitory neurons and schizophrenia. *Nature Reviews Neuroscience, 6*(4), 312–324.

Lisman, J., & Buzsaki, G. (2008). A neural coding scheme formed by the combined function of gamma and theta oscillations. *Schizophrenia Bulletin, 34*(5), 974–980.

Lisman, J. E., & Idiart, M. A. (1995). Storage of 7 ± 2 short-term memories in oscillatory subcycles. *Science, 267*(5203), 1512–1515.

Llinas, R. R. (1988). The intrinsic electrophysiological properties of mammalian neurons: insights into central nervous system function. *Science, 242*(4886), 1654–1664.

Luo, H., & Poeppel, D. (2007). Phase patterns of neuronal responses reliably discriminate speech in human auditory cortex. *Neuron, 54*(6), 1001–1010.

Mathewson, K. E., Gratton, G., Fabiani, M., Beck, D. M., & Ro, T. (2009). To see or not to see: prestimulus alpha phase predicts visual awareness. *Journal of Neuroscience, 29*(9), 2725–2732.

Mazzoni, A., Brunel, N., Cavallari, S., Logothetis, N. K., & Panzeri, S. (2011). Cortical dynamics during naturalistic sensory stimulations: experiments and models. *Journal of Physiology, Paris, 105*(1–3), 2–15.

Mesulam, M. M. (1981). A cortical network for directed attention and unilateral neglect. *Annals of Neurology, 10*(4), 309–325.

Miller, G. A. (1956). The magical number seven plus or minus two: some limits on our capacity for processing information. *Psychological Review, 63*(2), 81–97.

Miltner, W. H., Braun, C., Arnold, M., Witte, H., & Taub, E. (1999). Coherence of gamma-band EEG activity as a basis for associative learning. *Nature, 397*(6718), 434–436.

Moghaddam, B. (2003). Bringing order to the glutamate chaos in schizophrenia. *Neuron, 40*(5), 881–884.

Montemurro, M. A., Rasch, M. J., Murayama, Y., Logothetis, N. K., & Panzeri, S. (2008). Phase-of-firing coding of natural visual stimuli in primary visual cortex. *Current Biology, 18*(5), 375–380.

Moore, T., & Armstrong, K. M. (2003). Selective gating of visual signals by microstimulation of frontal cortex. *Nature, 421*(6921), 370–373.

Morillon, B., Lehongre, K., Frackowiak, R. S., Ducorps, A., Kleinschmidt, A., Poeppel, D., et al. (2010). Neurophysiological origin of human brain asymmetry for speech and language. *Proceedings of the National Academy of Sciences of the United States of America, 107*(43), 18688–18693.

Mormann, F., Fell, J., Axmacher, N., Weber, B., Lehnertz, K., Elger, C. E., et al. (2005). Phase/amplitude reset and theta–gamma interaction in the human medial temporal lobe during a continuous word recognition memory task. *Hippocampus, 15*(7), 890–900.

Nirenberg, S., & Meister, M. (1997). The light response of retinal ganglion cells is truncated by a displaced amacrine circuit. *Neuron, 18*(4), 637–650.

Onton, J., Delorme, A., & Makeig, S. (2005). Frontal midline EEG dynamics during working memory. *Neuroimage, 27*(2), 341–356.

Onton, J., & Makeig, S. (2009). High-frequency broadband modulations of electroencephalographic spectra. *Frontiers in Human Neuroscience, 3*, 61.

Osipova, D., Hermes, D., & Jensen, O. (2008). Gamma power is phase-locked to posterior alpha activity. *PLoS One, 3*(12), e3990.

Palva, S., & Palva, J. M. (2007). New vistas for alpha-frequency band oscillations. *Trends in Neurosciences, 30*(4), 150–158.

Pavlides, C., Greenstein, Y. J., Grudman, M., & Winson, J. (1988). Long-term potentiation in the dentate gyrus is induced preferentially on the positive phase of theta-rhythm. *Brain Research, 439*(1–2), 383–387.

Pfurtscheller, G. (2001). Functional brain imaging based on ERD/ERS. *Vision Research, 41*(10–11), 1257–1260.

Pijnenburg, Y. A., v d Made, Y., van Cappellen van Walsum, A. M., Knol, D. L., Scheltens, P., et al. (2004). EEG synchronization likelihood in mild cognitive impairment and Alzheimer's disease during a working memory task. *Clinical Neurophysiology, 115*(6), 1332–1339.

Poeppel, D. (2003). The analysis of speech in different temporal integration windows: cerebral lateralization as 'asymmetric sampling in time'. *Speech Communication*, 41(1), 245–255.

Rampp, S., & Stefan, H. (2006). Fast activity as a surrogate marker of epileptic network function? *Clinical Neurophysiology*, 117(10), 2111–2117.

Ray, S., & Maunsell, J. H. (2011). Different origins of gamma rhythm and high-gamma activity in macaque visual cortex. *PLoS Biology*, 9(4), e1000610.

Ray, S., Niebur, E., Hsiao, S. S., Sinai, A., & Crone, N. E. (2008). High-frequency gamma activity (80–150 Hz) is increased in human cortex during selective attention. *Clinical Neurophysiology*, 119(1), 116–133.

Romei, V., Brodbeck, V., Michel, C., Amedi, A., Pascual-Leone, A., & Thut, G. (2008). Spontaneous fluctuations in posterior alpha-band EEG activity reflect variability in excitability of human visual areas. *Cerebral Cortex*, 18(9), 2010–2018.

Romei, V., Gross, J., & Thut, G. (2010). On the role of prestimulus alpha rhythms over occipito-parietal areas in visual input regulation: correlation or causation? *Journal of Neuroscience*, 30(25), 8692–8697.

Rutishauser, U., Ross, I. B., Mamelak, A. N., & Schuman, E. M. (2010). Human memory strength is predicted by theta-frequency phase-locking of single neurons. *Nature*, 464(7290), 903–907.

Saalmann, Y. B., Pigarev, I. N., & Vidyasagar, T. R. (2007). Neural mechanisms of visual attention: how top-down feedback highlights relevant locations. *Science*, 316(5831), 1612–1615.

Saalmann, Y. B., Pinsk, M. A., Wang, L., Li, X., & Kastner, S. (2012). The pulvinar regulates information transmission between cortical areas based on attention demands. *Science*, 337(6095), 753–756.

Sadeh, B., & Knight, R. T. (2012). Phase-amplitude cross-frequency coupling during visual processing measured with scalp EEG. Program No. 746.09. *2012 Neuroscience Meeting Planner*. Washington, DC: Society for Neuroscience, 2012. Online.

Sanchez-Vives, M. V., & McCormick, D. A. (2000). Cellular and network mechanisms of rhythmic recurrent activity in neocortex. *Nature Neuroscience*, 3(10), 1027–1034.

Sauseng, P., Klimesch, W., Heise, K. F., Gruber, W. R., Holz, E., Karim, A. A., et al. (2009). Brain oscillatory substrates of visual short-term memory capacity. *Current Biology*, 19(21), 1846–1852.

Sauseng, P., Klimesch, W., Stadler, W., Schabus, M., Doppelmayr, M., Hanslmayr, S., et al. (2005). A shift of visual spatial attention is selectively associated with human EEG alpha activity. *European Journal of Neuroscience*, 22(11), 2917–2926.

Schack, B., Vath, N., Petsche, H., Geissler, H. G., & Moller, E. (2002). Phase-coupling of theta-gamma EEG rhythms during short-term memory processing. *International Journal of Psychophysiology*, 44(2), 143–163.

Schroeder, C. E., & Lakatos, P. (2009). Low-frequency neuronal oscillations as instruments of sensory selection. *Trends in Neurosciences*, 32(1), 9–18.

Siegel, M., Donner, T. H., & Engel, A. K. (2012). Spectral fingerprints of large-scale neuronal interactions. *Nature Reviews Neuroscience*, 13(2), 121–134.

Siegel, M., Warden, M. R., & Miller, E. K. (2009). Phase-dependent neuronal coding of objects in short-term memory. *Proceedings of the National Academy of Sciences of the United States of America*, 106(50), 21341–21346.

Spencer, K. M., Nestor, P. G., Niznikiewicz, M. A., Salisbury, D. F., Shenton, M. E., & McCarley, R. W. (2003). Abnormal neural synchrony in schizophrenia. *Journal of Neuroscience*, 23(19), 7407–7411.

Stam, C. J., Jones, B. F., Nolte, G., Breakspear, M., & Scheltens, P. (2007). Small-world networks and functional connectivity in Alzheimer's disease. *Cerebral Cortex*, 17(1), 92–99.

Stam, C. J., Montez, T., Jones, B. F., Rombouts, S. A., van der Made, Y., Pijnenburg, Y. A., et al. (2005). Disturbed fluctuations of resting state EEG synchronization in Alzheimer's disease. *Clinical Neurophysiology*, 116(3), 708–715.

Stam, C. J., van der Made, Y., Pijnenburg, Y. A., & Scheltens, P. (2003). EEG synchronization in mild cognitive impairment and Alzheimer's disease. *Acta Neurologica Scandinavica*, 108(2), 90–96.

Stern, E. A., Bacskai, B. J., Hickey, G. A., Attenello, F. J., Lombardo, J. A., & Hyman, B. T. (2004). Cortical synaptic integration in vivo is disrupted by amyloid-beta plaques. *Journal of Neuroscience*, 24(19), 4535–4540.

Sternberg, S. (1966). High-speed scanning in human memory. *Science*, 153(3736), 652–654.

Szczepanski, S. M., Parvizi, J., Auguste, K. I., Kuperman, R. A., & Knight, R. T. (2012). Dynamic fronto-parietal interactions facilitate spatial attention: Evidence from electrocorticography. Program No. 728.05. *2012 Neuroscience Meeting Planner*. Washington, DC: Society for Neuroscience, 2012. Online.

Tort, A. B., Komorowski, R. W., Manns, J. R., Kopell, N. J., & Eichenbaum, H. (2009). Theta-gamma coupling increases during the learning of item-context associations. *Proceedings of the National Academy of Sciences of the United States of America*, 106(49), 20942–20947.

Tort, A. B., Kramer, M. A., Thorn, C., Gibson, D. J., Kubota, Y., Graybiel, A. M., et al. (2008). Dynamic cross-frequency couplings of local field potential oscillations in rat striatum and hippocampus during performance of a T-maze task. *Proceedings of the National Academy of Sciences of the United States of America*, 105(51), 20517–20522.

Uhlhaas, P. J., Linden, D. E., Singer, W., Haenschel, C., Lindner, M., Maurer, K., et al. (2006). Dysfunctional long-range coordination of neural activity during Gestalt perception in schizophrenia. *Journal of Neuroscience*, 26(31), 8168–8175.

van Dijk, H., Schoffelen, J. M., Oostenveld, R., & Jensen, O. (2008). Prestimulus oscillatory activity in the alpha band predicts visual discrimination ability. *Journal of Neuroscience*, 28(8), 1816–1823.

van Putten, M. J. (2003). Nearest neighbor phase synchronization as a measure to detect seizure activity from scalp EEG recordings. *Journal of Clinical Neurophysiology*, 20(5), 320–325.

Vellutino, F. R., Fletcher, J. M., Snowling, M. J., & Scanlon, D. M. (2004). Specific reading disability (dyslexia): what have we learned in the past four decades? *Journal of Child Psychology and Psychiatry*, 45(1), 2–40.

Volgushev, M., Chistiakova, M., & Singer, W. (1998). Modification of discharge patterns of neocortical neurons by induced oscillations of the membrane potential. *Neuroscience*, 83(1), 15–25.

von Stein, A., & Sarnthein, J. (2000). Different frequencies for different scales of cortical integration: from local gamma to long range alpha/theta synchronization. *International Journal of Psychophysiology*, 38(3), 301–313.

Voytek, B., Canolty, R. T., Shestyuk, A., Crone, N. E., Parvizi, J., & Knight, R. T. (2010). Shifts in gamma phase-amplitude coupling frequency from theta to alpha over posterior cortex during visual tasks. *Frontiers in Human Neuroscience*, 4, 191.

Ward, L. M. (2003). Synchronous neural oscillations and cognitive processes. *Trends in Cognitive Sciences*, 7(12), 553–559.

Worden, M. S., Foxe, J. J., Wang, N., & Simpson, G. V. (2000). Anticipatory biasing of visuospatial attention indexed by retinotopically specific alpha-band electroencephalography increases over occipital cortex. *Journal of Neuroscience*, 20(6), RC63.

Wynn, J. K., Light, G. A., Breitmeyer, B., Nuechterlein, K. H., & Green, M. F. (2005). Event-related gamma activity in schizophrenia patients during a visual backward-masking task. *American Journal of Psychiatry*, 162(12), 2330–2336.

Yizhar, O., Fenno, L. E., Davidson, T. J., Mogri, M., & Deisseroth, K. (2011). Optogenetics in neural systems. *Neuron*, 71(1), 9–34.

Yuval-Greenberg, S., Tomer, O., Keren, A. S., Nelken, I., & Deouell, L. Y. (2008). Transient induced gamma-band response in EEG as a manifestation of miniature saccades. *Neuron*, 58(3), 429–441.

Index

Printed and bound by CPI Group (UK) Ltd, Croydon, CR0 4YY

15/10/2024

01774801-0001